ESSENTIAL PSYCHOTHERAPIES

WITHDRAWN

ESSENTIAL PSYCHOTHERAPIES

Theory and Practice

THIRD EDITION

Edited by
Stanley B. Messer
Alan S. Gurman

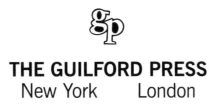

THE GUILFORD PRESS
New York   London

© 2011 The Guilford Press
A Division of Guilford Publications, Inc.
72 Spring Street, New York, NY 10012
www.guilford.com

Printed in the United States of America

This book is printed on acid-free paper.

Last digit is print number: 9   8   7   6   5   4   3   2

Library of Congress Cataloging-in-Publication Data

Essential psychotherapies : theory and practice / edited by Stanley B. Messer,
    Alan S. Gurman. -- 3rd ed.
      p. ; cm.
    Includes bibliographical references and indexes.
    ISBN 978-1-60918-197-0 (hardcover : alk. paper)
  1. Psychotherapy. I. Messer, Stanley B. II. Gurman, Alan S.
  [DNLM: 1. Psychotherapy--methods. 2. Mental Disorders--therapy. WM 420]
  RC480.E69 2011
  616.89'14--dc22

                                 2011008383

To our children—

Elana and Tova Messer,
Leora Mitzner,
and
Jesse and Ted Gurman

About the Editors

Stanley B. Messer, PhD, is Dean of the Graduate School of Applied and Professional Psychology at Rutgers, The State University of New Jersey, where he was Chairperson of the Department of Clinical Psychology for 9 years. He is interested in the application of psychodynamic theory and research to the brief and integrative therapies and has contributed to the debate on evidence-based practice. The author or editor of a number of books and many articles and book chapters, Dr. Messer is currently Associate Editor of the online journal *Pragmatic Case Studies in Psychotherapy* and serves on several other editorial boards. He is an American Psychological Association Fellow in the Society of Clinical Psychology, the Society of Theoretical and Philosophical Psychology, and the Division of Psychotherapy. Dr. Messer maintains a private practice in Highland Park, New Jersey.

Alan S. Gurman, PhD, is Emeritus Professor of Psychiatry at the University of Wisconsin School of Medicine and Public Health in Madison. A pioneer in the development of integrative approaches to couple therapy, he has edited and written many influential books; is a past two-term editor of the *Journal of Marital and Family Therapy*; and is former President of the Society for Psychotherapy Research. Dr. Gurman has received numerous awards for his contributions to couple and family therapy, including the Distinguished Achievement in Family Therapy Research Award from the American Family Therapy Academy and the Distinguished Contribution to Family Psychology Award from the American Psychological Association. He is also a recipient of the Award for Distinguished Achievement in Teaching and Training from the Association of Psychology Postdoctoral and Internship Centers.

Contributors

Martin M. Antony, PhD, Department of Psychology, Ryerson University, Toronto, Ontario, Canada

Jeshmin Bhaju, PhD, Department of Psychiatry and Behavioral Sciences, Emory University School of Medicine, Atlanta, Georgia

Arthur C. Bohart, PhD, Department of Psychology, California State University, Dominguez Hills, California; Department of Psychology, Saybrook University, San Francisco, California

Virginia Brabender, PhD, Institute for Graduate Clinical Psychology, Widener University, Chester, Pennsylvania

Glenn M. Callaghan, PhD, Department of Psychology, San Jose State University, San Jose, California

Marianne P. Celano, PhD, Department of Psychiatry and Behavioral Sciences, Emory University School of Medicine, Atlanta, Georgia

Rebecca Coleman Curtis, PhD, Derner Institute of Advanced Psychological Studies, Adelphi University, Garden City, New York; William Alanson White Institute of Psychiatry, Psychoanalysis and Psychology, New York, New York

Kimberly A. Dienes, PhD, Department of Psychology, Roosevelt University, Chicago, Illinois

William C. Follette, PhD, Department of Psychology, University of Nevada, Reno, Nevada

Arthur Freeman, EdD, ScD, ABPP, Department of Behavioral Medicine, Midwestern University, Downers Grove, Illinois

Jerry Gold, PhD, Derner Institute of Advanced Psychological Studies, Adelphi University, Garden City, New York

Alan S. Gurman, PhD, Department of Psychiatry, University of Wisconsin School of Medicine and Public Health, Madison, Wisconsin

Irwin Hirsch, PhD, William Alanson White Institute of Psychiatry, Psychoanalysis and Psychology, New York, New York

Michael F. Hoyt, PhD, Kaiser Permanente Medical Center, San Rafael, California

Nadine J. Kaslow, PhD, Department of Psychiatry and Behavioral Sciences, Emory University School of Medicine, Atlanta, Georgia

Stanley B. Messer, PhD, Graduate School of Applied and Professional Psychology, Rutgers, The State University of New Jersey, Piscataway, New Jersey

Mark A. Reinecke, PhD, ABPP, ACT, Department of Psychiatry and Behavioral Sciences, Northwestern University, Chicago, Illinois

Lizabeth Roemer, PhD, Psychology Department, University of Massachusetts, Boston, Massachusetts

Ann Sauer, PhD, Department of Behavioral Medicine, Midwestern University, Downers Grove, Illinois

Kirk J. Schneider, PhD, Adjunct Faculty, Saybrook University, and the Existential–Humanistic Institute, San Francisco, California

George Stricker, PhD, Department of Clinical Psychology, Argosy University, Washington, DC

Susan Torres-Harding, PhD, Department of Psychology, Roosevelt University, Chicago, Illinois

Jeanne C. Watson, PhD, Department of Adult Education and Counselling Psychology, Ontario Institute for Studies in Education, University of Toronto, Toronto, Ontario, Canada

David L. Wolitzky, PhD, Department of Psychology, New York University, New York, New York

Contents

PART I. INTRODUCTION

1. Contemporary Issues in Psychotherapy Theory, Practice, and Research: 3
   A Framework for Comparative Study
   Stanley B. Messer and Alan S. Gurman

PART II. PSYCHOANALYTIC APPROACHES

2. Contemporary Freudian Psychoanalytic Psychotherapy   33
   David L. Wolitzky

3. Relational Psychoanalytic Psychotherapy   72
   Rebecca Coleman Curtis and Irwin Hirsch

PART III. BEHAVIORAL AND COGNITIVE APPROACHES

4. Behavior Therapy: Traditional Approaches   107
   Martin M. Antony and Lizabeth Roemer

5. Cognitive Therapy   143
   Kimberly A. Dienes, Susan Torres-Harding, Mark A. Reinecke, Arthur Freeman, and Ann Sauer

6. Behavior Therapy: Functional–Contextual Approaches   184
   William C. Follette and Glenn M. Callaghan

PART IV. EXPERIENTIAL AND HUMANISTIC APPROACHES

7. Person-Centered Psychotherapy and Related Experiential Approaches   223
Arthur C. Bohart and Jeanne C. Watson

8. Existential–Humanistic Psychotherapies   261
Kirk J. Schneider

PART V. SYSTEMS-ORIENTED APPROACHES

9. Family Therapies   297
Nadine J. Kaslow, Jeshmin Bhaju, and Marianne P. Celano

10. Couple Therapies   345
Alan S. Gurman

PART VI. OTHER INFLUENTIAL MODELS OF THERAPEUTIC PRACTICE

11. Brief Psychotherapies   387
Michael F. Hoyt

12. Integrative Approaches to Psychotherapy   426
George Stricker and Jerry Gold

13. Group Psychotherapies   460
Virginia Brabender

Author Index   494

Subject Index   506

PART I

INTRODUCTION

CHAPTER 1

Contemporary Issues in Psychotherapy Theory, Practice, and Research
A Framework for Comparative Study

Stanley B. Messer
Alan S. Gurman

This book presents the core theoretical and applied aspects of essential psychotherapies in contemporary clinical practice. In our view, essential psychotherapies are those that form the conceptual and clinical bedrock of psychotherapeutic training, practice, and research rather than those that may be generating momentary enthusiasm but are soon likely to fade from the therapeutic scene. We believe there are two quite distinct categories of essential psychotherapies. First are those approaches whose origins are found early in the history of psychotherapy, although all of these have been revised and refined considerably over time. Examples of such foundational and time-honored approaches are Freudian-derived psychoanalytic psychotherapy; existential–humanistic, person-centered and experiential models; behavior therapy; and group therapy. Second are the psychotherapies developed more recently that have had a strong influence on practice, training, and research, and are likely to have staying power. Examples are the relational, cognitive, family, couple, brief, and integrative therapies, and the functional–contextual approach to behavior therapy.

The first two editions of *Essential Psychotherapies* have become a primary source for comprehensive presentations of the most prominent contemporary influences in the field of psychotherapy. Although there are literally hundreds of differently labeled "psychotherapies," the great majority are only partial methods, single techniques, or minor variations on existing approaches. We believe that they can be subsumed by about a dozen quite distinguishable types.

As editors, we have challenged our contributing authors to convey not only what is basic and core to their ways of thinking and working, but also what is new and forward-looking in theory, practice, and research. Our contributors, all eminent scholars and practicing clinicians, have helped to forge a volume that is well suited to exposing advanced undergraduates, beginning graduate students, and trainees in all the mental health professions to the major schools and methods of modern psychotherapy. Because the chapters were written by cutting-edge representatives of their therapeutic approaches, there is something genuinely new in these presentations that will be of value to more experienced therapists as well.

As in the first two editions, each chapter offers a clear sense of the history, current status, assessment approach, techniques, and research on the therapy being discussed, along with its foundational ideas about personality and psychological health and dysfunction. As both academicians and practicing psychotherapists, we endorse the adage that "there is nothing so practical as a good theory" (Lewin, 1951, p. 169). Each chapter balances the discussion of theory and practice and emphasizes the interaction between them.

Before detailing our organizing framework for the chapters in this book, three comments about its contents are in order. First, while *Essential Psychotherapies* provides substantive presentations of the major schools of psychotherapeutic thought and general guidelines for practice, it does not emphasize, per se, treatment prescriptions for specific disorders or "special populations." Included, however, are examples of such applications, especially within the behavioral and cognitive approaches. Whereas forces in the contemporary world of psychotherapy support a rather broad movement to specify particular techniques for particular problems and types of persons, we continue to believe that the majority of practitioners approach their work from the standpoint of theory as it informs general strategies and techniques of practice. Optimally, such techniques and interpersonal stances have survived in the crucible of systematic research and can be considered supported or validated. In other words, we believe that there is an interplay among theory, practice, and research that encompasses what we know about empirically supported treatments and techniques, as well as those aspects of the psychotherapy relationship that have a marked effect on the success of therapy (e.g., Friedlander, Escudero, & Heatherington, 2006; Norcross, 2011).

Second, there is considerable energy being devoted to the development and refinement of integrative approaches to psychotherapy (see Stricker & Gold, Chapter 12, this volume). While valuing the search for integrative principles and common factors that transcend particular therapies (e.g., Gurman, 2008; Messer, 2009), we support the continuing practice of teaching relatively distinct schools or systems of psychotherapy. We agree with Feldman and Feldman (2005) that "for therapists to offer a truly balanced and systematic integration, they need to be well versed in the core concepts and techniques of a variety of orientations and conscious of the strengths and limitations of each perspective" (pp. 398–399).

Third, we believe that therapists' personalities increase their attraction to certain approaches and diminish their interest in others. As Gurman (1983) has emphasized, "The choice of a favorite method of psychotherapy . . . is always very personal" (p. 22). Fortunately, the field of psychotherapy provides enough variety of concepts and modes of practice to match the personal predilections of any aspiring clinician.

THE EVOLUTION OF PSYCHOTHERAPY AND OF "ESSENTIAL PSYCHOTHERAPIES"

Despite the fact that the essential approaches are largely the same as when this volume first appeared in 1995, there have been some important changes in the landscape of psychotherapy. First, although Gestalt therapy and transactional analysis have left their imprint on current models, and were popular and prominent therapies in earlier times, they are less so today. As a result, there are no separate chapters devoted to them. Gestalt therapy, however, is addressed within Bohart and Watson's Chapter 7 (this volume) on person-centered and related experiential approaches. Due to the growth of various offshoots of behavior and cognitive therapy, such as dialectical behavior therapy, acceptance and commitment therapy, meditation and mindfulness, and so forth—sometimes known as the "third wave" of behavior therapy (Goldfried, 2011; Hayes, 2004)—we have added a chapter on these and other innovations. At the same time, we have reluctantly not included a separate chapter on postmodern approaches (Tarragona, 2009), because they have not penetrated the general practice of individual psychotherapy very deeply. They have had a continuing influence on other modalities of therapy, however, especially those that are couple- and family-oriented, and these influences are addressed in the chapters here on couple and family therapy (Gurman, Chapter 10; Kaslow, Bhaju, & Celano, Chapter 9) as well as in the chapter on brief therapy (Hoyt, Chapter 11). The social constructionist philosophical outlook of these approaches, which emphasizes the ways in which human beings construe reality rather than viewing it as a fixed, objective entity, tend to downplay the role of the therapist as an "expert," view clients in nonpathologizing terms, decry the relevance of traditional diagnosis, and emphasize the role of social and cultural context in understanding people's suffering.

The various models of psychotherapy appearing here stem from different views of human nature, about which there is no universal agreement. Working from alternative epistemological outlooks (e.g., introspective [from within] vs. extraspective [from the outside]), these schools of therapy embrace quite different ways of getting to know clients. In addition, these therapies encompass distinct visions of reality or combinations thereof, such as tragic, comic, romantic, and ironic views of life (Messer & Winokur, 1984), which influence what change consists of and how much is considered possible. We believe that it is important for the field to appreciate and highlight the different perspectives and visions exemplified by each model or school of therapy even while respecting the search for common principles in theory and practice.

A FRAMEWORK FOR COMPARING THE PSYCHOTHERAPIES

It is not the answer that enlightens, but the questions.
—EUGENE IONESCO

Our theories are our inventions; but they may be merely ill-reasoned guesses, bold conjectures, hypotheses. Out of these we create a world, not the real world, but our own nets in which we try to catch the real world.
—KARL POPPER

As in the earlier editions of *Essential Psychotherapies*, we provided the authors with a comprehensive set of guidelines (presented below). These have proven useful in facilitating readers' comparative study of the major models of contemporary psychotherapy and may also be used by the student as a template for studying therapeutic approaches not included here. We believe that these guidelines include the basic and requisite elements of an adequate description of any type of psychotherapy.

In offering these guidelines to our authors, we aimed to steer a midcourse between providing the reader with sufficient anchor points for comparative study, while not constraining the authors' expository creativity. (See italics below for required content.) We believe that our contributors succeeded in following the guidelines, while describing their respective approaches in an engaging fashion. Authors were encouraged to sequence their material within chapter sections according to their own preferences. They were also advised that they need neither to limit their presentations to the matters raised in the guidelines nor address every point identified therein, but that they should address these matters if they were relevant to their treatment approach. Authors were also free to merge sections of the guidelines if doing so helped them communicate their perspectives more meaningfully. Those features we considered essential to include were highlighted. We believe that the authors' flexible adherence to the guidelines helped to make clear how theory helps to organize clinical work and facilitates case conceptualization. The inclusion of clinical case material in each chapter serves, in an important way, to illustrate the constructs and methods described previously.

Although most of our author guidelines remained unchanged from those in the first two editions, we made a few additions and modifications. We allowed more space for a section on "Research Support," adding the term *Evidence-Based Practice* to it. We asked the authors to be sure to address cultural factors (e.g., ethnicity, race, religion/spirituality, social class, gender) and to offer suggestions of DVDs and videotapes that illustrate each approach. We now present these author guidelines, along with our rationale for, and commentary on, each area. In this fashion, we hope to bring the reader up to date on continuing issues and controversies in the field.

HISTORICAL BACKGROUND

History is the version of past events that people have decided to agree on.
—NAPOLEON BONAPARTE

PURPOSE: To place the approach in historical perspective within the field of psychotherapy.

Points to consider:

1. Cite the *major influences that contributed to the development of the approach* (e.g., people, books, research, theories, conferences). What sociohistorical forces or *Zeitgeist* shaped the emergence and development of this approach (Victorian era, American pragmatism, modernism, postmodernism, etc.)?

2. What therapeutic forms, if any, were forerunners of the approach (psychoanalysis, learning theory, organismic theory, etc.)?

3. What were the types of patients for whom the approach was developed? Speculate as to why.

4. Cite the early theoretical concepts and/or therapy techniques.

People's lives can be significantly influenced for the better in a wide range of ways—for example, a parent adopts a new approach toward his defiant adolescent, a member of the clergy facilitates a congregant's self-forgiveness, an athletic coach or teacher serves as a life-altering "role model" for a student, and so on. Yet none of these, or other commonly occurring healing or behavior-changing experiences, qualifies as psychotherapy. *Psychotherapy refers to a particular process rather than just to any experience that leads to desirable psychological outcomes.* Written over four decades ago, Meltzoff and Kornreich's (1970) definition of psychotherapy is still quite apt, although their term *techniques* has to be seen as including relationship factors, and the phrase "judged by the therapist" must be broadened to include the client's perspective:

> Psychotherapy is . . . the informed and planful application of techniques derived from established psychological principles, by persons qualified through training and experience to understand these principles and to apply these techniques with the intention of assisting individuals to modify such personal characteristics as feelings, values, attitudes and behaviors which are judged by the therapist to be maladaptive or maladjustive. (p. 4)

Given such a definition of psychotherapy, we believe that developing an understanding and appreciation of the professional roots and historical context of psychotherapeutic models is an essential aspect of one's education as a therapist (Norcross, VandenBos, & Friedheim [2010] provide the most comprehensive accounts of the histories of all the major psychotherapy approaches to date). Lacking such awareness, a particular therapy might seem to have evolved from nowhere and for no known reason. An important aspect of a therapist's ability to help people change lies not only in his or her belief in the more technical aspects of the chosen orientation, as in the aforementioned definition, but also in the worldview implicit in it (Frank & Frank, 1991; Messer & Winokur, 1984). Having some exposure to the historical origins of a therapeutic approach helps clinicians comprehend such an implicit worldview.

In addition to appreciating the professional roots of therapeutic methods, it is enlightening to understand why particular methods, or sometimes clusters of related methods, appear on the scene in particular historical periods. The intellectual, economic, and political contexts in which therapeutic approaches arise often provide meaningful clues about the emerging social, scientific, and philosophical values that frame clinical encounters. Such values may have a subtle but salient impact on whether newer treatment approaches endure. For example, until quite recently, virtually all the influential and dominant models of psychotherapy were derived from three broad outlooks: psychoanalysis, humanism, and behaviorism.

In the last few decades in particular, however, two newer conceptual forces have shaped the landscape of psychotherapy in visible ways. The systems-oriented methods of family and couple therapy have grown out of an increasing awareness of the contextual embeddedness of all human behavior (Gurman & Snyder, 2010). Indeed, even the more traditional therapeutic approaches, such as those grounded in psychoanalytic thinking, have become more relational. Likewise, emerging integrative and brief psychotherapeutic approaches have gained recognition and stature in the last two decades, in part as a response to increased societal and professional expectations that psychotherapy demonstrate both its efficacy and its efficiency (Hoyt, Chapter 11 and Stricker & Gold, Chapter 12, this volume; Messer, Sanderson, & Gurman, 2003).

THE CONCEPT OF PERSONALITY

Children are natural mimics—they act like their parents
in spite of every attempt to teach them good manners.
—ANONYMOUS

PURPOSE: To describe within the therapeutic framework the conceptualization of
personality.

Points to consider:

1. What is the *theory of personality development* in this approach?
2. What are the *basic psychological concepts used* to understand patients?

All approaches to psychotherapy are attempts to change or improve some aspect of personality or problematic behavior. Yet *not all theories of therapy include a concept of personality, nor
do all theories of personality necessarily have a companion theory of change.* For example, one form
of personality theory is known as trait theory, the most prominent current form of which is
the "five-factor model" (Hofstee, 2003). The five factors or dimensions said to describe personality, as derived from factor-analytic studies, are Neuroticism, Extraversion, Openness
to Experience, Agreeableness, and Conscientiousness. There is no therapy or change process corresponding to this theory. On the flip side of the coin, and more pertinent to this
volume, is that some theories of therapy are not linked to a specific theory of personality. A
good example is behavior therapy, which accounts for consistency in people's behavior, with
concepts such as conditioned and operant learning, stimulus generalization, and modeling.
Although there are different definitions of what constitutes personality, three elements are
usually included:

1. Personality is not merely a collection of individual traits or disconnected behaviors,
   but is structured, organized, and integrated.
2. This structural criterion implies a degree of consistency and stability in personality
   functioning. Behavioral manifestations of that structure may vary, however, according to the situational context. This is due to behavior being a function of the interaction of personality and situational factors.
3. There is a developmental aspect to personality that takes into account childhood
   and adolescent experience; that is, personality emerges over time out of a matrix of
   biological and social influences.

There exists an intimate connection between personality theory and the factors posited to bring about change by any theory of psychotherapy. Psychoanalysis, for example,
emphasizes unconscious aspects of human functioning, including disguised motives,
ambivalence in all human relations, and intricate interactions among the structures of
mind, namely, id, ego, and superego. Thus, it is not surprising that an essential curative
factor in this theory is interpretation of motives, defenses, conflicts, and other hidden features of personality. A cognitive theory of personality, by contrast, is based on the assumption that mental structures determine how an individual comes to evaluate and interpret
information related to the self and others. In particular, this theory posits "scripts" (Abel-

son, 1981) or "schemas" (Neisser, 1967) that organize and determine individuals' behavior, affect and experience. Psychotherapy, within this approach, involves cognitive reeducation, in the course of which old, irrational, or maladaptive cognitions are unlearned and replaced by new, more adaptive ones. As well, areas of deficiency are remedied by the learning of new cognitive skills (see Dienes, Torres-Harding, Reinecke, Freeman, & Sauer, Chapter 5, this volume).

PSYCHOLOGICAL HEALTH AND PATHOLOGY

> Utopias will come to pass when we grow wings and all people
> are converted into angels.
>   —FYODOR DOSTOYEVSKI

PURPOSE: To describe the way in which psychological health and pathology are conceptualized within the approach.

Points to consider:

1. Describe any formal or informal system for *diagnosing or typing patients.*
2. *How do symptoms or problems develop? How are they maintained?*
3. Is there a concept of the *ideal or healthy personality* within this approach?

Much can go awry in the developing personality due to biological or psychosocial factors. Symptoms can result from contemporaneous stresses and strains or, more typically, from the interaction of a personality disposition with a current event that triggers emotional disturbance or maladaptive interpersonal behavior. *Although some theories avoid the use of language and labels that pathologize human experience, they still speak clearly about what constitutes maladaptive behavior.* Thus, even schools of therapy that do not formally judge the health of a person based on external criteria, such as symptoms or interpersonal difficulties, do attend to the consequences of behavior in terms of that person's welfare and interest.

It should be noted that psychological disorders possess no natural boundaries, only loose categorical coherence. This is not an instance in which nature is carved at its joints. All efforts to date have failed to identify objective features that underlie the various mental disorders as characterized by *Diagnostic and Statistical Manual of Mental Disorders* (DSM), the manual of psychiatric disorders (American Psychiatric Association, 2000). What people seem to agree on is their undesirability, which is more a moral than a scientific valuation (Woolfolk, 1998). In fact, *a therapy may reveal its esthetic and moral values by how it conceptualizes mental health and psychological well-being.* For example, "Psychoanalysis puts forth the ideal of the genital personality, humanistic psychology the self-actualized person, and cognitive-behavior therapy, the objective problem-solving human being" (Messer & Woolfolk, 1998, p. 257).

In other words, the terms of personality theory, psychopathology, and the goals of psychotherapy are not neutral. They are embedded in a value structure that determines what is most important to know about and change in an individual, couple, family, or group. Even schools of psychotherapy that attempt to be neutral with regard to what constitutes healthy (and, therefore, desirable) behavior and unhealthy (and, therefore, undesirable) behavior inevitably, if unwittingly, reinforce the acceptability of some kinds of client strivings more so than others.

Ways of assessing personality and pathology are closely linked to the underlying theory. If the latter focuses on unconscious factors, for example, asking about dreams and early memories may be considered a more fertile mode of assessment than self-report questionnaires (Messer & Wolitzky, 2007). In the following chapters, the reader is encouraged to look for the links among personality theory, the description of psychopathology, the manner of assessing these dimensions, and the kinds of changes that are sought.

THE PROCESS OF CLINICAL ASSESSMENT

> If you are sure you understand everything that is going on,
> you are hopelessly confused.
> —WALTER MONDALE

PURPOSE: To describe the methods used to gain understanding of an individual's (or couple's or family's) style or pattern of interaction, symptoms, and adaptive resources.

Points to consider:

1. What, if any, is the *role of standard psychiatric diagnosis* in your assessment? Does it influence treatment planning, or is it used primarily for administrative purposes?

2. *At what unit level(s) is assessment made* (e.g., individual, dyadic, systemic)?

3. *At what psychological levels is assessment made* (e.g., intrapsychic, behavioral, systemic)?

4. To what extent and in what ways are *cultural factors (e.g., ethnicity, race, religion/spirituality, social class, gender)* considered in your assessment?

5. Are any tests, devices, questionnaires, or structured observations typically used?

6. Is assessment separate from treatment or integrated with it (e.g., what is the temporal relation between assessment and treatment)?

7. Are the patient's strengths/resources a focus of your assessment? If so, in what way?

8. What other dimensions or factors are typically involved in assessing dysfunction?

The practicality of a good theory of psychotherapy, including ideas about personality development and psychological dysfunction, becomes evident as the therapist tries to make sense of both problem stability (how problems persist) and problem change (how problems can be modified). As indicated earlier in Meltzoff and Kornreich's (1970) classic definition of psychotherapy, the therapist is obligated to take some purposeful action in regard to his or her understanding of the nature and parameters of whatever problems, symptoms, complaints, or dilemmas are presented. Therapists typically are interested in understanding what previous steps patients have taken to resolve or improve their difficulties, and what adaptive resources the patient, and possibly other people in the patient's world, has for doing so. Moreover, the therapist pays attention to the cultural (ethnic, racial, religious, social class, gender) context in which clinically relevant concerns arise. Such contextualizing factors can play an important role in how the therapist collaboratively both defines the problem at hand and selects a general strategy for addressing the problem therapeutically. As Hayes and Toarmino (1995) have emphasized, understanding the cultural context in which problems are embedded can serve as an important source of hypotheses about what maintains problems and what types of interventions may be helpful. In this vein, Fontes (2008) has described how to conduct helpful interviews with culturally and linguistically diverse patients.

How therapists actually engage in clinical assessment varies from one approach to another (Eells, 2007), but all include face-to-face clinical interviews. The majority of therapists emphasize the immediate therapist–patient conversation as the source of such understanding. A smaller number of therapists also opt to complement such conversations with direct observations of the problem as it occurs (e.g., in family and couple conflict situations, or in cases involving anxiety-based avoidance of specific stimuli). In addition, some therapists regularly include in the assessment process a variety of patient self-report questionnaires or inventories and may also use structured interview guides, which are usually research-based instruments. Generally, therapists who use such devices have specialized clinical practices (e.g., focusing on a particular set of clinical disorders for which such measures have been specifically designed).

The place of standard psychiatric diagnosis in the clinical assessment phase of psychotherapy likewise varies widely. The overwhelming majority of psychotherapists of different theoretical orientations routinely consider the traditional diagnostic, psychiatric status of patients according to the criteria of the current edition of DSM (e.g., American Psychiatric Association, 2000), at least to meet requirements for financial reimbursement, maintenance of legally required treatment records, and other such institutional contingencies. Although engaging in such formal diagnostic procedures may provide a useful orientation to the general area of a patient's concerns, every method of psychotherapy has developed and refined its own, more fine-grained, idiosyncratic ways of understanding each individual patient's problem. Moreover, some newer approaches to psychotherapy argue that "diagnoses" do not exist "out there" in nature but merely represent the consensual labels attached to certain patterns of behavior in particular cultural and historical contexts. Such therapy approaches see the use of diagnostic labeling as an unfortunate and unwarranted assumption of the role of "expert" by therapists, which may inhibit genuine collaborative exploration between therapists and "patients" or "clients" (e.g., see Bohart & Watson, Chapter 7, and Schneider, Chapter 8, this volume). For such therapists, what matters more are the fluid issues with which people struggle, not the diagnoses they are given.

All things considered, the primary dimension along which clinical assessments vary is the intrapersonal–interpersonal one. Some therapy models emphasize "intrapsychic" processes, whereas others emphasize social interaction. In fact, there is a constant interplay between people's "inner" and "outer" lives. Emphasis on one domain "versus" another reflects an arbitrary punctuation of human experience that probably says as much about the theory of the perceiver as it does about the client who is perceived.

THE PRACTICE OF THERAPY

In theory, there is no difference between theory and practice.
In practice, however, there is.

—ANONYMOUS

PURPOSE: To describe the typical structure, goals, techniques, strategies, and process of a particular approach to therapy and their tactical purposes.

Points to consider:

A. Basic Structure of Therapy

   1. *How often* are sessions typically held?

   2. Is therapy *time-limited or unlimited*? Why? How long does therapy typically last? How long are typical sessions?

   3. Who is typically included in therapy? Are combined formats (e.g., individual plus family or group sessions) ever used?

   4. How structured are therapy sessions?

B. Goal Setting

   1. Are there *treatment goals that apply to all or most cases* for which the treatment is appropriate (see the section "Treatment Applicability and Ethical Considerations") regardless of presenting problem or symptom?

   2. Of the number of possible goals for a given patient group, *how are the central goals selected*? How are they prioritized? Who determines the goals of therapy? Are therapist values involved in goal setting?

   3. *Do cultural factors (e.g., race, religion, social class, ethnicity, gender) typically influence the setting of treatment goals?*

   4. Do you *distinguish between intermediate or mediating goals and ultimate goals*?

   5. Is it important that treatment goals be discussed with patients explicitly? If yes, why? If not, why not?

   6. At what level of psychological experience are goals established (are they described in overt behavioral terms, in affective–cognitive terms, etc.)?

C. Process Aspects of Treatment

   1. *Describe and illustrate with brief case vignettes major commonly used techniques and strategies.*

   2. How is the decision made to use a particular technique or strategy at a particular time? Typically, are different techniques used in different phases of therapy?

   3. Are "homework" or other out-of-session tasks used?

   4. What are the most commonly encountered forms of *resistance to change*? How are these dealt with?

5. What are both the most common and *the most serious technical errors* a therapist can make operating within his or her therapeutic approach?

6. Are psychotropic *medications ever used* (either by the primary psychotherapist or in collaboration with a medical colleague) within your approach? What are the indications–contraindications for their use?

7. On what basis is termination decided, and how is termination effected?

8. Have recent findings in neuroscience influenced important process aspects of your therapeutic approach?

Psychotherapy is not only a scientific and value-laden enterprise but also part and parcel of its surrounding culture. It is a significant source of our current customs and worldviews and thus possesses significance well beyond the interactions between clients and therapists. For example, when laypeople refer to Freudian slips, defenses, guilt complexes, conditioned responses, existential angst, identity crises, codependency, enabling partner, or discovering their true self, they are demonstrating the impact of psychological and psychotherapeutic categories on their vocabulary and cultural conversations. Similarly, when they explain their problems in terms of childhood occurrences, such as parental neglect, repressed memories, conditioned emotional reactions, or lack of unconditional positive regard, they are affirming that the institution of psychotherapy is much more than a technical, medical, or scientific endeavor. It helps to shape the very terms in which people think, and even constitutes the belief system they use to explain and make sense out of their lives (Messer & Woolfolk, 1998, 2010).

At the same time, psychotherapy is a sensitive barometer of those customs and outlooks to which the different modes of practice are responsive and incorporate within their purview. The relation between psychotherapy and culture, then, is one of reciprocal influence (Messer & Wachtel, 1997). For example, two currently important cultural phenomena affecting the practice of psychotherapy are the corporatization of the mental health service delivery system and the medicalization of how psychological disorder is treated. Regarding the former, the advent of managed health care has had a strong impact on the practice of psychotherapy (Cantor & Fuentes, 2008). Managed care itself was a response to rapidly rising health care costs and the efforts of large businesses to curtail them. Managed care organizations (MCOs) were created to handle health care for such large corporations and did so by charging a set dollar amount per month for each person they contracted to cover. The MCOs, which were assuming the health care financial risks, could only make a profit if costs were held down, thus producing a strong incentive to keep payments to health service providers to a minimum. What this typically meant was that MCOs would cover only a certain number of psychotherapy sessions, or a certain dollar amount per year. This, in turn, brought about the flourishing of brief or time-limited therapy and, simultaneously, decreased the affordability and attractiveness of longer-term therapies. As it happens, the more behavioral, cognitive, family, and couple therapies tend to be relatively short term in outlook (e.g., Gurman, 2001), whereas the psychoanalytic (both traditional and relational), existential, and experiential therapies are more open-ended. The former therapies are briefer because they are typically problem-focused and goal-oriented, whereas the latter are generally more exploratory and depth-oriented in their *modus operandi*. In this way, an economic issue has reverberated through the health care culture, supporting certain kinds of practice and diminishing others.

We wish to emphasize that this effect is not due primarily to scientific findings, clinical judgment, or popular demand but, rather, to the economic needs of American business and the nation at large. Although we value the practice of brief therapy (e.g., Gurman, 2005; Messer et al., 2003), we also believe that both short- and long-term therapy should be available as possible choices for patients according to professionally judged and documented need. To illustrate that the provision of long-term therapy in the United States is a possible option, we note that psychoanalysis is included in government health care coverage in Germany and has achieved considerable evidential support (Leichsenring & Rabung, 2008; Shedler, 2010).

Regarding the medicalization of mental health treatment, the language of medicine has long been prominent in the field of psychotherapy. We talk of "symptoms," "diseases," "disorders," "psychopathology," and "treatment." As Messer and Wachtel (1997) remarked, "It is a kind of new narrative that reframes people's conflicts over value and moral questions as sequelae of 'disease' or 'disorder,' thereby bringing into play the prestige (and hence curative potential) accruing to medicine and technology in our society" (p. 3). Modern psychotherapy started with Freud, who was a physician. Because the major practitioners of therapy were physicians for at least the first half of the last century, the language of medicine came naturally to them. In addition, they wished to see psychotherapy as an integral part of the medical profession. Quite aside from these historical influences, in the latter half of the 20th century and beginning of the 21st, there has been good reason to consider treatment of mental disorders as medical. There are now medications that have been at least moderately successful in treating various mental conditions, such as bipolar disorder, schizophrenia, major depression, and anxiety. The popular success and research backing of some medications has led some psychologists to lobby for attainment of prescription privileges. Were this to occur, it would have a huge impact on the practice of psychotherapy.

Medication for conditions such as anxiety, social phobia, and depression are now promoted on television directly to the consumer, with the promise of the pill removing a person's worries and blues. Thus, the drug companies have played their part in promoting a biological approach to mental disorder. Many such symptoms, however, are closely related to interpersonal conflicts and other problems in living, which are not so readily dispatched. Regarding the symptoms of depression, at least among outpatients, psychotherapy and medication are usually equivalent in the short run, with psychotherapy (often cognitive-behavioral therapy) reducing the risk of relapse. In the case of depression, research has shown that about three-fourths of the effect of medication is placebo or suggestion (Kirsch & Sapirstein, 1999), and that these effects seem to last for 80% of patients (Khan, Redding, & Brown, 2008).

A *meta-analysis* (a statistical approach that summarizes the results of many quantitative studies) indicated that for older adults, there was no difference in the effects of psychotherapy and medication in the treatment of depression (Pinquart, Duberstein, & Lyness, 2006). Similarly, brief forms of cognitive therapy, behavior therapy, psychodynamic therapy, and interpersonal therapy have all been shown to do as well as medication in alleviating depression, without side effects or the loss of empowerment that the former may entail (Cuijpers, van Straten, Andersson, & van Oppen, 2008; Hollon, Thase, & Markowitz, 2002). A recent meta-analysis concluded that it is only for the most severe depressive symptoms that antidepressant medication produces better results than placebo (Fournier et al., 2010). Some research indicates that there is an advantage to combining psychotherapy and medication in the treatment of depression, both regarding outcomes (de Jonghe, Kool, van Aalst, Dekker, & Peen, 2001) and in enhancing remission rates for chronic depression (Manber et al., 2008). Such findings may lead to a greater degree of integration of pharmacotherapy and psychotherapy in the future (Winston, Been, & Serby, 2005).

The spread of the biological way of understanding psychopathology, as well as the biological mode of treating emotional disorders, has had its effects on the practice of psychotherapy: Clients and therapists are more likely to consider having medication prescribed. Psychologists and other nonmedical therapists are collaborating more frequently with physicians in treating their patients. Courses in psychopharmacology are now routinely offered or even required in counseling, clinical, and clinical social work training programs. This trend has also been supported by MCOs, which consider medication a less expensive alternative to psychotherapy. Relatedly, recent advances in neuroscience, especially in the realm of "affective neuroscience" (e.g., Panksepp, 1998) and "interpersonal neurobiology" (e.g., Siegel, 1999), have demonstrated the brain's capacity for plasticity and change, providing a basis for some broad principles to guide psychotherapy with both individuals (e.g., Cozolino, 2002) and couples (e.g., Fishbane, 2007). But Levenson (2010) advises caution about prematurely concluding "that we can identify specific neurological processes and brain structures to explain precisely why and how our therapeutic interventions work" (p. 116). From our standpoint, it would be unfortunate if the range of essential therapies described herein were not taught and practiced, if the psychological outlook these essential therapies convey were not respected, and if the important kind of psychological help these therapies offer were made less available because of excessive exuberance toward biologizing our understanding of psychological suffering and change.

THE THERAPEUTIC RELATIONSHIP AND THE STANCE OF THE THERAPIST

You can do very little with faith, but you can do nothing without it.
—SAMUEL BUTLER

PURPOSE: To describe the stance the therapist takes with patients.

Points to consider:

1. How does the therapeutic relationship influence the outcome of therapy?

2. What techniques or strategies are used to *create a treatment alliance? Describe and illustrate.*

3. To what degree does the therapist overtly control sessions? *How active/directive is the therapist?*

4. Does the therapist assume responsibility for bringing about the changes desired? Is responsibility left to the patient? Is responsibility shared?

5. Does the therapist use self-disclosure? What limits are imposed on therapist self-disclosure? In general, *what role does the "person" of the therapist play in this approach? Describe and illustrate.*

6. Does the therapist's role change as therapy progresses? Does it change as termination approaches?

7. Is *countertransference or the therapist's experience of the patient* recognized or employed in any fashion?

8. What *clinical skills or other therapist attributes are most essential* to successful therapy in your approach?

In recent years, a great deal of effort has been expended to identify empirically supported treatments (ESTs) among the many existing forms of psychotherapy (e.g., Nathan & Gorman, 2007). Although such efforts can be useful for important public policymaking decisions, they tend to focus heavily on one particular domain of the therapy experience—the role and power of therapeutic techniques. Increasingly, EST-oriented efforts have been counterbalanced by efforts to investigate and understand the essential characteristics and effects of empirically supported relationships (ESRs; Castonguay & Beutler, 2006; Norcross, 2011). Such undertakings rest on a solid empirical basis for arguing that *the therapist as a person exerts at least moderate effects on the outcome of psychotherapy, and that these effects often outweigh those that are attributable to treatment techniques per se* (Wampold, 2001). Even symptom-focused therapy encounters, which rely substantially on the use of clearly defined change-inducing techniques, occur in the context of human relationships characterized by support and reassurance, persuasion, identification, and the modeling of active coping.

The kind of therapeutic relationship required by each approach to psychotherapy affects the overall "stance" the therapist takes to the experience (how the working alliance is fostered, how active and self-disclosing the therapist is, etc.). Thus, different therapeutic orientations appear to call forth (and call for) somewhat different therapist attributes and interpersonal inclinations. Therapists with a more or less "take charge" personal style may be better suited to practicing therapy approaches that require a good deal of therapist activity and structuring than to those requiring a more reflective style, and so on.

Given the presumed equivalence of effectiveness of the major methods of psychotherapy (Lambert & Ogles, 2004), it is not surprising that idiosyncratic personal factors influence therapists' preferred ways of practicing. Thus, it has been found that therapists generally do not advocate different approaches on the basis of their relative scientific status but are more influenced by their own direct clinical experience, personal values and philosophy, and life experiences (Norcross & Prochaska, 1983; Stewart & Chambless, 2007).

Finally, it is worthwhile to remember that therapeutic techniques themselves may significantly alter the nature of the therapist–patient relationship. Although all techniques are born within an originating "home theory," they are often "exported" for use within other frameworks. Messer (2001) has referred to this process as *assimilative integration*. Although helpful techniques may not lose their effectiveness when imported into a different therapy, introducing them is also a type of communication to the patient, whose response must then be taken into account.

CURATIVE FACTORS OR MECHANISMS OF CHANGE

The road is not the road, the road is how you walk it.
—JUAN RAMÓN JIMÉNEZ

PURPOSE: To describe the factors (or mechanisms of change) that lead to change and to assess their relative importance. Include research findings if possible.

Points to consider:

1. What are the proposed *curative factors or mechanisms of change* in this approach?

2. Do patients *need insight or understanding* in order to change? (Differentiate between historical–genetic insight and interactional insight.)

3. Are interpretations of any sort important and, if so, do they take history into account? If interpretations of any kind are used, are they seen as reflecting a psychological "truth" or are they viewed rather as a pragmatic tool for effecting change?

4. How important is the learning of new interpersonal skills as a curative element of change? When important, are these skills taught in didactic fashion, or are they shaped as approximations that occur naturalistically in treatment?

5. Does the therapist's personality or psychological health play an important part in bringing about change?

6. *How important are techniques as opposed to relational factors* for the outcome of therapy?

7. To what extent does the management of termination of therapy determine outcome?

8. What aspects of your therapy are *not* unique to your approach (i.e., are common to all or most psychotherapies)?

A current controversy in the psychotherapy research literature is whether change is brought about largely by specific ingredients of therapy or factors common to all therapies. The former usually refers to specific technical interventions, such as biofeedback, systematic desensitization, *in vivo* exposure, cognitive reframing, interpretation, or empathic responding, which are said to be the ingredient(s) responsible for client change. Quite frequently, these techniques are set out in detail in manuals to which the practitioner is expected to adhere in order to achieve the desired result. The specific ingredient approach is in keeping with the medical model insofar as one treats a particular disorder with a psychological technique (akin to administering a pill or employing a surgical technique), producing the psychological equivalent of a biological or physical effect. Its proponents tend to fall in the cognitive and behavioral camps, but at least in theory could hail from any of the psychotherapy schools. Followers of the EST movement are typically adherents of this approach, advocating specific modes of intervention for different forms of psychopathology.

Common factors refer to features of therapy that are not specific to any one approach. Because outcome studies comparing different individual therapies have found few differences among the therapies (Lambert & Ogles, 2004), it has been conjectured that this finding is due to the importance of therapeutic factors the various therapies have in common. Similar assessments have appeared in the realm of couple and family therapies (e.g., Sprenkle, Davis, & Lebow, 2009). Thus, instead of running horse race research to discern differences among the therapies, proponents argue that effort should be redirected to their commonalities. These include *client factors*, such as positive motivation and expectation for change; *therapist qualities*, such as warmth, ability to form a good alliance, and empathic attunement; *strategic processes*, such as providing feedback, exposing clients to the elements of the problem in thought or behavior, and helping them to acquire mastery; and *structural features* of the treatment, such as the provision of a rationale for the person's disorder and having a coherent theoretical framework for interventions (Grencavage & Norcross, 1990; Weinberger & Rasco, 2007).

Drawing on the common factors approach, Wampold (2001) developed what he refers to as a "contextual" model. In it, "the purpose of specific ingredients is to construct a coherent treatment that therapists believe in, and this provides a convincing rationale to clients. Furthermore, these ingredients cannot be studied independently of the healing context and atmosphere in which they occur" (Messer & Wampold, 2002, p. 22). In a sense, this is a common factors model that also takes account of the context in which those factors occur, namely, a healing atmosphere, and the employment of a specific theoretical model. In his important book, *The Great Psychotherapy Debate* (2001), Wampold has made the case for the centrality of common factors such as the therapy alliance, the therapist's allegiance to his or her theory or rationale for treatment, and the personality qualities and skill of the therapist. He reviews the evidence for the specific ingredients model and finds it wanting. Nevertheless, proponents have also presented convincing evidence in favor of the specific ingredients model (e.g., Baker, McFall, & Shoham, 2009; Chambless & Ollendick, 2001), especially as applied to health-related conditions (Barlow, 2004). One could argue that it is ethically incumbent upon practitioners to inform therapy consumers of the availability of such treatments.

Results indicate that four broad factors contribute to therapeutic efficacy, namely, therapist factors, patient or client factors, relationship factors, techniques, and their interaction (Castonguay & Beutler, 2006). Patient and therapist attributes, specific interventions, and quality of the therapeutic relationship each add something to the prediction of treatment outcome. According to one analysis of change factors, common factors account for 35%; therapist effects, 20%; and techniques, 5%; with the remaining 40% coming from extratherapeutic sources (Lambert, 2008). The latter include client characteristics, such as ego strength, and environmental factors, such as social support. Wampold (2001) also statistically analyzed psychotherapeutic effects and concluded that at least 70% are due to general effects, such as common factors (e.g., client/extratherapeutic, placebo), and less than 8% are due to specific techniques. In this sense, support was found for both the specific ingredients and common factors models, with the latter predominating.

TREATMENT APPLICABILITY AND ETHICAL CONSIDERATIONS

> All who drink this remedy recover in a short time, except those whom it does not help, who all die and have no relief from any other medicine. Therefore, it is obvious that it fails only in incurable cases.
>
> —GALEN

PURPOSE: To describe those patients for whom your approach is especially relevant and any ethical issues that are particular to your approach.

Points to consider:

1. For what *kinds of patients* is your approach particularly relevant?

2. For whom is your approach either *not appropriate* or of uncertain relevance?

3. Are there either inherent or likely limitations in the applicability of your approach to people of *diverse cultural backgrounds (e.g., as a function of ethnicity, race, religion/spirituality, social class, and gender)*?

4. When, if ever, would a referral be made for another (i.e., different) type of therapy?

5. Are there aspects of your approach that raise particular ethical issues?

In the end, questions about the applicability, relevance, and helpfulness of particular psychotherapy approaches to particular kinds of symptoms, problems, and issues are best answered through careful research on *treatment efficacy* (as determined via randomized clinical trials) and *effectiveness* (studies in practice settings). Testimonials, appeals to established authority and tradition, and similar unsystematic methods are insufficient to the task. Psychotherapy is too complex to track the interaction among, and impact of, the most relevant factors in therapeutic outcomes on the basis of only individual participants' perceptions. Moreover, the contributions to therapeutic outcomes of therapist, patient, relationship, and technique factors probably vary from one therapeutic method to another.

When Galen's observations (in the opening epigraph) about presumptively curative medicines are applied to psychotherapy nowadays, they are likely to be met with a knowing chuckle and implicit recognition of the inherent limits of all our treatment approaches. Still, *new therapy approaches rarely make only modest and restrained claims of effectiveness, issue "warning labels" for "customers" for whom their ways of working are either not likely to be helpful or may possibly be harmful, or suggest that alternative approaches may be more appropriate under certain conditions.*

If therapy methods continue to grow in number (and we see no reason to predict otherwise), the ethical complexities of the psychotherapy field may grow commensurately. There are generic kinds of ethical matters with which therapists of all orientations must deal; for example, confidentiality, adequacy of recordkeeping, duty to warn, respect of personal boundaries regarding sexual contact and dual relationships, and so forth. Yet more recent influential approaches, especially those involving multiperson clientele (e.g., couple and family therapy) raise practical ethical matters that do not emerge in more traditional modes of practice—for example, balancing the interests and needs of one person against the interests and needs of another, all the while also trying to help maintain the very viability of the patient system (e.g., marriage or family) itself (Gottlieb, Lasser, & Simpson, 2008).

Such potential influences of new perspectives on ethical concerns in psychotherapy are perhaps nowhere more readily and saliently seen than when matters involving cultural diversity are considered. Certainly, all psychotherapists must be sensitive in their work to matters of race, ethnicity, social class, gender, sexual orientation, and religion, adapting and modifying both their assessment and treatment-planning activities, and perspectives and active intervention styles as is deemed functionally appropriate to the situation at hand (Hayes & Toarmino, 1995). To do otherwise risks the witting or unwitting imposition of the therapist's values onto the patient, such as in the important area of setting goals for their work together.

In a poll conducted a decade ago by Norcross, Hedges, and Prochaska (2002), experts in the field of psychotherapy predicted that a culture-sensitive orientation would become one of the most widely employed points of view in the subsequent decade. Feminism, which shares many philosophical assumptions with multiculturalism (Gurman & Fraenkel, 2002), was also predicted to show an increasing impact on psychotherapy. This has certainly taken place. To begin with, the American Psychological Association (2003) issued a report in its flagship journal, the *American Psychologist*, on multicultural training, research, and practice, encouraging therapists to enhance their multicultural awareness and culture-specific strategies. Edited books on race, culture, feminism, spirituality, and gay issues, as they pertain to psychotherapy and counseling, have appeared, putting multiculturalism closer to the center than at the periphery of practice (Gielen, Draguns, & Fish, 2008; Moodley & Palmer, 2006; Sue & Sue, 2008). Research has followed suit, producing results such as the positive association between clients' ratings of therapist multicultural competence and those of the working alliance, therapist empathy, and satisfaction (Fuertes et al., 2006).

A renewed interest in the importance of spirituality and religion as aspects of human diversity is evident in the publication of a new American Psychological Association journal, *Psychology of Religion and Spirituality* (McMinn, Hathaway, Woods, & Snow, 2009). How these areas of human functioning can be fruitfully addressed in psychotherapy is also the subject of several recent books (e.g., Pergament, 2007; Sperry & Shafranske, 2005). That psychotherapy is at least as much a socially and culturally situated activity as a biologically driven one is elaborated in a series of papers on psychotherapy as practiced internationally (Wachtel, 2008).

The cultural perspective has usefully challenged many normative assumptions and practices in the general field of psychotherapy, forcing it to recognize the diversity of social and psychological experience, and the impact of relevant social beliefs that often confuse clinical description with social prescription. Critiques of various psychotherapies from these contemporary perspectives have sensitized therapists to the potential constraining and even damaging effects of a failure to recognize the reality of one's own necessarily limited perspective.

RESEARCH SUPPORT AND EVIDENCE-BASED PRACTICE

> If all the evidence as you receive it leads to but one conclusion, don't believe it.
>
> —MOLIÈRE

> The process of being scientific does not consist of finding objective truths. It consists of negotiating a shared perception of truths in respectful dialogue.
>
> —ROBERT BEAVERS

PURPOSE: To summarize existing research that supports the efficacy and/or effectiveness of your approach and generally describe the role of research in the typical practice of your approach.

Points to consider:

1. Describe the *nature and extent of empirical research that supports the efficacy and/or effectiveness* of your approach.

2. *If supportive research is not abundant, on what other bases* can the effectiveness of your approach be argued?

3. (How) do research findings on your approach typically get incorporated into clinical practice?

Psychotherapy Process and Outcome Research

Each chapter in this volume provides a snapshot of the *outcome research* backing its particular model of therapy. *The hundreds, if not thousands, of studies on the outcome of psychotherapy* are testament to investigators' efforts to place the field on a firm scientific footing. In recent times, a statistical process known as *meta-analysis* has been applied across a large number of these studies. This procedure compares the efficacy of a particular therapy to a wait-list control group, to another therapy, or to other treatment modalities, such as medication. Two major findings have emerged from these meta-analyses. The first is that being treated in psychotherapy is considerably more effective than not being treated. In fact, to be more precise, roughly four out of five people will be better off after being in therapy (Lambert & Ogles, 2004).

The second major finding is that there is little comparative difference in the effectiveness of the therapies that have been extensively practiced and researched, such as the ones discussed in this volume, even for such symptom-dominated problems as posttraumatic stress disorder (Benish, Imel, & Wampold, 2008) and substance abuse (Imel, Wampold, Miller, & Fleming, 2008). Time and again, the results of comparative studies have shown that when pitted against one another, each therapy is more effective than being on a wait list, but not better than any other standard therapy (e.g., Lambert & Ogles, 2004; Luborsky et al., 2002).

The other major kind of psychotherapy research is known as *process research*. Rather than focusing on the question of whether therapy works, it studies what takes place during the therapy, such as the nature of the techniques employed. A subset of process research is process-to-outcome research, which attempts to answer the question of how therapy works; that is, it relates process variables to change within a session or to therapy outcome (e.g., Ablon, Levy, & Katzenstein, 2006). For example, the effects of client factors (e.g., race, age, defensiveness, motivation), therapist factors (e.g., warmth, attunement, experience), different kinds of interventions (reflection, cognitive reframing, interpretations), and the interaction among these and other variables and their relation to outcomes are all part of process research. Thousands of such studies cannot be as neatly summarized as the field's outcome results. The reader will find further examples in the research sections or elsewhere in the body of the individual chapters.

Evidence-Based Practice: The Science and Practice of Psychotherapy

There is a long history of disconnection between psychotherapy practitioners and psychotherapy researchers (e.g., Norcross, Klonsky, & Tropiano, 2008). The latter typically criticize clinicians for engaging in practices that lack empirical justification (e.g., Baker et al., 2009), and clinicians characterize researchers as being out of touch with the complex realities of conducting psychotherapy (e.g., Zeldow, 2009). Unfortunately, such criticisms are not entirely unwarranted.

As already noted, the world of psychotherapy has seen an increased pressure placed on the advocates of particular therapeutic methods to document both the efficacy of their approaches through carefully controlled clinical research trials and the effectiveness of these methods via evaluations in uncontrolled, naturalistic clinical practice contexts (Nathan & Gorman, 2007). This movement to favor ESTs has even more recently been challenged by a complementary movement of psychotherapy researchers who assert the often overlooked importance of ESRs in therapy (Norcross, 2011).

The term EST refers to those treatments tested by randomized clinical trials (RCTs) for a specific diagnostic entity (e.g., social anxiety) while employing a treatment manual. The effort by the American Psychological Association Division (12) of Clinical Psychology to list the ESTs was intended to affirm that many psychological interventions for specific psychiatric disorders are as effective as psychopharmacological treatments, if not more so. Incidentally, a large majority of the ESTs on the Division 12 list were cognitive-behavioral in orientation.

The EST project quickly polarized psychologists into those who embraced it and asserted that it was unethical to practice any other treatment when an EST existed, and others who raised objections to ESTs gaining hegemony in the field, given their many limitations (e.g., Messer, 2004). These include the undue emphasis on techniques versus the centrality of relationship and other common therapeutic factors in therapy; neglect of client personality and therapist characteristics, which are known to affect outcomes; the time-limited nature of the treatments studied; the question of the applicability of ESTs to dually diagnosed patients or those without diagnoses; and neglect of patients of different racial, ethnic, and cultural backgrounds (LaRoche & Christopher, 2008).

Whereas the term EST refers to the results of research affirming the positive outcomes of a specific therapy, a broader term has come into use, namely, evidence-based (psychological) practice (EBPP or EBP). How does EBP differ from ESTs? The prestigious Institute of Medicine (2001) defined EBP as the integration of research (the emphasis in ESTs) with clinical expertise and patient values. Following suit, a report of an American Psychological Association Presidential Task Force on Evidence-Based Practice (2006) defined EBP as "the integration of the best available research with clinical expertise in the context of patient characteristics, culture and preferences" (p. 273). As the document explains, "ESTs start with the treatment and ask whether this treatment works for a certain disorder or problem under specified circumstances. EBPP starts with the patient and asks what research evidence (including relevant results from randomized clinical trials) will assist the psychologist to achieve the best outcome" (p. 273).

This definition is far friendlier to the important roles of clinicians and patients, and to the kinds of therapy that put more emphasis on relationship factors than techniques, such as psychodynamic, experiential, and other humanistic therapies (Messer & Wampold, 2002). At the risk of oversimplification, those who advocate an EST perspective tend to be associated with certain theoretical orientations (behavioral, cognitive, cognitive-behavioral; e.g., Barlow, 2004) and styles of practice (brief), and those who adopt an ESR perspective tend to be associated with other theoretical orientations (psychoanalytic and psychodynamic, person-centered, experiential, existential–humanistic; e.g., Messer, 2004), whereas other dominant approaches (integrative, family and couple, group) stand somewhere in the middle, akin to an EBP perspective (e.g., Gurman & Fraenkel, 2002).

Other American Psychological Association divisions besides Division 12 have promulgated their own principles of EBP, which take the larger, more integrative view (e.g., the Divisions of Psychotherapy [29] and Humanistic Psychology [32], and the Society of Counseling Psychology [17]), and set forth guidelines for facilitating a synergistic relationship between research and practice (e.g., the Division of Family Psychology [43]; Sexton et al., 2010). For more on the role of clinical expertise in EBP, see Goodheart (2006); on the necessity of taking patient/client preferences and values into account, see Messer (2006). Note that the books in which the latter two references appear thoroughly cover the dialogue and debate over EBP.

Regarding their role in daily practice, Zeldow (2009) points out that clinicians will always have to deal with uncertainty and uniqueness as they respond during therapy sessions in a moment-to-moment way, and will have to rely on not only empirical research but also their clinical judgment and values. Wolf (2009) sums it up well, stating that "both a scientific knowledge base and a model of clinical practice that value the judgment of the expert are necessary for psychology to be a learned profession" (p. 11). Can the field of psychotherapy foster more evidence-based practice without unduly constraining the kinds of evidence and expertise that are needed to inform it? That is, *can we create a truly scientific practice that is truly practice-friendly?*

CASE ILLUSTRATION

A good example is the best sermon.
—YANKEE PROVERB

PURPOSE: To illustrate the clinical application of this model by detailing the major assessment, structural, technical, and relational elements of the process of treating a person–couple–group viewed as typical, or representative, of the kinds of patients for whom this approach is appropriate.

Points to consider:

1. *Relevant case background (e.g., presenting problem, referral source, previous treatment history).*

2. *Description of relevant aspects of your clinical assessment: functioning, structure, dysfunctional interaction, resources, and individual dynamics/characteristics, including how you arrived at this description.*

3. *Description of the process and content of goal setting.*

4. *Highlight the major themes, patterns, and so forth, of the therapy over the whole course of treatment. Describe the structure of therapy, the techniques used, the role and activity of the therapist, and so forth.*

NOTE. Do not describe the treatment of a "star case," in which therapy progresses perfectly. Select a case that, while successful, also illustrates the typical course of events in your therapy.

The first psychotherapist to use case illustrations was none other than the founder of modern psychotherapy, Sigmund Freud. Here is what he wrote about the case history approach:

It still strikes me as strange that the case histories I write read like short stories and that, as one might say, they lack the serious stamp of science. I must console myself with the reflection that the nature of the subject is evidently responsible for this, rather than any preference of my own. . . . A detailed description of mental processes such as we are accustomed to find in the works of imaginative writers enables me, with the use of a few psychological formulas, to obtain at least some kind of insight into the course of that affliction [i.e., hysteria]. [The case histories provide] an intimate connection between the story of the patient's suffering and the symptoms of his illness. (Breuer & Freud, 1893–1895/1955, p. 160)

There are several advantages to the case report as a method for presenting the process of therapy. The therapist is in a privileged position to know what has happened over the course of therapy. A *case study* summarizes large quantities of case material in a richly textured, narrative fashion. Well-written cases bring material alive in a compelling way and bring us in on the unfolding sequence of events, major emergent themes, and results of the therapy. The treating therapist permits readers to participate in his or her sense of discovery and excitement in elaborating new ideas and techniques (Messer & McCann, 2005).

There are disadvantages to the case report as well, particularly from a scientific standpoint. First, it is one person's view only, albeit that of a trained observer. What is not recorded may be technical mistakes that are not remembered or are simply omitted to avoid guilt or shame (Spence, 1998). We cannot assume that accounts prepared for publication are veridical, because we know that memory is affected by wishes and confirmatory bias. The summary report, therefore, is not a substitute for the recording of actual dialogue between client and therapist, because the data are selected in terms of both what is reported and the inferences that are drawn by the reporting therapist.

Nevertheless, there have been several creative endeavors to employ case studies in such a way as to overcome these obstacles, at least partially. One employs a "hermeneutic single-case efficacy design" (Elliott et al., 2009). It uses a "mixture of quantitative and qualitative information to create a rich case record that provides both positive and negative evidence for the causal influence of therapy on client outcome" (p. 544). It searches for negative evidence to rule out competing explanations as to how events external to therapy might have caused client improvement. A second approach, known as "multiple case depth research" (Schneider, 1999), combines both case study methodology and in-depth experiential therapeutic principles. In its effort to achieve validity, it poses three questions: Are the data plausibly linked to theory? Is the theory generalizable? Is the conclusion plausibly disconfirmable?

A third approach, called the pragmatic case study method (Fishman, 2001), refers to systematic, qualitative case studies that capture the process and outcome of psychotherapy as practiced and written up under standardized headings. Such cases also include, where possible, a comparison of the individual with others via intake and outcome data on standardized quantitative measures. The overall aim is to maintain the clinical richness and creativity of the case study, while generating a database that permits cross-case comparisons and more generalized rules of psychotherapeutic practice. The pragmatic case study has been developed in an Internet-based journal called *Pragmatic Case Studies in Psychotherapy* (*pcsp.libraries.rutgers.edu/index.php/pcsp/about/pcspabout*), allowing open access and sufficient space for narratively rich case exposition. It remains to be seen to what extent such clinical, single-case research efforts will be generative and supplement more typical group-based empirical approaches.

CODA: INTEGRATION AND SPECIALIZATION IN PSYCHOTHERAPY

The modern trend toward integration in psychotherapy goes back at least to Dollard and Miller's (1950) classic, *Personality and Psychotherapy*, which sought to bring together the psychoanalytic and behavioral orientations. About midway through the period from Dollard and Miller's book until today Wachtel's (1977) highly influential *Psychoanalysis and Behavior*

Therapy appeared, followed by a revised edition, which encompassed a newer relational emphasis (Wachtel, 1997). This domain of psychotherapy has progressed over the years from a rather singular emphasis on the integration of particular therapeutic approaches to a parallel emphasis on the actual process and principles of integrating apparently disparate points of view and clinical methods (see, e.g., Messer, 2001).

Certainly, one of the main forces behind the "integration movement" has been empirical—that is, the repeated finding of rough equivalence of treatment outcomes among different approaches, leading to an increased interest in identifying the common factors involved in psychotherapeutic change, as discussed earlier. But empirical foundations notwithstanding, many integrative efforts have grown more out of conceptual and clinical concerns and questioning than out of research findings per se. This is an important attribute of the integration movement. Without it, there may evolve merely a series of rather arid integrations of formerly unconnected approaches, which, as the latest "products" of integration, take on lives of their own and merely add to the already very long list of identifiable psychotherapies. Moreover, the integrative movement necessarily always relies on the continued existence of original theories of therapy to serve as its own launching pad. Perhaps ironically, integrative development cannot continue without original theories remaining vital.

At the same time that the integration movement is likely to persist, there has certainly been a continuing parallel movement in the world of psychotherapy toward increased specialization. This specialization, a logical outgrowth of the EST movement, emphasizes models of therapy practice and training that place a premium on the application of highly specific treatment interventions to the remediation of highly specific disorders and problems (e.g., dialectical behavior therapy [Linehan et al., 2006] or transference-focused psychotherapy [Clarkin, Levy, Lenzenweger, & Kernberg, 2007] to treat borderline personality disorder.) It appears that significant numbers of recently trained psychotherapists are opting to specialize in their clinical work, often by focusing their clinical activities on the treatment of a specific range of patient problems or diagnoses. Ironically and dialectically, the field's push toward specialization may help fuel the movement toward integration.

SUGGESTIONS FOR FURTHER STUDY

PURPOSE: To aid the instructor in assigning relevant readings and/or DVDs/ videotapes as supplements to the text.

Points to include (plus one-sentence annotation for each reference)

1. *Two articles or accessible book chapters that provide detailed, extensive clinical case studies.*
2. *Two research-oriented articles or chapters, preferably one of which includes an overview of research findings or issues pertinent to your approach.*
3. Two DVDs or videotapes that demonstrate your therapeutic approach.

ACKNOWLEDGMENT

The authors thank Lisa Grinfeld for her assistance with this chapter.

REFERENCES

Abelson, R. P. (1981). Psychological status of the script concept. *American Psychologist, 36,* 715–729.

Ablon, J. S., Levy, R. A., & Katzenstein, T. (2006). Beyond brand names of psychotherapy: Identifying empirically supported change processes. *Psychotherapy, 43,* 216–231.

American Psychiatric Association. (2000). *Diagnostic and statistical manual of mental disorders* (4th ed., text rev.). Washington, DC: Author.

American Psychological Association. (2003). Guidelines on multicultural education, training, research, practice and organizational change for psychologists. *American Psychologist, 58,* 377–402.

American Psychological Association Presidential Task Force on Evidence-Based Practice. (2006). Evidence-based practice in psychology. *American Psychologist, 61,* 271–285.

Baker, T. B., McFall, R. M., & Shoham, V. (2009). Current status and future prospects of clinical psychology. *Psychological Science in the Public Interest, 9,* 67–103.

Barlow, D. H. (2004). Psychological treatments. *American Psychologist, 59,* 869–878.

Benish, S., Imel, Z. E., & Wampold, B. E. (2008). The relative efficacy of bona fide psychotherapies of post-traumatic stress disorder: A meta-analysis of direct comparisons. *Clinical Psychology Review, 28,* 746–758.

Breuer, J., & Freud, S. (1955). Studies on hysteria. In J. Strachey (Ed. & Trans.), *Standard edition of the complete psychological works of Sigmund Freud* (Vol. 2, pp. 1–305). London: Hogarth Press. (Original work published 1893–1895)

Cantor, D. W., & Fuentes, M. A. (2008). Psychology's response to managed care. *Professional Psychology, 39,* 638–645.

Castonguay, L. G., & Beutler, L. E. (2006). *Principles of therapeutic change that work.* New York: Oxford University Press.

Chambless, D. L., & Ollendick, T. H. (2001). Empirically supported psychological interventions: Controversies and evidence. *Annual Review of Psychology, 52,* 685–716.

Clarkin, J. F., Levy, K. N., Lenzenweger, M. F., & Kernberg, O. F. (2007). *American Journal of Psychiatry, 164,* 1–8.

Cozolino, L. (2002). *The neuroscience of psychotherapy.* New York: Norton.

Cuijpers, P., van Straten, A., Andersson, G., & van Oppen, P. (2008). Psychotherapy for depression in adults: A meta-analysis of comparative outcome studies. *Journal of Consulting and Clinical Psychology, 76,* 909–922.

de Jonghe, F., Kool, S., van Aalst, G., Dekker, J., & Peen, J. (2001). Combining psychotherapy and antidepressants in the treatment of depression. *Journal of Affective Disorders, 64,* 217–229.

Dollard, J., & Miller, N. E. (1950). *Personality and psychotherapy.* New York: McGraw-Hill.

Eells, T. D. (Ed.). (2007). *Handbook of psychotherapy case formulation* (2nd. ed.). New York: Guilford Press.

Elliott, R., Rhea, P., Alperin, R., Dobrenski, R., Wagner, J., Messer, S. B., et al. (2009). An adjudicated hermeneutic single-case efficacy design study of experiential therapy for panic/phobia. *Psychotherapy Research, 19,* 543–557.

Feldman, L. B., & Feldman, S. L. (2005). Commentary. In J. C. Norcross & M. R. Goldfried (Eds.), The future of psychotherapy integration: A roundtable. *Journal of Psychotherapy Integration, 15,* 392–471.

Fishbane, M. D. (2007). Wired to connect: Neuroscience, relationships, and therapy. *Family Process, 46,* 395–412.

Fishman, D. B. (2001). From single case to database: A new method for enhancing psychotherapy, forensic, and other psychological practice. *Applied and Preventive Psychology, 10,* 275–304.

Fontes, L. A. (2008). *Interviewing clients across cultures: A practitioner's guide.* New York: Guilford Press.

Fournier, J. C., DeRubeis, R. J., Hollon, S. D., Dimidjian, S., Amsterdam, J. D., Shelton, R. C., et al. (2010). Antidepressant drug effects and depression severity: A patient-level meta-analysis. *Journal of the American Medical Association, 303,* 47–53.

Frank, J. D., & Frank, J. B. (1991). *Persuasion and healing.* Baltimore: Johns Hopkins University Press.

Friedlander, M. L., Escudero, V., & Heatherington, L. (2006). *Therapeutic alliances with couples and families: An empirically informed guide to practice.* Washington, DC: American Psychological Association Press.

Fuertes, J. N., Stracuzzi, T. I., Hersch, M., Bennett, J., Scheinholtz, J., & Mislowack, A. (2006). Therapist multicultural competency: A study of therapy dyads. *Psychotherapy, 43,* 480–490.

Gielen, U. P., Draguns, J. G., & Fish, J. M. (2008). *Principles of multicultural counseling and therapy.* New York: Routledge.

Goldfried, M. R. (2011). Mindfulness and acceptance in cognitive behavior therapy: What's new? In J. Herbert & E. Forman (Eds.), *Acceptance and mindfulness in cognitive behavior therapy* (pp. 317–333). Hoboken, NJ: Wiley.

Goodheart, C. D. (2006). Evidence, endeavor, and expertise in psychological practice. In C. D. Goodheart, A. E. Kazdin, & R. J. Sternberg (Eds.), *Evidence-based psychotherapy: Where practice and research meet* (pp. 37–61). Washington, DC: American Psychological Association.

Gottlieb, M. C., Lasser, J., & Simpson, G. L. (2008). Legal and ethical issues in couple therapy. In A. S. Gurman (Ed.), *Clinical handbook of couple therapy* (pp. 698–717). New York: Guilford Press.

Grencavage, L. M., & Norcross, J. C. (1990). Where are the commonalities among the therapeutic common factors? *Professional Psychology: Research and Practice, 21,* 372–378.

Gurman, A. S. (1983). *Psychotherapy research and the practice of psychotherapy.* Presidential address, Society for Psychotherapy Research, Sheffield, UK.

Gurman, A. S. (2001). Brief therapy and couple/family therapy: An essential redundancy. *Clinical Psychology: Science and Practice, 8,* 51–65.

Gurman, A. S. (2005). Brief integrative marital therapy. In J. Lebow (Ed.), *Handbook of clinical family therapy* (pp. 353–383). New York: Oxford University Press.

Gurman, A. S. (2008). Integrative couple therapy: A depth-behavioral approach. In A. S. Gurman (Ed.), *Clinical handbook of couple therapy* (4th ed., pp. 383–423). New York: Guilford Press.

Gurman, A. S., & Fraenkel, P. (2002). The history of couple therapy: A millennial review. *Family Process, 41,* 199–260.

Gurman, A. S., & Snyder, D. K. (2010). Couple therapy. In J. Norcross, G. VandenBos, & D. Freidheim (Eds.), *History of psychotherapy* (2nd ed., pp. 485–496). Washington, DC: American Psychological Association.

Hayes, S. C. (2004). Acceptance and commitment therapy, relational frame theory and the third wave of behavioral and cognitive therapies. *Behavior Therapy, 35,* 639–665.

Hayes, S. C., & Toarmino, D. (1995, February). If behavioral principles are generally applicable, why is it necessary to understand cultural diversity? *Behavior Therapist, 18,* 21–23.

Hofstee, W. K. B. (2003). Structures of personality traits. In T. Millon & M. J. Lerner (Eds.), *Handbook of psychology: Vol. 5. Personality and social psychology* (pp. 231–254). New York: Wiley.

Hollon, S. D., Thase, M. E., & Markowitz, J. C. (2002). Treatment and prevention of depression. *Psychological Science in the Public Interest, 3,* 39–77.

Imel, Z. E., Wampold, B. E., Miller, S. D., & Fleming, R. R. (2008). Distinctions without a difference: Direct comparisons of psychotherapies for alcohol use disorders. *Journal of Addictive Behaviors, 22,* 533–543.

Institute of Medicine. (2001). *Crossing the quality chasm: A new health system for the 21st century.* Washington, DC: National Academy Press.

Khan, A., Redding, N., & Brown, W. A. (2008). The persistence of the placebo response in antidepressant clinical trials. *Journal of Psychiatric Research, 42,* 791–796.

Kirsch, I., & Sapirstein, G. (1999). Listening to Prozac but hearing placebo: A meta-analysis of antidepressant medication. In I. Kirsch (Ed.), *How expectancies shape experience* (pp. 303–320). Washington, DC: American Psychological Association.

Lambert, M. J. (2008, April). *Searching for the supershrink: What are the differences between therapists whose patients have outstanding and poor outcomes?* Keynote address presented at the Austrian Cognitive Behavior Therapy Association, Bad Aussee, Austria.

Lambert, M. J., & Ogles, B. M. (2004). The efficacy and effectiveness of psychotherapy. In M. J. Lambert (Ed.), *Bergin and Garfield's handbook of psychotherapy and behavior change* (5th ed., pp. 139–193). New York: Wiley.

LaRoche, M., & Christopher, M. S. (2008). Culture and empirically supported treatments: On the road to a collision. *Culture and Psychology, 14,* 333–356.

Leichsenring, F., & Rabung, S. (2008). Effectiveness of long-term psychodynamic psychotherapy: A meta-analysis. *Journal of the American Medical Association, 300*(13), 1551–1565.

Levenson, H. (2010). *Brief dynamic psychotherapy*. Washington, DC: American Psychological Association.

Lewin, K. (1951). *Field theory in social science: Selected theoretical papers* (D. Cartwright, Ed.). New York: Harper & Row.

Linehan, M. M., Comtois, K. A., Murray, A. M., Brown, M. Z., Gallop, R. J., Heard, H. L., et al. (2006). Two-year randomized controlled trial and follow-up of dialectical behavior therapy vs. therapy by experts for suicidal behaviors and borderline personality disorder. *Archives of General Psychiatry, 63*, 757–766.

Luborsky, L., Rosenthal, R., Diguer, L., Andrusyna, T. P., Berman, J. S., Levitt, J. T., et al. (2002). The dodo bird verdict is alive and well—mostly. *Clinical Psychology: Science and Practice, 9*, 2–12.

Manber, R., Kraemer, H. C., Arnow, B. A., Trivedi, M. H., Rush, A. J., Thase, M. E., et al. (2008). Faster remission of chronic depression with combined psychotherapy and medication than with each therapy alone. *Journal of Consulting and Clinical Psychology, 76*, 459–467.

McMinn, M. R., Hathaway, W. L., Woods, S. W., & Snow, K. N. (2009). What American Psychological Association leaders have to say about *Psychology of Religion and Spirituality*. *Psychology of Religion and Spirituality, 1*, 3–13.

Meltzoff, J., & Kornreich, M. (1970). *Research in psychotherapy*. New York: Atherton.

Messer, S. B. (2001). Assimilative integration [Special issue]. *Journal of Psychotherapy Integration, 11*, 1–154.

Messer, S. B. (2004). Evidence-based practice: Beyond empirically supported treatments. *Professional Psychology, 35*, 580–588.

Messer, S. B. (2006). What qualifies as evidence of effective practice?: Patient values and preferences. In J. C. Norcross, L. E. Beutler, & R. F. Levant (Eds.), *Evidence-based practice in mental health* (pp. 31–39). Washington, DC: American Psychological Association.

Messer, S. B. (2009). Common factors in psychotherapy: Three perspectives. *Applied and Preventive Psychology, 13*, 22–23.

Messer, S. B., & McCann, L. (2005). Research perspectives on the case study: Single-case method. In J. S. Auerbach, K. N. Levy, & C. E. Schaffer (Eds.), *Relatedness, self-definition, and mental representation: Essays in honor of Sidney J. Blatt* (pp. 222–237). New York: Routledge.

Messer, S. B., Sanderson, W. C., & Gurman, A. S. (2003). Brief psychotherapies. In G. Stricker & T. A. Widiger (Eds.), *Handbook of psychology: Vol. 8. Clinical psychology* (pp. 407–430). New York: Wiley.

Messer, S. B., & Wachtel, P. L. (1997). The contemporary psychotherapeutic landscape: Issues and prospects. In P. L. Wachtel & S. B. Messer (Eds.), *Theories of psychotherapy: Origins and evolution* (pp. 1–38). Washington, DC: American Psychological Association.

Messer, S. B., & Wampold, B. E. (2002). Let's face facts: Common factors are more potent than specific ingredients. *Clinical Psychology: Science and Practice, 9*, 21–25.

Messer, S. B., & Winokur, M. (1984). Ways of knowing and visions of reality in psychoanalytic and behavior therapy. In H. Arkowitz & S. B. Messer (Eds.), *Psychoanalytic therapy and behavior therapy: Is integration possible?* (pp. 53–100). New York: Plenum Press.

Messer, S. B., & Wolitzky, D. L. (2007). The psychoanalytic approach to case formulation. In T. D. Eells (Ed.), *Handbook of psychotherapy case formulation* (2nd. ed., pp. 67–104). New York: Guilford Press.

Messer, S. B., & Woolfolk, R. L. (1998). Philosophical issues in psychotherapy. *Clinical Psychology: Science and Practice, 5*, 251–263.

Messer, S. B., & Woolfolk, R. L. (2010). Philosophy of psychotherapy. In I. B. Weiner & W. E. Craighead (Eds.), *The Corsini encyclopedia of psychology* (4th ed., Vol. 3, pp. 1387–1389). New York: Wiley.

Moodley, R., & Palmer, S. (Eds.). (2006). *Race, culture and psychotherapy*. New York: Routledge.

Nathan, P. E., & Gorman, J. M. (Eds.). (2007). *A guide to treatments that work* (3rd ed.). New York: Oxford University Press.

Neisser, U. (1967). *Cognitive psychology*. New York: Appleton-Century-Crofts.

Norcross, J. C. (Ed.). (2011). *Psychotherapy relationships that work: Therapist contributions and responsiveness to patients* (2nd ed.). New York: Oxford University Press.

Norcross, J. C., Hedges, M., & Prochaska, J. O. (2002). The face of 2010: A Delphi poll on the future of psychotherapy. *Professional Psychology, 33*, 316–322.

Norcross, J. C., Klonsky, E. D., & Tropiano, H. L. (2008). The research–practice gap: Clinical scientists and independent practitioners speak. *Clinical Psychologist, 61*, 14–17.

Norcross, J. C., & Prochaska, J. O. (1983). Clinicians' theoretical orientations: Selection, utilization and efficacy. *Professional Psychology, 14*, 197–208.

Norcross, J. C., VandenBos, G., & Freedheim, D. (Eds.). (2010). *History of psychotherapy* (2nd ed.). Washington, DC: American Psychological Association.

Panksepp, J. (1998). *Affective neuroscience.* New York: Oxford University Press.

Pergament, K. I. (2007). *Spiritually integrated psychotherapy.* New York: Guilford Press.

Pinquart, M., Duberstein, P. R., & Lyness, J. M. (2006). Treatments for later-life depressive conditions: A meta-analytic comparison of pharmacotherapy and psychotherapy. *American Journal of Psychiatry, 163*(9), 1493–1501.

Schneider, K. J. (1999). Multiple-case research: Bringing experience-near closer. *Journal of Clinical Psychology, 55*, 1531–1540.

Sexton, T., Gordon, K. S., Gurman, A. S., Lebow, J. L., Johnson, S. M., & Holtzworth-Munroe, A. (2010). *Evidence-based treatments in couple and family therapy: Report of the Task Force on Evidence-Based Treatments in Family Psychology.* Division 43, American Psychological Association.

Shedler, J. (2010). The efficacy of psychodynamic psychotherapy. *American Psychologist, 65*, 98–109.

Siegel, D. (1999). *The developing mind: Toward a neurobiology of interpersonal experience.* New York: Guilford Press.

Spence, D. P. (1998). Rain forest or mud field: Guest editorial. *International Journal of Psychoanalysis, 79*, 643–647.

Sperry, L., & Shafranske, E. P. (Eds.). (2005). *Spiritually oriented psychotherapy.* New York: Guilford Press.

Sprenkle, D., Davis, S. D., & Lebow, J. C. (2009). *Common factors in couple and family therapy.* New York: Guilford Press.

Stewart, R. E., & Chambless, D. L. (2007). Does psychotherapy research inform treatment decisions in private practice? *Journal of Clinical Psychology, 63*, 267–281.

Sue, D. W., & Sue, D. (2008). *Counseling the culturally diverse.* New York: Wiley.

Tarragona, M. (2009). Postmodern/poststructuralist therapies. In J. L. Lebow (Ed.), *Twenty-first century psychotherapies* (pp. 167–205). New York: Wiley.

Wachtel, P. L. (1977). *Psychoanalysis and behavior therapy.* New York: Basic Books.

Wachtel, P. L. (1997). *Psychoanalysis, behavior therapy and the relational world.* Washington, DC: American Psychological Association Press.

Wachtel, P. L. (Ed.). (2008). Psychotherapy from an international perspective. *Journal of Psychotherapy Integration, 18*, 66–69.

Wampold, B. E. (2001). *The great psychotherapy debate: Models, methods and findings.* Mahwah, NJ: Erlbaum.

Weinberger, J. L., & Rasco, C. (2007). Empirically supported common factors. In S. G. Hofmann & J. L. Weinberger (Eds.), *The art and science of psychotherapy* (pp. 103–129). New York: Routledge.

Winston, A., Been, H., & Serby, M. (2005). Psychotherapy or psychopharmacology: Different universes or an integrated future? *Journal of Psychotherapy Integration, 15*, 213–223.

Wolf, A. W. (2009). Comment: Can clinical judgment hold its own against scientific knowledge?: Comment on Zeldow. *Psychotherapy, 46*, 11–14.

Woolfolk, R. L. (1998). *The cure of souls: Science, values and psychotherapy.* San Francisco: Jossey-Bass.

Zeldow, P. B. (2009). In defense of clinical judgment, credentialed clinicians, and reflective practice. *Psychotherapy, 46*, 1–10.

PART II

PSYCHOANALYTIC APPROACHES

Contemporary Freudian Psychoanalytic Psychotherapy

David L. Wolitzky

The aim of this chapter is to introduce the theory and practice of contemporary Freudian psychoanalysis and the psychoanalytic psychotherapy that derived from it. The term *psychoanalysis* refers to (1) a theory of personality and psychopathology, (2) a method of investigating the mind, and (3) a theory of treatment. I am concerned primarily with the theory of treatment but will need to present some of the basic theoretical concepts as the context for understanding the rationale for therapeutic intervention.

HISTORICAL BACKGROUND

Sigmund Freud (1856–1939) was the founder of psychoanalysis and the father of modern psychotherapy. Although he was confronted with the exigencies of the clinical situation, Freud's primary aspiration was to develop psychoanalysis as a theory of the human mind and to develop it secondarily as a therapeutic modality. Accordingly, his theoretical writings consume the bulk of the 23 volumes of his collected works, published as the definitive *Standard Edition of the Complete Psychological Works of Sigmund Freud* (Freud, Volume 1, 1891—Volume 23, 1940).

As a comprehensive theory of personality and psychopathology, psychoanalysis had a profound impact on 20th-century thought and culture, an impact unrivaled by any other conception of personality. Psychoanalytic theorizing has not only aimed at understanding and explaining the nature of psychopathology but has also addressed the broader domain of normal personality functioning and the development of personality. In this sense it can be regarded as a general psychology. As such, it ranges from neurobiological explanations of key aspects of mental life (e.g., cognition, affect, and motivation) to sociocultural, historical theorizing about the origins of society and the family. Attempts to understand art, literature, music, religion, and virtually all other aspects of human experience according to psychoanalytic principles (so-called *applied psychoanalysis*) have filled innumerable journals and books for more than a century.

The origins of psychoanalysis can be traced back to the last two decades of the 19th century, to the cultural context of turn-of-the-century Vienna. It has evolved during the course of the past century and spread throughout the world, particularly to the rest of Europe, the United States, and South America. Freud's life and the psychoanalytic movement he inspired and led have been the subject of a multitude of books and articles through the years.

In the past century, we saw many developments in psychoanalytic theory and practice. All of them took their point of departure from Freud by either extending or modifying a line of thought implicit or undeveloped in his work, or by rejecting essential Freudian assumptions yet referring to their alternative conceptions by the term *psychoanalytic*. Indeed, there have been many heated professional squabbles through the years about whether one should call certain "deviations" from the original theory and practice of psychoanalysis by that name. For instance, the so-called neo-Freudians (e.g., Adler, Jung, and Horney) have been called "deviant" in that each departs from Freud's emphasis on the importance of childhood sexuality. Whether a new school of psychoanalytic thought evolves and becomes assimilated into the mainstream of the prevailing psychoanalytic paradigms or becomes a "deviant" school often has more to do with the existing sociohistorical *Zeitgeist* than with the extent to which the theory advanced departs from Freud's views. A case in point is Kohut's (1971) self psychology, which departs in fundamental ways from basic Freudian tenets yet has not created the kinds of schisms that characterized earlier theoretical differences.

There is by now significant diversity within what has been termed "the common ground of psychoanalysis" (Wallerstein, 1990), meaning attention to the clinical phenomena of transference and resistance. However, even these phenomena are conceptualized differently by different psychoanalytic theorists. Thus, it is no longer accurate to refer to *the* psychoanalytic theory of personality or of treatment. Rather, we need to specify the particular theoretical perspective from which we derive our clinical approach. In this chapter, I focus primarily on the *contemporary Freudian approach to treatment*. This approach is heavily influenced by traditional Freudian theory, its ego-psychological extensions, and modifications of those views. Therefore, I will start with an account of Freud's core concepts, some of their extensions and modifications by later theorists, and their implications for treatment.

For present purposes, we can divide theoretical changes in psychoanalytic thinking into four main eras: (1) Freud's postulation of libidinal and aggressive instinctual drives as the prime movers of mental life; (2) the development of ego psychology, which focused on the defensive and coping devices used to deal with conflicted, often unconscious wishes; (3) the evolution of various versions of object relations theories, with their focus on needs for relatedness rather than gratification of sexual and aggressive wishes, and on the internalized representation of .interpersonal relationships; and (4) the advent of self psychology (Kohut, 1971, 1977, 1984), in which the cohesion and fulfillment of the self came to be regarded as the individual's primary aim (Pine, 1990). In the last two decades, we have witnessed the widespread influence of what broadly can be termed *American relational theory*. Developed mainly by Mitchell (1988), relational theories (which are discussed by Curtis & Hirsch in Chapter 3, this volume) are an amalgam of Sullivan's (1953) interpersonal theory and British object relations theories, primarily Fairbairn (1941) and Winnicott (1965). Relational theorists' point of departure from Freudian theory is captured in Fairbairn's (1952, p. 82) dictum that "libido is object seeking, not pleasure seeking," in other words, that we are more interested in relationships than in satisfying instinctual drives. In my view, this is a false dichotomy that has created much unnecessary controversy.

This chapter focuses primarily on the first and second eras of psychoanalytic theorizing and on the contemporary understandings of those views. This *contemporary Freudian* approach continues to adhere to most of the core propositions of Freud's clinical theories in the context of subsequent modifications and extensions of those theories. Current conceptualizations by and large dispense with Freud's metapsychological concepts such as "cathexis" and "psychic energies," because such concepts have little scientific basis and are far removed from the clinical situation. Given this brief, orienting context, we can now proceed to trace the evolution of the Freudian theory of treatment.

Prior to the development of any form of psychoanalytic therapy, the main methods of treating emotional and mental disturbances were rest, massage, hydrotherapy (warm baths), faradic therapy (the application of low-voltage electrical stimulation to areas of the body that were symptomatic), and hypnosis. As we shall see later, psychoanalysis evolved from attempts to treat symptoms via hypnosis (e.g., Charcot, 1882; Janet, 1907).

Freud, impressed by Charcot's demonstrations of hypnotic effects, became particularly interested in the potential of hypnotic suggestion as a therapeutic tool. The kinds of patients first treated by Freud were usually late adolescent women who presented with hysterical symptoms, that is, disturbances in the senses and/or the musculature, such as "blindness," paralyses, mutism, convulsive-like motor actions (e.g., trembling), and anesthesia (i.e., loss of or diminished sensation in one or more parts of the body). These symptoms came to be regarded as psychological when no organic basis for them could be found. It is quite likely that some organic conditions were mistaken for neurotic ones and vice versa.

At first, Freud tried the direct, hypnotic suggestion that the symptom(s) disappear, an approach that generally met with limited success. Some patients could not readily be hypnotized; in others, symptoms would dissipate but return. These early clinical experiences led Freud to become more curious about the causes and mechanisms of symptom formation and to search for more effective therapeutic methods. With regard to the latter, Freud sometimes used the so-called "pressure technique," in which he placed his hand on the patient's forehead and gave the strong suggestion that the patient would remember the original experience associated with the onset of the symptoms. These early variations in technique evolved into the method of *free association,* in which the patient is asked to say whatever comes to mind, without the usual editing and inhibition characteristic of typical social interactions.

The patient known as Anna O provided a critical turning point for Freud and for the development of psychoanalysis. Anna O was suffering from a variety of hysterical symptoms. She wanted the opportunity to talk and have a "catharsis"; this marked the birth of psychoanalysis as the "talking cure." Breuer and Freud (1895/1955) published their ideas about Anna O and other patients in *Studies on Hysteria,* the key idea contained in this work being that "hysterics suffer from reminiscences"; that is, a painful memory is dissociated from the mass of conscious experience and the "quota of affect" associated with that memory is converted to a bodily symptom. The release of the dammed-up affect via retrieving and talking about the memory allows for the "associative reabsorption" of the blocked idea and feelings, and causes the symptom to disappear.

In this early phase of his work, Freud's focus was on eliminating the symptom. Symptoms were regarded as circumscribed, disembodied foreign objects to be excised, not unlike an impacted wisdom tooth. The nature of the person in whom the symptoms resided was not considered important. However, Freud soon realized that patients' symptoms were meaningful expressions of their character and overall personality functioning. Over the next several decades, Freud evolved his theory of personality development and psychopathology, which took into account the interaction of biological and experiential factors, to explain both symptom formation and the development of character traits and defenses.

As he developed his *psychodynamic* point of view, Freud saw patients as being motivated by a desire not only to seek gratification of wishes but also to keep the wish and its associated affect out of awareness if it was regarded as dangerous and/or unacceptable. In this "drive-defense" model, *repression* (i.e., the motivated expulsion from consciousness and forgetting of the disagreeable idea or conflicted wish) is an attempt to repudiate or disavow impulses that are likely to be anxiety arousing or repugnant to one's sense of morality. Although repression and other defensive maneuvers (e.g., projection, denial, reaction formation) appear to banish threatening wishes, they do not destroy them, and they always weaken the personality by impairing its integrated functioning.

THE CONCEPT OF PERSONALITY

For Freud, the basic unit of study was the intrapsychic life of the individual, that is, the basic motives, wishes, anxieties, defenses, and regulatory capacities of the developing child, as seen primarily from the perspective of psychic conflicts within the person regarding the search for instinctual drive gratification.

What are the basic tensions one must reduce to avoid unpleasure and achieve instinctual gratification? Freud always postulated two major classes of instinctual drives. At first, the two drives were the sexual or *libidinal* and the self-preservative or *ego instincts*. Later, Freud theorized that the two major drives were the *libidinal* (or sexual) drive and the *aggressive* drive, both broadly conceptualized. According to the theory, a drive is the psychical representative of the instinct. It is a demand made on the mind for work. It impels the organism to mental and physical activity, the aim of which is to discharge the nervous system excitation produced by the drive. According to Freud's final theory, sexuality (broadly conceived as sensual) and aggression (also broadly conceived; e.g., competition) were the two basic human motivational wellsprings of behavior.

There are four main characteristics of an instinctual drive; it has a *source* (a bodily tension), an *impetus* (a degree of intensity), an *aim* (to lessen the drive tension), and an *object* (the means whereby the drive tension is reduced; e.g., sucking one's thumb or milk from mother's breast). The object is the most variable aspect of the drive (i.e., the drive can be more or less satisfied in a number of ways). Although the term *object* sounds quite impersonal and strange when applied to a person, it is used generally in psychoanalytic theory to indicate that wishes can be directed to inanimate objects and, especially, to so-called *internalized objects* (mental representations of the other). We do not directly observe drives but infer them on the basis of *drive derivatives* (i.e., wishes).

Freud believed that there were two basic tendencies governing mental life, the *pleasure principle* and the *reality principle*. According to the pleasure principle, the basic tendency of the organism is to maximize pleasure and to minimize pain, and to do so in as rapid and automatic a way as possible. Increases in endogenous excitation were regarded as unpleasant, whereas decreases were associated with pleasure. Reality forces the organism to give up sole reliance on the pleasure principle. For example, the hungry infant needs eventually to discriminate between a fantasy of being fed and actually eating, in other words, to operate according to the *reality principle*.

Freud's theory has a strong developmental emphasis, as seen in his *stages of psychosexual development*. These stages are the *oral, anal, phallic*, and *genital*. Each stage is influenced by the preceding ones and in turn influences subsequent stages. As the name implies, the *oral* stage centers on concerns with hunger, with the mouth as the chief bodily zone involved, but is conceived of more broadly as including maternal care and comfort. At this stage the primary fear is loss of the object—that is, of the mother as the supplier and regulator of the infant's needs. In the *anal* phase, the focus is on toilet training, and the major anxiety is loss of the parent's love. In the *phallic* phase, the boy is subject to *castration anxiety* (and the girl to *penis envy*), and in the *genital* stage, guilt is the major danger. Erikson (1950/1963) presented a psychosocial elaboration of Freud's psychosexual stages in which he emphasized the psychological experiences central to each psychosexual stage (e.g., describing the oral stage as the time when the infant first establishes a "basic trust" or "mistrust" of the social world).

The anticipation of the dangers in each psychosexual stage gives rise to *signal anxiety* and triggers a *defense* against a potentially full-blown, traumatic anxiety. For example, suppose a young boy has incestuous wishes toward his mother but believes and fears that such wishes are wrong and will lead to his castration by the father. The boy, who both loves his father and fears and resents him as an unwanted rival, now needs to defend against his sexual wishes toward his mother. This, of course, is the classic *Oedipal conflict* so central to traditional Freudian theory.

Two other key Freudian concepts deserve at least brief mention: *fixation* and *regression*. According to Freud, excessive frustration or satisfaction at each psychosexual stage could lead to a *fixation*, or rigid clinging to a particular mode of satisfaction characteristic of that stage. For example, excessive oral satisfaction (or frustration) could lead to the persistence of thumb-sucking long after it is age appropriate. *Regression* refers to the reinstatement of a mode of seeking satisfaction that is no longer age appropriate. If, for example, the birth of a sibling leaves the older sibling feeling terribly unloved, he or she might revert to thumb-sucking. Freud believed that the major modes of adaptation to the environment and to the regulation of tension states are well developed by the time a child is about 6 years old and change relatively little after that.

Additional core, interrelated propositions of traditional Freudian theory that contemporary Freudians still embrace include the following:

1. The principle of psychic determinism states that there is a lawful regularity to mental life; that is, even seemingly random or "accidental" mental phenomena have causes.

2. A substantial part of mental life takes place outside conscious awareness. Unconscious wishes and motives exert a powerful influence on conscious thought and behavior, and can explain seemingly random or "accidental behaviors" (e.g., slips of the tongue and many other kinds of parapraxes described by Freud, 1901/1960), in *The Psychopathology of Everyday Life*).

3. All behavior is motivated by a desire (a) to avoid being rendered helpless by excessive stimulation, and (b) to maximize pleasure and minimize pain (*the pleasure principle*).

4. Inner conflict is inevitable and ubiquitous; all behavior reflects efforts at effecting a compromise among the various components of the personality, principally one's desires for

instinctual drive gratification (sexual and aggressive) and the constraints against such grat-ification (physical reality, social constraints, and superego prohibitions). This idea takes its fullest form in Freud's (1923/1961, 1926/1959) structural theory of id, ego, and superego.

Freud's clinical observations led him to the idea that the main inner *conflicts* were ones between the person's impulses and his or her internalized notions of right and wrong, as well as their assessments of the risks and dangers of becoming aware of or expressing the concealed impulses. Accordingly, he grouped psychological aspects and forces in the mind into three main agencies of the mind—the id, the ego, and the superego. The *id* refers to our sexual and aggressive instinctual strivings. The *superego* has two aspects, our internal-ized values (i.e., our conscience) and our ego ideals (our criteria for feeling good about ourselves). The *ego* is described in terms of a variety of functions (e.g., judgment, plan-ning, reality testing, coping and defensive strategies) that work together to determine the cost–benefit of expressing particular id urges. In a healthy, functioning person these three aspects of personality blend harmoniously with one another.

Although textbooks continue to present the standard Freudian view of id, ego, and superego, among many contemporary Freudians, this conceptualization has given way in recent years to one in which all mental activity is viewed as a *compromise formation* (Brenner, 1994). This term describes the mind as functioning to give expression to the person's wishes while taking into account the potential anxiety, fear, and guilt the free expression of wishes might engender.

5. Anxiety in small doses (i.e., *signal anxiety*) is a danger signal that triggers defen-sive measures designed to avoid awareness and/or behavior geared toward gratification of unconscious wishes, in order to avoid an anticipated full-blown traumatic experience of anxiety that would totally overwhelm the ego and flood the organism with an unmanage-able amount of excitation.

6. The principle of *multiple determination* (sometimes misleadingly called "overdetermi-nation") refers to the facts of divergent and convergent causality; that is, the same motive can give rise to myriad behaviors, and a given behavior is a function of multiple motives.

Psychoanalytic ego psychology was developed, in part, as a corrective to an excessive emphasis on sexual and aggressive motives. Aspects of ego psychology were implied by Freud but fully developed by Anna Freud (1937), Hartmann, Kris, and Loewenstein (1946), and others. As seen by these theorists, ego capacities (e.g., cognition, delay of gratification, reality testing, and judgment) can be involved in conflict but later function as "conflict-free spheres of the ego." This theoretical thrust was an attempt to flesh out the ego's role in adaptation and to make theoretical room for behaviors, interests, and motives that are not always embedded in conflict or simply indirect expressions or sublimations of sexual or aggressive wishes.

Mahler's (1968) studies of separation–individuation and Jacobson's (1964) work on the self have contributed significantly to our understanding of the development of the self-hood, a topic largely ignored in early psychoanalytic writings. In more recent years, issues of self-esteem and disturbances in the sense of self have been a prominent focus of psycho-analytic theorizing, particularly in borderline and narcissistic conditions (Kernberg, 1975; Kohut, 1971). These theoretical developments owe much to Freud's papers *On Narcissism* (1914/1957) and *Mourning and Melancholia* (1917/1958) which contain numerous implica-tions for our conceptions of psychosis, character development, identification and loss, and object relations.

PSYCHOLOGICAL HEALTH AND PATHOLOGY

Behavior is dysfunctional or pathological to the extent that the *compromise formations* among the constituents of the personality (wishes, moral standards, preferred modes of defense, judgments about reality, etc.) are *maladaptive*; that is, they create more pain than pleasure, bring the person into significant interpersonal conflict, create undue anxiety and/or guilt and depressive affects, lead to significant inhibitions in personal functioning, and thereby impair the person's capacity to love and/or work. In this view, there is no sharp demarcation between "normal" and "abnormal" functioning.

The appearance of symptoms or the development of ego inhibitions is an indication of ineffective coping with inner conflict. For example, the onset of *agoraphobia* (fear of open spaces) can represent the person's failed defense against the anxiety attached to desires to separate and function in a more autonomous manner, desires that may be experienced as arousing sufficient separation anxiety for the person to seek the seeming safety of home. The onset of hysterical blindness in a mother who harbors hostile wishes toward her son, who then has a bad accident because his mother was not watching him, may be understood, in part, as self-punishment for her hostile wishes. In another example, impotence in a male in relation to certain women, but not others, may be due to the fact that the women with whom the impotence occurs are unconsciously regarded as incestuous objects, and the impotence is an inhibition of unacceptable, anxiety-ridden Oedipal wishes.

The formation of symptoms is based on wishes regarded as dangerous and/or unacceptable that are too strong, and/or defenses that are too weak to contain the wishes in a sufficiently disguised form. The outbreak of psychological symptoms is an expression of the "return of the repressed." In this "drive-defense" model, symptoms vary with respect to the extent to which they show evidence of the underlying wish and its attempted gratification (e.g., obsessive thoughts of stabbing someone) or show more clearly the defensive side of the conflict (e.g., hiding all the knives in the house).

The maintenance of symptoms is due to the primary and secondary gain they provide. The *primary gain* is the relative freedom from anxiety and other dysphoric affects (Brenner, 1982) that is achieved while partially satisfying a wish in a compromise form. *Secondary gain* refers to the fringe benefits of a symptom (e.g., "justifiable" escape from normal responsibilities and feeling that one's dependency needs are more legitimate).

The same drive-defense model also is used as part of the explanation for development of personality or character styles. By *personality* or *character* I mean the unique psychological organization (of traits, conflicts, defensive and coping strategies, attitudes, values, cognitive style, etc.) that characterizes the individual's stable, enduring modes of adaptation across a wide range of conditions encountered in his or her "average expectable environment" (Hartmann, 1939). With regard to the drive-defense model, a pattern of noncommitment in relationships, for example, might protect the person against the feared consequences of emotional and romantic intimacy in instances in which such intimacy might give rise to claustrophobic anxiety, which in turn might be based on a sense of danger about what may be seen as a forbidden *Oedipal triumph*. This term refers to any wish, attitude, or action that signifies (usually on an unconscious, symbolic level) the son's desire to win the competition with his father for his mother's love. Such desires typically are conflicted due in part to fear of the father's retribution in the form of disapproval, rejection, and castration. To avoid these anxieties, the person might choose to enter relationships that are at some level "known" to preclude the possibility of a serious commitment. When this pattern is repeated, the person might have the conscious experience of feeling frustrated and puzzled at the failure of any of his relationships to last, without being aware of the underlying dynamic conflict.

Over the years, there has been increasing interest in studying character and character pathology (e.g., Baudry, 1989; Reich, 1933). In part, this interest is due to the apparently growing number of patients who present with character disorders, particularly narcissistic and borderline personalities, rather than symptom neuroses, and to the idea that dealing with symptoms in treatment is less effective if one fails to address the personality in which they are embedded. Maladaptive patterns of dealing with conflict tend to become rigidified and repeated in vicious cycles, as in the case I present later. By definition, personality structure changes at a slow rate. This is one reason that meaningful personality change through psychotherapy generally takes a long time.

THE PROCESS OF CLINICAL ASSESSMENT

The unit of study is the individual or, more specifically, the problematic aspects of his or her personality functioning. Although the clinician will want to know a great deal about the individual's actual adaptive and maladaptive functioning in different social contexts (family, friends, work groups, etc.), the main relevance of this information is its value in understanding the intrapsychic world of the individual.

The primary means of conducting the assessment of the individual's personality and psychopathology is through a series of clinical interviews, on the basis of which the clinician assesses the prospective patient's suitability for psychoanalytic treatment (Messer & Wolitzky, 2007). In the course of the clinical interview, the therapist attempts to form an initial picture of the patient's current and past level of functioning, including the nature, onset, duration, intensity, and fluctuation of symptoms. The therapist also begins to get a sense of the patient's character style, his or her principal defenses and regulation of affect, intactness of reality testing, self-esteem issues, quality of interpersonal relationships, and the core unconscious conflicts presumed to underlie manifest aspects of behavior. The clinician also is interested in the the psychodynamic significance of current stresses faced by the prospective patient and factors influencing the patient's decision to seek treatment. Part of this broad assessment of functioning includes an appraisal of the person's ego interests, areas of and capacity for pleasure, personality strengths, achievements, and the current reality situation.

In the course of eliciting this information, the clinician also appraises the prospective patient's suitability for treatment. Among the main qualities evaluated are the person's motivation for change; ego resources, including capacity to regress in the service of the ego (e.g., to engage in fantasy); access to and tolerance of affects; capacity to form a good therapeutic alliance, and degree of *psychological mindedness*. The latter refers to the patient's capacity for self-reflective awareness, an introspective tuning in on one's inner experiences. Because analysis requires that the patient oscillate between verbalizing his or her subjective experience and, in collaboration with the analyst, reflecting on the multiple meanings of those experiences, an inability or disinclination to view experience and behavior in psychological terms does not bode well for this form of treatment. One reason some of the initial clinical interviews are relatively unstructured is to allow for this kind of assessment.

In addition to the kinds of assessments mentioned, the analyst should also assess whether he or she has particular personality conflicts, personal biases (e.g., with respect to value systems), or other factors that might preclude the possibility of maintaining the objectivity and therapeutic conditions necessary to be helpful to the patient. If there are such potential problems, referral to another clinician is indicated.

Referrals for psychological testing are relatively rare, both at the stage of the initial assessment and later on. Such a referral is more likely when there is little treatment progress or marked unclarity regarding diagnosis (e.g., if organicity or a learning disability is suspected).

Finally, the therapist needs to assess whether matters of money, time, and/or immediate crises in the patient's life would interfere significantly with the feasibility of a sustained, unhurried analytic process. In the event that such factors are present to a strong degree, an alternative approach is recommended (e.g., a delay in the beginning of treatment; crisis intervention; and/or a more supportive, less challenging therapy).

There is no universally accepted, formal psychoanalytic system for diagnosing different varieties of dysfunction (Messer & Wolitzky, 2007). Originally, Freud focused primarily on three symptom pictures: hysterical, obsessional, and phobic. Other psychiatric syndromes soon received attention (e.g., depression, paranoid conditions, bipolar disorder, schizophrenia, and perversions). In recent years, narcissistic and borderline conditions have been the focus of intense interest, because such patients are increasingly common in psychoanalytic practice.

Psychoanalysts today generally have little use for the official psychiatric diagnostic system, the *Diagnostic and Statistical Manual of Mental Disorders* (DSM-IV; American Psychiatric Association, 2000). This view is partly due to the following;

1. Successive versions of the DSM have become increasingly atheoretical and less sympathetic to a psychoanalytic viewpoint.
2. Many analysts do not place much value on an initial, formal diagnosis beyond the gross classification of the patient as psychotic, borderline, or neurotic.
3. Many, if not most, patients seen in private analytic practices rarely meet all DSM-IV criteria for a given diagnostic category but frequently approximate, especially as the treatment unfolds, the criteria for several diagnoses; in other words, rarely do we see pure types and, in any case, the focus is more on the underlying dynamics than on the changing symptom picture.
4. A purely descriptive classification that does not attempt to address etiological and dynamic factors is of limited interest or clinical utility to psychoanalytic clinicians.

To address the limitations of DSM-IV (e.g., as a merely descriptive, atheoretical classification scheme), psychoanalytic clinicians devised the *Psychodynamic Diagnostic Manual* (PDM; PDM Task Force, 2006). The PDM provides a more comprehensive assessment of personality, including more of a focus on the patient's inner life. In addition to categories for manifest symptom patterns (S axis) and personality patterns (P axis), there is an assessment of the patient's mental functioning (M axis). The M axis includes, for example, an assessment of the patient's defensive patterns, capacity for relationships and intimacy, capacity for affective experience, and psychological mindedness. These qualities are considered important for understanding the patient's personality and planning treatment.

There have been several other psychoanalytically based attempts to form diagnostic assessments of dysfunction based on dynamic and structural features of personality functioning, particularly when the diagnostic formulation has implications for specific modifications and variations in psychoanalytic approaches to treatment. For example, Kernberg (1975), a highly influential analyst who has concentrated on borderline personality organization, has made notable contributions to the diagnosis of different levels of psychic struc- ture and pathology. His aim has been to understand these conditions from an integrated theoretical perspective that combines British object relations theories, ego psychology, and the work of Mahler (1968) and Jacobson (1964), who were interested in the developmental course of self–object (i.e., self–other) differentiation.

THE PRACTICE OF THERAPY

Basic Structure of Therapy

In what follows, I confine myself to an account of the practice of psychoanalytic treatment as it is usually thought of in relation to neurotic and some high-functioning patients with bor- derline personality disorder. I do not discuss the modifications that are made for patients with seriously borderline and narcissistic disorders, nor do I consider specific treatment approaches to particular syndromes (e.g., panic disorder, schizophrenia).

Some introductory comments are in order prior to a discussion of the basic structure of therapy. First, it is inaccurate to refer to *the* contemporary Freudian approach to treat- ment, because even among those who identify themselves as contemporary Freudians, one can delineate a range of positions. The traditional, conservative wing of Freudians adheres mainly to traditional Freudian theory, with its emphasis on a purely interpretive focus on sexual and aggressive conflicts, and unconscious fantasies as these are expressed in the transference. Technical neutrality (i.e., not taking sides in the patient's conflicts), relative anonymity, and abstinence (i.e., not gratifying transference wishes) are stressed as neces- sary for the flowering and interpretation of the transference. A second group of Freudians advocates a focus on the moment-to-moment interplay of impulse and defense at the surface of consciousness and encourages the patient to become an observer of his or her defensive maneuvers and the motives for them (Gray, 1994). A third line of thought reflects a strong appreciation of the importance of the therapeutic relationship in facilitating the analytic process with all patients but particularly with the more disturbed and difficult-to-reach patient who finds it difficult to develop "analytic trust," to realize that he or she is a presence in the analyst's mind (Ellman, 1998). Thus, as Ellman notes, the contemporary Freudian landscape ranges from the fairly "classical" approach of interpreting unconscious conflicts in terms of Freud's structural model (id, ego, superego) to Brenner's (1994) related idea of compromise formation among the components of psychic conflict, to a major focus on help- ing the patient becomes an observer and interpreter of his or her own defensive operations (the ego psychological model), to the vital importance of the analyst as a new, benign object who can facilitate the resumption of developmental growth (the self and object Freudians), an approach that goes back to Ferenczi's (1926) work and is expressed in other writings (e.g., Strachey, 1934; Stone, 1961; Loewald, 1960; Modell, 1976).

Second, psychoanalytic approaches to treatment can be arrayed on a continuum from what has been called "expressive," "exploratory," "insight-oriented," or "interpretive" at one end to an explicitly "supportive" approach that features reassurance, praise, advice, and encouragement instead of interpretations of transference and defense at the other. It should be noted that even in expressive therapy there are inherently supportive elements (e.g., listening with interest, being nonjudgmental) that not only help build a treatment alliance that makes patients more receptive to interpretations but also can be therapeutic in their own right. Schachter and Kachele (2007) advocate what they call "psychoanalysis- plus," that is, the deliberate, albeit judicious, use of explicitly supportive interventions in the context of all psychoanalytic treatment.

Third, there has been a lot written about the distinction between *psychoanalysis* and *psychoanalytically oriented psychotherapy*. There are some who make a sharp, qualitative distinction between these two forms of treatment and others who stress their similarities and overlap. In the past, the distinction has rested mainly on external criteria, such as frequency of sessions and the use of the couch. More recently (Gill, 1994) the distinction is based on the main intrinsic criterion of the degree of sustained transference-focused interpretations. Compared with psychoanalytic therapy, psychoanalysis is characterized by more frequent transference interpretations and fewer explicitly supportive interventions.

For those who favor the distinction, the implication is that whenever it is applicable, psychoanalysis, rather than psychoanalytic therapy, is the treatment of choice. It is regarded as a deeper, more thorough approach to the patient's problems. Other forms of treatment (e.g., dynamically based supportive psychotherapy) mix the "pure gold of psychoanalysis" with the "copper of suggestion" (Freud, 1905/1953, p. 260; Freud, 1919/1955). Thus, the common clinical maxim that has guided psychoanalytically oriented clinicians is to be as supportive as necessary and as exploratory as possible, that is, to minimize suggestion, advice, and reassurance and to focus on interpretations leading to insight, whether one is conducting psychoanalysis or psychoanalytic therapy. Thus, the range of psychoanalytic therapies can be regarded on a continuum, with psychoanalysis at one end, psychoanalytic psychotherapy in the middle, and supportive therapy at the other end.

In psychoanalysis today, sessions typically are held three or four times per week, for 45 or 50 minutes, over a period of many years. Psychoanalytic psychotherapy and supportive therapy usually takes place at a frequency of once or twice a week in the face-to-face position. It can last as long as psychoanalysis or may be as short as 12 sessions (e.g., Messer & Warren, 1995).

The powerful and innovative feature of psychoanalysis proper is the attempt, paradoxical in nature, to use the therapist's authority (derived in part from the patient's positive transference) to promote patient autonomy by freeing the patient from excessive reliance on suggestion and authority. Analysts have been particularly sensitive to this issue in light of the origins of psychoanalysis in Freud's initial experiments with hypnotic suggestion. Concern about capitalizing on suggestion is less the case in psychoanalytic psychotherapy, and even less in supportive treatment, where the therapist deliberately uses his or her authority and employs direct suggestions more freely.

As noted earlier, there are inherently supportive elements even in psychoanalysis (e.g., a caring, benign therapeutic relationship, as well as the implicit suggestion to think or act in a certain way, that accompanies both interpretive and noninterpretive interventions. For example, the therapist statement "You are being rather harsh with yourself" implies that the patient need not be so self-critical). It is difficult to disentangle the therapeutic benefits of support, both implicit and explicit, from those that derive from insight. In more recent years, there has been at least a partial disillusionment with insight as the primary vehicle of therapeutic change, and an increased emphasis on the healing powers of the relationship per se, especially with more disturbed patients.

In what follows, I focus primarily on psychoanalysis, with the understanding that most of what I say is more or less applicable to psychoanalytic psychotherapy.

Conduct of the Sessions

After the initial consultation sessions and arrangements for the therapy (e.g., frequency of sessions, fee), the sessions are deliberately unstructured. The analyst invites the patient to *free-associate*, that is, to say whatever comes to mind. Thus, the patient determines the content of the session. The more freely and openly the patient talks, and the more he or she is able and willing to suspend the normal inhibitions and editing processes that are part and parcel of our usual dialogue with others, the more self-disclosing the person becomes, and the easier it will be for previously repressed or suppressed feelings and thoughts to come to the surface for analytic scrutiny and understanding. The rationale for use of the couch is that being in a supine position and not seeing the analyst will facilitate the turning of attention inward rather than responding to visual cues emitted by analyst (e.g., facial expressions). Of course, even on the couch the patient is alert to nonverbal and paralinguistic features of the analyst's behavior. To whatever extent necessary, the analyst spells out the rationale for the suggested procedures and conditions of the treatment. This can include not only the rationale for the use of the couch and free association but also the analyst's role as a catalyst for the patient's self-explorations; the reasons for generally not answering questions immediately or directly; the understanding of the patient–therapist relationship as, in many respects, a microcosm of the patient's interactions with others; and so on.

The goal of encouraging the patient to free-associate is a mediating or process goal. It allows both patient and analyst to observe when and how the patient engages in defensive maneuvers in the face of actual or anticipated anxiety, or other dysphoric affect. In this manner, the patient gets an increasingly clear sense of how his or her mind works, and how these workings are shaped by unconscious factors, and by anxiety and defenses.

Rarely is a time limit imposed on the therapy. The main exception is brief, psychoanalytically oriented treatment, in which the initial treatment contract makes clear that the therapy comprises a fixed number of sessions or a fixed time period (see Messer & Warren, 1995, for an account of the variety of short-term psychoanalytically oriented psychotherapies). There also are a variety of psychoanalytically informed therapies that I do not discuss in this chapter, including child, couple, family, and group therapies.

In individual treatment, significant others in the patient's life typically are not seen by the patient's therapist. Sometimes combined formats are used. For example, a patient in individual treatment may also be seen as part of couple, family, or group therapy. In these circumstances, it generally is not considered proper practice for the patient's individual therapist to treat the patient in one of the other modalities as well. To do so would interfere with the optimal development and attempted resolution of the transference.

Goal Setting

Stated in general terms, the ultimate goal of treatment is to increase adaptive functioning by ameliorating the disabling symptoms, crippling inhibitions, and maladaptive defenses and conflict solutions that have plagued the patient. As the patient gradually reduces the neurotic vicious cycles that characterized prior adaptive efforts, he or she experiences this change as involving an expanded sense of personal agency and freedom. Usually, this goal is assumed to be so basic and obvious as not to require explicit verbalization.

Successful outcome also involves a reduction in symptoms as a by-product of the resolution of conflicts. Some conflicts are not fully resolved, nor is the patient's life expected to be free of stress. Accordingly, in *Studies on Hysteria,* Freud stated that the treatment could be considered successful if it transformed "hysterical misery into common unhappiness" (Breuer & Freud, 1895/1955, p. 305). Although the patient's stated goal is relief of emotional distress and neurotic suffering, many patients also have an unconscious need to suffer. It is not surprising to a psychoanalytic clinician to observe that after a period of improvement in treatment the patient's functioning might deteriorate. Freud called this the *negative therapeutic reaction* and regarded it as a serious obstacle to improvement.

At first, Freud thought that the path to cure involved "making the unconscious conscious." His later epigrammatic statement of the goal of psychoanalysis, consistent with the replacement of the topographic theory (conscious, preconscious, unconscious) by the structural theory (id, ego, superego), was "where id was, there shall ego be" (Freud, 1933/1964, p. 80). In other words, awareness was still considered a necessary but now a no longer sufficient condition for change The patient must also be able to accept and to integrate previously disavowed, split-off aspects of his or her personality.

Research support for this view is found in a series of studies by Luborsky and his colleagues (e.g., Luborsky & Crits-Christoph, 1990). They examined treatment protocols to identify core conflictual relationship themes (CCRTs) based on an assessment of relationship episodes described by the patient. A CCRT consists of a *wish* expressed by the patient, the *response* by the person to whom the wish is directed, and the patient's *reaction to the response* of the other. Patients typically show a few key CCRTs that remain fairly stable over the course of treatment in the sense that the same themes continue to be expressed. What changes is that the patient handles his or her issues in a more adaptive manner and with less subjective distress.

Process Aspects of Treatment

The main strategy in the conduct of psychoanalytic treatment is the analysis of transference reactions and resistances that emerge from the patient's "free associations." Compared with psychoanalysis proper, in *psychoanalytic* psychotherapy there is relatively less focus on the transference.

Transference

Freud first mentioned transference in *Studies on Hysteria* (Breuer & Freud, 1895/1955), calling it a "false connection," because the patient's reaction could not be adequately accounted for by the present situation. Freud assumed that it derived from unresolved childhood conflicts related to the parents. He saw transference as both a powerful obstacle to and an essential factor in the treatment. The value of transference reactions is that they can bring to light, with strong emotion, the patient's hidden and forgotten unacceptable impulses, conflicts, and fantasies. At the same time, patients naturally resist awareness of these kinds of mental contents, particularly when they are directed to the person of the therapist. However, the emotional reliving of childhood conflicts with the analyst can bring the patient's problems into bold relief, and repressions can be lifted in the context of emotionally vivid and meaningful experiences centered on the analyst.

As a useful, working definition of transference, one can cite Greenson (1967). *Transference* is the "experience of feelings, drives, attitudes, fantasies, and defenses toward a person in the present which do not befit that person but are a repetition of reactions originating in regard to significant persons of early childhood, unconsciously displaced onto figures in the present" (p. 155). In describing transference as a new edition of an old object relationship, Freud (1912/1953) observed that the repetition need not be literal, just that it express the same conflicts.

Transference reactions to emotionally significant persons in the present are fairly ubiquitous and are not restricted to experiences in analysis. In fact, in everyday life, they often are a source of considerable difficulty in interpersonal relationships. What is distinctive about psychoanalytic treatment is that they are *analyzed*. What enables transferences to be analyzed is the patient's cooperation and collaboration in the analytic work, a collaboration that itself is motivated by positive transference. As Freud (1940/1964, p. 175) put it, the positive transference "becomes the *true motive force* of the patient's collaboration. . . . He leaves off his symptoms and seems apparently to have recovered merely for the sake of the analyst."

Freud originally classified transference reactions into three kinds: the *positive* (erotic) transference, the *negative* (hostile), and the *unobjectionable* (i.e., aim-inhibited or nonerotic) positive transference necessary for cooperating and collaborating in the analytic work (an attitude that, as we see later, is the basis for the therapeutic (Zetzel, 1956) or working alliance (Greenson, 1965). The other characteristics of transference reactions, which essentially follow from Greenson's definition, are that they show evidence of inappropriateness, tenacity, and capriciousness. In this sense, whatever element of veridicality they may contain, transference reactions are considered inaccurate, distorted attributions about the emotional experience, behavior, intentions, and other aspects of the analyst's behavior. However, as noted earlier, Gill (1994) states that it is important to realize that so-called "transference" reactions are not created out of "whole cloth" but are triggered by real qualities of the analyst. Therefore, he argues that transference reactions should not be considered "distortions" but as the patient's experience of the analyst.

The intense concentration of the patient's core conflicts on the person of the analyst in the form of feelings, fantasies, and marked preoccupation in an increasingly regressive manner has been termed the *transference neurosis*. In more recent years, there is controversy about how frequently a full-blown transference neurosis occurs, as opposed to *transference reactions,* and how necessary a transference neurosis is for a good therapeutic outcome. Today, the term *transference neurosis* is not commonly used, and fewer analysts consider it necessary for effective analytic work.

The term *regressive transference* refers to the enhanced activation of childhood conflicts and attitudes in relation to the analyst. It should be noted (Macalpine, 1950) that the patient's readiness for the emergence of a regressive transference is facilitated by certain features of the analytic situation (e.g., the relative anonymity of the analyst, the withholding of deliberate transference gratifications, the invitation to free-associate, and the supine position of the patient).

In the traditional Freudian account, the analysis of the transference reveals the *infantile neurosis* (the central conflicts of childhood, whether or not they were clinically manifest at that time). Currently, analysts focus at least as much on the "here-and-now" transference. Bringing the past into the present in the form of transference is simultaneously a new experience, not simply the reenactment of earlier experiences. One way to think about the "new" and the "old" in the therapeutic relationship is that the patient needs to experience the analyst as an "old" object in order for the transference to form and take hold, and as a "new" object in order for the patient to collaborate with the analyst, and to understand and to resolve the transference.

Resistance

As the patient attempts to free-associate, there inevitably will be indications of *resistance* both to the awareness of warded-off mental contents and to the behavioral and attitudinal changes that might be attempted, based on such awareness. *Resistance,* following Gill (1982), can be defined as defense expressed in the transference, though Freud (1901/1960) defined it more broadly as anything that interferes with the analysis.

Because the patient fears the anxiety and/or depressive affect (e.g., humiliation, shame, and guilt) that is anticipated as an accompaniment to the awareness of certain wishes and fantasies, particularly those that involve the analyst, the natural tendency is to defend against and to avoid becoming aware of those mental contents. At the same time, the analytic situation has been deliberately designed to maximize the possibility of such awareness.

Resistance can and does take many forms, both blatant (e.g., a deliberate refusal to say what is on one's mind) and subtle (e.g., filling every silence quickly out of fear that the analyst may be critical of "resistance"). The last example highlights the fact that the patient's resistance is usually connected to the analyst, and these transference resistances are the major focus of analytic attention. As Freud (1912/1953) said, "The resistance accompanies the treatment step by step. Every single association, every act of the person under treatment must reckon with the resistance and represents a compromise between the forces that are striving towards recovery and the opposing ones" (p. 103). In other words, the patient is simultaneously motivated to express and to conceal wishes, fantasies, and conflicts associated with dysphoric affects.

Patients (and, unfortunately, also many therapists) think of resistance as something bad, as something to be overcome. This pejorative connotation doubtless derives from the early days of psychoanalysis, in which Freud used hypnosis, pressure techniques, and the insistence on complete candor ("You *must* pledge to tell me *everything* that comes to mind") in the initial formulation of the "fundamental rule" of free association. Thus, resistance naturally and inevitably includes "opposition to free association, to the procedures of analysis, to recall, to insight, and to change" (Eagle & Wolitzky, 1992, p. 124). Gill (1982) spoke of resistance to the awareness of transference and resistance to the resolution of transference. At the same time, resistances are designed to protect the patient against anxiety and the fear of change, that is, to maintain the familiar status quo, however painful. Finally, it should be noted that the affirmative, as well as the obstructive, aspects of resistance need to be recognized. For instance, resistance can be used in the service of forestalling a feared regression, asserting the patient's autonomy, or protecting the therapist from one's destructive impulses.

The underlying sources of the clinical manifestations of resistance, according to Freud (1937), include the constitutional strength of the instinctual drives, rigid defenses, and powerful, repetitive attempts to seek particular, familiar forms of drive gratification (what Freud called the "adhesiveness of the libido"). A major focus of psychoanalysis and psychoanalytic psychotherapy is the *interpretation* of transference and resistance, our next topic.

Interpretation

Interpretation (particularly, though not exclusively, of the transference) leading to insight has long been regarded as *the* major curative factor in psychoanalytic treatment. In recent years, however, many analysts have given considerable weight to the curative properties of the noninterpretive elements in the therapeutic relationship (e.g., therapist empathy and implicit support), particularly with more disturbed patients. *Interpretation,* broadly conceived, refers both to meanings attributed to discrete aspects of the patient's behavior and experience, and to constructions that attempt to offer a more comprehensive account of larger portions of the patient's history and behavioral patterns.

Schematically stated, the optimal interpretation, though not necessarily presented comprehensively at one time, would take the form "What you are doing (feeling, thinking, fantasizing, etc.) with me now is what you also are doing with your current significant other (spouse, child, boss, etc.), and what you did with your father (and/or mother) for such and such reasons and motives and with such and such consequences." In the convergence of the past and the present (both in the treatment relationship and in other current relationships), the recognition of repetitive, pervasive, and entrenched patterns of relating and of personal functioning can have maximum emotional and cognitive impact. This three-way convergence, referred to as the "triangle of insight" (Malan, 1976), is likely to carry greater emotional conviction.

Although interpretation of transference resistances is considered to be "the single most important instrument of psychoanalytic technique" (Greenson, 1967, p. 97), other interventions usuallly are necessary prerequisites to interpretation. For example, confrontation and clarification are preparatory to interpretation. *Confrontation* points to the fact of resistance (e.g., "I notice that when you are reminded of your mother, you quickly change the subject"). *Clarification* refers to exploration of why the patient is resisting (e.g., "Talking about your mother that way seems to have made you uncomfortable"). This line of inquiry blends into interpretations of the unconscious fantasies and motives for the resistance (e.g., "You think that wishing to be alone with your mother was wrong and that I will chastise you for feeling that way"). A detailed exposition of these techniques can be found in Greenson (1967).

The overarching therapeutic strategy is to foster and flexibly maintain the conditions necessary for interpreting the transference. It is believed that a good working alliance (defined later) and an "optimal" degree of transference gratification–frustration will facilitate the desired oscillation between the patient's self-observation and expression of feeling, and the analysis of defense and transference. However, there will be occasions, particularly with the so-called "nonclassical" analytic patient, when the therapist knowingly and advisedly employs nonanalytic interventions, including advice, active support, suggestions, and so on.

Among some contemporary Freudians (e.g., Gray, 1994), the emphasis has not been on directly interpreting the unconscious wishes underlying the transference but on interpreting defenses against awareness and/or the resolution of the transference. So-called *defense analysis* focuses on the ways in which the patient attempts to ward off anxieties and fears. Most analysts today agree that defense analysis should start at the "surface" and proceed gradually to "deeper" levels, like peeling the layers of an onion. As the patient becomes a better observer of his or her own defensive behavior, the patient often will be able to access previously warded-off mental content without much interpretive help from the analyst (Gray, 1994). Some theorists (e.g., Weiss & Sampson, 1986) stress that feeling safe as a result of the analyst passing tests posed by the patient also enables the patient to access his or her own previously warded-off mental contents, with little or no interpretation from the analyst.

Despite the increased flexibility of analytic technique and open acknowledgment of the inevitably interactive, two-person nature of the analytic relationship, contemporary Freudians, like their more traditional predecessors, cannot seem to shake the image of being aloof, authoritarian, and technique driven (Fiscalini, 2004). However, contemporary Freudians, readily agree that any analyst who is wooden in style and lacking in spontaneity, while slavishly and inflexibly adhering to a set of preselected clinical techniques and theories, is not likely to be effective.

These days, clearly, everything that transpires between the patient and therapist, including interpretations, is part of an ongoing interaction. As Oremland (1991) reminds us, the distinction is really between interactions that emphasize interpretations and interactions that do not. Thus, interpretations are particular kinds of interactions. It is safe to say that virtually all contemporary Freudian psychoanalysts have discarded the original model of the analyst as a "blank screen" in favor of the view of the therapeutic relationship as an ongoing, two-person transference–countertransference matrix in which patient and analyst issues are enacted.

Given the inherently interactive nature of the relationship, the analyst needs to be alert to ruptures in the therapeutic alliance, the dynamics of the transference–countertransference enactments, as well as the patient's experience of the analyst's interpretations. The Freudian analyst is as interested in these aspects of the process as in the content of any interpretation. For example, does the patient seem to experience an interpretation as an instance of feeling empathically understood, and how does he or she feel if it is not such an instance? Is the fact and/or the content of an interpretation experienced as a humiliation, a gift, a sexual penetration, or all of the above? Freudian analysts appreciate the recursive nature of the transference (i.e., that often the patient and the analyst are enacting the very theme about which they are talking).

A few final comments are in order before I leave the topic of interpretation. The shifting cultural attitude away from a positivistic, objective, knowable reality toward a more relativistic, pluralistic, constructivist stance has had a significant impact on psychoanalysis, particularly with regard to its views of interpretation. This change has been referred to as the "hermeneutic turn" in psychoanalysis. From this perspective, interpretations are regarded much more as co-constructions by analyst and patient than as discoveries of an underlying psychic reality. Lines of interpretation are considered to be as much a reflection of the analyst's preferred story lines and narratives as they are veridical readings of the patient's psychic reality (Schafer, 1992). In part, this view is an antidote to an analytic stance in which the analyst thinks he or she possesses something akin to interpretive infallibility, a countertransference danger that can plague any analyst, regardless of theoretical persuasion (Eagle, Wolitzky, & Wakefield, 2001).

Process of Therapy

According to Freud, psychoanalysis can be likened to chess; the opening moves and the end game are fairly standard, but the long middle phase is not predictable and is open to many variations. In psychoanalytic treatment, clinicians distinguish between an opening phase, the extended, middle phase of "working through," and the termination phase.

The Opening Phase: Attention to the Working or Therapeutic Alliance

The primary emphasis in the opening phase of treatment is on the establishment of rapport and a good working relationship, the importance of which was recognized early on in Freud's notion of the "unobjectionable positive transference." Subsequently, this aspect of the therapeutic relationship has been called the "working alliance" (Greenson, 1965), the "therapeutic alliance" (Zetzel, 1956), and the "helping alliance" (Luborsky, 1984). Although there are differences in these similar-sounding concepts, for present purposes I regard them as equivalent and restrict myself to Greenson's conception. (For a review of the psychodynamic theory, empirical research, and practice implications related to the therapeutic alliance, see Messer & Wolitzky, 2010).

According to Greenson (1967), the *working alliance* is the "relatively non-neurotic, rational relationship between patient and analyst which makes it possible for the patient to work purposefully in the analytic situation" (p. 45). The patient achieves this attitude when feeling safe and accepted in the analyst's presence. Being in a stable, nonjudgmental, predictable relationship focused mainly on the patient's needs contributes to the "background of safety" (Sandler, 1959) that enables the patient to communicate his or her thoughts and feelings more openly. It also fosters an identification with, or at least an adoption of, the clinician's analytic stance. This collaborative spirit of inquiry and understanding, which is part of the alliance between the analyst's analytic attitude and the patient's reasonable, self-observing ego, is not a once-and-for-all achievement but one that is inevitably disrupted by the patient's transference reactions, as well as the therapist's countertransference reactions.

Analytic interventions, as well as silence, can be experienced as narcissistic injuries caused by the patient's sense of the analyst's failure of empathy. Ruptures in the alliance are not only inevitable but are also seen as important and necessary spurs to the therapeutic process, because, when recognized, they create the opportunity for repair and the reestablishment of the alliance. From this perspective, the treatment can be thought of as a series of ruptures and repairs that ultimately strengthen the therapeutic bond. Thus, although the ruptures might arouse negative feelings and shake the patient's trust in the analyst, the repairs can restore and solidify it. The patient learns that a relationship can survive some pain and misunderstanding when the analyst is a fair and decent person.

An unwitting transference–countertransference enactment in which the patient and therapist are drawn into and engage in neurotically based interactions, without awareness, is the most common cause of a disruption in the alliance. The rupture can take the form of subtle avoidance and withdrawal or it may be overtly confrontational (e.g., questioning the analyst's competence). In recent years, we have seen an extensive theoretical and research literature on the alliance (e.g., Safran & Muran, 2000).

Some Freudian analysts (e.g., Brenner, 1979) have cautioned that an emphasis on promoting and maintaining the alliance runs the risk of providing the patient with unanalyzed transference gratification and is thus counterproductive. However, virtually all analysts would agree that the patient's capacity to listen to, reflect on, and make effective use of transference interpretations requires the presence of a good working relationship. In empirical studies of psychoanalytic psychotherapy, Luborsky and Crits-Christoph (1990) have found that the strength of the helping alliance, measured early in treatment, is a statistically significant, if not overly robust, predictor of treatment outcome.

How does one foster the treatment alliance? The primary answer is that one listens empathically and nonjudgmentally; is alert to detecting and managing countertransference reactions; explains, to the extent necessary, the rationale for the rules and the framework of the treatment (e.g., why one does not routinely answer questions); and offers interpretations with proper timing, tact, and dosage. By the latter, I mean that the therapist develops a sense of the patient's optimal level of anxiety and his or her vulnerabilities to narcissistic injury (blows to self-esteem). The therapist functions in a way that is aimed at not traumatically exceeding these levels. These considerations take precedence over any technical rules for handling the opening phase of treatment (or any phase, for that matter). Thus, the usual technical precepts of analyzing defenses before impulses, beginning with the surface, allowing the patient to determine the subject of the session, and so on, are all liable to be suspended if clinical judgment so dictates.

Given this perspective, the most common and serious technical errors a therapist can make are really not technical per se but stem from countertransferential attitudes and interventions that reflect rigid, arbitrary, unempathic responsiveness to the patient and thereby fail to respect the patient's individuality, integrity, autonomy, and anxiety tolerance. Any specific, discrete technical error (e.g., intervening too rapidly and fostering premature closure instead of giving the patient the opportunity to express his or her feelings and thoughts more fully) is considered problematic but relatively minor when compared to the danger of retraumatization that can occur if the therapist acts in the manner previously described. Thus, common technical errors, such as failing to leave the initiative with the patient; frequent interruptions and questions (especially those that call for a simple "yes" or "no" rather than encouraging exploration); offering farfetched, intellectualized or jargon-filled interpretations; an excess of therapeutic zeal; attitudes of omniscience and grandiosity; dogmatism; the need to be seen as clever; engaging in power struggles with the patient; failure to begin or end the session on time; and being punitive or overly apologetic all derive their potentially adverse effects from the extent to which they express undetected and therefore unmanaged countertransference (to be discussed later).

Some analysts recommend explicit techniques for fostering the alliance. For example, the therapist can use words that promote a sense of collaboration and bonding. Thus, instead of "What did you mean by that?", the analyst could say, "Let's try to understand what that meant." This kind of statement encourages an identification with the analytic attitude of reflection on the meaning of one's experience and behavior. Sterba (1934) offered the distinction between the "experiencing ego" and the "observing ego." In an effective working alliance, the patient oscillates between reporting his or her experience through free-associations (the *experiencing ego*) and periodically stepping back to observe and reflect on these experiences (the *observing ego*). This "split in the ego" is essential to the work of self-discovery.

The Middle Phase: Working Through

In the extended, middle phase of treatment, the focus is on the analysis of transference and resistance, with the aim of having patients "work through" their long-standing conflicts. *Working through* refers to "the repetitive, progressive and elaborate explorations of the resistances which prevent insight from leading to change" (Greenson, 1967, p. 42).

In the early days of psychoanalysis, Freud reported some dramatic "cures" in which hysterical symptoms disappeared, at least temporarily, following the recall of the traumatic memories of the experiences that first gave rise to the symptoms. Patients, even fairly sophisticated ones, often have the fantasy that a single, blinding insight will free them to take the path previously not taken because it was unseen or too frightful to pursue. In fact, as patients become aware of their core conflicts, they appreciate that they have been repeatedly reenacting many variations of the same theme in ways that they regard as vital, even though such actions also cause them pain and suffering. Becoming aware of one's patterns of maladaptive living in the context of the transference, recalling their similarity to childhood reactions and modes of relating to significant others, and realizing the unconscious fantasies on which they are based usually is a slow, painstaking, "two steps forward–one step back" process.

Resistance to change often can be slow to dissolve. Maintaining the status quo commonly is seen as the safest course. Fear and guilt concerning the consequences of change (e.g., feeling that one does not deserve to be happy, that changing means abandoning or being disloyal to a parent, and the reluctance to relinquish long-cherished fantasies and beliefs) continue to be analyzed in their various, often subtle forms, so that the secondary, as well as the primary, gain of the symptoms or neurotic patterns may be lessened.

Thus, repeated exploration and elaboration of the patient's key, unconscious conflicts and the defenses against them as they become expressed in the context of the therapeutic relationship, and in other aspects of the patient's life, are the core of the analytic process. The analytic process can be viewed as consisting of numerous sequences of (1) the patient's resistance to awareness and to change, (2) the analyst's interpretation of the resistance, and (3) the patient's responses to the interpretation, all in the context of transference–countertransference enactment.

The End Phase: Termination

With the exception of brief psychodynamic therapy (Messer & Warren, 1995), relatively little has been written regarding termination compared with the literature on other aspects of treatment. It is generally agreed that termination should not be forced (as in setting a specific time limit), unilateral, premature, or overdue. It has been claimed that a poorly planned and handled termination phase can practically destroy an otherwise good analysis.

As the work proceeds, therapist and patient periodically assess the degree of progress made toward achieving the therapeutic goals. Ideally, the idea of termination emerges naturally in the minds of both participants as they recognize that the therapeutic goals (both those articulated at the start and ones that developed later on) have been essentially met, and that the treatment has therefore reached the point of diminishing returns. Unfortunate but realistic reasons for termination include the judgment that little or no progress has been made over a significant period of time.

Actual termination ideally is planned to commence at some specified time after a mutual decision has been reached. The rationale for a planned termination phase rather than an abrupt ending includes the idea that separation from the analyst is a significant psychological event that will evoke feelings, fantasies, and conflicts that resonate with earlier separations from or losses of significant others. It is not unusual that once a target date for termination is set, feelings along these lines emerge, feelings that previously had been latent or not dealt with before termination became a looming reality. Even when the patient initiates the idea of termination, it is not unusual for the analyst's agreement to terminate to be experienced as a rejection and abandonment. In addition, the temporary return of symptoms in the termination phase is not uncommon, often as an expression of separation fears ("See, I'm not ready to stop treatment").

In summary, the optimal criteria for termination are the reduction of the transference, the achievement of the main treatment goals, an acceptance (or at least tolerance) of the futility of certain strivings and childhood fantasies, an increased capacity for love and work (Freud's succinct statement of the goals of analysis), a reduction in the intensity and poignancy of core conflicts, the attainment of more stable and less maladaptive coping patterns and interpersonal relationships, a reduction in symptoms, and the development of a self-analytic capacity. This latter quality is considered an important new ego function, built on the patient's psychological mindedness and on his or her identification with and internalization of the analyst's analytic attitude. It should help the person during the posttermination consolidation of the analytic work and subsequently as well. Patient and analyst part with the understanding that the door is open for a return for more analytic work at some time in the future. The analyst goes on analyzing into the last session. Self-understanding is never complete or final. Treatment does not resolve conflict completely, nor is it expected to immunize the patient completely from future psychological difficulties.

THE THERAPEUTIC RELATIONSHIP AND THE STANCE OF THE THERAPIST

The analyst's stance is best described as one in which the primary aim is to maintain an analytic attitude (Schafer, 1983) that will facilitate and maintain a positive working alliance and make analytic work possible. A major component of the *analytic attitude* is the analyst's genuine interest in helping the patient, expressed, in part, through the creation of a safe, caring, nonjudgmental therapeutic atmosphere.

Analytic Neutrality

Analytic neutrality is considered an essential feature of the proper analytic attitude. *Neutrality* is here understood *not* in the sense of indifference to the patient but in the sense of *not* taking sides in the patient's conflicts. In other words, the analyst attempts to be objective in the context of offering an empathetic understanding of the patient. This stance has also been called benevolent neutrality or technical neutrality. As stated by Anna Freud (1954), the analyst attempts to adopt a position equidistant among the id, ego, and superego.

In addition, the analyst respects the uniqueness and individuality of the patient and does not attempt to remake the patient to fit any particular image or set of values. The analyst does not exploit the patient to meet his or her own needs. The analyst does not try to rescue the patient, to play guru, to become engaged in power struggles with the patient, or to seek the patient's adulation; nor does he or she feel critical or impatient toward the patient. The analyst appreciates that patients both seek and are frightened by the prospect of change, and that ambivalence is a ubiquitous feature of human experience.

This description may begin to sound like an impossible ideal. It should be kept in mind that it is an ideal to be aspired to, with the recognition that one can only approximate it and should not be unduly self-critical when the approximation is inevitably less than one would wish. It should, however, direct the analyst to reflect on factors that might be interfering with the maintenance of neutrality.

Therapeutic neutrality does not prohibit the therapist from some ordinary human interactions, such as saying "hello" and "good-bye" to a patient or wishing the patient well on the eve of an important experience (childbirth, graduation, marriage, surgery, etc.). At the same time, while not enjoined from engaging in such natural reactions, some analysts would not say "I look forward to seeing you," even if they genuinely meant it. Here there is still the residual issue of the optimal balance between analyzing the patient's needs and wishes, and gratifying some of the patient's needs and perhaps not going on to explore the meanings of the patient's behavior. Brenner's (1979) objection to the emphasis on the therapeutic alliance was based on this concern, but it appears to be less of a concern among current analysts.

Because therapy entails the interaction of two personalities there cannot be a truly "uncontaminated" transference. The analyst, of course, gives cues, witting and unwitting, about his or her personality and values from the location and furnishing of the office, the manner of dress, and so forth. However, there is still a large realm of nondisclosure that allows many degrees of freedom for the patient to "construct" the analyst. The patient's appreciation of his or her own needs and motives for making particular attributions or selective readings of the analyst will be more emotionally convincing to the extent to which it is not based on obvious reality cues. This is also the rationale for the analyst's relative anonymity and abstinence (withholding of explicit transference gratifications; e.g., praise). Freudian analysts are concerned that the temporary satisfaction of transference wishes might reduce the patient's motivation for treatment or for self-reflection, and make analysis of the transference and the resistances all the more difficult. This is not to say that there are no gratifying aspects to the patient's experience of the analytic process. On the contrary, several silent factors inherent in the situation can be powerful sources of satisfaction and security. Foremost among these elements is the sense of steady support that comes from the sustained, genuine interest of a benign listener over a long course of regular and frequent contacts. This sense of support has been referred to as a *holding environment* (Winnicott, 1965). This term is a metaphor derived from Winnicott's view that the analytic setting bears a similarity to features of the mother–child interaction, in which the child is not only literally held as a means of soothing but is also cared for and loved more generally, and comes to rely on the provision of this protection, which engenders a sense of safety and security.

What enables the analyst to provide a good holding environment, one that includes a shifting but optimal balance or abstinence and responsiveness with respect to the patient's transference wishes? To answer this question, I next discuss the concepts of empathy and countertransference.

Empathy

Based on the amalgam of past clinical experience, knowledge of human development, general models of human behavior, and particular psychoanalytic theories, the analyst tries to listen, as Freud recommended, with "evenly hovering attention" (i.e., not with a preset bias toward certain kinds of material) and will later organize the material in particular ways to develop a working mental model of the patient. This crucial, nonjudgmental listening process is guided by the analyst's empathy. *Empathy* involves a partial, transient identification with the patient, in which the analyst attempts to apprehend in a cognitive–affective manner what it is like for the patient to experience his or her outer and inner world in a particular manner. In other words, the analyst tries to enter the patient's experiential world by imagining, both cognitively and affectively, what the patient's subjective experience is like. The analyst oscillates between relating to patients in this way and stepping back periodically as an observer and reflecting on why patients seem to be experiencing their inner world in a particular manner. These reflections serve as the basis for the private clinical inferences made by the analyst that then lead to the actual interpretations made to the patient. Offered with proper timing, tact, and dosage, interpretations attempt to convey both empathic understanding and explanation of patients' difficulties. (For a detailed analysis of the nature of empathy and its role in therapy, see Eagle & Wolitzky, 1997).

Countertransference

Countertransference can be thought of as empathy gone awry; that is, to the extent that the analyst's feelings or actions toward, and understanding of, the patient are influenced by the analyst's unconscious, unresolved conflicts and attitudes and/or conscious biases, the analyst is not being objective and is thereby not functioning in the best interests of the patient.

At first, countertransference was thought of as the direct counterpart to the patient's transference (i.e., as the analyst's transference to the patient's transference, or to the patient more generally). By this definition, countertransference was regarded as an unconscious, undesirable, potentially serious obstacle to effective treatment. Freud (1910/1957) held that the therapist's countertransference limited the degree to which the patient could progress in treatment. Some authors (e.g., Langs, 1982) go so far as to assert that *all* treatment failures are due to unrecognized and/or unmanaged countertransference reactions.

In more recent years, influenced in large part by work with more disturbed patients, the concept of countertransference has been broadened to include all the analyst's emotional reactions to the patient, whether conscious or unconscious, and the analyst's transference reactions to not only the patient's transference but also the patient's personality, as well as reactions to being in the role of analyst. Some authors (e.g., Weiner & Bornstein, 2009) make a distinction between *specific* and *generalized* countertransference. The former refers to an analyst's reactions that are unique to a particular patient and triggered when some aspect of the patient or what the patient says triggers unresolved issues in the analyst that lead to positive (e.g., overly nurturing) or negative (e.g., hostile) reactions to the patient; the latter refers to reactions that tend to be present in all, or most, cases treated by a particular analyst (e.g., a strong need to be idealized).

The broader definition of countertransference has been called "totalistic," in contrast to the earlier "classical" definition (Schlesinger & Wolitzky, 2002). The therapist's emotional reactions, whether based primarily on his or her own conflicts or due mainly to the fact that the patient's behavior would likely evoke the same reaction in virtually all analysts, came to be regarded both as inevitable and as potentially quite useful, indeed vital to understanding the patient. The therapist's reactions, when subjected to self-reflection, can point to feelings that the patient might be "pulling for" from the therapist and therefore can serve as one important guide to the interpretations offered by the therapist. However, an analyst needs to be careful and not assume automatically that just because one is feeling a certain way, the patient is trying to evoke that particular reaction. To make such an automatic assumption (as one unfortunately encounters in some recent psychoanalytic literature) is to ignore the possibility that it is primarily one's own conflict-based countertransference that is responsible for what one thinks the patient is trying to make one feel.

As noted previously, even though the analyst has been analyzed, countertransference–transference enactments are inevitable. What is considered crucial is to be able to recognize the co-constructed nature of such enactments before they become too intense, disruptive, or traumatic for the patient, and to step back, reflect on, and use one's awareness in the service of understanding and interpretation. Some countertransference reactions are direct and blatant, but most are subtle and therefore potentially more insidious. Even some blatant countertransference-based reactions that are not readily recognized by the analyst might be brought to the analyst's attention by the patient.

Transference–countertransference enactments are episodic or chronic patient–therapist interactions (e.g., victim–perpetrator) that express unresolved conflicts or unsatisfied needs. To the extent that the asymmetrical structure of the analytic situation allows the therapist to be somewhat less emotionally vulnerable than the patient, the therapist's unresolved issues can be in relative abeyance during the sessions. And to the extent that the therapist is alert to his or her countertransference, the frequency and intensity of enactments will be induced more by the patient than by the therapist. At the same time, even when initiated primarily by the patient, the therapist often will be drawn into an enactment.

The prescription for dealing with countertransference reactions is self-analysis, informed by the analyst's own prior training analysis and clinical supervision, and, if necessary, supplemented by consultations with colleagues and/or by the analyst's resumption of his or her own therapy. The presumption is that undetected (and therefore unmanaged) countertransference reactions always have a detrimental impact on the treatment. The literature is replete with clinical vignettes demonstrating that a bogged-down analysis resumed its forward thrust following the analyst's awareness of a countertransference trend and the new interpretation to which it gives rise. Although these accounts generally are persuasive, it is not clear how much, and what kinds of, undetected countertransference the average patient could in fact tolerate and still have a reasonably successful analysis.

Also unclear, and fairly controversial, is the issue of countertransference disclosure. In other words, to what extent and under what circumstances should the analyst disclose to the patient the fact of his or her countertransference and perhaps include the presumed basis for it? Some analysts, more typically those with a relational orientation, regard it as essential for the egalitarian spirit of the analytic process and for affirming the patient's sense of reality, whereas others feel that it could unnecessarily burden the patient and should be employed quite sparingly.

Virtually all therapists do agree that the analytic ideal requires that self-analysis be a constant, silent, background accompaniment to the conduct of each analytic session (Schlesinger & Wolitzky, 2002). Attention to one's own experience can provide vital data concerning fruitful lines of exploration.

CURATIVE FACTORS OR MECHANISMS OF CHANGE

Since the inception of psychoanalysis, there has been continual discussion and debate concerning its curative ingredients. By now, it is clear that no single factor can be said to be the major element in therapeutic change for all patients. Although there are few formal statements of the necessary and sufficient conditions for therapeutic change, there is a general consensus that the conditions conducive to positive outcomes include the following: (1) a person who (a) is suffering emotionally, (b) is motivated to change, (c) shows some degree of psychological mindedness, (d) has sufficient ego strength and frustration tolerance to endure the rigors of the treatment, and (e) has a decent enough history of gratifying, trusting interpersonal relationships to form and maintain a reasontable working alliance in the face of the inevitable difficulties involved in the treatment; and (2) a therapist who (a) can provide a safe atmosphere and be an effective catalyst for the patient's self-exploration, (b) can facilitate and maintain the working alliance in the face of its inevitable strains and ruptures, (c) is relatively free of unmanaged countertransference reactions, and (d) provides accurate, empathically based interpretations of transference and extratransference behaviors with the timing, tact, and dosage necessary to facilitate insight into the unconscious conflicts that influence the patient's symptoms and maladaptive patterns of behavior.

Broadly speaking, the curative factors created by the listed conditions have been divided into two main categories—insight and the relationship. This is potentially a somewhat false distinction, because insight based on interpretation takes place in the context of the patient–therapist relationship. Thus, an interpretation leading to an emotionally meaningful insight can be, and often is, simultaneously experienced as a profound feeling of being understood (perhaps the strongest expression of a solid "holding environment"). Nonetheless, the distinction between insight and relationship factors is retained in an attempt to assign relative influence to the element of enhanced self-understanding versus the therapeutic benefits of the relationship per se. Among the benefits of the latter, one can include the support inherent in the therapeutic relationship; the experience of a new, benign relationship with a significant person (i.e., one who does not re-create the traumatic experiences the patient suffered in relation to the parents); and identification with the analyst and the analytic attitude, which includes a softening of superego self-punitiveness and feeling understood, supported, and a sense that one's emotional upheavals can be safely "contained" by the analyst, even when the analyst's interpretive efforts arouse some degree of anxiety.

Among most contemporary Freudian analysts, especially those who maintain a more or less traditional view, these relationship elements are mainly regarded as necessary but secondary background factors that give interpretations their mutative power. Echoing the views of Kohut's (1971) self psychology, as well as those of object relations theorists, other contemporary Freudian therapists regard the relationship as directly therapeutic in its own right. These Freudian therapists are sympathetic to Kohut's (1984) view that the main impact and virtue of interpretations is that they strengthen the empathetic bond between patient and therapist.

Some writers have suggested that a comprehensive theory of curative factors would have to consider that the relative therapeutic efficacy of insight and relationship factors might depend on the type of patient being treated ("anaclitic" [dependent] vs. an "introjective" [self-critical]; Blatt, 2008) and the stage of treatment. A generalization also found in the literature is that, relatively speaking, patients whose early history was marked by serious disturbances in the mother–child relationship would benefit more, relatively speaking, from the healing aspects of the relationship, whereas patients who struggle primarily with Oedipal problems would find insight a more potent factor.

There are many examples in the literature of the relative emphasis on the patient–therapist relationship and on insight as curative factors. A good contemporary example of an emphasis on the healing power of often silent, unarticulated aspects of the relationship is seen in the writings of the Boston Process Group (e.g., Lyons-Ruth, 1998). Basing their work on studies of early infant–mother interaction and processes of attunement to therapist and patient subjective states, these authors look for analogous processes in the psychoanalytic situation. One of their key concepts is "implicit relational knowing" (Lyons-Ruth, 1998) that derives from shared "moments of meeting." These "moments" of attunement constitute new ways of being together. An example might be the patient's realization that the analyst is genuinely interested in listening to and responding to what the patient is saying, and by this interest the analyst is expressing the attitude that the patient is a person of worth. This experience contrasts with the patient's internalized way of relating to those perceived to be in authority. For instance, a patient recalls that the clear, explicit rule, particularly at the family dinner table, was that his parents expected silence from the children during dinner unless specifically addressed and asked to speak. As an adult in treatment, this patient can have the experience of the analyst as a new object and engage in new, experiential learning; that is, he or she can realize that it is permissible, even desirable, to speak freely to an interested listener. This experience does not preclude interpretation (e.g., "I have the feeling that you fell silent just now because you were not sure that I was really interested in what you were starting to say, and that this feeling reminds you of how it felt at the family dinner table when you felt you were getting the message that you should be seen but not heard"). The implicit message in this interpretation is that the analyst is in fact interested in what the patient has to say. Whether such messages generally are better conveyed implicitly and/or noninterpretively is an interesting empirical question.

A major example of the emphasis on insight rather than on the therapeutic relationship is seen, for example, in the work of Gray (1994), who advocates "close process monitoring." In this approach, the analyst is particularly alert to moments in the session when the patient's associations and behavior suggest that anxiety signals have become active and defenses have been instigated to ward them off. The patient is encouraged to become an observer of this process and (implicitly) to refrain from instituting defensive operations in order to uncover the warded-off, anxiety-laden mental contents. Insight into unconscious conflicts is still the goal, but the analyst is less active in interpreting these conflicts than was the case in the past. Those, like Gray, who see themselves as facilitators of the patient's self-analysis, find it especially important to minimize the role of suggestion in the treatment.

TREATMENT APPLICABILITY AND ETHICAL CONSIDERATIONS

Patients typically seek psychoanalysis or psychoanalytic psychotherapy for reasons they seek other forms of therapy (e.g., actual or anticipated changes in or loss of important personal relationships, setbacks in one's career or life transitions, disturbing anxiety and depressive symptoms, the unavailability of usual social or emotional supports). When stressful life changes occur in a context of chronic, unresolved conflicts, the resulting state of disequilibrium can result in symptoms that prompt the person to seek treatment.

Social Class

Psychotherapy in general, and psychoanalysis in particular, has long been criticized as limited to a small segment of the population. The so-called YAVIS syndrome refers to the typical psychotherapy patient as Young, Affluent, Verbal, Intelligent, and Successful. Psychoanalytic patients have been depicted as those who are wealthy and without significant personal problems (i.e., "the worried well"; Doidge, 1999; Kaley, Eagle, & Wolitzky, 1999). According to this view, psychoanalysis is a personal journey of self-exploration for the narcissistically self-indulgent rather than an experience of encounter with painful truths about oneself by individuals who are troubled and dysfunctional in their relationships and work. This is not an entirely accurate view (Doidge, 1999). While attempts were made early on to apply psychoanalytic understanding to work with underprivileged and disadvantaged populations (e.g., Aichorn, 1935; Altman, 1995), by and large it is true that unmodified, intensive psychoanalytic treatment in this country is an expensive proposition, particularly in these days of managed care, with its limited insurance coverage for long-term psychotherapy.

Types of Patients and Patient Pathology

Patient Populations

Freud never intended that psychoanalysis would have a broad range of application, and he realized that to be employed more widely it would require significant modification. Over the years, psychoanalytically oriented approaches have been developed for the treatment of children, adolescents, couples, groups, and families. A separate chapter would be required to begin to do justice to the range and complexity of the factors involved in these treatment applications.

Range of Pathology

Although originally geared to neurotics, psychoanalytic treatment, in one variation or another, was tried in patients with schizophrenia (Federn, 1952; Searles, 1965). In more recent years, however, the practice of dynamic psychotherapy, and particularly psychoanalytic therapy, with patients with schizophrenia seems to have diminished substantially in favor of drug therapy and other forms of intervention (e.g., supportive therapy, social skills training, behavior therapy, family therapy, and community treatment programs). Nevertheless, there still are a few residential treatment centers in which psychoanalytic therapy is practiced with seriously disturbed patients, some of whom have schizophrenia but most of whom have severely borderline personalities. Blatt and Ford (1999) reported substantial therapeutic gains with long-term, intensive, psychoanalytically oriented treatment of seriously disturbed, treatment-resistant inpatients. The psychoanalytic treatment of severe borderline and narcissistic conditions is more frequently carried out on an outpatient basis (Kernberg et al., 1989).

Cultural Factors

Psychoanalytic psychotherapy has certain inherent features and values that set boundaries on its range of application. For example, cultural factors can influence the degree to which patients have a sense of comfort and legitimacy in self-disclosure, particularly when there are cultural taboos against saying anything negative about one's loved ones. Collectivist cultures tend not to value an individual approach and might well find group, family, or community approaches more compatible (Markus & Kitayama, 1998). Psychoanalytic treatment encourages the free expression of emotions, so cultures that value restraint of emotion would find this central feature incompatible. People from some cultures are less inclined to take the initiative and expect the therapist to be more active and to provide more structure than is typical in psychoanalytic treatment. Finally, sociocultural differences between patient and therapist also need to be considered, because a therapist who is not sensitive to cultural differences will have a more difficult time understanding a patient from a different culture.

In summary, it probably is fair to say that virtually all of psychoanalysis proper is applied to fairly well-educated, upper-middle-class individuals in major urban centers who do not rely primarily on third-party payments and can afford private fees, even if it means having one to three sessions per week instead of the four or five that were more common in the past. But for accounts of modified psychoanalytic treatment with disadvantaged populations, see Altman (1995).

Ethical Considerations

Although practitioners have a natural inclination to recommend to patients the kind of treatment they have been trained to conduct, ethical considerations require caution. For example, standard psychoanalysis is not the treatment of choice for patients whose reality situation is so dire and overwhelming as to preclude prolonged, leisurely introspection, nor should it be recommended to someone whose sole aim is to overcome a specific habit (e.g., smoking). In general, the ethical issues relevant to psychoanalysis are those germane to psychotherapy in general (e.g., not exploiting the patient's emotional vulnerability). Needless to say, the therapist should adhere to the highest professional and ethical standards, and refrain from exploiting the patient in any way.

Matching Patients with Therapeutic Modalities and with Therapists

Matching patients with therapists and therapeutic modalities takes place on an informal basis during the course of the initial consultations. For example, some therapists feel poorly suited to work with certain kinds of patients, while some patients are likely to benefit more from cognitive-behavioral treatment than from psychoanalytic treatment.

RESEARCH SUPPORT

For most of its history psychoanalysis has based its theories and assessments of treatment outcome almost exclusively on the case study method. Few analysts were trained in research methodology, yet conducting an analysis was seen as simultaneously doing research. Conceptions of therapeutic action were based on accumulated "clinical experience" and an amalgam of the received wisdom of supervisors and teachers, theoretical preferences, and common sense.

It is only in recent years, with the popularity of psychiatric drugs, rival therapies, and the influence of managed care, that analysts have begun to heed the call for accountability and to supplement clinical insights and claims with more systematic, empirical, methodologically sophisticated inquiries focused on the process and outcome of treatment.

The first ambitious long-term treatment and long-term follow-up study (Wallerstein, 1986) was the Menninger Foundation Psychotherapy Research Project (PRP). In the PRP study, patients were seen in either psychoanalysis ($N = 22$) or psychoanalytic psychotherapy with supportive elements ($N = 20$). About 60% of patients in each group showed at least moderate improvement that was durable over time. About half of the 42 patients showed positive therapeutic changes even without evidence of having obtained insight into their core conflicts.

In the last few years, there has been an impressive proliferation of more methodologically sophisticated empirical research on the process and outcome of psychoanalytic treatment. Fonagy's (2002) compendium of treatment research contains a review of some 80 different studies conducted all over the world, as far away as New South Wales. Most of the studies cited by Fonagy are naturalistic, without control groups or randomized assignment of patients (although this requirement is debatable), and other *desiderata* of an ideal research design. However, some of the studies do include the important feature of evaluation at various time points, including long-term follow-up, and many of them reported favorable results. For example, Sandell and colleagues (2000) reported that (1) outcomes for psychoanalysis were superior to those for analytically oriented psychotherapy; (2) classical analysts achieved better results with psychoanalysis than with psychotherapy; (3) psychoanalytic psychotherapy and psychoanalysis, compared with various kinds of short-term treatments and a no-treatment control group, showed greater symptom reduction and social adjustment at 1- and 2-year follow-up; (4) benefits of treatment over seven time periods of evaluation, compared to a waiting-list control, increased over the period prior to treatment to long-term follow-up, from roughly 30 to 55% for the psychotherapy group (with effect sizes ranging from 0.4 to 0.6) and from 10 to 75% for the psychoanalysis group (with effect sizes ranging from 0.4 to 1.5, a very large effect size); and (5) better results were achieved by more experienced psychoanalysts, especially females, and with greater session frequency during treatment.

These data provide some encouragement for the claims made by analysts on the basis of their clinical experience. Together with other studies summarized in the open door review (Fonagy, 2002), it is reasonable to state overall that the majority of these studies report positive results for psychoanalysis and psychoanalytic psychotherapy.

Since the last edition of this volume, additional methodological improvements have permitted further significant research progress in more clearly demonstrating the benefits of both long- and short-term psychoanalytic treatment (Leichsenring & Rabung, 2008; Shedler, 2010). In the most recent review of research in psychodynamic therapy, Shedler states that such treatment now has substantial empirical support. He notes that

> effect sizes for psychodynamic therapy are as large as those reported for other therapies that have been actively promoted as "empirically supported" and "evidence based." In addition, patients who receive psychodynamic therapy maintain therapeutic gains and appear to continue to improve after treatment ends. Finally, nonpsychodynamic therapies may be effective in part because the more skilled practitioners utilize techniques that have long been central to psychodynamic theory and practice. The perception that psychodynamic approaches lack empirical support does not accord with available scientific evidence and may reflect selective dissemination of research findings. (p. 98) (see also Mundo, 2006; Yager, 2008).

Thus far, there is no evidence that superior therapy outcomes are more likely as a function of the theoretical orientation of the analyst. This important question might be explored in the next decade. In addition, we can expect to see a further burgeoning of interest in tracking changes in regional brain activity in relation to changes in psychotherapy (e.g., Linden, 2006). Finally, there likely will be significant additional research on the process of therapy, a research literature that I cannot review here (e.g., the nature and frequency of transference interpretations, and alliance ruptures and repairs in relation to treatment outcome).

Before concluding with a case illustration, it will be helpful to present a condensed, overall statement of the *contemporary Freudian theory of therapeutic action*. The reader can consider the summary below as a framework for reading the case illustration that follows. Based on the theories and concepts presented, I can say that the optimal process and outcome of psychoanalytic psychotherapy involves the following:

1. The patient is introspective and psychologically minded, with adequate reality testing. He or she is suffering from symptoms and maladaptive character traits (i.e., pathological compromise formations) based on currently repressed conflicts (and developmental deficits) that are influenced by wishes and fantasies (e.g., Oedipal wishes) originating in early childhood.

2. These conflicts become expressed in the context of the therapeutic relationship, particularly in the form of transference and resistance.

3. The expressions of these conflicts is facilitated by (a) a relatively unstructured, safe, situation that fosters free associations and open communication; (b) the analyst's free floating, evenly hovering attention; and (c) a "neutral" (i.e., unbiased) nonjudgmental, empathetic attitude in the context of a good therapeutic alliance.

4. The process proceeds on the principle of optimal frustration of transference wishes on the grounds that this stance of abstinence, and the analyst's relative anonymity, will help the patient experience and gain insight into the intrapsychic basis of his or her inner conflicts and interpersonal problems, helped along by the analyst's well-timed, empathic, interpretations, and the patient's "working through" of previously unresolved conflicts.

5. The noninterpretive aspects of the patient–analyst relationship can have significant therapeutic value in their own right. These include (a) the patient's experience and internalization of a new, benign relationship with a nonjudgmental parental figure, which helps reduce the harshness of the patient's superego; (b) the steady, implicit support of someone who listens empathically and understands the patient's feelings and struggles in the context of a safe atmosphere (or "holding environment"); and (c) the patient's identification with the analyst and the analytic attitude of delayed action in favor of respectful reflection on one's emotional experiences.

6. Noninterpretive verbal interventions are used sparingly in exploratory therapy. These include suggestion, advice, praise, confrontation, and therapist self-disclosure.

7. The preceding conditions are facilitated to the extent that the ongoing transference–countertransference enactments of the two participants are such that the analyst, by virtue of awareness and management of the countertransference, is adept at learning about the patient's dynamics, serving as a catalyst for the patient's insight, and recognizing and repairing the inevitable ruptures in the therapeutic alliance, thereby building "analytic trust" (Ellman, 2007). In this connection, it is said that the patient has to experience the analyst as an "old object" for the transference to develop, and as a "new object" for it to be analyzed and resolved.

8. Contemporary Freudian analysts are not a homogeneous group. They vary in numerous ways, including the degree to which they (a) emphasize the "here and now" versus extratransference and so-called "genetic" transference interpretations; (b) incorporate concepts from self psychology and object relations perspectives; (c) stress the therapeutic alliance, and its ruptures and repairs, as an important curative element in treatment; (d) intentionally disclose aspects of their countertransference; and (e) embrace the idea that the analytic process involves an ongoing enactment of the core issues of both participants.

9. At this point, all Freudian analysts, as well as those of other psychoanalytic persuasions, probably would agree on the need for a multiple-factor model to explain therapeutic action.

CASE ILLUSTRATION

At the request of the editors, I have not selected a case that proved to be an outstanding success, but one that showed a moderate degree of improvement at termination. Obviously, I can only present a highly condensed account of selected aspects of the case.

Mr. T started treatment at the age of 24, having been referred by his university counseling service. He was on the verge of being dropped from the university for an increasingly long string of incompletes that began in his freshman year (age 18) and snowballed, such that he was adding new incompletes at a faster rate than he was undoing the backlog of those he had already accumulated. He showed marked procrastination in not only his academic work but also in every realm of his life (paying bills late, missing trains because he arrived late, etc.).

The patient grew up in an upper-middle-class family in a Midwestern suburb. He felt clearly favored over his brother, 2 years his senior. His father, a person of seemingly indefatigable energy, was a successful attorney who also was actively involved in the life of his community. The boy was awed and envious when witnessing the respect and esteem accorded his father. His admiration of and identification with his father was one important basis for (1) his feeling that he wanted to be similarly recognized, as well as his serious doubts that he would ever be held in such high regard, and (2) his belief that to devote his energies exclusively to only *one* major goal or project was to forgo the possibility of successfully competing with his father, who was competent in his multiple pursuits.

The patient's mother led him to believe he was special, and that he had not only the ability and the potential but also the *obligation* to achieve greatness as an adult. These messages contributed to the patient's sense of having a special destiny that he ought to fulfill. Together with the model of mastery provided by his father, the patient's sense of a duty to perform, combined with his perfectionistic strivings, motivated him to overextend himself and contributed to his severe procrastinating behavior. His procrastination also expressed his underlying resentment of and rebellion against the external and internalized pressure to succeed. Thus, Mr. T never completed any project until faced with a truly unavoidable and serious deadline. Not surprisingly, Mr. T felt himself to be the passive victim of an unremitting barrage of environmental impingements and hassles (e.g., bills and taxes that he was expected to pay on a timely basis) and interpersonal expectations that he experienced as onerous obligations (e.g., being on time for therapy sessions and for dates with friends or women).

Mr. T experienced his mother as an extremely demanding, controlling, manipulative, opinionated, intolerant, and unempathic person who derived sadistic pleasure from taking advantage of her power over him. For example, he complained that she often would be the last mother to arrive when picking him up after school; he waited helplessly while all the other students left.

Given the entrenched nature of Mr. T's problems, his characterological difficulties, and his vulnerability to feelings of depression and frustration, in a context of psychological mindedness, intact reality testing, capacity for relatedness, and generally good ego resources, I recommended, after three or four initial interviews, that we embark on psychoanalysis at a frequency of four sessions per week. I reviewed with him the material and the themes of the initial interviews and summarized the main presenting issues he seemed to want to explore: his severe procrastination and his problems managing his time; his feelings of anxiety, depression, and low self-esteem; his turbulent, sticky relationship with his mother; and his difficulties with women (e.g., frequent power struggles), his problems in concentration, his need to take on more than he could handle, and the problems generated by this tendency (always feeling behind and having to play "catch-up," resenting any and all obligations, etc.).

We then turned to the contractual aspects of our working relationship; we agreed on a fee and arranged a schedule. I informed him about my usual vacation times and told him about my fee policy regarding missed sessions, namely, that I would charge him for missed sessions but would try to arrange makeup sessions when I could. I then offered a brief description of how I thought we could best work together. Because he had no prior experience in treatment I invited Mr. T to feel free to say what came to mind. I told him that it would help our work if, unlike what happens in ordinary conversation, he could suspend the usual editing or withholding of any thoughts or feelings that he might regard as tangential, irrelevant, or embarrassing. I added that my role would be to facilitate his self-exploration by making comments and observations from time to time. I explained the rationale for the use of the couch, which he accepted readily. I asked whether he had any questions for me, but he claimed not to have any at the moment.

The treatment began with his elaboration of the themes and issues that emerged in the initial interviews. In the interest of brevity, I restrict my account almost exclusively to his problems with time and with concentration. Fairly quickly, these issues began to be expressed in his relationship with me. For instance, the patient had a great deal of difficulty getting to the sessions on time. Not infrequently, he would arrive *exactly* at the midpoint of the session, seemingly without conscious intent to do so. On a couple of occasions he arrived with 2 or 3 minutes left, explaining that the idea of missing the session altogether was more troubling than the frustration of traveling 40 minutes each way for 2 or 3 minutes of his session with me. Once on the couch, he showed little awareness that the end of the session was approaching, continuing to talk in a way that made my stopping the session feel to both of us like an intrusive interruption rather than a somewhat natural ending.

Time was a bitter enemy in *every* aspect of Mr. T's life. He would resist doing things until he inevitably was coerced into action, even though he consciously hated being coerced. In addition to his precarious academic standing based on his long list of incompletes, his telephone and electrical service were regularly threatened with termination for delinquent payment of bills; he was never on time to a date, a dance, a concert, or any other activity, even those about which he was enthused.

Transitions from one activity to another were extremely difficult for Mr. T. He recalled that, as a child, he had a strong resistance to going to sleep, exceeded by his even more powerful resistance to getting up on time to go to school. For Mr. T, simply to be awake and conscious was to feel automatically a profound sense of the impingement of reality demands. He complained of an aversive sense of burden and responsibility in relation to all his unfinished daily tasks, to say nothing of the grand accomplishments on his future agenda. So profound were his yearnings to be free of these pressures that to stand up straight and carry himself erect, as opposed to being in a slouched or supine position, often felt extremely effortful and was experienced as a hardship to be endured and resented.

The patient experienced the passage of time, during which he managed to avoid chores, school assignments, or other obligations, as a welcome, albeit temporary reprieve from feeling coerced. He realized that his ability to resist the passage of time was an expression of his need for freedom. Because his procrastinating stance was an invitation to others to pressure him, it was hard for him to relax. His sense of his mother constantly nagging him was never far from his awareness.

Material relevant to the patient's problems with time emerged over many months and became one main focus of the treatment. These problems were intimately intertwined with his problems in concentration. Stated succinctly, to pay attention, to concentrate, felt painfully coercive to him. The patient did not have a basic deficit in attention, because he could concentrate well, but only when he was doing what he wanted to do, although even then he soon felt that concentrating was burdensome and his attention wandered.

I turn now to some of the technical precepts that guided my overall approach to this patient and to a demonstration of the actual interventions derived from these precepts. By my patient listening, my periodic, general requests for associations (e.g., "What comes to mind?"), and by occasional specific but open-ended questions designed to elicit further associations ("Any other thoughts or feelings about what you just said?"), I attempted to understand and to collaborate with him in the interpretation of the probable meanings of his behavior and experiences in relation to his chronic lateness and his difficulties in concentration as expressions of unconscious, core conflicts originating in childhood and reenacted in his relationship with me.

For example, some months into the analysis, I pointed out to the patient that he had been late a lot, something that, of course, he knew. He replied that it was difficult for him to get anywhere on time, that I should therefore not take it personally, and that he did not keep track of time enough to focus on when he would have to leave to show up on time for the session. The tone of his remarks suggested to me that he took my observation as a criticism. Rather than respond directly to the content of what he said, I focused on the affect implied in his reply. The technical precept guiding this choice was the idea of emphasizing the implicit, affective aspects of the "here and now" transference, in this instance, the issue of how he experienced my comment.

From the perspective of technique, my reference to his lateness is what Greenson (1967) would call a *confrontation,* albeit mild from my perspective. It conveys the message "Both the fact of your repeated lateness and your affective–cognitive response to my calling attention to it are matters of psychological import that we might profitably examine together."

By inquiring whether he might have experienced my observation as a criticism I was engaging in the technical intervention that Greenson calls *clarification.* As indicated earlier, confrontation and clarification are preparatory to *interpretation,* which searches for the *meanings* of behavior and experience. My confrontation and clarification already hint at the possibility of a transference reaction. At the same time, I wanted to maintain a positive working alliance by suggesting that we collaborate in examining our interchange. As the therapist, I also needed to be aware of why and how I chose to intervene at that time and with my particular choice of words and their tone. What countertransferential attitudes, affects, and conflicts might have been activated in me, including the questions of how *I* felt about his lateness (e.g., Was I irritated and sounding critical in the content, tone, syntax, or other aspects of my remarks? Did waiting for him trigger particular issues in my personality and experiences? In what ways might we be reenacting with one another the dynamics of our earlier relationships? Could my feelings lead to a rupture in the therapeutic alliance?).

Not surprisingly, the patient replied that he did feel somewhat chastised by my comment and that it reminded him of a similar reaction to the female therapist he saw initially and who referred him to me. He claimed that she actually chided him for lateness to his sessions with her. At this point, I had to consider whether I, too, although I did not chide him overtly (having taken his story about his prior therapist as a warning), was silently annoyed at him. As best as I could tell, I had mixed feelings about his frequent lateness. On the one hand, there were times I was mildly annoyed and imagined how his habitual lateness could be irritating to others, which stimulated me to think that he might have wanted to give me a taste of how he felt when his mother was late in picking him up from school. At the same time, I realized that a part of me was sometimes glad he was late, so that I could check my phone messages. My reaction, which stirred some feelings of guilt, made me question whether I was encouraging his lateness in some subtle way.

Mr. T's thoughts next turned to his mother and her almost invariable lateness in picking him up from elementary school in the afternoon. He felt angered at what he felt was the power differential and double standard in their relationship; she constantly chided him for being late in getting ready for school, yet she apparently had no compunction about keeping him waiting in all sorts of situations (e.g., she would drag him to stores and would take her time shopping, while he waited impatiently and with much frustration). After listening to him elaborate these memories and feelings, I asked him to consider the possibility that one meaning of his lateness with me might be a desire to keep me waiting as his mother had kept him waiting, to right the humiliating, infuriating wrong that he felt she had imposed upon him. I suggested that his understandable desire for revenge was expressed by reversing roles and being late with others (myself included) as she was with him. (There were other layers of meaning to his lateness [e.g., his need to feel special, to remain in a passive state and have all his needs fulfilled] that we explored later on in the treatment.) In making these kinds of interpretations I also communicated the view that while he bitterly resented his mother's accusations and criticisms, he also felt that they had a certain degree of merit, and that this contributed to his feeling that he was being a "bad boy."

Variations and elaborations of this line of *interpretation* were offered repeatedly in contexts in which issues of control, autonomy, and a sense of obligation were prominent in the patient's associations and in a host of childhood memories, as well as in his current behavior. For instance, he would graciously accept a dinner invitation, but as the hour of his expected arrival approached, he increasingly felt the invitation to be a burden. What began as a freely chosen, pleasant anticipation became transformed into an onerous obligation that aroused resentment. He felt similarly about our sessions.

As indicated earlier, the patient's problems with time were closely linked to his difficulties in concentration. For example, it was evident that Mr. T had a great deal of difficulty listening to my comments and interpretations. Not infrequently, he would remark, "Could you say that again? I completely lost track of what you said." Rather than simply repeat what I had said, which I did at the beginning of treatment, I asked him what came to mind about his not retaining it in the first place. He replied,

> "As you know, I've always had trouble paying attention to what I'm doing. I can't concentrate and often don't realize that I'm not concentrating until some time later. If I'm reading an assigned chapter in a textbook, I find that after a few pages I turn to some unassigned portion of the text and start to read without much less problem in concentration or in remembering what I read. Of course [*said with a knowing chuckle*], if the unassigned portion became the assignment, I would wander to some other part and forget what I had read. I engage in my 'shutdown procedure' without realizing it at the time."

I then said, "It seems that you often experience what I say in here as carrying the demand that you pay attention and do your 'homework' here immediately. Perhaps that resonates with your feelings about submitting to your mother's demands." The patient, struggling to retain my comment, replied that he did feel that expecting him to pay attention to what I had to say was coercive. In this context, as earlier in relation to the issue of time and being kept waiting by his mother, he again recalled ignoring his mother's entreaties that he do his homework as well as struggles with his mother around keeping his room neat and clean. The patient spontaneously acknowledged that there was something gratifying in defying what he felt was required or expected. For example, he again recalled times when his mother thought that he was in his room studying, while he was playing instead, feeling good (but also guilty) about getting away with something.

We were able to see that not hearing what I said was not some meaningless, momentary memory lapse but a significant here-and-now transference marker of his conflict between obedience and defiance. When I spoke, his mind "wandered to the unassigned portion," and he engaged in his "shutdown procedure" with me. His emotional insights into the nature, origins, and pervasiveness of this conflict were facilitated by so-called "genetic" transference interpretations, which linked his resistance to aspects of the analytic process to struggles with his mother.

It should be emphasized that what I am describing here is a *tiny* fragment of a long, often arduous process. It is not that patient and analyst suddenly arrive at one all-encompassing, blinding insight in which everything heretofore cloudy and obscure gels, such that long-standing conflicts suddenly become fully and forever resolved. This image, still a common fantasy, is a holdover from the rapid, usually short-lived, dramatic "cures" in the early days of psychoanalysis that followed immediately upon the retrieval of an unconscious, traumatic memory. In fact, the analytic process is one in which insights are gained, lost, and regained. There are strong resistances against translating insight into action. This is why analysts talk about the importance of *working through*. At times, working through is written about as though it were a special process or phase within the analysis. It is more accurate to say that working through *is* the analysis, as analyses usually are characterized by variations on a few central themes.

In summary, the diagnostic picture that emerged over the course of treatment was that Mr. T had an obsessive–compulsive character structure, with narcissistic, depressive, and passive–aggressive features. Dynamically, his core conflicts centered on (1) his passive wishes in relation to his mother and his guilt over such wishes, as well as his autonomous strivings to free himself from enmeshment with his mother; (2) his rage at, and desire to defy, maternal authority on the one hand, and his feeling that he should obediently yield to it in order to be a "good boy" and win her love and approval on the other; and (3) his Oedipal rivalry with his father, contributing to his grandiose wishes to be mother's favorite through some great achievement, along with his identification with and love for his father and his desire not to hurt him. Although these conflicts interacted with one another in synergistic ways, his internalized struggle with his mother was the most significant conflict and the one that contributed most to his impaired functioning. This is why I focus on this aspect of his personality in this brief presentation.

The reenactment, eventual understanding, and working through of the conflicts in the transference in a context of empathy, support, and a basically sound therapeutic alliance, which went through cycles of rupture and repair, contributed to the patient's much greater sense of personal agency and to an increase in his self-esteem based on a diminution of the superego pressures that he fulfill his alleged potential for greatness. The repairs of our alliance ruptures increased his sense of trust in me and his ability to differentiate our relationship from his relationship with his mother. One could say that he had to perceive me as an "old object" (i.e., as similar to his mother) for the transference to develop, and as a "new object" (different than his mother) for the transference to be analyzed and for him to have a "corrective emotional experience."

Eventually, Mr. T's battles with time diminished. He made considerable progress in coming to terms with his rage against his mother, and his fear and guilt about relinquishing her as a manipulative, persecutory internal presence. There was a reduction in his guilt over his indirectly expressed resentments and a corresponding decrease in his passive–aggressive defiance of external demands. He also came to uncouple the idea of his success with the notion of his father's demise. In these (and other) ways, he freed himself to take more genuine control over his own life.

The treatment lasted for 8 years. The patient finished college, obtained an advanced degree, and, after several turbulent relationships with women that were modeled on the conflicts in his relationship with his mother, he became engaged to a woman who was refreshingly different from his mother. However, relative to others, he still had a lower threshold for feeling coerced and still showed some inclination to procrastinate.

SUGGESTIONS FOR FURTHER STUDY

This chapter is intended as an introduction to the topic. There are many other complex concepts and issues regarding theories and techniques of analytic therapy that I could not cover here. However, the interested student is encouraged to read further, and would do well to start with the references cited in the next section, as well as the next chapter in this book.

Recommended Reading

Gabbard, G. (2004). *Long term psychodynamic psychotherapy—a basic text.* Washington, DC: American Psychiatric Press.—An exposition of key concepts and principles of psychodynamic psychotherapy, with clinical vignettes.

Wolitzky, D. L., & Eagle, M. (1997). Psychoanalytic theories of psychotherapy. In P. L. Wachtel & S. B. Messer (Eds.), *Theories of psychotherapy: Origins and evolution* (pp. 39–96). Washington, DC: American Psychological Association.—An account of the theory and technical aspects of the main psychoanalytic approaches to treatment.

DVD

McWilliams, N. (2007). *Psychoanalytic therapy* (Systems of Psychotherapy Video Series). Washington, DC: American Psychological Association.

REFERENCES

Aichhorn, A. (1935). *Wayward youth.* New York: Viking Press.

Altman, N. (1995) *The analyst in the inner city: Race, class, and culture through a psychoanalytic lens.* Hillsdale, NJ: Analytic Press.

American Psychiatric Association. (2000). *Diagnostic and statistical manual of mental disorders* (4th ed., text rev.). Washington,DC: Author.

Baudry, F. (1989). Character, character type, and character organization. *Journal of the American Psychoanalytic Association, 37,* 655–686.

Blatt, S. J. (2008). *Polarities of experience.* Washington, DC: American Psychological Association.

Blatt, S. J., & Ford, R. Q. (1999). The effectiveness of long-term, intensive inpatient treatment of seriously disturbed, treatment-resistant young adults. In H. Kaley, M. N. Eagle, & D. L. Wolitzky (Eds.), *Psychoanalytic therapy as health care* (pp. 221–238). Hillsdale, NJ: Analytic Press.

Brenner, C. (1979). Working alliance, therapeutic alliance and transference. *Journal of the American Psychoanalytic Association, 27*(Suppl.), 137–157.

Brenner, C. (1982). *The mind in conflict.* New York: International Universities Press.

Brenner, C. (1994). Mind as conflict and compromise formation. *Journal of Clinical Psychoanalysis, 3*(4), 473–488.

Breuer, J., & Freud, S. (1895). Studies on hysteria. *Standard Edition, 2,* 1–305. London: Hogarth Press, 1955.

Charcot, J. M. (1882). Physiologie pathologique: Sur les divers états nerveux determines par l'hypnotization chez les hystèriques. [Pathological physiology: On the different nervous states hypnotically induced in hysterics]. *Comptas Rondus Academy of Science Paris, 94,* 403–405.

Doidge, N. (1999). Who is in psychoanalysis now?: Empirical data and reflections on some common misperceptions. In H. Kaley, M. N. Eagle, & D. L. Wolitzky (Eds.), *Psychoanalytic therapy as health care* (pp. 177–198). Hillsdale, NJ: Analytic Press.

Eagle, M., & Wolitzky, D. (1992). Psychoanalytic theories of psychotherapy. In D. K. Freedheim (Ed.), *History of psychotherapy: A century of change* (pp. 109–158). Washington, DC: American Psychological Association.

Eagle, M., & Wolitzky, D. L. (1997). Empathy: A psychoanalytic perspective. In A. C. Bohart & L. S. Greenberg (Eds.), *Empathy reconsidered* (pp. 217–244). Washington, DC: American Psychological Association.

Eagle, M., Wolitzky, D. L., & Wakefield, J. (2001). The analyst's knowledge and authority: A critique of the "new view" in psychoanalysis. *Journal of the American Psychological Association, 64*(2), 457–490.

Ellman, S. (1998). The unique contribution of the contemporary Freudian position. In C. S. Ellman, S. Grand, M. Silvan, & S. J. Ellman (Eds.), *The modern Freudians* (pp. 237–268). Northvale, NJ: Aronson.

Ellman, S. J. (2007). Analytic trust and transference love, healing ruptures and facilitating repairs. *Psychoanalytic Inquiry, 27*, 246–263.

Erikson, E. H. (1950). *Childhood and society* (rev. ed.). New York: Norton, 1963.

Fairbairn, W. R. D. (1941). A revised psychopathology of the psychosis and psychoneurosis. *International Journal of Psychoanalysis, 22*, 250–279.

Fairbairn, W. R. D. (1952). *Psychoanalytic studies of the personality.* London: Tavistock.

Federn, P. (1952). *Ego psychology and the psychoses.* New York: Basic Books.

Ferenczi, S. (1926). *Further contributions to the theory and technique of psycho-analysis.* London: Hogarth Press.

Fiscalini, J. (2004). *Coparticipant psychoanalysis.* New York: Columbia University Press.

Fonagy, P. (2002). An open door review of outcome studies in psychoanalysis. Available at *www.ipa.org.uk/research/complete.htm.*

Freud, A. (1937). *The ego and the mechanisms of defence.* New York: International Universities Press.

Freud, A. (1954). Problems of technique in adult analysis. *Bulletin of the Philadelphia Association for Psychoanalysis, 4*, 44–69.

Freud, S. (1891–1940). *The standard edition of the complete psychological works of Sigmund Freud* (Vols. 1–23). London: Hogarth Press.

Freud, S. (1901). The psychopathology of everyday life. *Standard Edition, 6*, 1–310. London: Hogarth Press, 1960.

Freud, S. (1905). On psychotherapy. *Standard Edition, 7*, 255–268. London: Hogarth Press, 1953.

Freud, S. (1910). The future prospects of psychoanalytic therapy. *Standard Edition, 11*, 139–151. London: Hogarth Press, 1957.

Freud, S. (1911). Formulations on the two principles of mental functioning. *Standard Edition, 12*, 218–226. London: Hogarth Press, 1958.

Freud, S. (1912). The dynamics of transference. *Standard Edition, 12*, 97–108. London: Hogarth Press, 1953.

Freud, S. (1914). On narcissism: An introduction. *Standard Edition, 14*, 73–102. London: Hogarth Press, 1957.

Freud, S. (1917). Mourning and melancholia. *Standard Edition, 14*, 237–258. London: Hogarth Press, 1958).

Freud, S. (1919). Lines of advance in psychoanalytic therapy. *Standard Edition, 17*, 135–144. London: Hogarth Press, 1955.

Freud, S. (1923). The ego and the id. *Standard Edition, 18*, 12–66. London: Hogarth Press, 1961.

Freud, S. (1926). Inhibitions, symptoms and anxiety. *Standard Edition, 20*, 77–174. London: Hogarth Press, 1959.

Freud, S. (1933). The dissection of the psychical personality. *Standard Edition, 17*, 57–81. London: Hogarth Press, 1964.

Freud, S. (1937). Analysis terminable and interminable. *Standard Edition, 23*, 216–253. London: Hogarth Press, 1964.

Freud, S. (1940). An outline of psycho-analysis. *Standard Edition, 23*, 144–207. London: Hogarth Press, 1964.

Gill, M. M. (1982). *Analysis of transference.* New York: International Universities Press.

Gill, M. M. (1994). *Psychoanalysis in transition: A personal view.* Hillsdale, NJ: Analytic Press.

Gray, P. (1994) *The ego and the analysis of defense.* Northvale, NJ: Aronson.

Greenberg, J., & Cheselka, O. (1995). Relational approaches to psychoanalytic psychotherapy. In A. S. Gurman & S. B. Messer (Eds.), *Essential psychotherapies* (pp. 55–84). New York: Guilford Press.

Greenson, R. R. (1965). The working alliance and the transference neurosis. *Psychoanalytic Quarterly, 34,* 155–181.

Greenson, R. R. (1967). *The technique and practice of psychoanalysis* (Vol. 1). New York: International Universities Press.

Hartmann, H. (1939). *Ego psychology and the problem of adaptation.* New York: International Universities Press.

Hartmann, H., Kris, E., & Loewenstein, R. M. (1946). Comments on the formation of psychic structure. In Papers on psychoanalytic psychology (*Psychological Issues, 4,* Monograph No. 14, pp. 27–55). New York: International Universities Press.

Jacobson, E. (1964). *The self and the object world.* New York: International Universities Press.

Janet, P. (1907). *The major symptoms of hysteria.* New York: Macmillan.

Kaley, H., Eagle, M. N., & Wolitzky, D. L. (Eds.). (1999). *Psychoanalytic therapy as health care.* Hillsdale, NJ: Analytic Press.

Kernberg, O. (1975). *Borderline conditions and pathological narcissism.* Northvale, NJ: Aronson.

Kernberg, O. F., Selzer, M. A., Koenigsberg, H. W., Carr, A. C., & Appelbaum, A. H. (1989). *Psychodynamic psychotherapy of borderline patients.* New York: Basic Books.

Kohut, H. (1971). *The analysis of the self.* New York: International Universities Press.

Kohut, H. (1977). *The restoration of the self.* New York: International Universities Press.

Kohut, H. (1984). *How does analysis cure?* Chicago: University of Chicago Press.

Langs, R. J. (1982). Countertransference and the process of cure. In S. Slipp (Ed.), *Curative factors in dynamic psychotherapy* (pp. 127–152). New York: McGraw-Hill.

Leichsenring, F., & Rabung, S. (2008). Effectiveness of long-term psychodynamic psychotherapy: A meta-analysis. *Journal of the American Medical Association, 300*(13), 1551–1565.

Linden, D. E. (2006). How psychotherapy changes the brain—The contribution of functional neuroimaging. *Molecular Psychiatry. 11*(6), 528–538.

Loewald, H. (1960). On the therapeutic action of psychoanalysis. *International Journal of Psycho-Analysis, 43,* 16–33.

Luborsky, L. (1984). *Principles of psychoanalytic psychotherapy: A manual for supportive–expressive (SE) treatment.* New York: Basic Books.

Luborsky, L., & Crits-Christoph, P. (1990). *Understanding transference: The CCRT method.* New York: Basic Books.

Lyons-Ruth, K. (1998). Implicit relational knowing: Its role in development and psychoanalytic treatment. *Infant Mental Health, 19*(3), 282–289.

Macalpine, I. (1950). The development of the transference. *Psychoanalytic Quarterly, 19,* 501–539.

Mahler, M. (1968). *On human symbiosis and the vicissitudes of individuation: Vol. I. Infantile psychosis.* New York: International Universities Press.

Malan, D. (1976). *The frontier of brief psychotherapy.* New York: Plenum Press.

Markus, H. R., & Kitayama, S. (1998). The cultural psychology of personality. *Journal of Cross-Cultural Psychology, 29,* 63–87.

Messer, S. B., & Warren, C. S. (1995). *Models of brief psychodynamic therapy: A comparative approach.* New York: Guilford Press.

Messer, S. B., & Wolitzky, D. L. (2007).The psychoanalytic approach to case formulation. In T. D. Eells (Ed.), *Handbook of psychotherapy case formulation* (2nd ed., pp. 67–104). New York: Guilford Press.

Messer, S. B., & Wolitzky, D. L. (2010). A psychodynamic perspective on the therapeutic alliance: Theory, research and practice. In J. C. Muran & J. P. Barber (Eds.), *The therapeutic alliance: An evidence-based guide to practice* (pp. 97–122). New York: Guilford Press.

Mitchell, S. (1988). *Relational concepts in psychoanalysis.* Cambridge, MA: Harvard University Press.

Modell, A. H. (1976). "The holding environment"and the therapeutic action of psychoanalysis. *Journal of the American Psychoanalytic Association, 24,* 285–307.

Mundo E. (2006). Neurobiology of dynamic psychotherapy: An integration possible? *Journal of the American Academy of Psychoanalytic Dynamic Psychiatry, 34*(4), 679–691.

Oremland, J. (1991). *Interpretation and interaction.* Hillsdale, NJ: Analytic Press.

Pine, F. (1990). *Drive, ego, object, and self.* New York: Basic Books.

PDM Task Force. (2006). *Psychodynamic diagnostic manual.* Silver Spring, MD: Alliance of Psychoanalytic Organizations.

Pulver, S. E. (1995). The technique of psychoanalysis proper. In B. E. Moore & B. D. Fine (Eds.), *Psychoanalysis: The major concepts* (pp. 5–25). New Haven, CT: Yale University Press.

Reich, W. (1933). *Character analysis: Principles and techniques for psychoanalysis in practice and training* (3rd ed.). New York: Orgone Institute Press.

Safran, J. D., & Muran, J. C. (2000). *Negotiating the therapeutic alliance: A relational treatment guide.* New York: Guilford Press.

Sandell, R., Blomberg, J., Lazar, A., Carlsswon, J., Broberg, J., & Schubert, J. (2000). Varieties of long-term outcome among patients in psychoanalysis and long-term psychotherapy: A review of findings in the Stockholm Outcome of Psychoanalysis and Psychotherapy Project (STOPP). *International Journal of Psychoanalysis, 81*(5), 921–942.

Sandler, J. (1959). *The background of safety.* Paper presented at the 21st Congress of the International Psychoanalytic Association, Copenhagen, Denmark.

Schachter, J., & Kachele, H. (2007). The analyst's role in healing: Psychoanalysis-plus. *Psychoanalytic Psychology, 24,* 429–444.

Schafer, R. (1983). *The analytic attitude.* New York: Basic Books.

Schafer, R. (1992). *Retelling a life.* New York: Basic Books.

Schlesinger, G., & Wolitzky, D. L. (2002). The effects of a self-analytic exercise on clinical judgment. *Psychoanalytic Psychology, 19*(4), 651–685.

Searles, H. (1965). *Collected papers on schizophrenia and related subjects.* London: Hogarth Press.

Shedler, J. (2010). The efficacy of psychodynamic psychotherapy. *American Psychologist, 65*(2), 98–109.

Sterba, R. (1934). The fate of the ego in analytic therapy. *International Journal of Psycho-Analysis, 15,* 117–126.

Stone, L. (1961). *The psychoanalytic situation: An examination of its development and essential nature.* New York: International Universities Press.

Strachey, J. (1934). The nature of the therapeutic action of psychoanalysis. *International Journal of Psycho-Analysis, 15,* 127–159.

Sullivan, H. S. (1953). *The interpersonal theory of psychiatry.* New York: Norton.

Wallerstein, R. S. (1986). *Forty-two lives in treatment: A study of psychoanalysis and psychotherapy.* New York: Guilford Press.

Wallerstein, R. S. (1990). Psychoanalysis: The common ground. *International Journal of Psycho-Analysis, 71,* 3–20.

Weiner, I. B., & Bornstein, R. F. (2009). *Principles of psychotherapy* (3rd ed.). New York: Wiley.

Weiss, J., & Sampson, H. (1986). *The psychoanalytic process: Theory, clinical observation, and empirical research.* New York: Guilford Press.

Winnicott, D. W. (1965). *The maturational processes and the facilitating environment.* London: Hogarth Press and Institute of Psycho-Analysis

Yager, J. (2008) The emerging evidence base for psychodynamic psychotherapies. *Journal Watch Psychiatry, 15*(1), 4.

Zetzel, E. R. (1956). Current concepts of transference. *International Journal of Psycho-Analysis, 46,* 39–52.

CHAPTER 3

Relational Psychoanalytic Psychotherapy

Rebecca Coleman Curtis
Irwin Hirsch

HISTORICAL BACKGROUND

Relational approaches to psychoanalytic psychotherapy represent a paradigm shift consistent with other developments in science and the humanities in the 20th century. One of the benefits is that this approach allows a rapprochement with current mainstream cognitive and social psychology. It is difficult to describe relational approaches in a unitary way. What is inherent in the concept is the view that each individual asked to describe it will present a subjective perspective that differs somewhat from that of the next "expert."

Freud developed the psychoanalytic method in a culture that increasingly looked to science as a source of orientation in a world where technology and industrialization had led to major changes in people's lifestyles. The science of the 19th century was that of *objective observation*. The observer of mental processes in psychoanalysis was to be this sort of neutral, impartial scientist at work, like an archeologist looking for deeper and deeper layers of unconscious facts in the patient's mind. *Essentialism* and *positivism* are other terms characterizing the natural science model that reflect much of psychoanalytic thinking for at least the first half of the 20th century. Essentialism refers to the idea that organisms have a natural biological essence, and positivism, to the idea that science can discover true propositions.

Images of the world were jolted in the 1920s and 1930s by Einstein's relativity theory, quantum physics, and Heisenberg's uncertainty principle. Quantum physics emphasized interconnections and mutual interactions, and Heisenberg demonstrated that phenomena were always affected by being measured. The ideal of the totally objective observer in the hard sciences was demonstrated to be impossible. If the observer were also a participant in the world of particle physics, then the psychoanalyst was certainly a participant in interactions with a patient, and his or her influence would have to be taken into account in that situation as well. Nonetheless, this ethos did not filter down to psychoanalysis until the late 1940s, heralded then by Harry Stack Sullivan's (1953) model of the therapist as both an observer and an unwitting participant in the dyad.

The ideas of the individual as embedded in relationships and the therapist as a participant–observer were taken up in the United States by Sullivan in his development of what was first called *interpersonal psychiatry*. Unlike many psychoanalysts who worked with rather well-functioning patients, Sullivan developed many of his ideas from working with males with schizophrenia. Sullivan joined forces with several prominent psychoanalysts who were also interested in social and cultural influences on personality development—Horney (1926), Fromm (1951, 1964), Fromm-Reichmann (1959a), and Thompson (1942) and eventually formed with the three latter therapists what became know as the interpersonal school of psychoanalysis. Thompson (as well as Melanie Klein) had been analyzed by Freud's colleague Ferenczi. Ferenczi, known as an analyst's analyst, was sent difficult patients other analysts could not help. Whereas Freud was considered the "father" of psychoanalysis, Ferenczi was considered the "mother." He was known for his focus upon early developmental and often pre-Oedipal, nonverbal interactions between mother and child, prioritizing such engagement over Freud's emphasis on innate drive states as the building blocks of human personality. Ferenczi also experimented with various new techniques, including conceptualizing the psychoanalytic relationship as mutually constructed. Ferenczi and Sullivan both had considerable influence on the development of relational psychoanalysis, the former more indirectly, through his impact on analysands such as Thompson, Klein, and Balint. Thompson became a consolidating figure within the interpersonal school, while Klein and Balint were key to the development of different aspects of object relations theory. Although there are important differences among these traditions, all basically share the view that relationships with caretakers are the most central features in any effort to understand development of personality. With respect to the therapeutic relationship, all three traditions highlight various ways, beyond objective observation, that therapists both unwittingly and purposefully interact with their patients (Hirsch, 1987). Perhaps partly because some of these analysts were working with more disturbed patients than those of their classical counterparts, they deviated early on from the standard Freudian technique of the time.

Around the same time that Sullivan was developing his interpersonal psychiatry in the United States, Fairbairn (1952) in Great Britain was arguing that people are primarily motivated to seek other people. This position, too, was in contrast to the classical Freudian belief that people are motivated primarily by sexual and aggressive drives, and derivatives of these drive states. He developed, simultaneously with but independent of Klein and Balint, an "object relations theory of psychoanalysis," drawing from the philosophical tradition of "subjects" (people) and the "objects" they observed. For Fairbairn, the term *objects* referred to the internalization of experiences with other people—what cognitive psychologists might call internalized "representations" of others.

In 1983, Gill published a paper arguing for a "person" point of view, in contrast to Freud's energy discharge model of the mind. He proposed the term *person* because *interpersonal* carried too heavily the weight of Sullivanian thinking, and *object relations* failed to distinguish between the work of Klein, in which an instinct-oriented model was still present to a degree, and the work of Balint and Fairbairn, in which the relations with early caretakers were dominant. Also, in 1983, Greenberg and Mitchell published a volume titled *Object Relations in Psychoanalytic Theory*. They argued that a paradigm shift had taken place in psychoanalysis, such that relations with others "constitute the fundamental building blocks of mental life" (1983, p. 3), in contrast to Freud's emphasis on the unfolding of biologically based, prewired psychosexual stages of development. All of the approaches Greenberg and Mitchell included under the "relational" umbrella have in common the focus upon relationships, external and internalized, as the primary way of understanding human development and personality organization. Although the clearest expression of this paradigm initially came in the work of Sullivan and Fairbairn, other key psychoanalytic theorists, such as Winnicott (1964), are viewed as moving psychoanalysis toward this emphasis, some without breaking completely with their Freudian framework. Levenson (1972), a major contributor to the interpersonal tradition, had already described paradigm shifts from Freud's work-machine model, to the information/communication model, and from this to the organismic model found in biology, where every element has connections with many other elements, so that influence can flow in several directions. Levenson emphasized the interpersonal entanglements into which the analyst could be drawn by the patient. Far from the objective scientist or the "blank screen" of the Freudian analyst, the therapist in the interpersonal/relational approach was a subjectivity of its own, interacting with the other subjectivity—the patient.

Greenberg and Mitchell (1983) suggested that the interpersonal approach of Sullivan and his colleagues (Horney, Fromm, Fromm-Reichman, and Thompson) lacked a well-developed theory of intrapsychic processes, whereas the varieties of object relations approaches (Winnicott, Fairbairn, and Klein) lacked sufficient focus on modes of describing actual interpersonal relations. These approaches complement each other, with the interpersonal tradition originally focused more upon external relations (and realities) and the object relations tradition focused more upon internalized relationships. By this time in history, however, both traditions address and have integrated the fundamental notion that unconscious processes or internalized worlds consist largely of internalized relational configurations (Mitchell, 1988, 1993).

In the United States, Kohut (1971, 1984) also developed many ideas that were in considerable harmony with Ferenczi's original view of the analyst as an empathic observer, and with theories of development that have much in common with object relations theorists such as Balint and Winnicott. Stolorow and others (Orange, Atwood, & Stolorow, 2001) have tried to extend Kohut's self psychology and integrate it into the intersubjective ethos long held by interpersonal psychoanalysts and their contemporary relational counterparts (Benjamin, 1998).

In 1991, the new journal, *Psychoanalytic Dialogues: A Journal of Relational Perspectives*, became a forum for comparing and contrasting the numerous traditions that lie within the large relational umbrella: interpersonal, varieties of object relational (Fairbairn, Winnicott, and Klein), self psychological, intersubjective, and postmodern feminist thinking. The relational approach continues to inspire excitement, with the International Association for Relational Psychoanalysis and Psychotherapy founded by Stephen Mitchell, holding its first meeting in 2002, with subsequent meetings in Italy, Greece, and Israel.

Relational approaches have been influenced by other intellectual trends in the 20th century, particularly postmodernism, constructivism, relativism, and perspectivism. Recently, views of self-organizing processes have been derived from theories about how order can emerge out of chaos. Living systems change to fit in with the environment. Psychological change involves fluctuations in response to differing external realities to the extent that a "tipping point" is reached, resulting in a new psychological organization. The self as a dynamic system has been discussed extensively by Piers, Muller, and Brent (2007).

CONCEPTS OF PERSONALITY

Because relational approaches draw from some very disparate theoretical frameworks, there is not a unified concept of personality. Generally, it is thought that individuals develop relatively stable patterns of being in the world. Their ways of being are intimately connected to the internalization of identifications with significant caretakers, much of which lies outside the boundary of consciousness. Many relational therapists believe that people tend to construct unconsciously their contemporary world to conform to the familiarity of past experience (cf. Cushman, 1995; Hoffman, 1998).

The particular approach of Sullivan centered around what he called the *self-system* (whereas other theorists might discuss concepts such as psychic structure or "character"). For Sullivan (1953), personality is the entire functioning of a person. The *self* refers to the organization of experience within the personality and is largely a composite of internalized experiences with others. Anxiety-free experiences as an infant with the caretaker, usually the mother, lead to the experience of the *good me*, whereas anxiety-filled experiences lead to the *bad me*. Some experiences, however, are so traumatic that they can not be integrated at all. These experiences Sullivan refers to as the *not me*. They are experiences felt as dread or as horror, such as in a nightmare. Concerns with the lack of integration of positive and negative experiences in persons suffering from disorders of the self are a central theme in many relational writings.

Although Winnicott had differentiated a static *true self* from a *false self*, most relational analysts view the self as socially constructed; that is, people are seen as having different thoughts, feelings, and ways of acting in the presence of different people and when alone in different contexts. All of these multiple self-states are viewed as real, including one or more that may be oriented toward pleasing others, instead of being considered "false" (Mitchell, 1993). The person is never conceived of as an isolated being in relational thought: "There is no such thing as a baby," Winnicott stated, "only a nursing couple" (1964, p. 88). Winnicott was trying to convey the idea that there are properties of a dyad that transcend the attributes of each individual person. Similarly, relational analysts refer to their approach as a *two-person psychology*, because these properties of the relationship between two people must always be taken into account in efforts to understand the individual. Ogden (1994), a contemporary Kleinian analyst, for example, has referred to the space between the analyst and the patient as the "analytic third"; in other words, the reflective space of psychoanalysis is another presence in the room. Other relational analysts, such as Altman (1995), have suggested that the surrounding culture is always present as a third party in the relationship between two people.

Sullivan's theory of personality was very influenced by developments in the cognitive science of his time. His model of the self is not dominated by the repression of unacceptable impulses, as in Freudian psychology. Instead, he posits a lack of connection, or dissociation of experiences that would be so conflictual as to be overwhelming if held in consciousness simultaneously. Such awareness may be disorganizing because it is incongruous with the current and stable organization of experience.

Experiences that are out of awareness or unconscious are critically important to relational psychoanalysts, as they are to psychoanalysts of all traditions. Recently relational analysts have expanded their ways of thinking about unconscious processes to include many experiences of which people are unaware, beyond dynamic unconscious experiences that are unattended or forgotten because they are threatening (Curtis, 2009). These processes are similar in some ways to what cognitive psychologists refer to as procedural memory, and implicit perceptual and memory processes. Donnel Stern (1997) has also referred to "unformulated experiences" that a person has never consciously articulated.

For Sullivan, the self-system developed out of a sense of anxiety. Anxiety may lead to selective inattention regarding experiences that are inconsistent with a person's dominant views or ways of being. To the extent that the person is anxious, his or her flexibility in attending to incongruous information and responding becomes more rigidified. For Fairbairn as well, the representations of the self developed out of anxiety.

A dissociative view of the mind prevails in relational thinking (cf. Bromberg, 1998; Curtis, 1996; Davies & Frawley, 1993). Fairbairn (1929/1994), in his medical thesis, argued that repression is a specific type of dissociation. Dissociated states may manifest themselves by physical symptoms, such as tics or somatic symptoms. Trauma may lead to a dissociation of experiences, such that a person may seem numb or intellectualized when discussing a traumatic event, all the while experiencing signs at other times that something is amiss. People do not feel conflicted about dissociated experiences, because they are not aware of them simultaneously with other states. Experiences that are "repressed" or pushed out of awareness, on the other hand, are experienced as conflictual at the moment of repression. Internal conflict, nonetheless, is an ever-present aspect of the human condition. The wish to risk knowing oneself and to change as a person is in ubiquitous conflict with the wish to remain ignorant of one's self and maintain a stable, albeit restricted, equilibrium.

In place of Freud's sexual and aggressive motivations as the central force that moves people, Sullivan conceptualized the need to satisfy tendencies toward security, tenderness (intimacy), and lust. When these needs cannot be met, they may undergo what he called a "malevolent transformation," leading to aggression and perhaps cruelty. Overall, in relational theories, aggression is not seen as instinctual. It is viewed as learned, stemming from either frustration or identification with a familiar aggressor. To the extent that the parent is empathic and able to take the baby's perspective or to reflect on the baby's functioning (Stern, 1985), the child is likely to feel soothed when anxious, and be more likely eventually to satisfy its desires. Infant researchers, such as Beebe, Jaffe, and Lachmann (1992) have observed that caretakers who can match the rhythm of their infants in a sort of dance-like interaction are able to help the baby regulate her or his emotions.

Sexuality, though instinctually based, is viewed as an important medium in which relational struggles are played out. The form of one's sexuality is developed through relational interaction. Sexuality provides the imaginative elaboration of bodily functions. It is a "powerful medium in which emotional connection and intimacy is sought, established, lost, and regained" (Mitchell, 1988, p. 107).

Relational analysts have been among the strongest critics of Freudian theories regarding the development of sexuality since Freud expressed them. Horney (1926) and Thompson (1942) both criticized his notions of female sexuality, arguing that penis envy was related not to biological differences but to the cultural advantages given to men. Castration anxiety in the literal sense has been seen as more related to the real, threatening statements given to boys in Freud's turn-of-the-century European culture, than as a universal phenomenon per se. However, "castration" fears, in the sense of feelings of threat and/or helplessness, are seen as universal. Stoller (1985) argued that castration anxiety was "existence anxiety" (p. 20n), and that men "do not fear loss of genitals per se (castration anxiety) as much as they fear to lose their masculinity and, more fundamentally, their sense of maleness" (p. 35). "Masochistic" tendencies in women have been viewed as a consequence of a lack of recognition of a girl's subjectivity by the father, not as a consequence of an adjustment to a sense of having been "castrated" (Benjamin, 1988).

Relational analysts think that the development of heterosexuality needs as much explanation as the development of homosexuality or bisexuality; there are no universal causalities for either. In addition, homosexuality and bisexuality are viewed as normal variants, not as pathological. This is also true for much of other sexual behavior, which historically had been referred to as "perversions" (Dimen, 2001; Drescher, 1998).

Aggression comes from being aggressed upon and from frustration, not from an inborn drive that must be discharged. People have the impulse to hurt when they are harmed, but if empathy is learned through the experience with a loving caretaker, the impulse to hurt another can be contained. Although all people have aggressive feelings, when loving feelings outweigh aggressive ones, relationships are easier to maintain. The desire to hurt others by people who have been neglected or harmed is not to be underestimated (Harris, 1998).

Relational theory has sometimes been criticized for reducing human motivation to a single drive—that for relationships. Yet Greenberg (1991), for example, has posited two broad categories of basic relational needs—one for security or safety, and the other for effectance. This thinking is built on the work of Fromm (1964), who described a universal human conflict between enmeshment in what is safe and familiar, and the wish to expand oneself—to separate from what is known and familiar. Both Fromm's and Greenberg's thinking is important to many relational therapists and reflects a dimension of experience that transcends simply relationship seeking.

A theory of five motivational systems in the work of Lichtenberg, Lachmann, and Fosshage (1992) has been incorporated into much of relational thinking. These five systems are the need for (1) physiological requirements, (2) attachment and affiliation, (3) exploration and assertion, (4) responding aversively through withdrawal and antagonism, and (5) sensual enjoyment and sexual excitement. Relational analysts are more likely to think about desires than about drives (Benjamin, 1988). Desire is "experienced always in the context of relatedness" (Mitchell, 1988, p. 3). Curtis (2009) has suggested two broad categories of desire—physical and psychological—or physical survival and survival of the meaning-making system.

Personality formation begins in the early stages of infancy, or even in the uterus. Relational analysts have embraced the work of attachment researchers, such as the psychoanalyst Bowlby (1969), who posited that infants develop expectations that others will be available to them emotionally to the same extent as the early caretaker. Infants and their caretakers communicate nonverbally by "eye contact, proxemics, conversational rhythms, games and signaling" (Beebe et al., 1992, p. 66). The infant develops expectancies of characteristic interaction sequences that become generalized in the first year of life, at the time when the ability to abstract information develops. Stern (1985) referred to the infant's capacity to internalize interactions and to generalize them, similar to what Bowlby had called *internalized working models*. The unconscious organizing structures early in life are believed to play a major role in the way other people are integrated into one's life. The open communication patterns of securely attached children and their parents provide a greater ability to revise working models of self and others flexibly than do more closed patterns of communication.

These internalized interactional patterns provide a model of development that is largely drawn from infant research, and it is quite different from much of Freudian developmental theory. Still, it is acknowledged that there are often self-critical and self-punitive tendencies among children reared by benign parents. Aggressive fantasies on the part of the child may produce guilt when parents are benign. Some relational analysts have been drawn to Kleinian theories of development, theories that place a central emphasis on innate aggression and its projection. Mitchell (1988) and others have noted that Klein's theories were taken not from the observations of normal infants and children, but from interactions of older and more disturbed children.

Although Oedipal dynamics, a central theme in the Freudian tradition, are examined and may well be a significant source of conflict, problems in living arise for a larger variety of reasons. For example, personality continues to develop during the elementary school years, when the formation of a close friendship may mitigate or modify earlier troubled engagements with caretakers. Relational theory assumes that conflicts within the personality are inevitable. Symptoms are rooted not only in conflicts between wishes and fears, or between people and society, but also in conflictual relational configurations that have been internalized from a life history of self–other interaction. Detailed descriptions of the dynamics of various personality disorders, such as obsessionalism, narcissism, paranoia, and borderline personality, can from a relational perspective be found in the *Handbook of Interpersonal Psychoanalysis* (Lionells, Fiscalini, Mann, & Stern, 1995).

Freudian psychoanalysis largely ignored the effects of traumas in the world at large, and relational psychoanalysis from its inception, but especially in the last decade, has looked at how life-threatening and out of the ordinary experiences affect personality (Boulanger, 2007; Davies & Frawley, 1993). Relational psychoanalysis, on the other hand, in moving away from the Freudian emphasis on sexuality, has dedicated considerable attention in the last decade to the body (Gentile, 2007; Knoblauch, 2005) and mind–body connections (or the lack thereof). In response to the prevalence of eating disorders, factors leading people to turn to food as opposed to others for comfort have become another focus (Gentile, 2007; Petrucelli & Stuart, 2001). Similarly, issues of addiction, heretofore neglected by psychoanalysts, have become a subject of attention (Burton, 2005; Director, 2005). In all of these areas, newer understandings of how people dissociate (or disconnect) are prominent. Experiences that are not held in consciousness simultaneously with others must be brought into consciousness so that traditional views of conflict in psychoanalysis then come to the fore.

It should be pointed out that relational psychoanalysis has moved away, in the past decade especially, from thinking so much in terms of traditional personality styles to consideration of new forms of relational organization (i.e., the ways people act and feel in the presence of particular other people and in particular situations; Lyons-Ruth, 2006). Relational analysts have been influenced to a large extent by infant research and the effects of nonverbal processes on personality development (Stern, 2008). Such effects had been ignored by Freudian psychoanalysis and were not known very well until recently. These processes have been studied in particular by the Boston Change Process Study Group (Stern, 2008) and other infant researchers, such as Beebe et al. (1992). Also, supporting the role of unconscious, implicit factors in personality change, a review of eight studies regarding the relationship between insight and outcomes in psychotherapy demonstrated only marginal support for the classical idea that insight is related to better therapeutic outcomes (Gibbons, Crits-Christoph, Barber, & Schamburger, 2007).

PSYCHOLOGICAL HEALTH AND PATHOLOGY

Sullivan (1953) preferred the term *problems in living* over other nomenclatures for psychiatric disorders. Fromm criticized the conformist personality he saw in American culture and was scathing in his attack on the "marketing personality." McDougall (1990, p. 156) coined the term *normopath*, and Bollas (1987, p. 137) referred to the *normatic personality*;

both terms refer to people who conform to the values of a society to the extent that their individual vitality is stifled. Thus, the problems in living for relational psychoanalysts do not correspond neatly with the criteria in the fourth edition of the *Diagnostic and Statistical Manual of Mental Disorders* (American Psychiatric Association, 2000). Nonetheless, relational analysts do make assessments regarding the level of functioning, and may prescribe medication or refer patients for medication evaluations if they believe that psychotherapy alone is insufficient. They are, however, quite critical of the "disease" model inherited from medicine. They do not expect to uncover a pathogen—a single repressed wish, for example. Instead, they view personality patterns as having been largely learned in social situations, and as having been reasonable, adaptive ways of coping in those situations (e.g., attachment styles learned largely in infancy and childhood). (Obviously, the temperaments with which infants are born also play a role.) If troubled ways of being are learned, new ways of relating also can be learned. There exists inherent optimism in a way of thinking that emphasizes personality as a function of experiential learning, not as biologically driven.

Relational analysts make note of patients' strengths and help them become more aware of their strengths and how to appreciate them. At the same time, relational analysts look at the gaps in patients' resources and help them become aware of these deficits. A patient with an obsessive style, who avoids feelings and provides endless details, might be asked, for example, "What are you feeling?" or "Can you tell me what is the most important thing that happened?" Problems in relating to others are obviously often a core focus, for much of what can be called psychopathology is expressed in the broad arenas of love, work, and play.

Flexible ways of relating are signs of health, whereas rigid ways of being are signs of inhibition and anxiety. Symptoms do not simply reflect illness or pathology but are always viewed as communications (Phillips, 1988). According to Phillips, the healthy child has a "flexible repertoire of symptoms" (p. 50).

A number of relational analysts have made important contributions to the understanding of severe disturbances. In particular, Sullivan, Fromm-Reichmann, and Searles worked successfully with patients with schizophrenia before the advances of psychotropic medications. Fromm-Reichmann's patient Hannah Greenberg documented her treatment in a popular novel (1964) and the film *I Never Promised You a Rose Garden*. For Sullivan, the self in the patient with schizophrenia has lost control of awareness and has lost the sense of a consensually validated self. For Searles (1965), treating patients with schizophrenia simply as unformed or egoless people is profoundly condescending. Sullivan, Fromm-Reichmann, and Searles all subscribed to an ethos characterized by Sullivan's attitude that we are all more simply human than otherwise. They argue that although patients with schizophrenia are more difficult to work with, they are not essentially different from others.

The relational tradition has paid more attention to what has actually happened, and fantasy based on that experience, than classical psychoanalysis. Whereas Freud once theorized that many of the stories he heard of incest and the sexual abuse of women, for example, were wishes and fantasies, the interpersonalists and relational analysts believed the stories could be based on something that really occurred. Traumas, especially those stemming from betrayal by parents, relatives, and other people in positions of authority, affect feelings and expectations in current situations in ways that fantasies not founded upon experiences do not. Relational analysts, more so than their Freudian colleagues, are mindful of the impact of what actually happens, that is, the social and cultural contributions to problems in living.

Health does not simply represent having better feelings about oneself (self-esteem) and others. By allowing more experiences into awareness, a person may also notice more threatening experiences when they exist. Health means a greater tolerance for such anxiety-provoking experiences, in addition to tolerance for desired, exciting experiences. Psychic health, as much as anything, refers to the ability to assimilate new experience, to transcend the identifications and the constraints of the past.

THE PROCESS OF CLINICAL ASSESSMENT

Relational therapists make informal assessments of patients in all interactions, even as they are gathering a history of the patient. Assessments are made at both interpersonal and intrapsychic levels, consistent with the origins of the approach. Of particular note are the interactional styles, styles of coping and defense, the range of emotions, cognitive abilities, feelings about oneself and others, and conflicts and inhibitions that may block the patient from achieving his or her goals. Diagnostic categories are known to the therapist, but categories eliminate the unique qualities of the individual that are of interest to the relational therapist. Such categories are used to the extent that they are required for records and are useful in summarizing characteristics of the patient, but they are generally viewed as too restrictive and stereotyping, especially in regard to personality disorders (Westen, 2002).

Assessments are made at individual, dyadic, and systemic levels. Although the individual is the primary focus of attention, the therapist is monitoring continually what transpires in the therapeutic dyad, and is cognizant of the cultural context as well. If the therapist thinks that couple or family therapy would be of benefit, such treatment (usually with a different therapist) is recommended, often in addition to individual treatment.

The events and feelings preceding a problem, the overall context in which it occurs, and any secondary gains the problem may provide are given serious consideration. A detailed inquiry is made into any problems that require specialized treatment, such as substance abuse. In the case of potential danger to self and others, inquiry into matters related to the likelihood of such events is conducted, and a judgment is made as to optimal treatment. Relational therapists working in a hospital or clinic setting utilize any formal assessments (e.g., psychological tests) usually conducted in that setting. Therapists in private practice refer patients for psychological, neuropsychological, or medical assessments when appropriate.

THE PRACTICE OF THERAPY

In the practice of psychotherapy, relational analysts draw from the rich literature of case studies and theory in psychoanalysis, although their practice may differ somewhat from that of their classical forebears. The relational emphasis is distinct from that of some other contemporary approaches, particularly psychotherapies that focus largely on symptom reduction. For relationalists, the unique experiences and meanings of people's existence are of very special interest. This contrasts with an interest in the *general* characteristics of all patients with a particular psychiatric diagnosis, and with the application of a standard technique that is relevant to everyone. Every therapist, every patient, and every dyad is unique. Indeed, most relational therapies prefer the term *approach* to the more technical word *technique*. Still, a short-term psychotherapy derived from Sullivan's interpersonal psychotherapy (Klerman, Weissman, Rounsaville, & Chevron, 1984) has the general approach of increasing interpersonal relations. This therapy, originally for depression, while not psychoanalytic in its approach, is being used very widely for a number of disorders, including bingeing, overeating, and borderline personality disorder.

Basic Structure of Therapy

Relational therapists usually prefer to meet with patients more than one time each week, although often this is not possible. Rarely would a relational therapist set a time limit, unless the therapist's work is consistent with one of the models of brief therapy (see Hoyt, Chapter 11, this volume). Most relational therapists would hope for frequent sessions with the patient in order that the interpersonal interactions with others that the patient finds problematic emerge with the therapist (transference). These problematic interactions may take some time to occur, or a meaningful level of intimacy may be slow to develop. Although the treatment is most likely to be individual therapy, family or group therapy may be used in conjunction with individual treatment. Despite sessions generally being unstructured, the relational therapist becomes more active if life-threatening or treatment-threatening issues occur.

Goal Setting

Traditionally, the goal of psychoanalytic treatment has been to increase awareness and through this process to effect a broadening of the organization of experience, so that a person is more flexible and less rigid. Enrichment of experience takes priority over symptom reduction, and optimal functioning in the areas of love, work, and play are of interest to relational therapists, as they are to all psychoanalytic therapists. In many ways, the precise goals of the therapy are not known in advance, because the hope is that the patient will open up to new experiences and, in this process, formulate new goals. Ultimately, however, the patient sets the goals, and the patient is certainly free to choose less ambitious aims than what most analytic therapists prefer.

If the therapist has reservations about a goal the patient expresses, he or she has an obligation to express a dissenting opinion or attempt to arrive at a mutually compatible goal. The relationally oriented therapist has a responsibility to explain in the first set of meetings something about the way he or she works if the patient comes from a background that is likely devoid of such knowledge. For example, if the patient comes to the therapist saying that he would like to work more hours each week and is already working an 80-hour week, the therapist might question this goal and suggest an alternative, such as exploring what makes working that many hours so important.

Despite the ambitious aims of most analytic therapies, patients will often want help, first and foremost, with symptom reduction. Increased awareness of when the symptom occurs, what covaries with it, and what other problems the symptom might reduce or disguise likely will help with symptom reduction. Addressing life-threatening and treatment-threatening behaviors will take priority over other goals. Certain other behavioral problems may also take priority, such as a substance abuse problem that will neutralize any benefit that psychoanalytic therapy may offer. Relational analysts vary in the extent to which they refer a patient for behavioral and other auxiliary treatments, or integrate such treatments into their own approach.

Relational therapists consider what the symptoms may communicate, how they have been adaptive, what they may symbolize, and with what they may coincide. A man who presents with a problem of premature ejaculation may have impulse control problems in other areas; a man who has retarded ejaculation may procrastinate elsewhere. The partner may be anxious and/or undermine the patient's confidence. The man may prefer not to be involved with this partner, or he may prefer a partner of another sex. To the extent that therapists conceive of the presenting problem as embedded in a larger picture, they will listen to the patient's communications with an open mind, or inquire in a more structured manner, so as to have a more nuanced picture of the whole person.

In helping the patient achieve whatever goals he or she has articulated, the therapist also has ideas about how best to achieve these goals. As already noted, the therapist will likely have in mind the traditional psychoanalytic goal of helping the patient work, love, and play more freely. Sullivan stated that treatment is aimed at "increasing a patient's skill in living" (1953, p. 175). Relational analysts will have in mind a variety of desired outcomes, such as tolerance of uncertainty and emotions, arousal of curiosity, greater awareness of one's impact upon others, increased capacity for self-reflection, mourning of losses and lost possibilities, separation from embeddedness in the past, and finding richer meaning in life. *Self-actualization*, a term developed by humanistic psychologists, is one way to characterize the broadest aim of most psychoanalytic psychotherapists.

In many cases, the patient will prioritize the treatment goals. The therapist, however, may think it likely that the patient's goals are linked with other goals that the patient has not considered important. For example, a woman who wishes to stop her bingeing and purging may insist that she does not wish to have closer personal relationships. The therapist may be wondering, however, how the patient can stop turning to food for comfort without an alternative, and might suggest that the food is her most comfortable "relationship." The relational therapist is likely thinking about the overall possible adaptive purposes a symptom may be serving, and that an attempt to remove the symptom without the patient developing an alternative way of fulfilling a longing or desire may not be effective. In this way the relational therapist is not simply trying to remove the symptom, without understanding its meaning.

Process Aspects of Treatment

Free association, interpretation, inquiry, empathy, observation, and analysis of defense and transference are some of the major types of interventions used by relational therapists. Therapists likely will be more active with more disturbed patients. Traditionally, psychoanalysts have tried to facilitate a patient in coming up with his or her own solutions to problems through increased awareness, and less rigid and defensive ways of being. But psychotherapy is inherently interactional. Psychoanalysts have attempted to avoid "transference cures," or having the patient simply adopt the therapist's ways of being or belief system out of liking, identification with, and/or respect for the therapist. Traditionally, techniques such as reassurance and particularly suggestion were to be avoided largely because of the danger of influencing patients to conform to the values of the therapist. Because relational analysts are very aware of the interactive nature of the therapeutic relationship, however, they recognize that some of these processes may inevitably seep into the interaction. Indeed, even therapist questions may contain an element of suggestion. For example, the question "How is it that you didn't pay your taxes?" suggests that it might have been a good idea to pay taxes. Reassurance is often given nonverbally with an "uh-huh," and further commentary on a topic that may be of interest to the therapist. Among the more insidious aspects of therapy is the possibility that patients change in accordance with therapists' desires alone.

History Taking and Inquiry

Some relational analysts begin therapy by gathering a thorough developmental history, including the background of the parents and grandparents, such as their place of birth, ethnicity, race, and religion. Also noted are the way the parents met, birth order of siblings, childbirth, preschool years, and relationships through childhood and adolescence. Sullivan suggested that therapists conduct a "detailed inquiry" into all of the areas of the patient's life, though this need not occur in the beginning of treatment and may, indeed, be quite gradual. For most, it is important to strike a balance between therapeutic reserve and impassioned interest. Curiosity is a vital therapist quality. The relational therapist may ask questions to examine not only what the patient says but also what he or she omits. The therapist's inferences about what may be taking place are also posed as questions. The therapist may ask, "Could it be that . . . ?" or say, "I wonder if. . . . "

Silence and Free Association

Most relational therapists are concerned with giving the patient space, so that the patient's own experience and ways of interacting can emerge. This is accomplished largely through the process of patients' free association, unless the lack of structure leads to a detrimental degree of anxiety. One of the strengths of a psychoanalytic approach is that the patient's unique and idiosyncratic way of perceiving the world is encouraged by a therapeutic attitude that emphasizes reserve. By remaining in the background the therapist allows the patient to emerge into the foreground.

Sullivan cautioned therapists that too much anxiety would impede treatment. The therapist should not interfere too much with the patient's *security operations*, lest the patient become more rigid or paralyzed by overwhelming anxiety. For this reason, an atmosphere of safety and predictability is created, with a clear frame of treatment in terms of the starting and ending times of sessions and, if possible, a regular meeting time each week. The therapist is often thinking of creating an environment in which the patient can feel *held* or *contained,* to use Winnicott's terms. In this tradition, the therapist attempts to be neither neglectful nor impingeing. Sullivan suggested, similar to findings by learning theorists, that a moderate level of anxiety or arousal is also desired in the therapy situation. Too little arousal does not lead to much new learning, and too much arousal leads to performance of the already dominant response, in this case, the previously learned maladaptive response. In this relatively nonstructured situation, the patient's own unique experiences are most likely to come into relief. The therapist notes the sequence of topics discussed, attempting to help to provide concrete, vivid examples if the patient tends toward generalities and abstractions.

Relational analysts acknowledge that they are often providing a *corrective emotional experience,* a term first used by Alexander and French (1946). Many types of experiences can lead to change, and elements of the relationship may be curative in and of themselves (Thompson, 1950). Those who speak of the relationship as *mutative* usually refer to a sequence of unwittingly living through old and "bad" experience with the patient, examining this experience, and evolving something new. At best, this new experience becomes internalized by the patient. Fromm-Reichmann (1959a) has been very clear, however, that childhood deprivations cannot be remedied in treatment simply by giving the adult what the child lacked. Mitchell (1988) also cautioned against what he called the "developmental tilt" in psychoanalysis—the idea that simply providing an experience with the good type of parental figure the patient did not have as a child will repair the early deficiencies. Unfortunately, meaningful change is not that easy. Epstein (1977) has suggested that therapists often wish to be the good parent the patient did not have, but it is unwittingly in being the "bad parent" that the patient is most helped. Salubrious new experience can only develop in a context where old experience is first repeated, mourned, and let go.

Analysis of Defense and Resistance

Resistance to change, and therefore to the therapeutic process, is universal. Every patient who comes to treatment wishes both to change and to remain embedded in her or his old world. Remaining stationary requires limiting awareness of dissociated internal experience. Anxiety is likely whenever what was dissociated in the first place is reactivated in the therapeutic process. The therapist's task is to help the patient feel safe enough to experience these dissociated aspects of self in a way that begins their integration into self-experience. The extent to which relational therapists point out how the patient is avoiding experience varies, yet Curtis, Field, Knaan-Kostman, and Mannix (2004) found that when interpersonal analysts rated which of 68 analyst behaviors they had found most helpful in their own analysis, the item "helped me experience feelings I was avoiding" was rated the most helpful. Some therapists, in acknowledgment of the patient's sense of vulnerability, simply wait for the defenses to wither away.

Fosshage (1997) has differentiated what he calls "empathic-centered" and "other-centered" listening. Therapists vacillate between these two perspectives at times—either reflecting empathic immersion in the patients' point of view (e.g., Kohut, 1971) or taking the position of the other (being the observer of the patient; e.g., Wolstein, 1975). By empathizing patients' experiences and reflecting these experiences, however, the therapist actually may be joining the patient's defenses or resistance. For example, the therapist, in the "empathic-centered" mode might reflect the patient's experience with parents and say: "Yes, you should take care of your parents at your own expense. That is a moral thing to do."

Another form of resistance is called "resistance to the awareness of transference" (Gill, 1982). Some patients resist the idea that patterns that have occurred with other people outside the treatment are occurring with the therapist. For therapists hoping to use the important leverage of the session's here-and-now situation, this form of resistance necessitates that the therapist persistently point out interactional phenomena, until patients are able to see how a pattern is occurring in their relationship.

Analysis of Transference

The aim of transference analysis is an illumination of the patient's subjective reality. Although the patient brings into the relationship with the therapist expectations from previous relationships, it is not assumed that the patient is totally distorting reality and/or that the therapist knows the objective "truth" about reality. The analyst is not believed to be a "blank screen" onto which the patient simply projects his or her own views of reality, but is instead another subjectivity, albeit a reserved one. The patient's experiences are explored not simply as distortions but as selective attention to real characteristics of the analyst. Given the relative ambiguity of the therapist's reserved stance, the patient may selectively attend to various aspects of the therapist and have many different feelings.

As patterns of interaction and selective attention emerge that have worked to reduce anxiety for the patient in the past, the patient may not only see the therapist in ways that he or she has viewed an important person in the past but also elicit responses from the therapist that have been elicited from others. In this way, patients' transferences often become actualized, reflected in the core relational notion that people tend to construct their contemporary world to conform to the past. In the interpersonal tradition, when the therapist is accused of being cold and uncaring, the therapist needs to inquire with true curiosity how he might be cold. Lichtenberg, Lachmann, and Fosshage (1996) referred to this process as "wearing the attribute," implying that it is plausible that the therapist may indeed be acting icily, thereby repeating jointly with the patient interactions from the latter's past. As treatment progresses, patients may become attuned to not only aspects of the therapist that reflect their old relational processes but also interactions that reflect something new (Levenson, 1983). Greenberg (1986) makes this point succinctly: "If the analyst cannot be experienced as a new object, analysis never gets under way; if he cannot be experienced as an old one, it never ends" (p. 98).

Mutual Enactment

Many contemporary analytic therapists no longer believe that therapists are able to be neutral. Therapists also unconsciously enact their subjectivity in the context of an intersubjective relationship, and countertransferential enactments are inevitable, much as are transferential enactments. The concept of participant–observer liberated many therapists from the unrealistic expectancy of achieving a most literal therapeutic neutrality and objectivity (e.g., Mitchell, 1997). From this newer point of view, analytic therapists should attempt to be both neutral and objective, and to refrain from purposefully influencing patients, while simultaneously recognizing that revealing aspects of their own personalities is inevitable.

Countertransference, subjectivity, unwitting participation, and enactment all can refer to more or less the same phenomenon—unconsciously based interaction that is unintended yet unavoidable. Once viewed as feelings that patients are unlikely to notice, therapist countertransference, for better or for worse, is now considered to be expressed in the form of subtle nonverbal, tonal, and attitudinal actions that inevitably have impact on patients. These countertransferential feelings may be consciously experienced affects or lie outside the therapist's awareness. In either case they inevitably register consciously or unconsciously with patients.

The concept of mutual enactment follows logically from this intersubjective way of thinking about analytic therapeutic process. One of the ways that therapists express the unconscious aspects of their countertransference is in the context of what some have referred to as actualization of patients' transferences. This is not as complicated as it may sound initially. For example, I (IH) found myself often bored and disinterested with a very withdrawn and reserved man. He entered therapy to address his chronic underachievement in work and failure to develop enduring love relations. His life history was highlighted by increasing disinterest in him on the part of his parents as each of three younger sisters was born. His father in particular was inattentive and, when he was involved, tended to be impatient and critical. This extremely intelligent man developed a pattern of emotional withdrawal, in order to hibernate from disappointing interactions, and severe underachievement, both to elicit attention and to pay back in a passive–aggressive manner his highly educated parents for their insensitivities toward him. My patient brought these relational patterns into his current world, and of course, into the transference–countertransference matrix. He withdrew from me and sabotaged our efforts, and I unwittingly responded by reciprocal withdrawal and my own anger-based disinterest. In some fundamental ways my patient's life history was relived in therapy—relived through not only transference enactment but also an unconscious, enactment with his therapist. At some point, I hope, either the patient or the therapist becomes aware of such unwitting mutual interactions and addresses them in the verbal realm of the therapy.

This rather simple, everyday example captures the essential aspects of what many relational therapists believe is an ongoing part of every therapeutic relationship. What is talked about in the therapy actually begins to be relived between the two participants, and there is always a significant element of unconscious process on both sides. The *actualization of the transference* refers to patients' living out their core internalized experience in a context where the therapist, always unwittingly, lives out the reciprocal role of the significant others in the patient's life history. In other words, I became like the critical and disinterested parents for him, expressing unwittingly a facsimile of his key life experience with significant others. It should be no surprise that my patient developed relationships in his current life outside of therapy that resembled both his life history and his relationship with me. This, of course, is why he so egregiously sabotaged his own work and induced both his supervisors and his lovers to become angry and impatient, and ultimately to withdraw and to fire or leave him. The aim of therapy is to view this interaction *in vivo*, discuss it, and by so doing arrive at a new configuration. If all works well in therapy, this new and explored interaction becomes part of the patient's internal experience, altering both his expectancies about life and the way he constructs his life.

Every patient who enters psychotherapy is expressing a wish to change, although there exists a part that wishes to repeat the past (i.e., stay loyal to the "internalized family"). Therapists get drawn into reliving old and maladaptive interactions, that is, mutual enactments, and this seemingly unfortunate occurrence may be turned into therapeutic gold when it is recognized and examined. As Levenson (1983) has said, therapists must become part of the problem before they can help patients separate from their internalized pasts.

Interpretation

Although a relational therapist may suggest a possible meaning to feelings, thoughts, or events, such a communication is viewed as only a hypothesis rather than a truth about the patient's mental life. Interpretations may be provided in order to deconstruct or to reframe the patient's usual understanding. They are provided in a collaborative manner to help patients make more sense of their lives and to expand consciousness. Interpretations explain current life by examining historical antecedents. They reflect the fundamental psychoanalytic value that self-awareness is preferable to mystification. To understand the way that one is helps a person feel that he or she is controlled not by external forces but by conflicts that currently lie within his or her psyche.

Analysis of Dreams

Dreams hold special significance for relational analysts (Blechner, 2001), just as they have for other psychoanalysts, from Freud forward. The interpersonalist Fromm (1951) traced the importance of dreams through history and described the lack of value given to them in Western industrialized cultures. Lawrence (1998) has revived Fromm's tradition of discussing dreams in groups, in a process he calls "social dreaming." Freud, of course, believed dreams to be the "royal road to the unconscious." Relational analysts are especially curious about the connection of the dream to the patient's life. The dream is viewed as an urgent message to oneself to examine something that might lead to trouble if unexamined. In the context of psychoanalytic therapy, often transferential implications to the dream may reveal feelings that have arisen in the therapeutic interaction but have yet to be addressed. Other relational analysts may investigate the different experiences of the self represented in the dream using the Gestalt technique of asking the patient to "become" each object and person in the dream.

Encouraging Experiences in the Moment

Relational therapists might ask patients to imagine being in a situation in the moment to help them experience it fully. Comments such as "Imagine being there right now" are used. Such interventions are especially likely when the patient is describing an event but having difficulty recalling parts of it, or when the patient is avoiding the affect associated with the event. Similarly, relational therapists may emphasize experiences going on in the moment with the therapist, referred to as "now moments."

Technical Errors

Since relational approaches can vary so much from one tradition to another, within each tradition, and from one practitioner to another, it is often difficult to agree on what is and is not a technical error. The term *error* suggests that there are right and wrong ways of conducting therapy. This relational flexibility is quite liberating for therapists, yet there is always the risk that such an attitude can be exploited by an "anything goes" approach. Nonetheless, psychoanalytic therapists of most persuasions agree about basic boundary issues, such as a set amount of time for each session; stability of fee among patients; no social contact outside of therapy hours; and avoidance of advice giving or imposition of the therapist's values.

Aside from issues related to basic boundaries, some common possibilities for therapist error are as follows: imposition of a preferred theory on the patient's verbalizations, thereby failing to understand the unique individuality of each patient; a rush to interpretation, before the patient has the chance to express him- or herself fully; failure to inquire about patient statements; withholding observations that may be illuminating; imposing so many observations that the patient becomes the secondary party in the interaction; assuming or insisting that a particular interaction is transferential despite the patient's insistence that it is not; failing to address transferential material when it may be vividly present in the interaction.

Another common error is the provision of an intellectual explanation or understanding without an experience-near or emotional insight. In most instances, such activity avoids the necessary emotional encounter required for meaningful change to occur. Still another error is frequently pointing out problematic behaviors or defenses, to the extent that the patient feels unduly criticized. It is important for all therapists to acknowledge how particular interactional patterns that have developed were adaptive—the only ones possible in a past situation—or how they were indeed rewarded in previous situations.

By becoming highly active, a relational therapist may foreclose the space and ambiguity for the patient's idiosyncratic perceptions and experiences to emerge, including transferential ones. If the therapist is too inactive, then the patient may become repetitive or "stuck" longer than if the therapist had intervened. It is difficult to determine in advance which approach will benefit the patient more, and there is no uniform prescription for how to relate to all patients.

Wachtel (1993) has described a number of "errors" in the therapist's wording of communications and ways for therapists to express themselves in a more helpful fashion. It is less blaming, for example, to point out how a defense was useful in the past than to say simply that a patient is being defensive in a particular way. Wachtel (1997) has also described some ways to avoid what he considers "errors" from a relational perspective by using techniques from nonpsychoanalytic approaches, as have Frank (1999) and Curtis (2009), in using behavioral techniques when patients avoid approaching feared situations.

Termination

Termination depends upon achieving the patient's goals, although the particular style of termination is reflective of and coordinates with the interaction up to that point. Therapeutic goals often change; at times, the goals initially set are achieved but new goals emerge. Although a particular patient may still have goals to pursue with the help of a therapist, patient and therapist at some point may realize that the patient is able to pursue these goals largely on his or her own. In regard to psychoanalysis, Witenberg (1976) stated, "Analysis never terminates. It is visits-to-the-analyst that terminate" (p. 336). In other words, a goal of any analytic therapy is to help the patient become his or her own therapist. Certainly the therapist can provide an opinion about the advisability of termination, but the decision ultimately rests with the patient.

Termination brings up feelings of attachment, separation, and loss. Sometimes symptoms reappear when a termination date is set. Because intense feelings may arise, a termination date is set well in advance. Some relational therapists taper off sessions, in order for patients to see how they manage on their own. Others may schedule a final appointment a month or so after the second-to-last meeting. Therapists help patients focus upon what they have done themselves in order to bring about change. At termination, the patient's previous stressors and dominant and new ways of responding may be reviewed (Curtis, 2002). Some therapists inquire as to what was helpful and hurtful in the treatment.

THE THERAPEUTIC RELATIONSHIP AND STANCE OF THE THERAPIST

An intense therapeutic relationship is considered essential to change. Otherwise, the therapist would not be able to help a patient face fears and wishes that have been too frightening to face during a whole lifetime. By trial and error, the relational therapist must find a balance between the safety of the old and the danger of the new. An alliance is created between patient and therapist through rapport, empathy, support, reflection, and the patient's sense of being known. A good example of a supportive comment is that of Fromm-Reichmann (1952/1959b, p. 181) when working with a very disturbed woman, steeped in her own feces in her room as an inpatient. The patient, apparently envious of Fromm-Reichmann, saw the label inside Fromm-Reichmann's coat from the best department store in Washington, DC. The patient commented, "Best, best, best—you have the best of everything." Fromm-Reichmann supportively answered, "I hope you'll be shopping again soon at Garfinkel's" (referring to a fancier store in Washington).

Different relational approaches have different basic stances; most conceive of the relationship as mutual but asymmetrical (Aron, 1996). Mutuality does not imply equality. The relationship is considered mutual because there is inevitably mutual influence, recognition, and empathy. The relationship remains asymmetrical, however, because the therapist does not purposefully disclose personal information anywhere near to the extent that the patient does. If the therapist were to take on a role similar to that of the patient, the relationship would blur into one similar to a friendship.

Countertransference

Conscious countertransferential feelings are often a therapist's strongest source of data in efforts to understand patients (Wolstein, 1975). As subjective as such data are, a therapist is in a prime position to speculate about the way patients are with others, by experiencing the feeling of otherness in the context of the therapeutic dyad. To give an example, one lonely man entered therapy with the complaint that women seemed unresponsive to him. It quickly became apparent to me (IH) that everything about this man's demeanor smacked of coldness, aloofness, and self-absorption. Although of the same gender as he, I assumed that the women he pursued found him equally off-putting. Using my own feelings of boredom, disinterest, and reciprocal withdrawal, I pointed out to him how I perceived him, suggesting that prospective girlfriends might be feeling something similar. Had I not been aware of my feelings and their import, I might have acted out my countertransferential disinterest, and essentially abandoned my patient emotionally. Countertransferential awareness provided the dual reward of controlling the possibility of abandoning my patient and making him aware of the way he related to others. Some relational therapists are more cautious than others about sharing their countertransferential observations, believing that such input might be experienced as too imposing.

Another type of countertransference is discussed by those therapists influenced by Klein (1957/1975), referred to as either "Kleinians" or Kleinian object relationists. They emphasize a type of countertransference termed *projective identification* (Bion, 1967), in which the therapist has feelings "projected" into him or her by the patient, because they are too frightening for the patient to tolerate. Once the therapist becomes aware of the projected feeling with which the patient identifies, he or she can both reduce the patient's anxiety by experiencing the feeling with less anxiety and better know the patient firsthand by experiencing the same feeling. When people simply "project," the targeted person does not change. Projective identification is differentiated from projection in that the targeted person, in this case the therapist, actually feels what is "projected" onto him or her.

Here is an illustration of this process. For a number of years, I (IH) worked with a highly articulate and intelligent college professor, who spent a portion of his session time berating me for my inadequacies in not helping him, and attempting to humiliate me for the many weaknesses he perceived me to have. His presenting complaint was an inability to feel happy, regardless of his achievements and his sexual conquests. My patient's way of relating to me closely resembled the way his father had interacted with him. Throughout his childhood, he was the butt of his father's sadistic teasing and put-downs. This persecution was unceasing, lasting until the day his father died. I feared that my patient would remain this way with me until one of us died. My patient could not be happy because he internalized his father's sadistic and competitive assaults, and no one could tolerate a close relationship with him because he identified with his hateful father. My primary feeling state when with this man resembled the way he felt with his father. My patient showed me firsthand what it was like to be him, and to live with his hidden sense of abject humiliation. This gave me a very clear sense of what it was like inside my patient's skin, beneath his most defensive attacking ways. I was then able to convey to him what I imagined he felt and what it was like to live with his father. My ability to conceptualize this enabled me both to refrain somewhat from retaliation and to withstand his assaults. As one might imagine, this interactional pattern did not cease with a single interpretation, although it helped give both of us a framework to make more sense of my patient's life, and it aided me in not drowning in my patient's attempted humiliations.

Countertransference tends to be less central in the tradition that represents the Winnicottian (Winnicott, 1964) stream under the relational umbrella (vs. the interpersonal and Kleinian object relations theories just discussed), since the basic therapeutic model is conceived of as a mother–child dyad, or a "holding environment." With regard to countertransferential feelings, therapists are normally advised to serve as "containers" for their patients' difficult affects, until the patients prove ready to experience consciously and regulate such feelings.

The newer tradition of self psychology (Kohut, 1984) bears great similarity to the Winnicottian object relationists in its basic view of the patient–therapist interaction. From this perspective, the primary therapeutic intention is toward empathic immersion in the patient's experiences. Empathy is the food that the patient lacks, and by providing enough consistency, the attuned therapist allows the patient to come closer to her or his potential. Self psychologists are well aware that perfect empathic attunement is impossible, and lapses in attunement are both inevitable and potentially beneficial in that they can be examined therapeutically. As in the holding environment, patients are expected to be hurt and/or angry when the therapist fails.

Every relational perspective holds that therapists are always "countertransferring," and that affective neutrality is impossible. Given this assumption, awareness of countertransference is always preferable to absence of awareness, even when such feelings are not revealed by the analyst directly.

Self-Disclosure

Relational analysts may disclose their feelings with a patient or provide other information, usually after asking the patient the reasons for the question. Tauber and Green (1959) made the controversial suggestion that an analyst might decide to tell a patient a dream the analyst had about the patient. For example, one morning before a patient came in, the therapist (RC) woke up dreaming that the patient brought a bag of golf clubs to the session. The therapist did not mention the dream to the patient in that session, but continued to think about it. Not getting anywhere that seemed to make any sense in that session, the therapist decided to mention it to the patient at the following session. The patient responded immediately, "I think of golf as what people do when they have nothing else to do. I've been taking it easy in here, lately. That is what your dream is about."

Davies (2004) and Ehrenberg (1992) have addressed the potential value of judicious affective countertransference disclosures. Davies gave the following example of such disclosure. A patient had been pushing to schedule a session earlier during the coming week. Davies was getting annoyed. The patient stated, "You're cold and unfeeling and ungiving. You've never been there for me, not ever. I mean, sometimes you pretend, but it's just skin-deep. Down deep inside you, where I can see, it's just ice. The least you could do is admit it" (p. 715). Davies responded, "Sometimes we hate each other, I think. Not always. Not even usually. But sometimes we can get to this place together. I guess we're gonna have to see where we can get from here. Neither of us likes it much. It just is" (p. 716). Among relational therapists, self-disclosure exists as one option, with some therapists self-disclosing fairly liberally, whereas others rarely, if ever, do so.

CURATIVE FACTORS OR MECHANISMS OF CHANGE

New experiences and the development of new meanings of experiences are the major factors leading to change according to the relational approach (Curtis, 2009). Although new experiences include an increase in awareness of that which was previously unconscious, they often include a new relational configuration with the therapist as well. Some relational theorists think that the relationship in and of itself may be curative. In order to examine here-and-now interactions, certainly a fair degree of warmth and empathy is called for on the part of the therapist. The therapist must not, however, act in a way that is so kind and gratifying that it deprives the patient of the freedom to feel anger that will likely arise in the context of a more ambiguous and reserved therapeutic situation.

Gill (1982) criticized his contemporaries for spending too much time on the past, when the real leverage in psychoanalysis, he believed, came from discussions of the relationship between the two therapy coparticipants. Since that time, there has been an increasing focus upon the analysis of transference, with most relational analysts noting that the analyst has transferences as well and can therefore never be simply an objective observer of the patients' transferences.

Early in the history of the interpersonal–relational tradition, many interpersonalists emphasized the analysis of other relationships over analysis of the transference. Sullivan had noted that it was too anxiety provoking, especially for disturbed patients, to discuss the relationship in the "here and now." Therefore, therapists could help patients deal with experiences in other relationships in their lives and by so doing, at least in some cases, patient and therapist might communicate implicitly about their own relationship. In contrast, Searles (1965) worked with patients with schizophrenia in a way that brought explanation of the transference–countertransference matrix into the very center of the work. He is among a group of analysts that helped shift the focus from extratransferential relationships to the here and now of the therapeutic interaction. That said, relational therapists can be quite different from one another and may have very different emphases in their work. For instance, strengthening the "healthier components" of a patient's personality by being supportive of adaptive qualities is considered a major curative factor. For some, engaging in this manner may enable the patient to cope better with his or her deficiencies and defects.

Analytic therapists have always relied on insight to bring about change. Insight may be about the relationship with the therapist, about matters outside the relationship, and especially about the impact of life history on current functioning. Such insights at best are not simply cognitive realizations—they are profoundly emotional, especially when focused on the here-and-now relationship between the two therapeutic participants. Most relational therapists consider insight alone as a curative factor to belong to the classical Freudian model. In the relational paradigm, change results not from a focus on insight into "the truth" but from the expansion of awareness of a wider set of interactional patterns and experiences. The patient has new experiences of self and others as hidden or disavowed aspects are noticed and reclaimed. Incorporation of these experiences into the person's self-representation is also considered an expansion of awareness. Increased tolerance of uncertainty and anxiety allows conflictual ways of being to be held in awareness simultaneously. Living with paradox may be seen as one sign of "health." Consistent with dynamic systems theory, new self-organizing processes and meanings emerge from previously unformulated experiences.

Mourning lost possibilities is considered to be another curative factor by relational psychotherapists. Many patients must grieve the loss of good relationships with parents, or aspects of family relationships on which they missed out. Patients may also have missed opportunities that must be mourned, or they may benefit from coming to grips with the reality that all choices foreclose other possibilities. When impossible goals are fully mourned, more energy is available for the possible ones.

Expansion of awareness, openness to new experiences, new meanings of experiences, and new self-organization occur in a situation of safety. Some analysts have called such a state "regression." The word *regression* is misleading, however, in that a person does not "regress" to an earlier level, but instead feels such a sense of safety with the therapist that he or she feels held or contained (Balint, 1968). In this relaxed state, all may be experienced—rational and irrational. Worst fears are experienced in a state of relative safety. Unfulfilled desires are tolerated. Those who never will be satisfied are mourned. The anxiety regarding the uncertainty of whether desires will be fulfilled is also tolerated. For some relational analysts, this experience is akin to that of love—not of romantic or brotherly love, but more that of the Greek *agape*, which refers to the idea of a god's love for his or her children. Reports by relational analysts revealed that what was most helpful in their own treatments was the therapist helping them to become aware of experiences they were avoiding, and to experience irrational thoughts and feelings (Curtis et al., 2004).

TREATMENT APPLICABILITY AND ETHICAL CONSIDERATIONS

Relational psychoanalytic therapy is applicable to a wide variety of patients, including very disturbed patients. As with any verbal therapeutic endeavor, it is most likely to be effective with patients who are self-reflective, verbal, and willing to examine their own contributions to their problems in living. Psychoanalytic therapists, however, adjust their interventions with patients who are not ideal candidates for analytic therapy, and engage in a form of treatment that may lead up to psychoanalysis. For example, with patients who externalize their problems or who are narcissistic, the therapist may need to emphasize reflective and empathic modes of intervention. With children or patients who are less verbal, modifications in the technique are required (e.g., the therapist might decide to talk more with a seriously disturbed patient who is mute). For patients who may come from a cultural background in which it is inconceivable that a professional will not provide professional direction or advice, the therapist may want to grant the patient's wishes to some extent, and attempt to examine the consequences of these interventions later. Wachtel, (1997), Frank (1999), and Curtis (2009) have described using adjunctive therapies in relational treatments. Relational therapists have adjusted their approach in working with inner-city (Altman, 1995; Wachtel, 1999), bilingual or deaf patients, and those with addictions. The concepts of dissociation and multiple self-states have been found to be useful in applying a psychoanalytically informed approach to such patients.

If a patient comes for treatment exclusively for a specific behavioral problem, such as substance abuse, a phobia, sexual misconduct, or smoking, the patient might be referred for a behavioral treatment dealing specifically with this problem (see Antony & Roemer, Chapter 4, this volume). A therapist might decline to treat a child alone, however, if the child would benefit more with the whole family in treatment.

Relational therapists must be clear with patients seeking symptom reduction about the manner in which they work and the length of time treatment may take. Problems ensue if the therapist overvalues fantasy and fails to inquire or be sufficiently concerned about external realities (e.g., losing a job or physical health). Relational therapists face ethical considerations, similar to other types of therapists, namely the lack of knowledge of techniques from other theoretical orientations that may be more effective for particular problems, or the overuse of an approach they prefer even when they know that other approaches have been shown to be more effective. A body of research suggests that symptoms dominated by substance abuse may be best alleviated through treatments established by groups such as Alcoholics Anonymous or by a period of residential treatment, and that phobias caused by traumatic experiences are best treated with behavioral therapies. Even Freud recommended behavioral exposure for phobias (1918/1953). In additional areas of dysfunction, where many research findings have suggested that a biological component plays a large role (e.g., bipolar disorder, schizophrenia), most believe that medications must be employed in addition to "talk therapy." Some relational therapists, indeed, are disinclined to employ psychoanalytic therapy in such situations where research literature indicates that other approaches have been effective. Relational therapists view all symptoms in the whole context of personality.

RESEARCH SUPPORT

Although there is considerable recent support for the effectiveness of psychoanalytic treatments (Leichsenring & Rabung, 2008; Levy & Ablon, 2009; Shedler, 2010; Wolitzky, Chapter 2, this volume), these studies tend not to include "relational" psychoanalytic psychotherapy in particular. Randomized controlled trials have supported efficacy for psychoanalytic treatments for depression, anxiety, panic, somatoform disorders, eating disorders, substance-related disorders, and personality disorders (Leichsenring, 2009). Furthermore, long-term psychoanalytic psychotherapy of at least 50 sessions was superior to various other short-term treatments in 23 studies with comparison groups for patients who met criteria for Axis I or Axis II disorders for overall outcome, target problems, and personality functioning (Leichsenring & Rabung, 2008). In Sweden, in a study not included in the Leichsenring and Rabung meta-analysis, Sandell et al. (2000) followed over 400 patients in analytically based psychotherapy over 3 years. Some of the analysts in this study likely held an object relations orientation. This study showed progressive improvement in measures of symptoms and morale the longer the patients were in treatment. It is interesting to note that the use of a classical analytic stance, that is, the nongratifying style Freud advocated, was found to be counterproductive. In another review of the efficacy of psychodynamic treatments according to the standards of the Society of Clinical Psychology, Gibbons, Crits-Cristoph, and Hearon (2008) concluded that psychodynamic treatments were efficacious for major depressive disorder and opiate dependence with patients who were also on medication, and likely efficacious as a monotherapy for both.

In the United States, most of the research on psychoanalytic therapies has been conducted on brief treatment (Messer, 2001). Messer and Warren (1995) have categorized a number of such short-term therapies as relational approaches. Interpretation of the patient's core conflictual relationship theme in Luborsky's supportive–expressive therapy has been found to be related to better outcomes (Crits-Christoph, Cooper, & Luborsky, 1988), including improvement in symptoms (Barber, Crits-Christoph, & Luborsky, 1996). A study of a brief interpersonally oriented psychodynamic therapy derived from this approach showed symptom remission in patients with general anxiety disorder (Crits-Christoph, Safran, Samstag, & Winston, 2005). Although this research was not designed from within the "relational" approach to psychoanalysis, the outcome data support it. Muran, Safran, Samstag, and Winston (2005) reported evidence that brief relational therapy is as effective as cognitive-behavioral and ego-psychological (supportive) treatment for patients with whom therapists find it difficult to establish a therapeutic alliance. And, of course, considerable research demonstrates the importance of the relationship itself (Norcross, 2002).

The interpersonal psychotherapy (Klerman et al., 1984) of 15-week duration has been found to be effective in numerous studies of depression, including those with older adults and adolescents. In a recent meta-analysis, it was found to be as effective as other therapies for depression and eating disorders (Kotova, 2005), and there is also support for its use with social phobias and posttraumatic stress disorder. In regard to personality disorders, a randomized controlled trial found significant positive changes in people with a diagnosis of Cluster C personality disorders (anxious, avoidant) treated with short-term dynamic therapy or cognitive therapy (Svartberg, Stiles, & Seltzer, 2004). It should be noted that the applicability of the results of these very brief therapies for long-term relational therapy is unknown.

Shedler (2010) has pointed out that there is additional support for links between psychoanalytic process and successful outcomes, whether or not investigators identified the processes as derived from psychoanalysis. There is also considerable support for relational models of the mind, personality, and change. Relational theory, to some extent, has developed as a consequence of this knowledge. In recent years, cognitive psychologists have published many studies supporting the idea of implicit, or what they call "nonconscious," factors in attention and memory (Westen, 1998). Whereas there is support for psychoanalytic ideas about defensive attention and memory, knowledge about the Freudian idea of *repression per se* is inconclusive (Curtis, 2009). There is, however, much more support for the concept of *dissociation* (Kihlstrom, Barnhardt, & Tataryn, 1992), a broader idea about disconnections (explained earlier in this chapter). Relational ideas about the mental representations of self, other, and relationships are similar to those found in a large body of research by social and cognitive psychologists (Westen, 1998).

Although not specific to relational psychoanalytic approaches alone, there is also research evidence for the existence of transferential processes (Glassman & Andersen, 1999). Whereas the evidence regarding the effectiveness of transference interpretations is mixed, positive therapy outcome has been found to be related to accurate transference interpretations in low dosages for high-functioning patients (Messer, 2001; Ogrodnicuk & Piper, 1999). Progress in therapy was also found to be related to therapist adherence to a psychodynamic focus formulated in object relations terms (Messer, Tishby, & Spillman, 1992). Transference-focused psychotherapy, although not derived from a relational perspective but central to it, has been found to be effective for borderline personality disorder (Levy, Wasserman, Scott, & Yeomans, 2009). In a study of transference-focused dialectical behavioral and supportive therapies, with 30 patients assigned to each treatment for 40 sessions, only transference-focused and supportive therapies showed reductions in impulsivity, and only transference-focused therapy showed reductions in irritability and verbal and direct assaults (Clarkin, Levy, Lenzenweger, & Kernberg, 2007).

Attachment research has been very influential in relational theories of development (Mitchell, 2000). The study of attachment processes within the psychoanalytic tradition began with the work of John Bowlby (1969, 1988). Bowlby, along with Sullivan and Fairbairn, was excluded from what was then mainstream psychoanalysis. Bowlby (1969) challenged Freud's view that hunger led infants to seek out their caretakers, describing instead an autonomous instinctual attachment system relatively independent of the drives related to hunger, sex, and aggression. For Bowlby, the need for attachment was primary, whereas for Freud it was secondary.

Attachment patterns have been studied by Ainsworth (Ainsworth, Blehar, Waters, & Wall, 1978) in infants, by Main (2001), and by a plethora of other researchers using a variety of measures of adult attachment styles (cf. Cassidy & Shaver, 2008). Various patterns of insecure attachment styles have been linked with many forms of psychopathology (Parkes, Stevenson-Hine, & Marris, 1991). Both attachment style (Fonagy, 2001; Levy, Meehan, Kelly, Reynoso, Weber, Clarkin, et al., 2008) and representations of self and other (Blatt, Auerbach, & Behrends, 2008) have been found to change during psychotherapy, which is consistent with the relational psychoanalytic approach. Mentalization-based therapy, a psychodynamic therapy rooted in attachment and cognitive theories and requiring limited training, helps patients become more aware of their own and others' mental states in order to address their difficulties. Mentalization-based therapy showed a steeper decline in all significant problems in an 18-month treatment, including suicide attempts and hospitalizations for patients with borderline personality disorder, than did structured clinical management in a randomized controlled trial (Bateman & Fonagy, 2009).

CASE ILLUSTRATION

Scott, age 26 when he started treatment, presented a symptomatic history of poorly controlled anger, initially in the form of adolescent brawling, and expressed more currently in extreme impatience, intolerance, arrogance, and provocative argumentativeness. His physically violent, bullying behavior culminated in his suspension from high school for part of his senior year, despite being near the top of his class in grade point average. Although he gained admission to an Ivy League college, his suspension cost him acceptance to his most coveted school. After he finished college, Scott accepted training positions at one, then another top tier investment banking firm. In both instances his technical performance was exemplary, yet he was fired for his surly and belligerent manner. He began therapy depressed about his unemployed status, wishing to prevent further self-destructive aggression.

Scott was extremely ambitious, placing far greater import on his career than on his love life. He acknowledged that his very short temper had interfered with romantic involvements with women, and that he had not yet had a long-term love relationship. This did not particularly disturb him, since he had a network of male buddies with whom he drank, gambled, and competed in sports; he rarely felt lonely. His relations with his parents were fractious. They were quite involved with one another, although this was punctuated by frequent and ugly verbal brawls and periods of estrangement. It was his mother who urged him to consider psychotherapy. Scott was a most reluctant patient, having little predisposition toward self-reflection and cessation of destructive action. Despite his very high intelligence, he lived in a universe of action and reaction. Thinking about highly personal things was viewed as inefficient at best, or as soft and effeminate at worst.

Scott, an only child, was Central American by birth, abandoned in the street by his mother, and adopted from an orphanage at about 1 year of age by upper-class European American parents in California. He was short, squat, and browned-skinned, with distinct

Native Indian features. He was raised with privilege in an affluent suburb by parents he described as basically devoted and loving. He noted that his father, a successful business-man, is a highly competitive person, loses his temper readily, argues frequently, and holds fierce grudges. His mother, who is a housewife, has a rich social life that is focused around country club activity and philanthropic causes. Scott described her as a beautiful and vain woman who places strong emphasis on physical appearance. Both parents noticed early their adopted son's high intelligence and expected from the beginning that he would be a high achiever.

Scott showed virtually no interest in his own personal or cultural heritage and never traveled to Central America or researched his biological beginnings. He was rarely con-scious of his racial characteristics except when rebuffed by the tall, light-skinned, blond women he uniformly desired. Parenthetically, Scott's mother is fair in complexion, and taller by 3 inches than he. Scott's early dreams in therapy were replete with imagery sug-gesting both a strong sense of difference and the inclination toward hypervigilance based on danger. In his first dream after entering therapy, he spoke of being in a room where it was his task to kill scorpions that were continuously emerging from cracks in the walls of his costly Manhattan apartment. Despite his lack of overt curiosity about his origins, the scorpions in his dreams, more likely in Central America than in Manhattan, for example, suggested that in his unconscious life, he lived between his two worlds.

My (IH) earliest contacts with Scott left me feeling shut out, intimidated, and angered. It took many telephone messages finally to speak and make an initial appointment with him. When we did meet, I found Scott cold, terse, and impatient with my initial question-ing. He was business-like, neither reflective nor curious, rarely elaborated on answers to my queries, and did not initiate dialogue. It looked as if he could not wait to leave the session, and he appeared bored and restless. After asking what it was like to be with me and getting a noncommittal answer, I observed that it seemed to me that he was generally angered and/ or bored by my presence—barely tolerant of my existence. He replied that he was neither, but that this experience was simply uncomfortable and unfamiliar. When I pressed, refer-ring to the evidence for my statement (e.g., his terseness, restlessness, disengagement, and annoyed and bored facial expressions), he became angry, declaring that he had already answered what I had asked, and asking why I was trying to provoke him.

My informal assessment of Scott after 1–2 months of twice weekly analytic psychother-apy, was of a young man who dealt with his anxieties and vulnerabilities largely through denial and aggressive activity. I assumed that Scott's pervasive anger and competitiveness reflected a partial identification with his father, feelings of being physically unappealing to his mother, and an unconscious effort to avoid emotional recognition of feelings associated with his having been abandoned, orphaned and adopted. Scott felt a sense of well-being to the extent that he engaged successfully in the male world of sports, academic, or business competition. Literally or figuratively beating another man helped him avoid recognition of his internal sense of profound tenuousness and fragility, the legacy of early rejection fol-lowed by the vulnerability of adoption. He felt that he was his parents' biological child and tried hard not to recognize that he looked different, denying the almost inevitable adop-tee's anxieties of once again being unloved or discarded.

Scott appeared throughout his life to engage in self-destructive actions, and by so doing, to repeat his core experience of being abandoned. This occurred most dramatically in his being kicked out of high school, in his recent firings, and, on a more everyday level, through initiating parental rejection via argument and initiating sexual abandonments through the choice of girls and women who would be unlikely to find him appealing. The absence of a viable career at the time of the initial consultation represented a great threat to him. Minus external success and avenues for competitive achievement, Scott was having difficulty avoiding the affective experience of depression, and fear of aloneness and abject weakness and helplessness.

The absence of romantic love in his life was more salient to Scott when he lost his work—the area of life that helped him maintain his psychological equilibrium. With both deficient love and work relationships, Scott was beginning to feel depressed and anxious that the world he built, which was based on denial and acting out, would come falling down upon him. His key internal conflict revolved, on the one hand, around attachment to an internalized past highlighted by abandonment and impoverished experience, and fear of being orphaned by his adoptive parents, and, on the other, the wish to embrace securely his new world of opportunity. Scott's inability to address his extraordinary vulnerability, terror, and absence of caretaking guaranteed that he would unconsciously repeat or live out these themes in his contemporary life. His extreme aggressiveness both protected him from experiencing vulnerability, and guaranteed that the abandonments of the past would be repeated. Scott unconsciously controlled his abandonments by bringing them on himself.

Although Scott was indeed quite emotionally distant, speaking with my recalcitrant patient about his life in a way that was new to him nonetheless appeared to translate into some quick, palpable results. I was very pleased that after only 2 months of therapy Scott found a good job and seemed to be controlling his anger and brusqueness with colleagues. However, it was not long after this development that his sense of urgency about therapy diminished, and he began to become more overtly bored and disinterested in our venture. In our sessions there was abundant silence. After a couple of months more of this trying work, Scott failed to show up for a session without calling. I was convinced that he had quit. When he arrived for his next session Scott said that he had had an emergency business meeting. When I asked why he had not called, he stated that he knew he was going to see me again in 2 days anyhow. The next time he canceled, he called in advance and asked for an alternate time. I returned his message, asking him to confirm the time I offered and his more than one-day-late return message was barely understandable: "Hi, that's OK." He did not leave his name on the message or engage in any other social amenity. When I questioned him about taking so long to call back, and then not leaving his name on my answering machine, he was dismissive and said that I was wasting his time with such small and petty interests. He was most likely simply busy at work, he said.

At about this time Scott began to yawn increasingly and more noisily during sessions. My own feelings ranged from a sense of invisibility to identifying with the high school kids he had beaten up; to the angry, retaliatory feeling that I was with someone uncivilized, whom I would like to have disappear. I asked whether he was aware of his increasingly loud and uncovered yawns, and he responded that he must be suffering the effects of long work hours and early morning sessions. I then told Scott that his manner on the telephone, the yawning, and his general absence of social decorum was striking and that, given his social background, this might have psychic significance. I added that I thought he was trying to get me to boot him out of treatment. To my surprise at the time, these observations were not met with a totally slammed door. Though Scott was still combative, this series of interactions proved to be a turning point in our 5-year psychotherapy.

Scott's conflicts around attachment to his core identity as an abandoned child in an impoverished and violent society, and his fear of fully recognizing these vulnerabilities and terrors, continued to have an impact on his life even as we addressed these issues. We spoke of his father's intense temper, piecing together how such rage provoked fears that he had not before articulated, of being both abandoned and physically injured. He began very tentatively to address his feeling that his mother found him physically unattractive. In addition to identifying with Scott's deepest fears and humiliations, I often felt the other side of the equation—the wish that he would go away, or at times, even die. He provoked enormous rage in me, and I continually struggled not to withdraw emotionally, not to ask him to leave treatment during periods when he missed sessions or otherwise withdrew and/ or demeaned me. Addressing his evocation of such feelings, we gradually arrived at Scott's becoming aware of his own stimulus value (i.e., what it is like to engage with him). It helped Scott see, for example, how he both intimidated and enraged his parents, and provoked his bosses to fire him. Indeed, Scott did drop out of therapy for brief periods over the 5 years, and such interludes dovetailed with his feeling vulnerable to and sensing my wishes to abandon him.

This sequence tended to run as follows: Scott appears involved with me and working productively; I feel a reciprocal warmth and affection; Scott misses sessions and/or becomes verbally sadistic with me; I interpret this sequence of vulnerability and attack to him; Scott angrily walks out of a session, saying he'll never return, or he just fails to show up for a number of sessions and does not return my calls. Sequences like this occurred six or seven times over our 5 years together, though less frequently in our final year. I credited Scott's feeling reasonably understood by me, and my relative resilience in the face of his assaults, for his returning to see me after each time he quit. Nonetheless, the durability of our therapy was touch and go for the better part of it.

Scott's life outside sessions, unsurprisingly, paralleled our relationship. He continued to clash periodically with, and to behave arrogantly and nastily to, colleagues and bosses alike, which resulted in his eventually losing the job he found shortly after he started therapy. Indeed, he was fired from still another good job before he settled in and persisted with his current one. In parallel, Scott's relationship with his parents remained volatile until near the end of psychotherapy. At one point his rage was so intense that his parents did not speak with him for 4 months. This breach and others tended to coincide with Scott's being frightened by his growing awareness of feelings of dependence and weakness, and his rageful and highly provocative response to such affects. Scott's love life remained barren until very near the end of therapy, when he began to date a young woman who appeared to be a good match for him. Prior to this, Scott would inevitably engage with women in one of two ways: He would pursue tall, blond, slender women who showed absolutely no interest in him, or he would begin to date a woman who seemed to like him, but soon turn on her in a nasty and abusive manner.

Scott and I agreed to terminate therapy at a time when his relational patterns had improved. He was getting along better with others, a change, I thought, reflected in his internal relational configurations. If his changes were judged to be only behavioral or external, then there would be little optimism that there was potential for these changes to endure meaningfully. But near termination, Scott seemed more inclined toward self-reflection; less inclined toward action; and more open, vulnerable, and generous with me, his parents, a girlfriend, and his coworkers. His rage and protective yet self-destructive provocations subsided considerably. He remained, however, a moody young man with whom it was often difficult for others to be. As might be expected, some of Scott's most abrasive ways were manifest in the transference, as we began to discuss termination. Fortunately, we were able to say goodbye on a note of relatively mutual warmth and affection. Scott is not a new person. He is someone who has faced some of his dreaded vulnerabilities and is open to a wider range of affective experiences with others, and within himself.

Over the course of therapy, Scott became far more curious about his history and more willing to face painful and theretofore unconscious experience. He traveled to his country of origin, although, to my knowledge, has not yet tried to find his biological parents. He stated that his father's rages scared him as a child and provoked fears of once again being placed for adoption. Scott spoke of a vague sense that his mother seemed affectionately inhibited with him—that she did not seem to appreciate his male body as did the moms of some of the kids with whom he grew up. He was able to discuss feeling pained by this, though, as a child, he did everything possible to prevent his becoming aware of such affects. More and more he recognized how defensive his anger was, and how it often served both to compensate for weakness and vulnerability, and to provoke the very abandonment he feared would occur. He was able to tell me that he now sometimes allows himself to own his origin as a Central American peasant, and to speculate that some of his physically violent behavior reflected his then unarticulated connection with how he imagined his biological parents to be. Scott's evolution as a person reflects the value of a therapy that emphasizes examination of the here-and-now interaction between patient and therapist as central to the development of new internalized experience.

CURRENT AND FUTURE TRENDS

There have been increasing concerns within relational psychoanalysis that the taboo against spirituality, initiated by Freud in his rejection of the conventional religious beliefs of his time, contributes to alienation and depression. Similarities between relational psychoanalysis and meditation techniques, especially Buddhism, have been noted at least since the publication of *Zen Buddhism and Psychoanalysis* (Fromm, Suzuki, & De Martino, 1960). In recent years the areas of similarity and difference in these processes of allowing whatever thoughts and feelings to come into the mind have been examined with increasing frequency (e.g., Langan, 2006; Rubin, 2009; Safran, 2003). Both traditions deal with increasing awareness and the realities of human suffering, and ways to endure and/or overcome it. They both consider issues of desire and restraint, and the effects of unbridled passion. Winnicott's idea of the false self has been viewed as being akin to the problems of the excessive concerns of the ego in Buddhism. Both see some form of aggression against and destruction of former patterns of organization as a precursor of creativity (Epstein, 2005). The interpretive tradition of psychoanalysis is also similar in some respects to that of the Judeo-Christian legacy. For example, the story of the Garden of Eden has been seen in psychoanalysis as symbolizing a step forward of humankind in awareness of not only good and evil, and consciousness of our own consciousness, but also knowledge of sexuality and its powerful forces, as well as the entrance of human beings into a wider system of language and the norms that guide society (Aron, 2005).

The experiences of people with gay, lesbian, and bisexual orientations, not previously viewed in psychoanalytic literature as healthy sexual choices, are being integrated into the understanding of "normal" development and of therapeutic practice. Considerable work has also been done by relational analysts to understand that the psychological experience of whiteness as similar to and distinguished from other racial and multiracial backgrounds (cf. Altman, 2006; Leary, 1999; Muran, 2007).

The focus of Western culture on efficiency, productivity, and their measurement is somewhat antithetical to the contemplative, reflective nature of psychoanalytic approaches, and their valuing of the subtle examination of relationships and of inner life. As Aron stated in a recent interview with Safran (2009), "People still want to be listened to in depth and always will" (p. 116). To the extent that human fulfillment remains important, patients will likely turn to reflective approaches such as psychoanalytic psychotherapy in their attempts to enjoy more fully their love relationships, work, and play.

SUGGESTIONS FOR FURTHER STUDY

Recommended Reading

Lionells, M., Fiscalini, J., Mann, C. H., & Stern, D. B. (1995). *Handbook of interpersonal psychoanalysis.* Hillsdale, NJ: Analytic Press.—Includes a complete review of all aspects of interpersonal psychoanalysis—basic psychological processes, development, psychopathology, therapy process, and technique.

Mitchell, S. A., & Aron, L. (Eds). (1999). *Relational psychoanalysis: The emergence of a tradition.* Hillsdale, NJ: Analytic Press.—Includes seminal articles regarding relational psychoanalysis.

Safran, J. D., & Muran, J. C. (2000). *Negotiating the therapeutic alliance: A relational treatment guide.* New York: Guilford Press.—Provides an overview of research on the therapeutic alliance and offers a model of brief relational psychotherapy.

Westen, D. (1991). Social cognition and object relations. *Psychological Bulletin, 109,* 429–455.—Review of research supporting the relational conceptualization of representations of self, others, and social causality.

DVDs

Safran, J. (2008). *Relational psychotherapy* (Systems of Psychotherapy Video Series). Washington, DC: American Psychological Association.

Wachtel, P. (2008). *Integrative relational psychotherapy* (Systems of Psychotherapy Video Series). Washington, DC: American Psychological Association.

REFERENCES

Ainsworth, M. D. S., Blehar, M., Waters, E., & Wall, S. (1978). *Patterns of attachment.* Hallsdale, NJ: Analytic Press.

Alexander, F., & French, T. M. (1946). *Psychoanalytic therapy.* New York: Ronald Press.

Altman, N. (1995). *The analyst in the inner city: Race, class, and culture through a psychoanalytic lens.* Hillsdale, NJ: Analytic Press.

Altman, N. (2006). Black and white thinking: A psychoanalyst reconsiders race. In R. Moodley & S. Palmer (Eds), *Race, culture and psychotherapy: Critical perspectives in multicultural practice* (pp. 139–149). New York: Routledge/Taylor & Francis Group.

American Psychiatric Association. (2000). *Diagnostic and statistical manual of mental disorders* (4th ed., text rev.). Washington, DC: Author.

Aron, L. (1996). *A meeting of minds: Mutuality in psychoanalysis.* Hillsdale, NJ: Analytic Press.

Aron, L. (2005). The tree of knowledge: Good and evil conflicting interpretations. *Psychoanalytic Dialogues, 15,* 681–707.

Balint, M. (1968). *The basic fault.* London: Tavistock.

Barber, J. P., Crits-Christoph, P., & Luborsky, L. (1996). Effects of therapist adherence and competence on patient outcome in brief dynamic psychotherapy. *Journal of Consulting and Clinical Psychology, 64,* 619–622.

Bateman, A., & Fonagy, P. (2009). A randomized controlled trial of outpatient mentalization-based treatment versus structured clinical management for borderline personality disorder. *American Journal of Psychiatry, 1666,* 1355–1364.

Beebe, B., Jaffe, J., & Lachmann, F. M. (1992). A dyadic systems veiw of communication. In N. Skolnick & S. Warshaw (Eds.), *Relational approaches to psychoanalysis* (pp. 61–82). Hillsdale, NJ: Analytic Press.

Benjamin, J. (1988). *Bonds of love: Psychoanalysis, feminism and the problem of domination.* New York: Pantheon.

Benjamin, J. (1998). *The shadow of the other: Intersubjectivity and gender in psychoanalysis.* Florence, KY: Routledge/Taylor & Francis.

Blatt, S. J., Auerbach, J. S., Behrends, R. S. (2008). Change in the representations of self and significant others in the treatment process: Links between representation, internalization, and mentalization. In E. L. Jurist, A. Slade, & S. Bergner (Eds.), *Mind to mind: Infant research, neuroscience, and psychoanalysis* (pp. 225–263). New York: Other Press.

Blechner, M. J. (2001). *The dream frontier.* Hillsdale, NJ: Analytic Press.

Bion, W. R. (1967). Notes on memory and desire. *Psychoanalytic Forum, 2,* 271–280.

Bollas, C. (1987). *The shadow of the object: Psychoanalysis of the unthought known.* New York: Columbia University Press.

Boulanger, G. (2007). *Wounded by reality: Understanding and treating adult onset trauma.* Hillsdale, NJ: Analytic Press.

Bowlby, J. (1969). *Attachment and loss* (Vol. 1). New York: Basic Books.

Bowlby, J. (1988). *A secure base.* New York: Basic Books.

Bromberg, P. (1998). *Standing in the spaces.* Hillsdale, NJ: Analytic Press.

Burton, N. (2005). Finding the lost girls: Multiplicity and dissociation in the treatment of addictions. *Psychoanalytic Dialogues, 15,* 587–612.

Cassidy, J., & Shaver, P. (2008). *Handbook of attachment: Theory, research, and clinical applications* (2nd ed.). New York: Guilford Press.

Clarkin, J. F., Levy, K. N., Lenzenweger, M. F., & Kernberg, O. F. (2007). The Personality Disorders Institute/Borderline Personality Disorder Foundation randomized control trial for borderline personality disorder. *American Journal of Psychiatry, 164,* 922–928.

Crits-Christoph, P., Cooper, A., & Luborsky, L. (1988). The acccuracy of therapists' interpretations and the outcome of dynamic psychotherapy. *Journal of Consulting and Clinical Psychology, 56,* 490–495.

Crits-Christoph, P., Gibbons, M. B. C., Narducci, J., Schamberger, M., & Gallop, R. (2005). Interpersonal problems and the outcome of interpersonally oriented psychodynamic treatment of GAD. *Psychotherapy: Theory, Research, Practice and Training, 42,* 211–224.

Curtis, R. (1996). The "death" of Freud and the rebirth of free psychoanalytic inquiry. *Psychoanalytic Dialogues, 6,* 563–589.

Curits, R. (2002). Termination from a psychoanalytic perspective. *Journal of Psychotherapy Integration, 12,* 350–357.

Curtis, R. C. (2009). *Desire, self, mind and the psychotherapies: Unifying psychological science and psychoanalysis.* New York: Aronson.

Curtis, R. C., Field, C., Knaan-Kostman, L., & Mannix, K. (2004). What 75 analysts found helpful and hurtful in their own analyses. *Psychoanalytic Psychology, 21,* 183–202.

Cushman, P. (1995). *Constructing the self, constructing America: A cultural history of psychotherapy.* New York: Addison-Wesley.

Davies, J. M. (2004). Whose bad objects are these, anyway?: Repetition and our elusive love affair with evil. *Psychoanalytic Dialogues, 14,* 711–732.

Davies, J. M., & Frawley, M. G. (1993). *Treating adult survivors of childhood sexual abuse.* New York: Basic Books.

Dimen, M. (2001). Perversion is us?: Eight notes. *Psychoanalytic Dialogues, 11,* 825–860.

Director, L. (2005). Encounters with omnipotence in the psychoanalysis of substance users. *Psychoanalytic Dialogues, 15,* 567–586.

Drescher, J. (1998). *Psychoanalytic therapy and the gay man.* Hillsdale, NJ: The Analytic Press.

Ehrenberg, D. (1992). *The intimate edge.* New York: Norton.

Epstein, L. (1977). The therapeutic function of hate in the countertransference. *Contemporary Psychoanalysis, 13,* 442–460.

Epstein, M. (2005). A strange beauty: Emmanuel Ghent and the psychologies of East and West. *Psychoanalytic Dialogues, 15,* 125–138.

Fairbairn, W. R. D. (1952). *Psychoanalytic studies of the personality*. London: Routledge.

Fairbairn, W. R. D. (1994). Dissociation and repression. In E. F. Birtles & D. E. Scharff (Eds.), *From instinct to self: Selected papers of W. R. D. Fairbairn* (pp. 13–79). Hillsdale, NJ: Aronson. (Original work published 1929)

Fonagy, P. (2001). *Attachment theory and psychoanalysis*. New York: Other Press.

Fosshage, J. (1997). Countertransference as the analyst's experience of the analysand: Influence of listening perspectives. *Psychoanalytic Psychology, 12*, 375–391.

Frank, K. A. (1999). *Psychoanalytic participation: Action, interaction, and integration*. Hillsdale, NJ: Analytic Press.

Freud, S. (1953). Lines of advance in psychoanalytic theory. In J. Strachey (Ed.), *Standard edition of the complete psychological works of S. Freud, 17*, 159–168. (Original work published 1918)

Fromm, E. (1951). *The forgotten language*. New York: Rinehart.

Fromm, E. (1964). *The heart of man*. New York: Harper & Row.

Fromm, E., Suzuki, D. T., & De Martino, R. (1960). *Zen Buddhism and psychoanalysis*. Oxford, UK: Harper.

Fromm-Reichmann, F. (1959a). *Psychoanalysis and psychotherapy: Selected papers of Frieda Fromm-Reichmann* (D. M. Bullard, Ed.). Chicago: University of Chicago Press.

Fromm-Reichmann, F. (1959b). Some aspects of psychoanalytic psychotherapy with schizophrenics. In D. M. Bullard (Ed.), *Psychoanalysis and psychotherapy: Selected papers of Frieda Fromm-Reichmann* (pp. 176–193). Chicago: University of Chicago Press. (Original work published 1952)

Gentile, K. (2007). *Creating bodies: Eating disorders as self-destructive survival*. Mahwah, NJ: Analytic Press.

Gibbons, M. B. C., Crits-Christoph, P., Barber, J. P., & Schamburger, M. (2007). Insight in psychotherapy: A review of empirical literature. In L. G. Castonguay & C. Hill (Eds.), (pp. 143–165). Washington, DC: American Psychological Association.

Gibbons, M. B. C., Crits-Christoph, P., & Hearon, B. (2008). The empirical status of psychodynamic therapies. *Annual Review of Clinical Psychology, 4*, 93–108.

Gill, M. M. (1982). *Analysis of transference* (Vol. I). New York: International Universities Press.

Gill, M. M. (1983). The point of view of psychoanalysis: Energy discharge or person? *Psychoanalysis and Contemporary Thought, 6*, 523–552.

Glassman, N. S., & Andersen, S. M. (1999). Activating transference without consciousness: Using significant-other representations to go beyond what is subliminally given. *Journal of Personality and Social Psychology, 77*, 1146–1162.

Greenberg, H. (1964). *I never promised you a rose garden*. New York: Holt.

Greenberg, J. R. (1986). Theoretical models and the analyst's neutrality. *Contemporary Psychoanalysis, 22*, 87–106.

Greenberg, J. R. (1991). *Oedipus and beyond: A clinical theory*. Cambridge, MA: Harvard University Press.

Greenberg, J. R., & Mitchell, S. A. (1983). *Object relations in psychoanalytic theory*. Cambridge, MA: Harvard University Press.

Harris, A. (1998). Aggression: Pleasures and dangers. *Psychoanalytic Inquiry, 18*, 31–44.

Hirsch, I. (1987). Varying modes of analytic participation. *Journal of the American Academy of Psychoanalysis, 15*, 205–222.

Hoffman, I. Z. (1998). *Ritual and spontaneity in psychoanalysis*. Hillsdale, NJ: Analytic Press.

Horney, K. (1926). The flight from womanhood: The masculinity complex in women as viewed by men and by women. *International Journal of Psychoanalysis, 12*, 360–374.

Kihlstrom, J. F., Barnhardt, T. M., & Tataryn, D. J. (1992). The psychological unconscious: Found, lost, and regained. *American Psychologist, 47*, 788–791.

Klein, M. (1975). *Envy and gratitude and other works: 1946–1963*. New York: Delacorte Press.

Klerman, G. L., Weissman, M. M., Rounsaville, B. J., & Chevron, E. S. (1984). *Interpersonal psychotherapy for depression*. New York: Basic Books.

Knoblauch, S. (2005). Body rhythms and the unconscious: Toward an expanding of clinical attention. *Psychoanalytic Dialogues, 15*, 883–896.

Kohut, H. (1971). *The analysis of the self: A systematic approach to the treatment of narcissistic personality disorders*. Madison, CT: International Universities Press.

Kohut, H. (1984). *How does analysis cure?* Chicago: University of Chicago Press.

Kotova, E. (2005). A meta-analysis of interpersonal psychotherapy. *Dissertation Abstracts International B: The Sciences and Engineering, 66*(5), 2828.

Langan, R. (2006). *Minding what matters.* Boston: Wisdom.

Lawrence, W. G. (Ed.). (1998). *Social dreaming @ work.* London: Karnac Press.

Leary, K. (1999). Passing, posing, and "keeping it real." *Constellations, 6,* 85–96.

Leischsenring, F. (2009). Psychodynamic psychotherapy: A review of efficacy and effectiveness studies. In R. A. Levey & J. S. Ablon (Eds.), *Handbook of evidence-based psychodynamic psychotherapy* (pp. 3–27). New York: Humana Press.

Leichsenring, F., & Rabung, S. (2008). Effectiveness of long-term psychodynamic psychotherapy: A meta-analysis. *Journal of the American Medical Association, 300*(13), 1551–1565.

Levenson, E. A. (1972). *The fallacy of understanding.* New York: Basic Books.

Levenson, E. A. (1983). *The ambiguity of change.* New York: Basic Books.

Levy, K. N., Meehan, K. B., Kelly, K. M., Reynoso, J. S., Weber, M., Clarkin, J. F., et al. (2006). Change in attachment patterns and reflective function in a randomized control trial of transference-focused psychotherapy for borderline personality disorder. *Journal of Consulting and Clinical Psychology, 74,* 1027–1040.

Levy, K. N., Wasserman, R. H., Scott, L. N., & Yeomans, F. E. (2009). Empirical evidence for transference-focused psychotherapy and other psychodynamic psychotherapy for borderline disorder. In R. A. Levy & J. S. Ablon (Eds.), *Handbook of evidence-based psychodynamic psychotherapy* (pp. 93–120). New York: Humana Press.

Levy, R. A., & Ablon, J. S. (Eds.). (2009). *Handbook of evidence-based psychodynamic psychotherapy.* New York: Humana Press.

Lichtenberg, J. D., Lachmann, F., & Fosshage, J. (1992). *Self and motivational systems: Toward a theory of psychoanalytic technique.* Hillsdale, NJ: Analytic Press.

Lichtenberg, J. D., Lachmann, F., & Fosshage, J. (1996). *The clinical exchange: Techniques derived from self psychology and motivational systems.* Hillsdale, NJ: Analytic Press.

Lionells, M., Fiscalini, J., Mann, C. H., & Stern, D. B. (1995). *Handbook of interpersonal psychoanalysis.* Hillsdale, NJ: Analytic Press.

Lyons-Ruth, K. (2006). The interface between attachment and intersubjectivity: Perspective from the longitudinal study of disorganized attachment. *Psychoanalytic Inquiry, 26,* 595–616.

Main, M. (2001). Categories of infant, child adult attachment: Attention stress. *Journal of the American Psychoanalytic Association, 48,* 1055–1096.

McDougall, J. (1990). *Plea for measure of abnormality.* New York: International Universities Press.

Messer, S. B. (2001). What makes brief psychodynamic therapy time efficient? *Clinical Psychology: Science and Practice, 8,* 5–22.

Messer, S. B., Tishby, O., & Spillman, A. (1992). Taking context seriously in psychotherapy research: Relating therapist interventions to patient progress in brief psychodynamic therapy. *Journal of Consulting and Clinical Psychology, 60,* 678–688.

Messer, S. B., & Warren, C. S. (1995). *Models of brief psychodynamic psychotherapy.* New York: Guilford Press.

Mitchell, S. A. (1988). *Relational concepts in psychoanalysis.* Cambridge, MA: Harvard University Press.

Mitchell, S. A. (1993). *Hope and dread in psychoanalysis.* New York: Basic Books.

Mitchell, S. A. (1997). *Influence and autonomy in psychoanalysis.* Hillsdale, NJ: Analytic Press.

Mitchell, S. A. (2000). *Relationality: From attachment to intersubjectivity.* Hillsdale, NJ: Analytic Press.

Muran, J. C. (2007). *Dialogues on difference: Studies of diversity in the therapeutic relationship.* Washington, DC: American Psychological Association.

Muran, J. C., Safran, J. D., Samstag, L. W., & Winston, A. (2005). Evaluating an alliance-focused treatment for personality disorders. *Psychotherapy: Theory, Research, Practice and Training, 42,* 532–545.

Norcross, J. C. (Ed.). (2002). *Psychotherapy relationships that work.* New York: Oxford University Press.

Ogden, T. (1994). *Subjects of analysis.* Northvale, NJ: Aronson.

Ogrodniczuk, J. S., & Piper, W. E. (1999). Use of transference interpretations in dynamically oriented individual psychotherapy for patients with personality disorders. *Journal of Personality Disorders, 13,* 297–311.

Orange, D. M., Atwood, G. E., & Stolorow, R. D. (2001). *Working intersubjectively: Contextualism in psychoanalytic practice.* Hillsdale, NJ: Analytic Press.

Parkes, C. M., Stenvenson-Hinde, J., & Marris, P. (1991). *Attachment across the life cycle.* London: Routledge.

Petrucelli, J., & Stuart, C. (2001). *Hungers and compulsions: The psychodynamic treatment of eating disorders and addictions.* Northvale, NJ: Analytic Press.

Piers, C., Muller, J. P., & Brent, J. (2007). *Self-organizing complexity in psychological systems.* Lanham, MD: Aronson.

Phillips, A. (1988). *Winnicott.* Cambridge, MA: Harvard University Press.

Rubin, J. (2009). Psychoanalytic reflections on spirituality. In B. Willock, R. C. Curtis, & L. C. Bohm (Eds.), *Taboo or not taboo?: Forbidden thoughts, forbidden acts in psychoanalysis and psychotherapy* (pp. 95–119). London: Karnac.

Safran, J. D. (Ed.). (2003). *Psychoanalysis and Buddhism: An unfolding dialogue.* Boston: Wisdom.

Safran, J. D. (2009). Interview with Lewis Aron. *Psychoanalytic Psychology, 26,* 99–116.

Sandell, R., Blomberg, J., Lazar, A., Carlsson, J., Bromberg, J., & Schubert, J. (2000). Varieties of long-term outcome among patients in psychoanalysis and long-term psychotherapy. *International Journal of Psychoanalysis, 81,* 921–942.

Searles, H. (1965). *Collected papers on schizophrenia and related subjects.* New York: International Universities Press.

Shedler, J. (2010). The efficacy of psychodynamic psychotherapy. *American Psychologist, 65,* 98–109.

Stern, D. (1985). *The interpersonal world of the infant.* New York: Basic Books.

Stern, D. (2008). The clinical relevance of infancy: A progress report. *Infant Mental Health Journal, 29,* 177–188.

Stern, D. B. (1997). *Unformulated experience: From dissociation to imagination in psychology.* Hillsdale, NJ: Analytic Press.

Stoller, R. (1985). *Observing the erotic imagination.* New Haven, CT: Yale University Press.

Sullivan, H. S. (1953). *The interpersonal theory of psychiatry.* New York: Norton.

Svartberg, M., Stiles, T., & Seltzer, M. H. (2004). Randomized controlled trail of the effectiveness of short-term dynamic psychotherapy and cognitive therapy for Cluster C personality disorders. *American Journal of Psychiatry, 161,* 810–817.

Tauber, E. S., & Green, M. (1959). *Prelogical experience.* New York: Basic Books.

Thompson, C. (1942). Cultural pressures in the psychology of women. *Psychiatry, 5,* 331–339.

Thompson, C. (1950). *Psychoanalysis.* New York: Grove Press.

Wachtel, P. M. (1993). *Therapeutic communication.* New York: Guilford Press.

Wachtel, P. M. (1997). *Psychoanalysis, behavior therapy, and the relational world.* Washington, DC: American Psychological Association.

Wachtel, P. M. (1999). *Race in the mind of America.* London: Routledge.

Westen, D. (1998). The scientific legacy of Sigmund Freud: Toward a psychodynamically informed psychological science. *Psychological Bulletin, 124,* 333–371.

Westen, D. (2002, April). *The nature and origins of character.* Paper presented at the annual meeting of the Psychoanalytic Division of the American Psychological Association, New York, NY.

Winnicott, D. W. (1964). *The child, the family, and the outside world.* Reading, MA: Addison-Wesley.

Winnicott, D. W. (1971). *Playing and reality.* Middlesex, UK: Penguin.

Witenberg, E. (1976). Termination is no end. *Contemporary Psychoanalysis, 12,* 335–338.

Wolstein, B. (1975). Countertransference: The analyst's shared experience and inquiry with his patients. *Journal of the American Academy of Psychoanalysis, 3,* 77–89.

PART III

BEHAVIORAL AND COGNITIVE APPROACHES

CHAPTER 4

Behavior Therapy
Traditional Approaches

Martin M. Antony
Lizabeth Roemer

Behavior therapy is not a unified approach to psychotherapy. In fact, in their *Dictionary of Behavior Therapy Techniques,* Bellack and Hersen (1985) list more than 150 different behavioral strategies for treating psychological problems. Behavior therapy includes a wide range of techniques, including exposure-based therapies for anxiety disorders, relaxation training, biofeedback, reinforcement-based treatments, assertiveness training, sensate focus for sexual dysfunction, "bell-and-pad conditioning" for bed-wetting, and many others. Modern behavioral treatments have also expanded to include cognitive strategies and, more recently, mindfulness- and acceptance-based approaches.

In addition, the theoretical assumptions of modern behavior therapy are also quite diverse. Behavior therapists differ with respect to the relative importance placed on factors such as environmental contingencies and the role of cognitions in understanding behavior. There is also disagreement regarding the importance of developing a unique, individualized, evidence-based treatment plan for each client versus relying only on standardized, session-by-session treatment protocols that have been subjected to randomized controlled outcome studies (Addis, Cardemil, Duncan, & Miller, 2006; Wilson, 1998).

Despite the differences among behavioral treatments, there are also a number of shared characteristics that distinguish behavioral treatments from other forms of psychotherapy. First, the emphasis in behavior therapy is on directly changing those relatively immediate factors that are thought to predispose, trigger, strengthen, or maintain problematic behaviors. Unlike some other forms of psychotherapy, in which the goal may be to help an individual to develop insight into the early developmental factors that may have initially contributed to a problem, behavior therapists work directly on problematic patterns of behavior by helping their clients to make changes, such as decreasing avoidance of feared situations (e.g., in phobias), eliminating compulsive rituals (e.g., in obsessive–compulsive disorder [OCD]), improving social skills (e.g., in schizophrenia), changing unhealthy eating patterns (e.g., in anorexia nervosa or obesity), or improving the quality of relationships (e.g., in distressed marriages). Behavioral treatments may also involve changing aspects of the environment that *reinforce* a particular problem. For example, if a child's behavioral problems appear to be reinforced by the parents' giving in to their son's or daughter's unreasonable demands whenever he or she has a tantrum, the parents may be taught alternative ways of responding to the child's screaming and crying. Similarly, someone who has withdrawn from almost all activities as a result of severe depression might be encouraged to begin to reintroduce various activities into his or her daily routine as a way of increasing the rewards that occur when a person is actively engaged in life.

Second, whereas therapists in traditional psychodynamic psychotherapy and person-centered psychotherapy tend to be relatively nondirective, behavior therapists tend to be quite directive, modeling or demonstrating alternative behaviors, encouraging the client to try particular exercises, and assigning between-session tasks at the end of each session. Behavioral treatments tend to emphasize the importance of learning new skills and changing behaviors that contribute to the individual's problems. In fact, clients sometimes point out the similarities between being in behavior therapy and being in school. Like formal education, behavior therapy tends to be focused on achieving particular goals, may include instruction and education, involves the completion of assignments between sessions, and is associated with repeated assessments to measure the extent to which goals are met.

The duration and setting of treatment can sometimes be quite different in behavior therapy than in other forms of therapy. First, behavior therapy is often brief, particularly when standard evidence-based protocols are followed. For example, in typical research studies on behavior therapy, treatment for anxiety disorders is often completed in as little as one session for a specific phobia (Zlomke & Davis, 2008) or 10–15 sessions for other anxiety disorders, such as panic disorder (Craske & Barlow, 2008) and social anxiety disorder (Antony & Rowa, 2008). The length of treatment may be longer in routine clinical practice, especially for cases in which the presenting problems are complex, or when the client wants to work on multiple problems. In addition, whereas most psychotherapies take place in the therapist's office during a 50-minute hour, behavior therapy sessions may last longer and may occur outside the therapist's office.

Finally, behavioral treatments are more strongly rooted in empirical research relative to other psychotherapies. As a result, the techniques used by behavior therapists change over time, as new information is learned about which techniques are most helpful, and which are unnecessary.

This chapter provides the reader with an understanding of the theory and practice of behavior therapy. Although modern behavior therapy is usually delivered as part of a comprehensive treatment package that also includes cognitive strategies, this chapter does not describe in detail the cognitive aspects of treatment, which can be learned in Dienes et al. (Chapter 5, this volume).

HISTORICAL BACKGROUND

Despite a few early papers describing exposure-based treatments for fear (e.g., Jones, 1924; Terhune, 1948), it was not until the 1950s and 1960s that interest in behavior therapy started to blossom, thanks to several researchers (e.g., Hans Eysenck, Cyril Franks, Arnold Lazarus, Isaac Marks, S. Rachman, Joseph Wolpe) working in South Africa, England, and the United States. Two conditions set the stage for the early popularity of behavior therapy. First, in the 1950s, basic research on learning theory-based explanations for clinical phenomena was becoming popular. For example, researchers with an interest in phobias were influenced by Mowrer's (1939) two-factor model, which explained phobias as being initially triggered by a traumatic *classical conditioning* experience (e.g., developing a fear of dogs after being bitten by a dog) and later maintained by *operant conditioning* or reinforcement for avoiding the feared stimulus (e.g., experiencing relief by avoiding dogs). Second, a number of clinical researchers (e.g., Eysenck, 1952) were becoming increasingly disenchanted with psychoanalysis, the dominant form of psychotherapy at the time. Eysenck and others criticized psychoanalysis for lacking research support and for being an ineffective treatment in many cases. The growing dissatisfaction with psychoanalysis, combined with the increasing interest in learning theory, set the stage for the birth of behavior therapy.

In the first professional publication to include *behavior therapy* (Lindsley, Skinner, & Solomon, 1953), the term described the application of an operant conditioning model to change problem behaviors in psychotic patients. Lazarus (1958) subsequently used the term to refer to Wolpe's procedures for treating neurotic clients by reciprocal inhibition (Wolpe, 1958), and shortly thereafter, other influential writers (e.g., Eysenck, 1960) used the term more broadly to refer to any treatments based on learning theory, and especially the principles of classical and operant conditioning. Beginning in the 1960s, the term *behavior modification* began to be used as well, particularly in the United States (e.g., Bandura, 1969; Ullmann & Krasner, 1965). Although the terms *behavior modification* and *behavior therapy* are sometimes used interchangeably, the term *behavior modification* has also been called on to describe treatment procedures that are specifically based on operant conditioning (e.g., token economy and aversive conditioning; O'Donohue & Krasner, 1995), and the term *behavior therapy* is more often used in discussions of the outpatient, clinic-based practice of behavioral approaches.

By the 1960s, behavior therapy was quickly being established as a bona fide approach to treating psychopathology. In 1963, the first major journal devoted to behavior therapy, *Behaviour Research and Therapy*, was founded by Eysenck, and 3 years later, the Association for Advancement of Behavior Therapy (AABT) was formed, with Cyril Franks as the founding president. Today, a large number of journals are devoted to behavior therapy, and AABT (now the Association for Behavioral and Cognitive Therapies) is the largest professional association in North America devoted to the study and practice of behavioral and cognitive therapy.

The domain of behavior therapy is no longer limited to treatments based on traditional learning theory and, increasingly, it is difficult to articulate the boundaries of this approach, because it is defined by those who practice it. Many behaviorally oriented clinicians now include a wide range of evidence-based techniques in their practices, including cognitive therapy, relaxation training, biofeedback, social skills training, and mindfulness-based strategies. In addition, almost all the journals that specialize in behavior therapy publish papers on a broad range of empirically supported psychological treatments. Although the variety of behavioral treatments has expanded over the years, the importance of using treatments that are supported by rigorous scientific study remains a hallmark of behavior therapy.

THE CONCEPT OF PERSONALITY

The notion of personality is based on the idea that individuals have characteristic patterns of feeling, thinking, and acting. Trait theories of personality suggest that, given a particular situation, different individuals respond in different ways, depending on the unique combination of personality traits we each possess. For example, some people (i.e., those with greater trait anxiety) are more likely than others to react with anxiety in a potentially threatening situation. In its most extreme form, trait theory places the cause of an individual's behavior in the person; that is, it is presumed that the individual's personality causes his or her behavior.

In contrast, behavioral theorists have tended to emphasize the role of context or situational factors in determining a particular individual's behavior. Walter Mischel (1984) is perhaps best known for demonstrating that people do not act consistently across situations, and that it is, in fact, difficult to predict accurately behavior based on measures of personality. For example, most people who report high levels of trait anger on personality measures are not angry in all situations. A person may be angry in one situation (e.g., being cut off while driving) and calm in other challenging situations (e.g., when a child spills his or her soup). From a behavioral perspective, as described here, it is the situation that determines behavior—not the presence or absence of particular personality traits.

On the surface, behavioral theory may seem to be at odds with a trait-based approach to understanding personality. However, the apparent differences probably have more to do with common misunderstandings about both approaches rather than actual differences. In fact, the two approaches are quite compatible. Most trait theorists acknowledge the role of context and situational factors in determining behavior. However, all other factors being equal, a trait approach would predict two different individuals to behave in characteristically different ways given the same situation. For example, an individual who is extraverted would be expected to be more social at a party than would an individual who is relatively introverted, assuming that all other factors (the person's mood, life stresses, the number of familiar people at the party, etc.) are equal for both individuals.

Similarly, most behaviorists would acknowledge that predisposing factors affect how an individual responds to particular situations, and that in some cases individuals respond similarly to a broad range of situations. However, behaviorists differ from other theorists in the way they define and explain these stable tendencies to respond to a wide range of situations in similar ways (i.e., personality). From a behavioral perspective, personality is defined in terms of an individual's behaviors, and behaviors are assumed to occur primarily as a result of an individual's learning history. So, to a behaviorist, an individual who is particularly introverted across a wide range of social situations might be introverted because he or she never learned any alternative ways to behave in these situations, or because being in social situations is not reinforcing for the individual.

Most behaviorists also acknowledge the role of biological constraints on learning. In other words, one's unique genetic composition, temperament, and other biologically determined factors are thought to influence the ways in which one learns, thereby influencing one's personality. When behavior therapists refer to an individual's learning history, they are typically including a broad range of experiences. For example, a number of repeated assaults in various public places could lead a person to fear being alone in public through a process of *classical conditioning* (i.e., the pairing of a neutral stimulus, such as being outside, with an event that naturally triggers a characteristic response, such as an assault). Through *stimulus generalization* (i.e., the spreading of the conditioned association to new situations that are similar to the situation where the trauma occurred), the individual might begin to feel unsafe in a wider range of situations, developing what one might consider an "anxious personality."

Although classical conditioning may contribute to the development of personality, operant conditioning is often thought to play an even larger role. B. F. Skinner (1974) suggested that behaviors, including those behaviors that make up a person's personality, are determined by patterns of reinforcement and punishment from the environment. According to this perspective (often referred to as *radical behaviorism*), someone who is generally dishonest, manipulative, and antisocial might have been reinforced for these behaviors in the past (e.g., spending time with friends who also engaged in these behaviors and reinforced the individual for engaging in these behaviors with praise, attention, and social connection), whereas someone who does not display these traits would likely not have been reinforced for these behaviors, and might even have been punished for behaving dishonestly.

From a behavioral perspective, other forms of learning are also thought to contribute to personality. For example, social learning theorists such as Albert Bandura discuss the role of *modeling* (observing others who exhibit a particular type of behavior) and its influence on behavior. Cognitive-behavioral theorists emphasize the causative role of an individual's beliefs and assumptions in determining behavior, as do social learning theorists. Our beliefs are thought to arise from various types of learning experiences, including classical conditioning events, operant conditioning, watching others behave in particular ways, or being exposed to various forms of information or misinformation from things that we hear, see, or read. According to cognitive-behavioral theory, one's cognitions mediate the relationship between one's learning history and one's behavior. In contrast, radical behaviorists see cognitions as a form of behavior influenced by one's learning history, just like any other behavior.

PSYCHOLOGICAL HEALTH AND PATHOLOGY

A behavioral approach to psychopathology does not judge behaviors as "healthy" or "unhealthy," separate from their context and their consequences. Instead, behaviors, whether deficient or excessive, are usually discussed with respect to whether they are *adaptive* or *maladaptive* in a particular cultural or social context. In this way, the definition of mental disorder from a behavioral perspective is consistent with the definition published in the text revision of the fourth edition of the *Diagnostic and Statistical Manual of Mental Disorders* (DSM-IV-TR; American Psychiatric Association, 2000). DSM-IV-TR defines a *mental disorder* as "a clinically significant behavioral or psychological syndrome or pattern that occurs in the individual and that is associated with present distress (e.g., a painful symptom), disability (impairment in one or more important areas of functioning) or with a significantly increased risk of suffering death, pain, disability, or an important loss of freedom" (p. xxxi). In other words, whether a pattern of behavior is considered pathological depends on the consequences of the behavior and not on the content or form of the behavior. This definition allows for appreciating differences between cultures and other groups. For example, a behavior that is considered normal in one culture or social group may be considered deviant in another culture or group.

Also, according to behavioral theory, adaptive and maladaptive behaviors are caused by the same basic learning processes. Differences between nonclinical manifestations of a problem and clinically relevant symptoms (e.g., normal sad moods vs. depression; occasional worry vs. generalized anxiety disorder) are typically thought to be quantitative, not qualitative, differences. In other words, the most important differences between an individual with clinical depression and a healthy individual who occasionally experiences sad mood are in the frequency, intensity, and consequences of the depression, not in the quality of the mood state.

THE PROCESS OF CLINICAL ASSESSMENT

Conceptual Issues in Behavioral Assessment

There are three general purposes of assessment in the context of behavior therapy—to understand an individual's problem, to plan treatment, and to measure change. In traditional behavior therapy, understanding a problem typically includes a comprehensive *functional analysis*. The process of functional analysis involves considering four different areas that can be summarized by the acronym SORC (stimulus–organism–response–consequence; Nelson & Hayes, 1986). The term *stimulus* refers to the antecedents of a problem behavior, including the controlling variables that trigger the behavior. For example, antecedents of problem drinking for a particular person may include factors such as being around drinking cues (e.g., friends who drink, places that serve alcohol, and smoking), life stresses (e.g., a hard day at the office), and having extra money to spend (e.g., payday). Variables having to do with the *organism* are those that are unique to the individual, including things such as physiological factors, temperament, learning history, expectancies, and other cognitive factors.

Describing the person's *responses* involves conducting a detailed analysis of the individual's behavior. For example, in the case of the individual who drinks excessively, the behavior therapist would likely want to know how frequently the person is drinking, how much the person drinks, and what the person is drinking. The assessment should identify problem *target behaviors* (e.g., behavioral *excesses* and *deficits* that will be the focus of change) as well as *alternative behaviors* (i.e., behaviors that can replace the problem behaviors). Finally, functional analysis involves examining the *consequences* of the behavior in order to understand the patterns of reinforcement and punishment from the environment that may be influencing the problem. For example, consequences of problem drinking may include positive effects, such as intoxication, reduced anxiety (an example of negative reinforcement through the reduction of an aversive internal state), and social support from one's drinking buddies, and negative effects, such as being late for work, relationship problems, and withdrawal symptoms the next morning. The results of a functional analysis may be used to develop an individualized treatment plan that will involve changing the triggers and reinforcing consequences for the problem behavior.

Behavior therapists differ in the extent to which to which they rely on idiographic or individualized assessments, such as functional analysis, versus using standardized assessment tools, such as symptom questionnaires or structured diagnostic interviews. In recent years, many behavior therapists have shifted away from traditional functional analysis toward a more symptom-focused assessment, with the goal of measuring the presence, absence, and severity of particular symptoms (panic attacks, depressed mood, drinking, binge eating, etc.), understanding the triggers for these symptoms, and establishing a diagnosis based on DSM-IV-TR criteria. Over the past few decades, effective behavioral treatments have been developed for a number of psychological disorders, and many of these have been empirically validated in the context of particular DSM-IV-TR diagnoses. Thus, knowing whether a particular person suffers from panic disorder or social anxiety disorder can inform decisions regarding the best treatment for the problem. In addition, insurance companies typically require a diagnosis in order to reimburse clients for psychological treatments—a practical reason why behavior therapists (and others) may have become more interested in diagnosis in recent years. Ideally, a comprehensive behavioral assessment should include aspects of both approaches, obtaining information about the types of symptoms a person is experiencing, and learning about any individual characteristics (patterns of reinforcement in the client's environment, cultural factors, etc.) that may have an impact on treatment.

From a behavioral perspective, a thorough assessment is thought to be essential for treatment planning. For example, the information obtained during the assessment is often used to establish the treatment goals. A client with OCD who reports washing her hands several hundred times per day might have a goal of reducing her hand washing to no more than 10 times daily. The assessment is also used to select appropriate treatment strategies. In this example, the assessment would involve making a list of situations that trigger a feeling of contamination and subsequent hand washing, and this list of situations would then be used to generate possible exposure practices (e.g., having the client touch various "contaminated" objects).

One way in which behavior therapy is different from most other forms of therapy is the importance placed on measuring outcome. A hallmark of behavior therapy is the use of empirically supported treatments and the measurement of treatment outcome for each client, using empirically supported assessment tools. Before treatment begins, measures are taken during a baseline period to establish the pretreatment level of symptoms. Ideally, measurement of the problem behaviors continues throughout treatment, followed by a thorough posttreatment assessment and occasional repeated assessments during follow-up.

Assessment Strategies Used in Behavior Therapy

Behavior therapists recognize that information obtained during an assessment is often inconsistent, depending on the way the information is collected. Therefore, a *multimodal* approach to assessment is typically recommended, in which a number of different sources of information (e.g., clients, family members, and teachers) and methods of collecting information are used in combination. Assessment tools used by behavior therapists may include methods such as behavioral observation, diaries, clinical interviews, self-report scales, and psychophysiological measures. Each of these approaches is discussed in this section.

Direct Behavioral Observation

Behavior therapists often use observation to assess their clients' symptoms directly. For example, a therapist who is interested in measuring the frequency of a young boy's disruptive classroom behaviors might ask the child's teachers to observe him and record each time he engages in particular target behaviors. Similarly, therapists who treat phobias behaviorally often use *behavioral approach tests* (BATs). A BAT involves instructing a client to enter a feared situation and measuring his or her responses, including subjective fear ratings (e.g., based on a scale ranging from 0 to 100, called a *subjective units of discomfort scale,* or SUDS), physical symptoms, overt behaviors, and anxious thoughts. Videotaping can also be a useful way of assessing behavior. For example, during social skills training, behavior therapists often use videotapes to record a client's performance and may play the tapes for the client as a tool for facilitating change in particular social behaviors.

Unobtrusive observation (i.e., observation in which the client is unaware that he or she is being observed) is most likely to provide a more typical sample of the client's behavior, because people tend to behave differently when they know they are being observed. Often, however, unobtrusive observation is either impractical or unethical. The effect on behavior of knowing that one is being observed can be minimized by observing the client for long periods (allowing time for the client to habituate to the presence of the observer), or by ensuring that the client is unaware of which specific behaviors are being measured during the observation period. In session, the therapist has an opportunity to observe a sample of the client's interpersonal behavior, although behavior observed during therapy may not generalize to other situations.

Monitoring Forms and Behavioral Diaries

Almost all behavioral treatments involve the monitoring of symptoms using a variety of diaries and other monitoring forms. For example, behavioral diaries are used to measure food intake in clients with eating disorders, panic attack frequency and symptoms in clients with panic disorder, and depressed mood in clients with depression. Diaries are also a helpful tool for facilitating compliance with homework during behavior therapy. For example, an individual being treated for a driving phobia might be asked to complete a diary each time he or she practices driving. The diary can provide information about the location and duration of the practice, the fear level experienced (based on the SUDS), any anxious behaviors or thoughts that were experienced, and the outcome of the practice.

Perhaps the biggest advantage of behavioral diaries is that they circumvent the problem of clients not recalling the details of their symptoms and experiences from the previous week. Having individuals record their experiences as they occur increases the likelihood that the information will be accurate. However, from a measurement standpoint, one disadvantage of behavioral diaries is the problem of reactivity. There is a considerable literature demonstrating that monitoring one's own behavior can lead to changes in behavior, particularly when the client first starts completing the diaries. For example, counting cigarettes smoked can lead to a reduction in smoking (McFall, 1970), and monitoring food intake in obese individuals can lead to a reduction in eating (Green, 1978), even before the actual treatment begins. Therefore, therapists should be aware that baseline symptoms and behaviors measured by diaries may not reflect the true baseline levels of these symptoms and behaviors.

Although reactivity limits the accuracy of baseline assessments of self-monitoring, it illustrates the usefulness of monitoring as part of an intervention. When clients begin systematically to notice their symptoms and the circumstances that precede and follow them, this process helps them to change problematic patterns of responding. This likely happens because monitoring (1) increases and expands awareness, so that clients are able to recognize patterns as they begin and see the consequences of their responses and the full context that surrounds their occurrence; (2) leads clients to approach their symptoms with curiosity and some amount of distance, rather than the judgment and criticism that is likely more typical; and (3) makes it easier to initiate behavior change, because early cues are detected.

Clinical Interviews

Like professionals who practice other forms of psychotherapy, behavior therapists use clinical interviews to collect important information about their clients, including the types of problems individuals are experiencing, relevant symptoms, behavioral manifestations of the problem (e.g., avoidance behaviors and binge eating), cognitive manifestations of the problem (e.g., dysfunctional beliefs), contributing factors and triggers, consequences of the problem, and treatment history. For much of the information collected, therapists must rely on unstructured clinical interviews, in which the clinician determines what questions to ask and how the resulting information will be used. The specific questions asked are, of course, determined by the types of information that the client provides.

Although they provide maximum flexibility, unstructured interviews are generally thought to be unreliable, leading different interviewers to obtain considerably different information. Therefore, behavior therapists prefer to use structured or semistructured interviews to supplement the information obtained during their unstructured clinical interviews. Structured and semistructured interviews address the issue of unreliability by standardizing the content, format, and order of questions, and the psychometric properties of these instruments are often well established. Generally, for the purpose of establishing a diagnosis in a clinical setting, semistructured interviews (e.g., the Structured Clinical Interview for DSM-IV [SCID-IV]; First, Spitzer, Gibbon, & Williams, 1996) are preferable to fully structured interviews, because they permit the interviewer to ask follow-up questions for clarification (after the standard question has been asked) (Summerfeldt, Kloosterman, & Antony, 2010).

Self-Report Scales

Literally thousands of self-report questionnaires and tests exist for measuring a wide range of problems. For example, Antony, Orsillo, and Roemer (2001) reviewed more than 200 evidence-based measures related to anxiety disorders alone. Ideally, a comprehensive behavioral assessment should include some client-administered measures to balance information obtained from clinician-administered scales, which can be influenced to a greater extent by interviewer biases. In addition, self-report scales have the advantage of being relatively cost-effective in that they are typically easy to score and do not require any clinician time to administer. An example of a popular self-report scale is the second edition of the Beck Depression Inventory (BDI-II; Beck, Steer, & Brown, 1996). This scale contains 21 items, takes a few minutes to complete, and provides a reliable and valid measure of depression severity. In addition, it includes questions that assess most of the official DSM-IV symptoms of depression (changes in appetite, loss of interest, suicidal thoughts, etc.); thus, it can be a useful way to confirm the results of a thorough diagnostic interview. In the behavioral treatment of depression, the BDI-II is often completed at each session, so the severity of depression can be tracked over the course of treatment.

Psychophysiological Assessment

Psychophysiological assessment involves measuring aspects of an individual's physiological functioning. This form of assessment is typically not used in routine clinical practice, but there are a number of situations in which it can be useful. For example, therapists and researchers who work with anxious clients sometimes measure the individual's heart rate as a physiological indication of fear. Changes in heart rate can be used to measure improvements over the course of treatment, along with more subjective measures such as self-report scales,

BATs, and clinical interview data. Similarly, individuals suffering from sleep disorders (e.g., insomnia) often undergo all-night electrophysiological monitoring of sleep, as measured by electroencephalography (EEG; measurement of brain activity), electro-oculography (EOG; measurement of eye movements), and electromyography (EMG; measurement of muscle activity) (Savard, Savard, & Morin, 2010). These measures are useful for the purpose of diagnosis in that they may help to distinguish among different sleep-related disorders.

THE PRACTICE OF THERAPY

Traditional behavior therapy emphasizes an idiographic approach to changing behavior. In other words, each client receives an individually tailored treatment, depending on the specific symptoms he or she reports and the particular variables that appear to be maintaining those symptoms. Increasingly, there has been a move toward the development of standardized treatment protocols that are designed to treat particular diagnostic categories, that contain particular behavioral and cognitive techniques, and that have been validated in controlled clinical trials. Although the movement toward using standardized treatments in clinical practice has been controversial (Addis et al., 2006; Wilson, 1998), this development has arisen for several reasons.

First, the emphasis placed on the identification and validation of empirically based treatments has helped to distinguish behavioral treatments from other forms of psychotherapy. In addition, the development of treatment manuals has facilitated the dissemination of effective psychological treatments, despite competition from psychotherapies with less empirical support, and pharmacological treatments, which are also marketed for particular diagnostic syndromes. Finally, managed care in the United States has demanded that clinicians deliver short-term treatments that work, and evidence-based psychological treatments have met those demands fairly well. There are a number of sources for information on empirically supported treatment manuals, including a website run by the Society of Clinical Psychology (2010) and books by Barlow (2008), Nathan and Gorman (2007), and O'Dononue and Fisher (2009).

In practice, differences between traditional ideographic approaches to treatment and more protocol-driven, symptom-focused approaches are often relatively small, especially when used by experienced behavior therapists. Most individualized treatment plans rely on strategies that are similar to those described in standard protocols. In addition, many standard protocols allow therapists to be flexible with respect to the strategies selected for particular clients.

In the rest of this section, we describe strategies commonly used in behavior therapy, including psychoeducation, exposure-based strategies, response prevention, operant strategies, behavioral activation, social and communication skills training, modeling, problem-solving training, relaxation-based strategies, mindfulness- and acceptance-based strategies, and emotion regulation skills training.

Psychoeducation

Most behavioral treatments include some form of psychoeducation, particularly during early sessions. Some of what is covered during the initial psychoeducation sessions includes discussion of a behavioral model for the problem being treated, a description of the treatment process, and an overview of the ways the treatment procedures are likely to have an impact on the problem. Psychoeducation should not involve lecturing to the client. Instead, it should involve a two-way discussion, in which the client is presented with new information and is also asked to provide feedback about the ways his or her symptoms are consistent (or inconsistent) with the model. Psychoeducation may also involve correcting misinformation that the client has picked up along the way and suggesting recommended readings about the target problem, or about effective methods for treating it.

For example, the initial session for a client being treated for a phobia of heights might include a general discussion of the nature of fear and phobias (e.g., that fear is a normal and healthy emotion that everyone experiences from time to time). The function of fear (to protect the individual from perceived danger) would also be discussed. The client would be reminded that the goal of treatment is not to remove all fear of heights (e.g., "It is helpful to be apprehensive in situations that are truly dangerous, such as standing on the edge of a cliff") but, rather, to bring the fear to a realistic level that no longer creates significant distress or impairment. The initial session might also include discussion of the role of anxious beliefs (e.g., "I will fall, be pushed, or jump from the high place") and avoidance of feared situations in maintaining the client's phobia, and would likely include an overview of the treatment strategies that will be used in therapy (Antony & Rowa, 2007). Although psychoeducation is an especially important feature during the initial phases of treatment, its use continued throughout treatment as well. For example, whenever a new therapy technique or assessment tool is introduced, it is important to discuss with the client how it is to be used and why it is being introduced. In addition, toward the end of treatment, therapist and client typically review strategies for maintaining improvements after therapy has ended. Psychoeducation makes the process of therapy transparent, so that the client is informed as to reasons for each intervention.

Exposure-Based Strategies

Some of the earliest behavioral treatments to be studied were based on the notion that exposure to feared objects and situations leads to a reduction in fear. Today, exposure is usually considered to be a necessary component of treatment for phobias, OCD, and other fear-based problems. In fact, in the case of certain specific phobias (e.g., spiders, needles), a single session of *in vivo* exposure is enough for the majority of sufferers to overcome their fear (Antony, McCabe, Leeuw, Sano, & Swinson, 2001; Zlomke & Davis, 2008). For other anxiety disorders, such as panic disorder and social anxiety disorder, exposure is an important component of a treatment protocol that typically includes a number of different strategies and occurs over a period of months.

Exposure Modalities

Exposure can be delivered in a number of different ways. In most cases, the method of choice is *in vivo exposure,* which involves exposing a person to his or her feared object or situation in real life. For example, an individual who fears driving is encouraged to drive; an individual who fears dogs is encouraged to be near and eventually handle dogs; and an individual with OCD who fears contamination is encouraged to touch things that he or she perceives as contaminated. In the case of social anxiety disorder, exposure practices may include role plays or simulated exposures as part of the treatment and are often combined with cognitive restructuring (i.e., challenging anxiety-provoking thoughts by examining the evidence for and against them) and sometimes social skills training.

A second manner by which exposure can be administered is in imagination. *Imaginal exposure* involves having a client imagine being in a feared situation. Although imaginal exposure can lead to a reduction in fear, it is typically not used for treating phobias, because it is not considered to be as powerful a method as *in vivo* exposure. There are two situations, however, in which imaginal exposure is considered appropriate: (1) for clients who are afraid of their own thoughts, images, or memories; and (2) for clients who are unable or unwilling to do *in vivo* exposure (e.g., a client with a specific phobia of storms who practices imaginal exposure between real thunderstorms).

A number of anxiety disorders are associated with a fear of thoughts, images, or memories. For example, individuals with OCD who have violent, religious, or sexual obsessions are often terrified of having thoughts they perceive as inappropriate or dangerous, and in these cases, the suppression of such thoughts is often thought to help maintain the OCD symptoms over time (Purdon, Rowa, & Antony, 2007). In such cases, teaching clients to bring on the frightening thoughts and images purposely, until they are no longer distressing, can be a useful way of decreasing OCD symptoms and may add to the effectiveness of *in vivo* exposure alone (Abramowitz, 1996). In addition, systematic imaginal exposure to the memories of a trauma can lead to a reduction in symptoms among people suffering from posttraumatic stress disorder (Riggs, Cahill, & Foa, 2006).

A third form of exposure, *interoceptive exposure,* essentially involves exposure to feared sensations. This method of exposure is used particularly when treating panic disorder, a problem in which individuals are usually frightened of the sensations associated with physical arousal and panic attacks (e.g., racing heart, dizziness, and breathlessness). Interoceptive exposure involves repeatedly exposing oneself to feared sensations using a series of exercises, such as hyperventilation (to induced lightheadedness and other symptoms), aerobic exercise (to induce racing heart and breathlessness), and spinning around (to induce dizziness) (Antony, Ledley, Liss, & Swinson, 2006). Over time, exposure to these and other exercises decreases the fear of panic symptoms that contributes to the occurrence of panic attacks and related symptoms by the process of *extinction* (Forsyth, Fusé, & Acheson, 2009).

A fourth modality by which exposure can be delivered is through virtual reality. *Virtual reality exposure* involves using three-dimensional, computer-generated images projected on the inside of a head-mounted display worn in front of the eyes. Several controlled studies have used virtual reality exposure to treat specific phobias (e.g., fears of heights, flying, driving, spiders), public speaking fears, and posttraumatic stress disorder. Recent meta-analyses (e.g., Powers & Emmelkamp, 2008) support the use of virtual reality exposure for anxiety disorders, and effect sizes for virtual reality exposure appear to be comparable to those for *in vivo* exposure. Head-to-head comparisons (e.g., Rothbaum et al., 2006) have also found virtual reality to be as effective as *in vivo* exposure for certain phobias.

Guidelines for Effective Exposure

How exposure is conducted appears to have a significant impact on the outcome of treatment (Abramowitz, Deacon, & Whiteside, 2011; Moscovitch, Antony, & Swinson, 2009). The following general principles should be considered.

• Exposure works best when it is *predictable* (i.e., the client knows what the exposure will involve and when it will occur) and under the client's *control* (i.e., the client is able to control the intensity and duration of the exposure) (see Moscovitch et al., 2009).

- Longer exposures lead to greater reduction in fear than do shorter exposures (e.g., Stern & Marks, 1973), and it is generally recommended that exposure practices should last long enough (sometimes up to 2 hours) for the client's fear to decrease, or until the client has learned that the feared consequence is unlikely to occur.

- Exposure should be intense enough to trigger a fear response, but it is not necessary (or probably even helpful) for the fear to be overwhelming (Foa, Blau, Prout, & Latimer, 1977).

- Exposure works best when practices are spaced close together, and daily, if possible (e.g., Foa, Jameson, Turner, & Payne, 1980). Because therapists typically cannot see their clients every day, completion of exposure practices between sessions is particularly important.

- Varying the stimulus across exposure practices appears to improve long-term outcome following exposure-based treatment (Rowe & Craske, 1998). For example, an individual being treated for a bridge phobia should drive over a number of different bridges to facilitate generalization of the fear reduction.

- Conducting practices in multiple contexts appears to protect clients better against experiencing a return of fear than conducting exposure in only one context (Gunther, Denniston, & Miller, 1998). For example, a client who fears spiders should practice exposure to harmless spiders in various places (therapist's office, basement, garden).

- Because distraction during exposure practices can sometimes interfere with a successful treatment outcome, particularly over the long term (e.g., Craske, Street, & Barlow, 1989), it is generally recommended that clients focus on the feared stimulus during exposure practices rather than distracting themselves, and thus avoiding the stimulus. In addition, it is typically recommended that other forms of subtle avoidance, such as relying on safety behaviors (e.g., driving well below the speed limit to decrease the impact of a possible accident), be reduced during exposure, although these behaviors may be useful during early exposure sessions (Rachman, Radomsky, & Shafran, 2008).

Exposure Hierarchies

To facilitate exposure, therapists and clients often generate an *exposure hierarchy*, which is a list of situations (usually 10–15) that an individual fears and avoids, rank-ordered from most difficult to least difficult. The hierarchy can then be used as a road map to guide the content of future exposure practices. The client starts with items near the bottom of the hierarchy and, as these are dealt with successfully, progresses to more and more difficult items until he or she is able to address the items near the top of the hierarchy with little fear. The hierarchy can also be used as an outcome measure by having the client rate his or her fear and avoidance levels for each item and repeating the ratings at each session (Katerelos, Hawley, Antony, & McCabe, 2008).

Response Prevention

Response prevention involves preventing behaviors that are designed to decrease anxiety, fear, or tension (e.g., compulsive hand washing), until the urge to perform these overprotective behaviors subsides. Conceptually, response prevention is a means of providing exposure experiences, and in practice, these two strategies are often used together. Although response prevention is used for a number of different problems, perhaps the most common use is in the treatment of OCD, where this method is also referred to as *ritual prevention*

(Franklin & Foa, 2007). In fact, the best supported psychological treatment for OCD is the combination of exposure to OCD triggers (e.g., contamination and frightening thoughts) and prevention of OCD rituals (e.g., checking, washing, and counting). Clients are encouraged to do whatever they can to prevent their rituals, until the urge to perform the ritual decreases. If a person feels unable to completely prevent a ritual, he or she might be asked to delay the ritual for progressively longer periods. Over the course of treatment, the urge to perform rituals usually decreases considerably and may be eliminated completely in some cases. Exposure and response prevention are supported by numerous studies for the treatment of OCD, and response prevention seems to contribute to successful treatment outcome over and above the effects of exposure alone (Foa, Steketee, Grayson, Turner, & Latimer, 1984; Franklin & Foa, 2007).

Operant Strategies

A basic tenet of behavioral theory is that consequences for behaviors either increase (*reinforce*) or decrease (*punish*) the likelihood that behaviors will recur. Reinforcement can be either *positive* (i.e., receiving a reward, such as a promotion at work or a gift, in response to a particular behavior) or *negative* (i.e., removing an aversive consequence in response to a particular behavior). An example of negative reinforcement is the reduction in distress that people experience after escaping from a feared situation. Similarly, positive punishment involves receiving an aversive consequence (e.g., electrical shock) following a particular behavior, whereas negative punishment involves the removal of something desirable (e.g., permission to borrow the family car) following a particular behavior.

Behavior is thus determined by environmental cues (signals technically known as *discriminative stimuli*) that indicate whether a behavior is likely to be rewarded or punished, and by previous history of reward or punishment for a given behavior in a given context. This model helps clients and therapists understand seemingly incomprehensible behavior (e.g., a heroin addict is responding to the strong negatively reinforcing contingency of removal of distress that follows heroin use, not purposely creating havoc in his or her family life). In addition, this model provides clear targets for clinical intervention through *contingency management* (i.e., arranging for different consequences to follow a given response). Applied behavior analysis incorporates these principles into comprehensive, individually focused treatment plans that typically emphasize reinforcing desired alternative behaviors, while reducing reinforcement of problematic behaviors (see Spiegler & Guevremont, 2010, for a review). These interventions have demonstrated efficacy across a wide range of presenting problems and settings (see Wallace & Najdowski, 2009, for a review).

Space permits only a brief overview of operant interventions here. An essential first step is a detailed assessment of the stimuli and consequences associated with target behaviors (including behaviors for which reduced frequency is desired, and those for which increased frequency is desired). Particular attention is paid to identifying the contingencies that are maintaining problematic behaviors. Efforts can then be made to eliminate *reinforcement* of problematic behavior and to introduce reinforcement of less frequent, desired behavior. For instance, a parent might be encouraged to ignore a child when he or she is yelling, then attend to the child when he or she begins speaking more quietly. When a desired behavior does not occur at all, *shaping* can be used to reinforce successive approximations of the desired behavior. Reinforcers should be identified for the specific individual, because not all consequences have the same effect for all individuals. A consequence is "reinforcing" (positively or negatively) only if it increases the likelihood of an individual's previous response.

Extinction (withdrawal of reinforcers) often helps to reduce the frequency of problematic behaviors, but in some cases punishment may also be used. Most commonly, *negative punishment* (or *response cost* procedures) is used. These procedures involve removal of available rewards contingent upon an undesired behavior; the most widely recognized examples are *time-out* procedures. In extreme cases (e.g., self-injurious behavior), *positive punishment* or *response-contingent aversive stimulation* (e.g., applying an unpleasant consequence, such as electrical shock, after a behavior is performed) may be used. However, numerous problems associated with these procedures (e.g., modeling of aggression, eliciting fear of the situation, failure to promote alternative responses, and lack of long-term efficacy) have led them to be used only infrequently. Pairing strategies for reducing behaviors with procedures aimed at increasing desirable behaviors provides clients with a sense of how to get what they want out of life and other people, rather than just teaching them how to avoid what they do not want (Nemeroff & Karoly, 1991).

In addition to altering *consequences* for clinically relevant behaviors, *cues* (i.e., discriminative stimuli) for behaviors can also be the targets of intervention. Individuals learn that responses in a specific context, with a specific stimulus present, yield certain consequences. These procedures involve bringing a target behavior under *stimulus control*. For instance, a client who is trying to lose weight (target behavior) might be encouraged to eat only in the kitchen (a discriminative stimulus), or only in response to hunger cues, thus reducing the stimuli that signal a response of eating. Similarly, individuals with insomnia might be instructed to engage in nonsleep behaviors (e.g., watching television, reading, eating) only in rooms other than the bedroom, in order to increase the strength of the association between bedroom cues and sleeping.

Although contingency management procedures are often applied in controlled environments, such as institutions or schools, these same principles can in fact be applied quite flexibly in many contexts. *Natural reinforcers* (those that occur in people's everyday environment), rather than artificial reinforcers, are more likely to lead to maintenance and generalization of behavior change. For example, responding with empathy and caring when a client shares a painful emotion is likely be more effective than a statement such as "Thank you for sharing that feeling with me." Even traditional "talk therapy" likely involves therapists unwittingly reinforcing certain classes of client behavior (e.g., emotional communication) and extinguishing other classes of behaviors (e.g., superficial conversation). Clients can also use *self-management* or *self-control* procedures to provide contingencies themselves. For instance, clients might put aside money not spent on cigarettes each day, then use that money to buy a reward for smoking abstinence. The stimulus control procedures described previously may also be considered self-management procedures—clients choose to engage in behaviors in certain contexts in order to strengthen certain habits (e.g., sleeping in the bedroom) and weaken others (e.g., by eating only in the kitchen).

Behavioral Activation

Behavioral activation (BA) therapy for depression (aimed at helping depressed individuals increase their contact with positive reinforcers and decrease patterns of avoidance and inactivity) was developed by Neil Jacobson and colleagues (e.g., Martell, Addis, & Jacobson, 2001; Martell, Dimidjian, Herman-Dunn, & Lewinsohn, 2010), though other BA protocols have also been developed (e.g., Lejuez, Hopko, & Hopko, 2001). An early dismantling study revealed that BA alone had comparable efficacy to cognitive therapy, which included both BA techniques and cognitive restructuring (Jacobson et al., 1996). Building on these findings, Jacobson and colleagues developed BA as a treatment in its own right. A recent randomized controlled trial found that BA is comparable to medication and cognitive therapy in the treatment of all levels of depression, with evidence for enhanced efficacy compared to cognitive therapy in the treatment of severe depression (Dimidjian et al., 2006).

BA focuses on factors external to the individuals as potential causal and maintaining factors for depression, and focuses its intervention on these factors. The emphasis in BA is on the inactivity characteristic of depressed individuals, leading to decreased contact with potential positive reinforcers, thus reducing opportunities for action to be reinforced. The inertia and withdrawal that are typical of depressed individuals serve a negatively reinforcing function, similar to the avoidance behaviors characteristic of anxiety disorders. Despite the short-term relief that likely results from inactivity (by reducing experiences with non-reinforcing environments), these avoidance behaviors can lead to secondary problems (e.g., occupational or relational difficulties) and also limit opportunities for contact with positive reinforcers. Furthermore, these avoidance patterns likely lead to disruptions in routines. Such disruptions are thought to play an etiological and maintaining role in depression (Ehlers, Frank, & Kupfer, 1988).

BA directly targets avoidance behavior and disruptions of routines. After establishing a therapeutic relationship and presenting the model of depression, the therapist emphasizes the goal of changing behavior rather than altering mood. Clients' tendency to believe they cannot engage in an action until they feel better is gently challenged by therapists requesting that clients try to engage in planned behaviors regardless of how they feel. Time is spent developing collaborative treatment goals.

A critical element of BA is its focus on functional analysis. Therapist and client explore the triggers for depressive episodes, the nature of depressive symptoms, how the client responds to depressive symptoms, and avoidant behaviors and disruptions of routines. Clients are taught to conduct their own functional analyses and encouraged to do so particularly after therapy ends in order to prevent relapse. Based on this functional analysis, the client and therapist develop targets for focused activation. Rather than encouraging activity generally, as many behavioral approaches do, BA focuses on idiographic identification of activities that the client believes will be beneficial. Monitoring forms are used to track actions, triggers, and consequences, and assignments are modified accordingly.

Avoidance behaviors are modified by helping clients identify the function of these behaviors (both the immediate relief and the longer-term problems) and choose alternative coping responses. The acronym TRAP is used to help identify triggers, responses, and avoidance patterns, whereas the acronym TRAC is used to help generate alternative coping responses to the same triggers and responses. Often alternative coping responses involve approach rather than avoidance behaviors. Attention is also paid to regulating routines and to integrating activation strategies into regular routines, in order to fully evaluate their impact. To maximize the impact of activation strategies, clients are encouraged to attend to their experience, particularly in their immediate environment, as they engage in activities. This is thought to increase the impact of present-moment contingencies and also to help circumvent ruminative thinking, which is thought to interfere with engagement in life.

Social and Communication Skills Training

Social skills and communication training involves teaching individuals or groups to communicate more effectively. This process may include learning basic skills, such as making eye contact, ordering food in a restaurant, standing an appropriate distance from others, and allowing others to speak without interrupting. Or it may involve learning more complex skills (e.g., being more assertive), becoming a more effective lecturer, developing improved dating skills, or performing more effectively in job interviews. Typically, social skills training includes strategies such as psychoeducation, modeling (e.g., having a teacher, therapist, or other individual demonstrate the behavior), behavioral rehearsal or role plays, and feedback. Clients may also be videotaped while role-playing a particular social interaction so they can later observe their performance.

Social skills training has been used across a large number of psychological and interpersonal problems. It is a standard psychological treatment for schizophrenia (e.g., Kurtz & Mueser, 2008) and is often included in the treatment of social anxiety (e.g., Herbert et al., 2005), and emotional and behavioral problems in children (e.g, Antshel & Remer, 2003). Adults with depression may also benefit from social skills training (Becker, Heimberg, & Bellack, 1987), and communication training is often included as a component of behavioral treatment for couples (e.g., Epstein & Baucom, 2002).

Modeling

Modeling was first described early in the history of behavior therapy by social learning theorists such as Albert Bandura (1969). Essentially, this procedure involves demonstrating a particular behavior in the presence of a client, usually before asking the client to perform the same behavior. Modeling may also be combined with reinforcing an appropriate response by the client. This procedure is often used in social skills training (e.g., demonstrating for a client appropriate responses during a job interview) and in teaching clients basic skills of living (cooking, dressing, etc.). Modeling is also often used in the treatment of phobias and other fear-based problems. For example, therapists often demonstrate by exposing themselves to a feared situation before asking the client to try the exposure practice.

Problem-Solving Training

Problem-solving training aims to teach clients to solve problems effectively, with the goal of reducing psychopathology and enhancing psychological and behavioral functioning (D'Zurilla & Nezu, 2010). Problem-solving training was first introduced in the early 1970s by by D'Zurilla and Goldfried (1971). According to the model, problem solving involves two components: (1) problem orientation and (2) problem-solving skills (also referred to as "problem-solving proper"). *Problem orientation* refers to an individual's appraisal of his or her awareness of problems that arise, as well as the appraisal of his or her ability to solve problems. This component of treatment includes strategies for overcoming obstacles in problem solving, fostering self-efficacy, recognizing problems when they arise, viewing problems as challenges, learning to understand the role of emotions, and learning to "stop and think" rather than react impulsively (D'Zurilla & Nezu, 2010). *Problem-solving skills* are the specific steps needed to solve problems effectively. This component of treatment teaches clients to solve problems using five steps: (1) problem definition and formulation, (2) generation of possible solutions, (3) selection of the best solutions, and (4) implementation of selected solutions and evaluation outcome (D'Zurilla & Nezu, 2010). Problem-solving training has been used successfully (either alone or as part of a multicomponent treatment package) in the treatment of a variety of conditions, including depression, stress, social anxiety, schizophrenia, and certain physical complaints, such as menstrual pain (Nezu, 2004).

Relaxation-Based Strategies

Relaxation training is often used in behavior therapy as either a stand-alone intervention or it is integrated into a multicomponent treatment package. The most extensively studied form of this intervention is progressive muscle relaxation (PMR; Bernstein, Borkovec, & Hazlett-Stevens, 2000; Jacobson, 1938), particularly within the context of applied relaxation, in which PMR is taught, and clients then learn how to use the relaxation response effectively in their daily lives (Bernstein et al., 2000). These interventions have demonstrated efficacy for generalized anxiety disorder and for certain health-related problems (e.g., hypertension, headache, chronic pain, insomnia, irritable bowel syndrome, and cancer chemotherapy side effects; Bernstein et al., 2000). Some studies also support the use of applied relaxation (typically combined with exposure-based strategies) for social anxiety disorder, agoraphobia, and certain specific phobias (Magee, Erwin, & Heimberg, 2009; Taylor, 2000). For some conditions (e.g., panic disorder), exposure-based approaches seem to contribute more to outcome than do relaxation-based strategies, whereas for other problems (e.g., generalized anxiety disorder), applied relaxation and cognitive-behavioral therapy yield comparable outcomes (Siev & Chambless, 2007).

Therapists commonly misapply relaxation-based strategies by focusing only on leading clients in a relaxation exercise and telling them to practice at home. Applied relaxation for anxiety (its most common use) involves three components, all of which are important. The first component is *early cue detection*. Using monitoring and both verbal and imaginal review of anxiety-provoking episodes from the previous week, therapist and client work together to identify early environmental, cognitive, physiological, and emotional cues for anxiety. By catching spirals of anxious responding at earlier and earlier points, when the anxiety is less pronounced, the client can eventually apply relaxation in a less aroused state, when it is most likely to be successful.

The second component of applied relaxation is *intensive relaxation practice*, beginning with PMR, in order to develop clients' ability to relax. Clients are taught that relaxation is a skill, just like any other skill, and therefore requires repeated practice in order to develop. Relaxation is presented as a process rather than an outcome, so that any increase in relaxing sensations is seen as progress. PMR (as described by Bernstein et al., 2000) involves instructing clients to attend progressively to 16 muscle groups, first briefly tensing them (5–7 seconds), then releasing them or "letting go" (30- to 60-second cycles). The tension cycles are provided to increase awareness of tense sensations in each muscle group and to provide momentum that enables a deeper level of relaxation. After completing the full cycle with the therapist (tensing each muscle group twice), clients practice twice a day between sessions. The process of relaxation is gradually shortened once a client has developed the ability to relax using a given strategy, until relaxation can be achieved rapidly through recalling the experience.

In the third component of applied relaxation (as described by Bernstein et al., 2000), the skills developed in the first two components are combined, so that the client can apply relaxation to his or her life. The client begins to practice applying relaxation (in its more condensed form) when he or she first detects an anxious cue, both in session and in daily life. The therapist first assists with in-session application by responding to apparent nonverbal cues of anxiety; over time, the client begins to detect cues him- or herself in session and apply relaxation.

Mindfulness- and Acceptance-Based Strategies

Several recently developed behavioral approaches to treating clinical problems explicitly emphasize cultivating acceptance of internal experiences, as opposed to efforts to change these experiences (Roemer & Orsillo, 2009). *Acceptance* involves "allowing, tolerating, embracing, experiencing, or making contact with a source of stimulation that previously provoked escape, avoidance, or aggression" (Cordova, 2001, p. 215). Acceptance-based strategies stem from theories and empirical findings that suggest clinical problems are often characterized by reactivity toward one's own internal experience (thoughts, feelings, images, sensations) and efforts to escape or avoid these experiences, which, although sometimes effective in the short term, often backfire (Hayes, Strosahl, & Wilson, 1999; Roemer & Orsillo, 2009). As such, the development of an alternative way of responding to internal experience (i.e., acceptance versus judgment, criticism, and avoidance) may promote more adaptive functioning.

Acceptance is, in a sense, an implicit aspect of traditional exposure-based treatments that encourage increased contact with, rather than avoidance of, internal and external stimuli (e.g., accepting rather than avoiding panic-related sensations in panic control treatment; Craske & Barlow, 2008). However, proponents of these acceptance-based behavioral therapies note that behavior therapy's traditional explicit focus on change may inadvertently overlook the importance of clients learning to give up some of their futile efforts of control (e.g., over their internal experiences [Hayes et al., 1999] or over their partner's behavior [Christensen, Wheeler, & Jacobson, 2008]) and learning to accept and validate their own experience (Linehan, 1993a). These clinical scientists have borrowed from Eastern and humanistic/experiential traditions in incorporating acceptance into their behavioral approaches to clinical problems. Acceptance should not be confused with resignation; these therapies all emphasize that an acceptance of things as they are does not preclude efforts to make changes in one's life—it may in fact facilitate making such changes.

Mindfulness-based strategies have been adapted for use in acceptance-based behavioral therapies to help clients to cultivate acceptance as opposed to avoidance (Linehan, 1993b; Segal, Williams, & Teasdale, 2002). *Mindfulness*, a concept drawn from Buddhist traditions and recently incorporated in psychological theory and therapy, has been defined as "an openhearted, moment-to-moment, nonjudgmental awareness" (Kabat-Zinn, 2005, p. 24). Rather than being seen as some kind of idealistic end state, mindfulness is a process that involves continually bringing one's attention to the present moment, again and again, while distractions continue to arise, taking one out of the present moment. As such, the practice of mindfulness involves continually developing the skill of noticing where attention is, responding with gentleness and compassion, and drawing attention back to the moment. Development of this skill has been proposed to facilitate regulation of emotions (Hayes & Feldman, 2004); to reduce depressive relapse by interrupting depressive ruminative spirals (Segal et al., 2002); to enhance cognitive, emotional, and behavioral flexibility (Shapiro, Carlson, Astin, & Freedman, 2006), and to facilitate adaptive responding to environmental contingencies (Roemer & Orsillo, 2009).

Treatments incorporate mindfulness practices that vary in length and content. In all approaches, mindfulness is practiced in session, using formal exercises to develop the ability to attend with compassion or kindly awareness. Clients are then encouraged to do formal practices (i.e., setting aside time to practice mindfulness, such as sitting meditation, yoga, or other, briefer practices) at home as well. Often clients are also encouraged to practice mindfulness informally, which involves bringing mindfulness to daily activities. Clients can first do this with neutral situations, such as washing dishes or walking to the bus stop, and gradually apply mindfulness in more emotionally charged situations, such as an argument with a partner. In this way, similar to applied relaxation, the skill of mindfulness practiced and strengthened in specific exercises is then applied more generally to living life.

Often mindfulness exercises begin with a focus on the breath, with clients noticing their breath as they inhale and exhale, without trying to change the way they are breathing. Other sensory exercises can then be added, such as eating a single raisin mindfully or listening to sounds mindfully. More challenging exercises involve mindfulness of emotions and thoughts, such as to imagine putting one's thoughts on a cloud as a way of cultivating a more decentered relationship to thoughts. A host of exercises is available from which clinicians may draw (e.g., Hayes et al., 1999; Roemer & Orsillo, 2009; Segal et al., 2002). Exercises should be carefully selected in order to facilitate development of the specific skills that are important for a particular client, stemming from the functional analysis of her or his presenting problem.

Acceptance and commitment therapy (ACT; Hayes et al., 1999) is an acceptance-based behavioral therapy developed from a radical behavioral model in which avoidance of internal experiences is seen as underlying many psychological disorders. A host of experiential exercises and metaphors are used to help clients to *defuse* from their internal experiences and see their thoughts and emotions as not defining them. Clients are also encouraged to begin to describe their experience differently, for instance, "I'm having the thought that I'm going to fail at this," rather than "I'm going to fail at this," in order to learn to be less fused with thoughts and reactions.

Acceptance (of internal responses) is cultivated in these treatment approaches with an explicit goal of promoting more flexible and optimal responding to situations. As such, ACT, and other acceptance-based behavioral approaches that draw from it, includes an explicit focus on behavioral change. Through exploring what is personally meaningful to clients (values clarification), therapists help clients identify *valued actions* that they have been avoiding in order not to experience distress, and clients begin to take action in these domains (Wilson & Murrell, 2004). This process is very similar to exposure, except that target actions are chosen because they are meaningful to the individual rather than anxiety-provoking (although there is certainly an overlap between the two). This focus on what is meaningful to clients may help to motivate them to approach contexts that they have habitually avoided. Continued mindfulness practice (or other acceptance-based strategies) helps clients to approach valued contexts even though distressing feelings and thoughts may arise.

Randomized controlled trials have revealed that treatments incorporating mindfulness and other acceptance-based strategies (along with other behavioral strategies) show promise in the treatment of depressive relapse, borderline personality disorder, substance use disorders, generalized anxiety disorder, psychotic disorders, and couple distress, although considerably more research is needed to determine active ingredients and mechanisms of action (see Roemer & Orsillo, 2009, for a review).

Emotion Regulation Skills Training

Many behavioral therapies either implicitly or explicitly help clients develop skills to more effectively recognize, understand, and respond to their own emotions (Mennin & Farach, 2007). Although regulation is sometimes thought of as involving only reduction in emotion responding, many theorists highlight the ways that enhancing or clarifying emotional responding, and promoting flexible behavioral responding in the presence of emotions, are also important aspects of emotion regulation (e.g., Gratz & Roemer, 2004; Mennin & Farach, 2007). The self-monitoring included in all behavior therapies helps clients to become more aware of their emotional responses, and the triggers and consequences to their emotions, and may also help them to be more aware of the complexity of their emotional responses. Exposure-based strategies can also be thought of as facilitating regulation of fearful and anxious responding. Also, the acceptance- and mindfulness-based strategies described earlier enhance emotion regulation skills (Hayes & Feldman, 2004) and are often included in treatments that explicitly target emotion regulation skills (e.g., Gratz & Gunderson, 2006; Mennin & Fresco, 2010).

Several clinical researchers have developed specific strategies to enhance emotion regulation skills as part of treatments for specific clinical presentations. The skills training component of dialectical behavior therapy (DBT; Linehan, 1993b) includes a module that focuses on emotion regulation skills that have been adapted for use across a number of clinical presentations, such as eating disorders, substance use disorders, and anxiety disorders. Emotion regulation therapy for generalized anxiety disorder includes emotion regulation skills training as part of its integrative approach to promoting effective, flexible emotional responding (Mennin & Fresco, 2010). Emotion regulation skills training has been incorporated into behavioral treatments for deliberate self-harm (Gratz & Gunderson, 2006), adult survivors of child sexual assault (Cloitre, Koenen, Cohen, & Han, 2002), and mood and anxiety disorders (Allen, McHugh, & Barlow; 2008; Ehrenreich, Goldstein, Wright, & Barlow, 2009); the first two approaches have received preliminary support in randomized controlled trials.

Interventions explicitly intended to enhance emotion regulation skills typically include an emphasis on helping clients to identify and clarify their emotional responses as they occur. Clients learn through monitoring, review, and imaginal rehearsal to differentiate among emotional responses, and to distinguish between *primary* emotional responses that are direct responses to environmental events and provide important information, and *secondary* emotional responses that may result from reactions to initial responses, or efforts to avoid emotions. Clients are also taught to identify and apply strategies that can help them to respond adaptively in the presence of intense emotional responding.

THE THERAPEUTIC RELATIONSHIP AND THE STANCE OF THE THERAPIST

In 1970, Lang, Melamed, and Hart published an article on an automated procedure for administering behavioral treatments for fear, concluding that "an apparatus designed to administer systematic desensitization automatically was as effective as a live therapist in reducing phobic behavior, suggesting that desensitization is not dependent on a concurrent interpersonal interaction" (p. 220). More recently, researchers have developed computer-based procedures for changing attentional biases that characterize many anxiety disorders (e.g., Amir, Beard, Burns, & Bomyea, 2009), suggesting that the therapeutic relationship may not be a necessary ingredient in behavioral interventions. Even self-help treatments based on behavioral principles often lead to improvement (den Boer, Wiersma, & van den Bosch, 2004).

Do these findings mean that the therapeutic relationship is unimportant in behavior therapy? Probably not. In most of the studies on self-help treatments, there is a confound: Clients are required to have regular contact with a clinician for the study assessments.

Self-help treatments for panic disorder may be less effective when they are used on their own, without occasional professional contact to monitor the client's progress and treatment compliance (Febbraro, Clum, Roodman, & Wright, 1999). In other words, the therapeutic relationship may be important even for self-help treatments.

There is now emerging evidence that therapist behaviors and the therapeutic relationship are relevant in behavioral treatments (Follette, Naugle, & Callaghan, 1996; Gilbert & Leahy, 2007; Keijsers, Schaap, & Hoogduin, 2000). For example, Keijsers, Schaap, Hoogduin, and Lammers (1995) concluded that therapist empathy, warmth, positive regard, and genuineness assessed early in treatment were predictive of a positive outcome following behavioral treatment for panic disorder and agoraphobia, as was the tendency for clients to rate their therapists as more understanding and respectful. Williams and Chambless (1990) found that individuals with agoraphobia who described their therapists as more confident, caring, and involved, improved more than those who did not describe their therapists in these ways. In addition, there is evidence that therapist style can affect a client's motivation during treatment for problem drinking, and that therapist styles that enhance motivation are particularly useful for alcoholics who are very angry and hostile (Miller, Benefield, & Tonigan, 1993).

For a long time, the therapeutic relationship has been underemphasized in behavioral writings and in the training of behavior therapists compared to many other forms of psychotherapy. Instead, researchers have tended to focus more on examining the efficacy of particular behavioral techniques, with little discussion of the context in which behavior therapy occurs. However, in recent years, therapists working within a behavioral framework have become increasingly interested in the role of the therapeutic relationship and in the effects of therapist behavior on the outcome of treatment (e.g., Gilbert & Leahy, 2007; Kohlenberg & Tsai, 2007). The therapist is potentially a powerful source of social reinforcement; thus, it makes sense from a behavioral perspective that the therapeutic relationship and therapist behavior play a role in the process and outcome of treatment.

CURATIVE FACTORS OR MECHANISMS OF CHANGE

Changes in Environmental Contingencies

A central factor thought to underlie change in behavior therapy involves the relationship between behavior and the environment. Given that behavior is thought to be functional (i.e., maintained by contingencies in the environment), behavior change is thought to result from alterations in environmental contingencies. This may take several forms. Most obviously, the individual's context may be altered to reduce reinforcement for problematic behavior and to increase reinforcement for desired behavior. This may be the case in parent training interventions in which the child's environment is directly altered, or in couple or family therapy in which the individuals' responses to one another are a target of intervention. Similarly, in self-management approaches, the client him- or herself may alter the contingencies in his or her environment.

Often the environment is not directly altered, but the client learns to engage in new behaviors that in turn are reinforced by existing environmental contingencies. For instance, in social skills training, it is expected that the individual will receive meaningful, natural social reinforcement for new skills, which increases the frequency of these newly learned behaviors. Similarly, *in vivo* exposure is likely to result in the client exhibiting new, nonavoidant behaviors (e.g., attending parties) that are then maintained by natural reinforcement from the environment. To maximize adaptive responding to new environments, behavior therapy focuses on helping clients to develop flexible behavioral repertoires (Goldiamond, 1974) rather than rigid behavioral patterns based on past learning. These flexible repertoires, along with a decreased emphasis on arbitrary verbal rules (i.e., rule-governed behavior; Hayes, Kohlenberg, & Melancon, 1989), are expected to promote continued adaptation after therapy has ended.

Emotional Processing and Inhibitory Learning

Exposure-based interventions were initially developed to *extinguish* fearful responses to classically conditioned stimuli. However, research has demonstrated that fearful associations are never unlearned (e.g., individuals can spontaneously recover "extinguished" fearful responses when they are reexposed to the unconditioned stimulus). Based on these findings, newer models suggest that exposure results in learning new, nonfearful associations to previously feared stimuli. According to Foa and Kozak's (1986) classic emotional processing model, fearful responses are altered when an individual fully accesses the associative fear network (including stimulus, response, and meaning elements of the fear) and incorporates new, nonthreatening information. Foa and Kozak reviewed research that supports the proposed importance of initial activation of the fear structure (indicated by physiological responding to the feared stimulus), as well as fear reduction within and across sessions for efficacious exposure therapy. However, a recent update of the theory noted that reductions in fearful responding within sessions may not in fact be necessary for new information to be incorporated (Foa, Huppert, & Cahill, 2006). Craske and colleagues (2008) reviewed inconsistencies in the data supporting these proposed indicators of successful exposure and suggested that exposure-based treatments are instead effective because they provide an opportunity for inhibitory learning (through the development of competing, non-threat-related associations) and the development of tolerance for fear and anxiety.

Cognitive Models

Many researchers have noted that exposure-based treatments may in fact lead to cognitive change for individuals, and this may be the mechanism of change. For instance, Mineka and Thomas (1999) suggest that exposure disconfirms clients' beliefs that they do not have control over anxiety-provoking situations. Similarly, both Zinbarg (1993) and Rachman (1996) note that exposure techniques may alter emotionally relevant cognitive representations. In other words, clients' experiences when engaging in previously avoided activities may challenge their beliefs that such behaviors are dangerous or impossible, leading them to be more likely to continue engaging in such behaviors. Behavioral experiments have long been an integral part of cognitive therapy, suggesting that a client's own experiences may provide particularly salient disconfirming data for clinically relevant cognitions. To date, no research has adequately addressed whether behavioral techniques are efficacious due to their facilitation of cognitive change. Although some data suggest that cognitive techniques do not significantly add to the efficacy of behavioral techniques for depression (e.g., Jacobson et al., 1996), this does not mean that the behavioral techniques do not have their effect due to cognitive change.

Changes in Clients' Relationship with Internal Experiences

The mindfulness- and acceptance-based behavioral approaches described earlier are based in models suggesting that, rather than internal experiences themselves being the problem, clients' critical, reactive, or "fused" (i.e., as though thoughts and feelings are permanent and self-defining) responses to these experiences and efforts to avoid them need to be the target of interventions (e.g., Hayes et al., 1999; Roemer & Orsillo, 2009; Segal et al., 2002). Many aspects of behavioral therapy, such as self-monitoring; early cue detection; and imaginal, interoceptive, and *in vivo* exposure; as well as aspects of cognitive therapy, such as identification of thoughts and generation of alternatives, may be effective because they reduce the degree to which thoughts, emotions, sensations, and memories are associated with threat, judgments, reactivity, and criticism. Behavioral and cognitive therapies may help clients to *decenter* (recognize thoughts as mental events rather than indicators of truth or the nature of the self) from their thoughts, and this may be a common mechanism of change across disparate strategies (e.g., Teasdale et al., 2002). This reduction in reactivity and avoidance may also be understood as an increase in tolerance of internal experiences (e.g., Craske et al., 2008) and is likely to be associated with enhanced emotion regulation skills (Mennin & Farach, 2007).

Biological Changes

Although it is commonly assumed that psychosocial interventions are efficacious through psychological mechanisms, recent research has indicated that psychosocial interventions can lead to biological changes. Most striking have been treatment findings in the OCD literature, in which successful behavior therapy has been associated with changes in glucose metabolic rates in the brain, comparable to changes found following pharmacotherapy (e.g., Saxena et al., 2009). Although this may mean that such biological changes are the mechanisms of change for behavior therapy, they may instead be correlates rather than causes of change.

TREATMENT APPLICABILITY AND ETHICAL CONSIDERATIONS

Applicability of Behavioral Treatments

Behavioral interventions have been applied to a wide range of presenting problems, including anxiety disorders, mood disorders, substance use disorders, serious mental illness (typically in combination with pharmacotherapy), eating disorders, personality disorders, childhood disorders (e.g., anxiety, conduct problems, and autism), and health problems. Behavioral interventions tend to be more effective when clients present with focal target problems (and these types of presentations have been the most commonly studied); however, functional analysis and behavioral principles can be adapted to address a wide range of more complex clinical presentations as well. Recent research has also begun to investigate the impact of behavioral interventions targeting a single disorder on comorbid disorders that are not necessarily the focus of treatment. In a number of cases, comorbid disorders tend to improve when a target problem (e.g., panic disorder) is treated, suggesting that the learning that takes place in these interventions may generalize to other, related problems (Craske et al., 2007).

Although the idiographic principles underlying behavior therapy make it particularly responsive to variability in client characteristics (e.g., gender, ethnicity, age, class, sexual orientation, and other individual-difference variables that may play an important role in understanding the function of specific behaviors and in expectations for therapy), the tendency to investigate efficacy of interventions using standardized protocols, with predominantly white samples, has provided only limited empirical knowledge of the applicability of these intervention techniques in clients from diverse backgrounds (as is true of all modes of therapy). Studies have nonetheless demonstrated the efficacy of these interventions across gender and a range of age groups (from children to older adults). And the few randomized controlled trials conducted on behavioral or cognitive behavioral therapies with clients from ethnic or racial minority backgrounds provide preliminary support for the efficacy of this approach. For instance, cognitive-behavioral therapies may be efficacious in the treatment of depression among Latino/a adults and youth, although improvements are often smaller in magnitude than those in trials with predominantly white clients (see Organista, 2006, for a review). A randomized controlled trial of group panic control treatment with African American women revealed significant symptomatic improvements among individuals who received the treatment (Carter, Sbrocco, Gore, Marin, & Lewis, 2003). A culturally adapted cognitive-behavioral therapy for Cambodian refugees with treatment-resistant posttraumatic stress disorder and panic attacks led to significant improvements in a broad range of symptoms in a randomized controlled trial (Hinton et al., 2005).

Despite these initially promising findings, as with all therapeutic approaches, clinicians need to consider cultural and sociological factors when providing behavior therapy to clients from diverse backgrounds. Fortunately, increasing attention to the need for attention to cultural factors in therapy has led to several useful resources to guide clinicians in providing behavioral or cognitive-behavioral therapies with clients from diverse backgrounds (e.g., Hays & Iwamasa, 2006; Martell, Safren, & Prince, 2004; Tanaka-Matsumi, Seiden, & Lam, 1996).

Ethical Issues

In addition to the ethical considerations associated with any form of psychotherapy, behavioral approaches raise some specific concerns that should be kept in mind. Given the focus on behavioral change, and the use of strategies that have an intentional impact on the likelihood of certain behaviors, people often express concern that behavior therapy can be coercive and impose change chosen by the therapist rather than the client. In fact, this is a consideration in all forms of therapy; contingencies are always present that are likely to affect clients' behavior. In behavior therapy, the goal of behavioral change is made explicit, and therapists collaborate with clients to ensure consensus on treatment goals. Progress and goals are continually assessed to provide repeated opportunities for clients to influence the course and direction of their therapy. Nonetheless, as in all therapies, therapists should attend to the power differential inherent in therapy and be sure that mutually agreed upon goals are in place.

Behavior therapy often involves activities that take place outside the clinic, such as riding the subway or elevators with clients. This change in context challenges traditional conceptualizations of the boundaries that surround therapy. For instance, a therapist might eat at a restaurant with a client or visit his or her home, activities that typically are forbidden in the context of a therapeutic relationship. It is important to be aware of the potential for these activities to be misconstrued by clients as evidence of a different sort of relationship. The clear rationale for the therapeutic utility of these activities assists in clarifying how they fall within the therapeutic rather than the social domain. Therapists must also be sensitive to any potential danger for clients during exposures, being sure at all times to maintain the safety of clients.

RESEARCH SUPPORT AND EVIDENCE-BASED PRACTICE

Without question, behavioral interventions (broadly defined) are the most studied, and therefore the best supported, psychological treatments for most psychological disorders (though there is evidence supporting other psychotherapies for particular disorders as well). The Society of Clinical Psychology (Division 12 of the American Psychological Association) maintains a website describing evidence-based treatments for a wide range of problems, and indicates whether each treatment is strongly supported by research, modestly supported by research, or controversial. At the time that this chapter was written, the site described a total of 60 treatments for specific psychological disorders. Thirty-eight of the 40 treatments listed as having strong support were behavioral interventions, and 11 of the 16 treatments listed as having modest support were behavioral (Society of Clinical Psychology, 2010). In other words, most evidence-based treatments endorsed on this list are behavioral and include strategies such as exposure-based approaches, cognitive interventions, behavioral family therapies, skills training, and other strategies for changing behavior.

Since behavior therapy was first developed in the 1950s, hundreds (if not thousands) of studies have evaluated its effectiveness and efficacy. For example, behavioral activation for depression (a treatment that involves increasing activity levels in people who are depressed) has been evaluated in at least 34 randomized controlled studies, and a recent meta-analysis found that behavioral activation is a well-established treatment for depression that works as well as other established approaches, such as cognitive therapy (Mazzuchelli, Kane, & Rees, 2009).

Another article reviewed 16 well-conducted meta-analyses of treatment studies on cognitive-behavioral therapy (Butler, Chapman, Forman, & Beck, 2006). This article only reviewed studies that included cognitive and cognitive-behavioral interventions, and did not include studies based only on traditional behavioral treatments. As noted earlier, behavioral strategies are typically combined with cognitive approaches for most problems. This review included 16 meta-analyses that included 9,995 participants across 332 studies. These studies included 562 comparisons covering 16 disorders or populations, including depression, anxiety disorders, schizophrenia, marital distress, anger, eating disorders, sexual offending, chronic pain, and internalizing disorders (e.g., anxiety, depression) in children. The review provided strong support for cognitive-behavioral treatment across a wide range of problems.

To assess the cost-effectiveness of cognitive-behavioral therapy, Myhr and Payne (2006) reviewed 22 health economic studies on cognitive-behavioral therapies for mood, anxiety, psychotic, and somatoform disorders. Evidence from studies conducted in the United States, United Kingdom, Australia, Canada, and Germany have generally found that cognitive-behavioral therapy, provided alone or in combination with pharmacotherapy, leads to improved outcomes and cost savings by reducing health care use.

With so many studies demonstrating the positive effects of behavioral treatments, a full review is beyond the scope of this chapter. A more thorough review is available elsewhere (e.g., Nathan & Gorman, 2007).

CASE ILLUSTRATION

Background Information and Pretreatment Assessment

Deborah was a 43-year-old woman who worked as a teacher. She was married and had two children. She reported having difficulties with social anxiety for as long as she could recall. The problem had been particularly bad since college, when she had to drop several courses due to anxiety over giving presentations. Although she could not recall how the problem began, she remembered a number of life events that seemed to lead to exacerbation of her anxiety. For example, during one particularly difficult year in high school, she remembered being teased on a regular basis and pretending to be ill on several occasions so she could stay home from school to avoid being around her classmates. She described her home life while growing up as relatively happy, although she also reported that her parents were critical at times, and that she often felt pressure from her parents to meet high standards in school and in other areas of her life.

As part of her initial assessment, Deborah received the SCID-IV (First et al., 1996). DSM-IV criteria were met for a principal diagnosis of social anxiety disorder (generalized), and a past diagnosis of major depressive disorder, triggered by the loss of a job 10 years earlier. She reported significant fear and avoidance of a wide range of social situations, including parties, public speaking (except when teaching her students), writing in public, speaking to people in authority, meeting new people, being assertive, and having conversations with others. She reported that her social anxiety had prevented her from making friends and returning to school to complete her master's degree. She finally decided to seek treatment after reluctantly agreeing to be the maid of honor at her sister's wedding, which was only 3 months away.

Deborah reported several characteristic thoughts that seemed to contribute to her social anxiety. Her primary concern in social situations was that she would appear stupid or incompetent in front of others, despite the fact that she almost always received positive feedback about her performance. Her anxious thoughts were particularly problematic at work and around people whom she did not know well. She became upset if she perceived even the slightest bit of rejection in these situations. However, she was quite comfortable around her family and her closest friends, and was rarely upset if they criticized her behavior. Deborah also reported a fear that she would seem boring, and that other people would not want to spend time with her if they had the opportunity to get to know her. When asked what types of factors affected her fear, Deborah mentioned that she was more anxious around others whom she perceived as better in some way (e.g., more competent, successful, or educated), whom she did not know well, or who appeared self-assured. She also reported being particularly anxious in brightly lit places (because others might notice her blushing or shaky hands) and in more formal situations.

At her initial assessment, Deborah completed a series of self-report scales, including the Social Interaction Anxiety Scale (SIAS; Mattick & Clarke, 1998) and the Social Phobia Scale (SPS; Mattick & Clarke, 1998) to measure her social anxiety, the Depression Anxiety Stress Scales (DASS; Lovibond & Lovibond, 1995) to measure depression and generalized anxiety, and several others. She also rated her fear and avoidance for each of 12 items from her exposure hierarchy, using scales ranging from 0 (*no fear; no avoidance*) to 100 (*maximum fear; complete avoidance*), and completed a BAT that involved trying to return a sweater to a department store. Deborah was able to wait in line at the store, but when she reached the front of the line, she was too anxious to approach the cashier to ask about returning the sweater.

Behavioral Conceptualization

Deborah's social anxiety seemed to be initially exacerbated by some negative events she had experienced in social situations. More recently, the anxiety appeared to be maintained by her avoidance of social situations and her exaggerated beliefs about the potential dangers of being around other people. A number of situations appeared to trigger Deborah's anxiety.

Treatment

Deborah received cognitive-behavioral group treatment, similar to that described by Heimberg and Becker (2002). Her group, which included six other clients, all with a principal diagnosis of social anxiety disorder, met for 12 weekly 2-hour sessions. The first two sessions included psychoeducation regarding the nature of social anxiety and its treatment. These sessions began with a discussion of the notion that anxiety and fear are normal emotions, and that attempts to avoid experiencing them can actually increase their frequency and intensity. In addition, the survival value of social anxiety and its associated symptoms was reviewed. Clients in the group were encouraged to recognize that not all social anxiety is problematic. At times, social anxiety can protect us from making mistakes that might otherwise be associated with severe negative social consequences. Clients were also encouraged to conceptualize their social anxiety in terms of three components: a *physical component* (e.g., blushing, shaking, and sweating), a *cognitive component* (e.g., unrealistic assumptions about social situations), and a *behavioral component* (e.g., avoidance and safety behaviors). The treatment strategies (see below) were reviewed, with an emphasis on how each technique can be used to target particular components of the problem. Assignments during these initial sessions involved monitoring anxiety symptoms in diaries and completing assigned readings, including introductory chapters from the *Shyness and Social Anxiety Workbook* (Antony & Swinson, 2008). Relevant readings from this book were assigned throughout the remaining sessions of treatment as well.

Subsequent sessions included primarily instruction in cognitive restructuring and exposure to feared situations (both during in-session simulated exposures and between-session *in vivo* exposures practiced for homework). Cognitive restructuring involved teaching the group to identify anxiety-provoking beliefs (e.g., "It is important for everyone to like me" and "If my hands shake during a presentation, people will think I am incompetent") and to consider more balanced or realistic interpretations regarding social situations, after evaluating the evidence for them. For her exposure practices, Deborah was encouraged to expose herself to situations in which she might, in fact, draw attention to herself or look incompetent in front of others. For example, she practiced purposely losing her train of thought during presentations, shopping and then returning items to stores, spilling water on herself in a restaurant, asking for directions, dropping her keys in public, and wearing her dress inside-out at the mall. Each client in the group, including Deborah, developed an individualized hierarchy used to guide his or her exposure practices. In addition to cognitive- and exposure-based strategies, one session of the group was spent discussing strategies for improving communication skills.

Outcome

Relative to the other members of the group, Deborah's progress was more gradual. However, she was particularly motivated and completed almost all of her between-session assignments. By the end of treatment, she was much less concerned about being judged by others, and she reported a reduction in the sensations of blushing and shaking. She had begun an evening course in pottery and reported having socialized a few times with her classmates.

Deborah was able to attend her sister's wedding and experienced only moderate levels of anxiety while carrying out her responsibilities as maid of honor. In addition, at the end of treatment she repeated the BAT. This time, she was able to return the sweater at the department store, with only minimal anxiety.

CURRENT AND FUTURE TRENDS

Because behavior therapy is grounded in a commitment to scientific inquiry, its practice is constantly evolving and changing. An integration of behavioral and cognitive techniques is more common than a separation of these two elements, so this is certainly a current (as well as a past) trend. In addition, researchers are investigating the potential utility of integrating other intervention strategies (both psychological and pharmacological) in order to maximize efficacy of interventions. For certain conditions, such as depression (Cuijpers, van Straten, Warmerdam, & Andersson, 2009), bipolar disorder (Miklowitz, 2009), and schizophrenia (Addington et al., 2005), combining psychological and pharmacological treatments appears to lead to improved outcomes over either approach alone. In contrast, for treating anxiety disorders, combined interventions do not appear to be more efficacious than either approach alone (Otto, Behar, Smits, & Hofmann, 2009). A potentially promising new area of pharmacological study involves the use of D-cycloserine (DCS), which been found to lead to enhanced extinction in animals, to facilitate exposure therapies for anxiety disorders; preliminary investigations in clinical samples appear promising (Norberg, Krystal, & Tolin, 2008). Researchers are examining the efficacy of integrating mindfulness- and acceptance-based techniques into behavioral treatments for a range of disorders (Roemer & Orsillo, 2009), as well as whether the addition of interpersonal and/or experiential elements to cognitive-behavioral therapies increases efficacy (e.g., Cloitre et al., 2002; Mennin & Fresco, 2010; Newman, Castonguay, Borkovec, & Molnar, 2004). We expect to learn more about the utility of psychotherapy integration in the coming years.

A recent trend concerns studying the effectiveness of behavioral interventions in clinical practice as opposed to research settings, which historically used narrow, nonrepresentative samples of clients with a given disorder. Recent studies typically use many fewer exclusion criteria and include more representative samples. In addition, behaviorists are conducting research in clinical settings to investigate the utility of treatments in the context where they will be applied. Initial findings on effectiveness are promising; a meta-analysis of effectiveness studies of cognitive-behavioral therapies for anxiety disorders found large effect sizes that were generally comparable to those from representative efficacy studies (Stewart & Chambless, 2009).

Finally, behaviorists are focused on developing interventions that target disorders not previously treated effectively, more diverse client samples, and comorbid clinical presentations. As described previously, researchers and clinicians are exploring how behavioral interventions can be used in a culturally sensitive manner, and whether these adapted interventions are efficacious. In addition, several protocols that have been developed specifically target comorbid and more complex clinical cases. DBT (Linehan, 1993a) specifically focuses on treating clients with multiple problems, as do ACT and other acceptance-based behavioral therapies, by targeting mechanisms thought to underlie a wide range of presenting problems. Protocols have also been developed to treat groups of clients with a range of anxiety disorders (Norton, Hayes, & Springer, 2008), anxiety and mood disorders (Allen et al., 2008) or eating disorders with comorbid mood and interpersonal problems (Fairburn et al., 2009). These efforts, combined with the focus on effectiveness, will help behavior therapists continue to develop interventions that can optimally treat the clients presenting for services.

SUGGESTIONS FOR FURTHER STUDY

Recommended Reading

Antony, M. M., & Roemer, L. (2011). *Behavior therapy*. Washington, DC: American Psychological Association.—Provides an up-to-date overview of behavior therapy.

Barlow, D. H. (Ed.). (2008). *Clinical handbook of psychological disorders* (4th ed.). New York: Guilford Press.—This edited volume provides detailed, session-by-session, evidence-based protocols for treating a wide range of psychological problems.

Butler, A. C., Chapman, J. E., Forman, E. M., & Beck, A. T. (2006). The empirical status of cognitive-behavioral therapy: A review of meta-analyses. *Clinical Psychology Review, 26,* 17–31.—An excellent overview of the evidence supporting behavioral treatments.

Kenny, W. C., Alvarez, K., Donohue, B. C., & Winick, C. B. (2008). Overview of behavioral assessment with adults. In M. Hersen & J. Rosqvist (Eds.), *Handbook of psychological assessment, case conceptualization, and treatment: Vol. 1. Adults* (pp. 3–25). Hoboken, NJ: Wiley.—Provides and excellent overview of behavioral assessment.

O'Donohue, W. T., & Fisher, J. E. (Eds.). (2009). *General principles and empirically supported techniques of cognitive behavior therapy*. Hoboken, NJ: Wiley.—Covers about 75 different behavioral and cognitive techniques.

Spiegler, M. D., & Guevremont, D. C. (2010). *Contemporary behavior therapy* (5th ed.). Belmont, CA: Wadsworth Cengage Learning.—Covers all major behavioral approaches, including historical perspectives, assessment, theory, strategies, and outcome.

DVD

Antony, M. M. (2009). *Behavioral therapy over time*. Washington, DC: American Psychological Association.—Includes six sessions of treatment with a client who has problems with compulsive hoarding.

REFERENCES

Abramowitz, J. S. (1996). Variants of exposure and response prevention in the treatment of obsessive–compulsive disorder: A meta-analysis. *Behavior Therapy, 27,* 583–600.

Abramowitz, J. S., Deacon, B. J., & Whiteside, S. P. (2011). *Exposure therapy for anxiety: Principles and practice*. New York: Guilford Press.

Addington, D., Bouchard, R.-H., Goldberg, J., Honer, B., Malla, A., Norman, R., et al. (2005). Clinical practice guidelines: Treatment of schizophrenia. *Canadian Journal of Psychiatry, 50*(Suppl. 1), 1S–57S.

Addis, M. E., Cardemil, E. V., Duncan, B. L., & Miller, S. D. (2006). Does manualization improve therapy outcomes? In J. C. Norcross, L. E. Beutler, & R. F. Levant (Eds.), *Evidence-based practices in mental health: Debate and dialogue on the fundamental questions* (pp. 131–160). Washington, DC: American Psychological Association.

Allen, L. B., McHugh, R. K., & Barlow, D. H. (2008). Emotional disorders: A unified protocol. In D. H. Barlow (Ed.), *Clinical handbook of psychological disorders: A step-by-step treatment manual* (4th ed., pp. 216–249). New York: Guilford Press.

American Psychiatric Association. (2000). *Diagnostic and statistical manual of mental disorders* (4th ed., text rev.). Washington, DC: Author.

Amir, N., Beard, C., Burns, M., & Bomyea, J. (2009). Attention modification program in individuals with generalized anxiety disorder. *Journal of Abnormal Psychology, 118*, 28–33.

Antony, M. M., Ledley, D. R., Liss, A., & Swinson, R. P. (2006). Responses to symptom induction exercises in panic disorder. *Behaviour Research and Therapy, 44*, 85–98.

Antony, M. M., McCabe, R. E., Leeuw, I., Sano, N., & Swinson, R. P. (2001). Effect of exposure and coping style on *in vivo* exposure for specific phobia of spiders. *Behaviour Research and Therapy, 39*, 1137–1150.

Antony, M. M., Orsillo, S. M., & Roemer, L. (Eds.). (2001). *Practitioner's guide to empirically based measures of anxiety.* New York: Springer.

Antony, M. M., & Rowa, K. (2007). *Overcoming fear of heights: How to conquer acrophobia and live a life without limits.* Oakland, CA: New Harbinger.

Antony, M. M., & Rowa, K. (2008). *Social anxiety disorder: Psychological approaches to assessment and treatment.* Göttingen, Germany: Hogrefe.

Antony, M. M., & Swinson, R. P. (2000). *Phobic disorders and panic in adults: A guide to assessment and treatment.* Washington, DC: American Psychological Association.

Antony, M. M., & Swinson, R. P. (2008). *The shyness and social anxiety workbook: Proven, step-by-step techniques for overcoming your fear* (2nd ed.). Oakland, CA: New Harbinger.

Antshel, K. M., & Remer, R. (2003). Social skills training in children with attention deficit hyperactivity disorder: A randomized-controlled trial. *Journal of Clinical Child and Adolescent Psychology, 32*, 153–165.

Bandura, A. (1969). *Principles of behavior modification.* New York: Holt, Rinehart & Winston.

Barlow, D. H. (Ed.). (2008). *Clinical handbook of psychological disorders* (4th ed.). New York: Guilford Press.

Beck, A. T., Steer, R. A., & Brown, G. (1996). *Manual for Beck Depression Inventory–II.* San Antonio, TX: Pearson Assessment.

Becker, R. E., Heimberg, R. G., & Bellack, A. S. (1987). *Social skills training treatment for depression.* Elmsford, NY: Pergamon Press.

Bellack, A. S., & Hersen, M. (Eds.). (1985). *Dictionary of behavior therapy techniques.* New York: Pergamon Press.

Bernstein, D. A., Borkovec, T. D., & Hazlett-Stevens, H. (2000). *New directions in progressive relaxation training: A guidebook for helping professionals.* Westport, CT: Praeger.

Butler, A. C., Chapman, J. E., Forman, E. M., & Beck, A. T. (2006). The empirical status of cognitive-behavioral therapy: A review of meta-analyses. *Clinical Psychology Review, 26*, 17–31.

Carter, M. M., Sbrocco, T., Gore, K. L., Marin, N. W., & Lewis, K. L. (2003). Cognitive-behavioral group therapy versus a wait-list control in the treatment of African American women with panic disorder. *Cognitive Therapy and Research, 27*, 505–518.

Christensen, A., Wheeler, J. G., & Jacobson, N. S. (2008). Couple distress. In D. H. Barlow (Ed.), *Clinical handbook of psychological disorders: A step-by-step treatment manual* (4th ed., pp. 662–690). New York: Guilford Press.

Cloitre, M., Koenen, K. C., Cohen, L. R., & Han, H. (2002). Skills training in affective and interpersonal regulation followed by exposure: A phase-based treatment for PTSD related to childhood abuse. *Journal of Consulting and Clinical Psychology, 70*, 1067–1074.

Cordova, J. V. (2001). Acceptance in behavior therapy: Understanding the process of change. *Behavior Analyst, 24*, 213–226.

Craske, M. G., & Barlow, D. H. (2008). Panic disorder and agoraphobia. In D. H. Barlow (Ed.), *Clinical handbook of psychological disorders: A step-by-step treatment manual* (4th ed., pp. 1–64). New York: Guilford Press.

Craske, M. G., Farchione, T. J., Allen, L. B., Barrios, V., Stoyanova, M., & Rose, R. (2007). Cognitive behavioral therapy for panic disorder and comorbidity: More of the same or less of more? *Behaviour Research and Therapy, 45*, 1095–1109.

Craske, M. G., Kircanski, K., Zelikowsky, M., Mystkowski, J., Chowdry, N., & Baker, A. (2008). Optimizing inhibitory learning during exposure. *Behaviour Research and Therapy, 46*, 5–27.

Craske, M. G., Street, L., & Barlow, D. H. (1989). Instructions to focus upon or distract from internal cues during exposure treatment of agoraphobic avoidance. *Behaviour Research and Therapy, 27,* 663–672.

Cuijpers, P., van Straten, A., Warmerdam, L., & Andersson, G. (2009). Psychotherapy versus the combination of psychotherapy and pharmacotherapy in the treatment of depression: A meta-analysis. *Depression and Anxiety, 26,* 279–288.

den Boer, P. C. A. M., Wiersma, D., & van den Bosch, R. J. (2004). Why is self-help neglected in the treatment of emotional disorders?: A meta-analysis. *Psychological Medicine, 34,* 959–971.

Dimidjian, S., Hollon, S. D., Dobson, K. S., Schmaling, K. B., Kohlenberg, R. J., Addis, M. E., et al. (2006). Randomized trial of behavioral activation, cognitive therapy, and antidepressant medication in the acute treatment of adults with major depression. *Journal of Consulting and Clinical Psychology, 74,* 658–670.

D'Zurilla, T. J., & Goldfried, M. R. (1971). Problem-solving and behavior modification. *Journal of Abnormal Psychology, 78,* 107–126.

D'Zurilla, T. J., & Nezu, A. M. (2010). Problem-solving therapy. In K. S. Dobson (Ed.), *Handbook of cognitive-behavioral therapies* (3rd ed., pp. 197–225). New York: Guilford Press.

Ehlers, C. L., Frank, E., & Kupfer, D. J. (1988). Social *zeitgebers* and biological rhythms: A unified approach to understanding the etiology of depression. *Archives of General Psychiatry, 45,* 948–952.

Ehrenreich, J. T., Goldstein, C. R., Wright, L. R., & Barlow, D. H. (2009). Development of a unified protocol for the treatment of emotional disorders in youth. *Child and Family Behavior Therapy, 31,* 20–37.

Epstein, N. B., & Baucom, D. H. (2002). *Enhanced cognitive-behavioral therapy for couples: A contextual approach.* Washington, DC: American Psychological Association.

Eysenck, H. J. (1952). The effects of psychotherapy: An evaluation. *Journal of Consulting Psychology, 16,* 319–324.

Eysenck, H. J. (1960). *Behavior therapy and the neuroses.* Oxford, UK: Pergamon Press.

Fairburn, C. G., Cooper, Z., Doll, H. A., Bohn, K., Wales, J. A., Palmer, R. L., et al. (2009). Transdiagnostic cognitive-behavioral therapy for patients with eating disorders: A two-site trial with 60-week follow-up. *American Journal of Psychiatry, 166,* 311–319.

Febrarro, G. A. R., Clum, G. A., Roodman, A. A., & Wright, J. H. (1999).The limits of bibliotherapy: A study of the differential effectiveness of self-administered interventions in individuals with panic attacks. *Behavior Therapy, 30,* 209–222.

First, M. B., Spitzer, R. L., Gibbon, M., & Williams, J. B. W. (1996). *Structured Clinical Interview for Axis I DSM-IV Disorders Research Version—Patient Edition* (SCID-I/P, ver. 2.0). New York: New York State Psychiatric Institute, Biometrics Research Department.

Foa, E. B., Blau, J. S., Prout, M., & Latimer, P. (1977). Is horror a necessary component of flooding (implosion)? *Behaviour Research and Therapy, 15,* 397–402.

Foa, E. B., Huppert, J. D., & Cahill, S. P. (2006). Emotional processing theory: An update. In B. O. Rothbaum (Ed.), *Pathological anxiety: Emotional processing in etiology and treatment* (pp. 3–24). New York: Guilford Press.

Foa, E. B., Jameson, J. S., Turner, R. M., & Payne, L. L. (1980). Massed versus spaced exposure sessions in the treatment of agoraphobia. *Behaviour Research and Therapy, 18,* 333–338.

Foa, E. B., & Kozak, M. J. (1986). Emotional processing of fear: Exposure to corrective information. *Psychological Bulletin, 99,* 20–35.

Foa, E. B., Steketee, G., Grayson, J. B., Turner, R. M., & Latimer, P. (1984). Deliberate exposure and blocking of obsessive–compulsive rituals: Immediate and long-term effects. *Behavior Therapy, 15,* 450–472.

Follette, W. C., Naugle, A. E., & Callaghan, G. M. (1996). A radical behavioral understanding of the therapeutic relationship in effecting change. *Behavior Therapy, 27,* 623–641.

Forsyth, J. P., Fusé, T., & Acheson, D. T. (2009). Interoceptive exposure for panic disorder. In W. T. O'Donohue & J. E. Fisher (Eds.), *General principles and empirically supported techniques of cognitive behavior therapy* (pp. 394–406). Hoboken, NJ: Wiley.

Franklin, M. E., & Foa, E. B. (2007). Cognitive behavioral treatments for obsessive compulsive disorder. In P. E. Nathan & J. M. Gorman (Eds.), *A guide to treatments that work* (3rd ed., pp. 431–446). New York: Oxford University Press.

Gilbert, P., & Leahy, R. L. (Eds.). (2007). *The therapeutic relationship in the cognitive behavioral therapies.* New York: Routledge.

Goldiamond, I. (1974). Toward a constructional approach to social problems. *Behaviorism, 2,* 1–84.

Gratz, K. L., & Gunderson, J. G. (2006). Preliminary data on an acceptance-based emotion regulation group intervention for deliberate self-harm among women with borderline personality disorder. *Behavior Therapy, 37,* 25–35.

Gratz, K. L., & Roemer, L. (2004). Multidimensional assessment of emotion regulation and dysregulation: Development, factor structure, and initial validation of the Difficulties in Emotion Regulation Scale. *Journal of Psychopathology and Behavioral Assessment, 26,* 41–54.

Green, L. (1978). Temporal and stimulus factors in self-monitoring by obese persons. *Behavior Therapy, 9,* 328–341.

Gunther, L. M., Denniston, J. C., & Miller, R. R. (1998). Conducting exposure treatment in multiple contexts can prevent relapse. *Behaviour Research and Therapy, 36,* 75–91.

Hayes, A. M., & Feldman, G. (2004). Clarifying the construct of mindfulness in the context of emotion regulation and the process of change in therapy. *Clinical Psychology: Science and Practice, 11,* 255–262.

Hayes, S. C., Kohlenberg, B. S., & Melancon, S. M. (1989). Avoiding and altering rule-control as a strategy of clinical treatment. In S. C. Hayes (Ed.), *Rule-governed behavior: Cognition, contingencies and instructional control* (pp. 359–385). New York: Plenum Press.

Hayes, S. C., Strosahl, K. D., & Wilson, K. G. (1999). *Acceptance and commitment therapy: An experiential approach to behavior change.* New York: Guilford Press.

Hays, P. A., & Iwamasa, G. Y. (Eds.). (2006). *Culturally responsive cognitive-behavioral therapy: Assessment, practice, and supervision.* Washington, DC: American Psychological Association.

Heimberg, R. G., & Becker, R. E. (2002). *Cognitive-behavioral group therapy for social phobia: Basic mechanisms and clinical strategies.* New York: Guilford Press.

Herbert, J. D., Gaudiano, B. A., Rheingold, A. A., Myers, V. H., Dalrymple, K., & Nolan, E. M. (2005). Social skills training augments the effectiveness of cognitive behavioral group therapy for social anxiety disorder. *Behavior Therapy, 36,* 125–138.

Hinton, D. E., Chhean, D., Pich, V., Hofmann, S. G., Pollack, M. H., & Safren, S. A. (2005). A randomized controlled trial of cognitive behavior therapy for Cambodian refugees with treatment resistant PTSD and panic attacks: A cross-over design. *Journal of Traumatic Stress, 18,* 617–629.

Jacobson, E. (1938). *Progressive relaxation.* Chicago: University of Chicago Press.

Jacobson, N. S., Dobson, K. S., Truax, P. A., Addis, M. E., Koerner, K., Gollan, J. K., et al. (1996). A component analysis of cognitive-behavioral treatment for depression. *Journal of Consulting and Clinical Psychology, 64,* 295–304.

Jones, M. C. (1924). A laboratory study of fear: The case of Peter. *Journal of General Psychology, 31,* 308–315.

Kabat-Zinn, J. (2005). *Coming to our senses: Healing ourselves and the world through mindfulness.* New York: Hyperion.

Katerelos, M., Hawley, L., Antony, M. M., & McCabe, R. E. (2008). The exposure hierarchy as a measure of progress and efficacy in the treatment of social anxiety disorder. *Behavior Modification, 32,* 504–518.

Keijsers, G. P. J., Schaap, C. P. D. R., & Hoogduin, C. A. L. (2000). The impact of interpersonal patient and therapist behavior on outcome in cognitive-behavior therapy: A review of empirical studies. *Behavior Modification, 24,* 264–297.

Keijsers, G. P. J., Schaap, C. P. D. R., Hoogduin, C. A. L., & Lammers, M. W. (1995). Patient–therapist interaction in the behavioral treatment of panic disorder with agoraphobia. *Behavior Modification, 19,* 491–517.

Kohlenberg, R. J., & Tsai, M. (2007). *Functional analytic psychotherapy: Creating intense and curative therapeutic relationships.* New York: Springer.

Kurtz, M. M., & Mueser, K. T. (2008). A meta-analysis of controlled research on social skills training for schizophrenia. *Journal of Consulting and Clinical Psychology, 76,* 491–504.

Lang, P. J., Melamed, B. G., & Hart, J. (1970). A psychophysiological analysis of fear modification using an automated desensitization procedure. *Journal of Abnormal Psychology, 76,* 220–234.

Lazarus, A. A. (1958). New methods in psychotherapy: A case study. *South African Medical Journal, 33,* 660–664.

Lejuez, C. W., Hopko, D. R., & Hopko, S. D. (2001). A brief behavioral activation treatment for depression: Treatment manual. *Behavior Modification, 25,* 255–286.

Lindsley, O. R., Skinner, B. F., & Solomon, H. C. (1953). *Studies in behavior therapy* (Status Report 1). Waltham, MA: Metropolitan State Hospital.

Linehan, M. M. (1993a). *Cognitive-behavioral treatment of borderline personality disorder.* New York: Guilford Press.

Linehan, M. (1993b). *Skills training manual for cognitive behavioral treatment of borderline personality disorder.* New York: Guilford Press.

Lovibond, S. H., & Lovibond, P. F. (1995). *Manual for the Depression Anxiety Stress Scales* (2nd ed.). Sydney: Psychology Foundation of Australia.

Magee, L., Erwin, B. A., & Heimberg, R. G. (2009). Psychological treatment of social anxiety disorder and specific phobia. In M. M. Antony & M. B. Stein (Eds.), *Oxford handbook of anxiety and related disorders* (pp. 334–349). New York: Oxford University Press.

Martell, C. R., Addis, M. E., & Jacobson, N. S. (2001). *Depression in context: Strategies for guided action.* New York: Norton.

Martell, C. R., Dimidjian, S., Herman-Dunn, R., & Lewinsohn, P. M. (2010). *Behavioral activation for depression: A clinician's guide.* New York: Guilford Press.

Martell, C. R., Safren, S. A., & Prince, S. E. (2004). *Cognitive behavioral therapies with lesbian, gay, and bisexual clients.* New York: Guilford Press.

Mattick, R. P., & Clarke, J. C. (1998). Development and validation of measures of social phobia scrutiny fear and social interaction anxiety. *Behaviour Research and Therapy, 36,* 455–470.

Mazzuchelli, T., Kane, R., & Rees, C. (2009). Behavioral activation treatments for depression in adults: A meta-analysis and review. *Clinical Psychology: Science and Practice, 16,* 383–411.

McFall, R. M. (1970). Effects of self-monitoring on normal smoking behavior. *Journal of Consulting and Clinical Psychology, 35,* 135–142.

Mennin, D. S., & Farach, F. (2007). Emotion and evolving treatments for adult psychopathology. *Clinical Psychology: Science and Practice, 14,* 329–352.

Mennin, D. S., & Fresco, D. M. (2010). Emotion regulation as an integrative framework for understanding and treating psychopathology. In A. M. Kring & D. M. Sloan (Eds.). *Emotion regulation and psychopathology: A transdiagnostic approach to etiology and treatment* (pp. 356–379). New York: Guilford Press.

Miklowitz, D. J. (2009). Pharmacotherapy and psychosocial treatments for bipolar disorder. In I. H. Gotlib & C. L. Hammen (Eds), *Handbook of depression* (2nd ed., pp. 604–623). New York: Guilford Press.

Miller, W. R., Benefield, R. G., & Tonigan, J. S. (1993). Enhancing motivation for change in problem drinking: A controlled comparison of two therapist styles. *Journal of Consulting and Clinical Psychology, 61,* 455–461.

Mineka, S., & Thomas, C. (1999). Mechanisms of change in exposure therapy for anxiety disorders. In T. Dalgleish & M. J. Power (Eds.), *Handbook of cognition and emotion* (pp. 747–764). Hoboken, NJ: Wiley.

Mischel, W. (1984). Convergences and challenges in the search for consistency. *American Psychologist, 39,* 351–364.

Moscovitch, D. A., Antony, M. M., & Swinson, R. P. (2009). Exposure-based treatments for anxiety disorders: Theory and process. In M. M. Antony & M. B. Stein (Eds.), *Oxford handbook of anxiety and related disorders* (pp. 461–475). New York: Oxford University Press.

Mowrer, O. H. (1939). Stimulus response theory of anxiety. *Psychological Review, 46,* 553–565.

Myhr, G., & Payne, K. (2006). Cost-effectiveness of cognitive-behavioural therapy for mental disorders: Implications for public health care funding policy in Canada. *Canadian Journal of Psychiatry, 51,* 662–670.

Nathan, P. E., & Gorman, J. M. (Eds.). (2007). *A guide to treatments that work* (3rd ed.). New York: Oxford University Press.

Nelson, R. O., & Hayes, S. C. (1986).The nature of behavioral assessment. In *Conceptual foundations of behavioral assessment* (pp. 3–41). New York: Guilford Press.

Nemeroff, C. J., & Karoly, P. (1991). Operant methods. In F. H. Kanfer & A. P. Goldstein (Eds.), *Helping people change: A textbook of methods* (4th ed., pp. 121–160). Needham Heights, MA: Allyn & Bacon.

Newman, M. G., Castonguay, L. G., Borkovec, T. D., & Molnar, C. (2004). Integrative therapy for generalized anxiety disorder. In R. G. Heimberg, C. L. Turk, & D. S. Mennin (Eds.), *Generalized anxiety disorder: Advances in research and practice* (pp. 320–350). New York: Guilford Press.

Nezu, A. M. (2004). Problem solving and behavior therapy revisited. *Behavior Therapy, 35,* 1–33.

Norberg, M. M., Krystal, J. H., & Tolin, D. F. (2008). A meta-analysis of D-cycloserine and the facilitation of fear extinction and exposure therapy. *Biological Psychiatry, 63,* 1118–1126.

Norton, P. J., Hayes, S. A., & Springer, J. R. (2008). Transdiagnostic cognitive-behavioral group therapy for anxiety: Outcome and process. *International Journal of Cognitive Therapy, 1,* 266–279.

O'Donohue, W. T., & Fisher, J. E. (Eds.). (2009). *General principles and empirically supported techniques of cognitive behavior therapy.* Hoboken, NJ: Wiley.

O'Donohue, W., & Krasner, L. (1995). Theories in behavior therapy: Philosophical and historical contexts. In *Theories of behavior therapy: Exploring behavior change* (pp. 1–22). Washington, DC: American Psychological Association.

Organista, K. C. (2006). Cognitive-behavioral therapy with Latinos and Latinas. In P. A. Hays & G. Y. Iwamasa (Eds.), *Culturally responsive cognitive-behavioral therapy: Assessment, practice, and supervision* (pp. 23–46). Washington, DC: American Psychological Association.

Otto, M. W., Behar, E., Smits, J. A. J., & Hofmann, S. G. (2009). Combining pharmacological and cognitive behavioral therapy in the treatment of anxiety disorders. In M. M. Antony & M. B. Stein (Eds.), *Oxford handbook of anxiety and related disorders* (pp. 429–440). New York: Oxford University Press.

Powers, M. B., & Emmelkamp, P. M. G. (2008). Virtual reality exposure therapy for anxiety disorders: A meta-analysis. *Journal of Anxiety Disorders, 22,* 561–569.

Purdon, C., Rowa, K., & Antony, M. M. (2007). Diary records of thought suppression attempts by individuals with obsessive–compulsive disorder. *Behavioural and Cognitive Psychotherapy, 35,* 47–59.

Rachman, S. J. (1996). Mechanisms of action of cognitive-behavior treatment of anxiety disorders. In M. R. Mavissakalian & R. F. Prien (Eds.), *Long term treatments of anxiety disorders* (pp. 49–69). Washington, DC: American Psychiatric Press.

Rachman, S., Radomsky, A. S., & Shafran, R. (2008). Safety behaviour: A reconsideration. *Behaviour Research and Therapy, 46,* 163–173.

Riggs, D. S., Cahill, S. P., & Foa, E. B. (2006). Prolonged exposure treatment of posttraumatic stress disorder. In V. M. Follette & J. I. Ruzek (Eds.), *Cognitive-behavioral therapies for trauma* (2nd ed., pp. 65–95). New York: Guilford Press.

Roemer, L., & Orsillo, S. M. (2009). *Mindfulness- and acceptance-based behavioral therapies in practice.* New York: Guilford Press.

Rothbaum, B. O., Anderson, P., Zimand, E., Hodges, L., Lang, D., & Wilson, J. (2006). Virtual reality exposure therapy and standard (*in vivo*) exposure therapy in the treatment of fear of flying. *Behavior Therapy, 37,* 80–90.

Rowe, M. K., & Craske, M. G. (1998). Effects of varied-stimulus exposure training on fear reduction and return of fear. *Behaviour Research and Therapy, 36,* 719–734.

Savard, J., Savard, M.-H., & Morin, C. M. (2010). Insomnia. In M. M. Antony & D. H. Barlow (Eds.), *Handbook of assessment and treatment planning for psychological disorders* (2nd ed.). New York: Guilford Press.

Saxena, S., Gorbis, E., O'Neill, J., Baker, S. K., Mandelkern, M. A., Maidment, K. M., et al. (2009). Rapid effects of brief intensive cognitive-behavioral therapy on brain glucose metabolism in obsessive–compulsive disorder. *Molecular Psychiatry, 14,* 197–205.

Segal, Z. V., Williams, J. M. G., & Teasdale, J. D. (2002). *Mindfulness-based cognitive therapy for depression: A new approach to preventing relapse.* New York: Guilford Press.

Shapiro, S. L., Carlson, L., Astin, J., & Freedman, B. (2006). Mechanisms of mindfulness. *Journal of Clinical Psychology, 62,* 373–386.

Siev, J., & Chambless, D. L. (2007). Specificity of treatment effects: Cognitive therapy and relaxation for generalized anxiety and panic disorders. *Journal of Consulting and Clinical Psychology, 75,* 513–522.

Skinner, B. F. (1974). *About behaviorism.* New York: Knopf.

Society of Clinical Psychology. (2010). *Website on research-supported psychological treatments.* Retrieved February 20, 2010, from *www.psychology.sunysb.edu/eklonsky-/division12/index.html.*

Spiegler, M. D., & Guevremont, D. C. (2010). *Contemporary behavior therapy* (5th ed.). Belmont, CA: Wadsworth Cengage Learning.

Stern, R., & Marks, I. (1973). Brief and prolonged flooding: A comparison in agoraphobic patients. *Archives of General Psychiatry, 28,* 270–276.

Stewart, R. E., & Chambless, D. L. (2009). Cognitive behavioral therapy for adult anxiety disorders in clinical practice: A meta-analysis of effectiveness studies. *Journal of Consulting and Clinical Psychology, 77,* 595–606.

Summerfeldt, L. J., Kloosterman, P., & Antony, M. M. (2010). Structured and semi-structured diagnostic interviews. In M. M. Antony & D. H. Barlow (Eds.), *Handbook of assessment and treatment planning for psychological disorders* (pp. 95–137). New York: Guilford Press.

Tanaka-Matsumi, J., Seiden, D.Y., & Lam, K. N. (1996). The Culturally Informed Functional Assessment (CIFA) Interview: A strategy for cross-cultural behavioral practice. *Cognitive and Behavioral Practice, 3,* 215–234.

Taylor, S. (2000). *Understanding and treating panic disorder: Cognitive-behavioural approaches.* Chichester, UK: Wiley.

Teasdale, J. D., Moore, R. G., Hayhurst, H., Pope, M., Williams, S., & Segal, Z. V. (2002). Metacognitive awareness and prevention of relapse in depression: Empirical evidence. *Journal of Consulting and Clinical Psychology, 70,* 275–287.

Terhune, W. S. (1948). The phobic syndrome: A study of eighty-six patients with phobic reactions. *Archives of Neurology and Psychiatry, 62,* 162–172.

Ullmann, L. P., & Krasner, L. (1965). *Case studies in behavior modification.* New York: Holt, Rinehart & Winston.

Wallace, M. D., & Najdowski, A. C. (2009). Differential reinforcement of other behavior and differential reinforcement of alternative behavior. In W. T. O'Donohue & J. E. Fisher (Eds.), *General principles and empirically supported techniques of cognitive behavior therapy* (pp. 245–255). Hoboken, NJ: Wiley.

Williams, K. E., & Chambless, D. L. (1990). The relationship between therapist characteristics and outcome of *in vivo* exposure treatment for agoraphobia. *Behavior Therapy, 21,* 111–116.

Wilson, G. T. (1998). Review: Manual-based treatment and clinical practice. *Clinical Psychology: Science and Practice, 5,* 363–375.

Wilson, K. G., & Murrell, A. R. (2004). Values work in acceptance and commitment therapy. In S. C. Hayes, V. M . Follette, & M. M. Linehan (Eds.), *Mindfulness and acceptance: Expanding the cognitive-behavioral tradition* (pp. 120–151). New York: Guilford Press.

Wolpe, J. (1958). *Psychotherapy by reciprocal inhibition.* Stanford, CA: Stanford University Press.

Zinbarg, R. E. (1993). Information processing and classical conditioning: Implications for exposure therapy and the integration of cognitive therapy and behavior therapy. *Journal of Behavior Therapy and Experimental Psychiatry, 24,* 129–139.

Zlomke, K., & Davis, T. E. (2008). One session treatment of specific phobias: A detailed description and review of treatment efficacy. *Behavior Therapy, 39,* 207–223.

CHAPTER 5

Cognitive Therapy

Kimberly A. Dienes
Susan Torres-Harding
Mark A. Reinecke
Arthur Freeman
Ann Sauer

Cognitive therapy has attracted substantial interest from mental health professionals during the 50 years since it was first ushered in by a 1956 symposium on information processing at MIT (Mahoney, 1977). Cognitive therapy came to prominence during the "cognitive revolution" and has progressed to a point where cognitively based therapies have moved to the forefront of professional interest. Cognitive therapy has become a meeting ground for therapists from diverse theoretical and philosophical positions, ranging from the psychoanalytic to the behavioral. Psychodynamic therapists find in cognitive therapy a dynamic core that involves working to alter tacit beliefs and interpersonal schemas. Behavioral therapists find a brief, active, directive, collaborative, psychoeducational model of psychotherapy that is empirically based and has as its goal direct behavioral change.

The merging of cognitive therapy and behavior therapy has become more the rule than the exception. Despite the link between cognitive and behavioral therapies, it is important to note some distinguishing factors. Behavior therapy focuses on learned behavior that arises from responses to an individual's environment. The target of these therapies is the "unlearning" of problematic behavior. Cognitive therapies, in contrast, focus on an individual's *beliefs* about the self, the world, and the future. The sources of pathology, and therefore the targets of therapy, are thoughts—maladaptive cognitions—that are frequently automatic and ingrained. Cognitive-behavioral therapies link these two approaches by targeting both problematic behaviors and maladaptive cognitions. Thus, the term *cognitive-behavioral therapy*, or CBT, subsumes cognitive approaches and has at times been used interchangeably with the term *cognitive therapy*. Empirical support in the form of randomized controlled outcome studies has led cognitive-behavioral therapies to be identified as empirically supported treatments for a range of conditions including depression, eating disorders, panic disorder, generalized anxiety disorder, obsessive–compulsive disorder, posttraumatic stress disorder, psychosis, and self-mutilation.

Contemporary cognitive therapy has become a broad-spectrum model of therapy and psychopathology, and has been applied to a wide range of problems, patient groups, and therapeutic contexts. CBT approaches have been described as particularly useful frameworks in work with individuals from diverse racial, ethnic, and cultural backgrounds. The emphasis on understanding environmental influences on behaviors and the individualized meaning of client symptoms allow for the integration of culturally specific beliefs, norms, behavioral expectations, and cultural supports in clinical conceptualizations of cognitions and behaviors (Hays, 2009). CBT approaches are useful when working with traditionally marginalized groups, such as people of color or individuals from lower socioeconomic backgrounds, because they minimize existing power differentials and facilitate empowerment through collaborative goal setting, psychoeducational components, agenda setting, and promotion of self-efficacy (Organista & Munoz, 1996). While the literature is limited, there is increasing support for the efficacy of CBT with ethnic/minority clients for diverse problems such as depression, generalized anxiety disorder, substance abuse, and posttraumatic stress disorder (Voss Horrell, 2008).

As cognitive models have developed they have become more specific, integrated, and differentiated. This has led to the development of alternative cognitive-behavioral "schools" or approaches, and to attempts to develop standards of clinical training in cognitive-behavioral psychotherapy. Cognitive models are essential components of comparatively more recent forms of therapy, such as acceptance and commitment therapy (ACT; Hayes, 2004) and mindfulness-based cognitive therapy (MBCT; Segal, Teasdale, & Williams, 2004).

Cognitive-behavioral strategies and techniques have "diffused" into wider practice. They have been integrated into therapeutic work by clinicians trained in other approaches. It is not uncommon to encounter clinicians who state that they conceptualize clients psychodynamically but selectively use cognitive techniques, reflecting increased acceptance of the usefulness of cognitive-behavioral models, or at least particular interventions. The more traditional understanding of cognitive therapy has changed as well to include an emphasis on the importance of the therapeutic relationship. Clinical warmth, empathy, and positive regard, core characteristics of client-centered psychotherapy, are now seen as forming a foundation for all effective psychotherapy (Bergin & Garfield, 2003). In a similar manner, cognitive strategies and techniques are becoming part of a general standard of care.

HISTORICAL BACKGROUND

Cognitive theory is founded on intellectual traditions dating to Stoic philosophers, such as Epictetus (1983), who in the first century commented, "What upsets people is not things themselves but their judgments about the things" (p. 13). Contemporary cognitive psychotherapy is founded upon the concept of *psychological constructivism,* which proposes that individuals are proactive and develop systems of personal meaning to organize their interactions with the world. Such knowledge (both personal and scientific) is relative insofar as it is based on personal and cultural epistemologies and may not be based on a knowable "objective" reality.

Contemporary cognitive psychotherapy reflects the confluence of several schools of thought and is an extension of the earlier work of Adler (1968), Bowlby (1985), Freud (1923), and Tolman (1949). The influence of psychodynamic theory on the evolution of cognitive psychotherapy is perhaps most apparent in the topographic model of personality and psychopathology that they share. Whereas Freud partitioned the psyche into the conscious, preconscious, and unconscious domains, with an individual's behavior primarily motivated by unconscious drives (the id), cognitive theorists partition cognitive processes into "automatic thoughts,""assumptions" and "schemas." More modern psychodynamic theories emphasize object relationships, or internal models of relationships, that closely resemble the cognitive concept of a relationship schema. Modern psychodynamic theories and cognitive models share a focus on individuals' basic assumptions that guide how they interact and operate.

Therapists such as Beck (1972), Ellis (1962), and Goldfried (Goldfried & Merbaum, 1973), were among the first to incorporate cognitive mediational constructs with behavioral theory. They focused on the role of social learning processes in the development of emotional problems and on the use of cognitive restructuring, the development of social problem-solving capacities, and the acquisition of behavioral skills in resolving them. The development of cognitive therapy accelerated during the 1970s. Early proponents argued for the incorporation of the findings of cognitive psychology into the behavioral model, expanding it from an S-R (stimulus–response) model for classical conditioning and an S-R-C (stimulus–response–consequence) model for operant conditioning to an S-O-R-C (stimulus–organism–response–consequence) model, into which cognitive control and cognitive constructs were incorporated. Over time, the focus on self-statements and "internal dialogue" shifted toward an examination of implicit meaning structures, because it appeared that clients perhaps were not able to report their internal dialogue, but were acting as if certain assumptions were true. Clients appeared to be using a cognitive information-processing model incorporating encoding, storage, and retrieval processes, some of which were not always within a person's awareness. Selective attentional processes and idiosyncratic encoding and retrieval processes appeared to underlie what was observed in therapy. In addition, the *schema construct*, developed within experimental developmental psychology and defined as cognitive representations of people, past experiences, and themselves, was incorporated into therapy (Goldfried, 2003).

Cognitive therapy is typically most closely identified with Aaron Beck (Beck, 1972; Scott & Freeman, 2010). He offered a continuity hypothesis, in which clinically significant difficulties represented extreme forms of normal emotional and behavioral functioning. He also utilized an information-processing paradigm, drawn from the cognitive research, which incorporated two critical elements: cognitive structures (schemas and automatic thoughts) and cognitive mechanisms (cognitive distortions). Regarding cognitive structures, Beck, Rush, Shaw, and Emery (1979) elaborated a model of automatic thoughts, intermediate assumptions, and core self-schemas in explaining the development and course of "depressogenic" thinking. Regarding cognitive mechanisms, they emphasized the influence of faulty schemas about self (self-schemas), the world, and others, which gave rise to and sustained faulty information processing, whereby clients distorted and filtered external environmental stimuli. This distorted processing of environmental information served to confirm the initial faulty schemas and general worldview of the client. The therapy, which incorporated both behavioral techniques (e.g., activity scheduling) and cognitive techniques (e.g., Socratic questioning), had as its goal changing the dysfunctional thought patterns and their underlying schemas.

Similarly, the now familiar ABC model of the relationships between "antecedent events," "beliefs," "behavior," and "consequences" for the individual, proposed by Ellis (1962; Ellis & Harper, 1961), suggested that neurotic or maladaptive behaviors are learned and directly related to irrational beliefs that people hold about events in their lives. Ellis developed a typology of common cognitive distortions, as well as a number of directive therapeutic techniques for changing them. Ellis's model assumes that by identifying and changing unrealistic or irrational beliefs, it is possible to alter one's behavioral or emotional reactions to events. Irrational beliefs are often tightly held and long-standing in nature, highly focused and, at times, confrontationally expressed interventions are necessary to dispute them. Ellis's therapeutic approach is active and pragmatic. Although the basic tenets of rational-emotive behavior therapy (REBT) have not, as yet, been subjected to extensive empirical scrutiny, Ellis's clinical techniques for challenging irrational beliefs are widely used.

Other theories elaborated on the role of cognitive mechanisms that contributed to the development of psychopathology. Meichenbaum (1977) described the role of internalized speech in the development of emotional disorders. Meichenbaum's techniques for "self-instructional training" via the rehearsal of "self-statements," modeling, and self-reinforcement have proven particularly useful in treating depressed or impulsive children. Similarly, Seligman (1975) proposed that individuals become depressed when they come to believe that they are unable to control important outcomes in their life (including both positive or reinforcing events and negative events or punishments). This "learned helplessness" model of depression was subsequently refined by Abramson, Seligman, and Teasdale (1978) in an "attributional reformulation" of the theory. Abramson, Metalsky, and Alloy (1989) went on to explore specific cognitive vulnerabilities to depression and especially pernicious "hopeless" reactions to negative events in cognitively vulnerable individuals.

Third-Wave Cognitive-Behavioral Therapies

More recently, newer models of therapy, while embedded in behavioral and cognitive traditions, also incorporate relatively new philosophical traditions and a shift of focus in therapeutic interventions. *Mindfulness* (nonjudgmental acceptance of cognitions and other internal experiences rather than cognitive restructuring), *contextualism* (a focus on emotional appraisal and regulation processes), a renewed emphasis on behavioral methods and techniques, and an emphasis on the function rather than the content of cognitions are all hallmarks of these new approaches (see Follette & Callaghan, Chapter 6, this volume). These models were developed in large part as a reaction to the perceived limited success of cognitive therapy in treating individuals with more intractable, chronic, or complex difficulties, such as people with personality disorders or chronic, relapsing depression, and others viewed as unsuitable candidates for traditional cognitive therapy (Young, Klosko, & Weishaar, 2003). While many of these therapies emphasize behavioral mechanisms, they also include a strong emphasis on cognitive processes.

Acceptance and Commitment Therapy

In the ACT model, psychopathology is believed to arise from a psychological inflexibility, as influenced by an overreliance on literal linguistic rules, and experiential avoidance that arises because some internal events, such as thoughts and feelings, are perceived as aversive or are evaluated negatively (e.g., feeling anxious is perceived to be "bad" because it is assumed to arise from negative events; Hayes, 2004). ACT holds that individuals should become aware of and examine their thoughts, and, in essence, change the relationship they have with their thoughts—not confuse their thoughts with reality—and not to judge, evaluate, or attempt to modify their cognitions (like traditional cognitive therapy), but simply to observe and accept their cognitions and feelings. Goals include increased mindfulness, promotion of distancing from one's cognitions (e.g., seeing one's thoughts as "just thoughts"), observation of cognitions and emotions in a nonjudgmental way, and exploration of values and development of commitment to engage actively with the external world and work toward having a meaningful, authentic life. Cognitive changes in ACT are believed to occur through several mechanisms, the most important of which is distancing. Though a source of debate, some (e.g., Arch & Craske, 2008) have argued that ACT shares many similarities with cognitive therapy processes and mechanisms, including the examination of cognitive events and development of new associations to one's thoughts. However, unlike traditional cognitive therapy, ACT specifically rejects cognitive restructuring because the focus is on addressing the *function*, not the content, of the cognition.

Mindfulness-Based Cognitive Therapy

MBCT, developed to treat chronic or long-standing major depressive disorder (Segal et al., 2004), builds upon Beck's model of cognitive therapy by elaborating on the process by which schemas and a client's overlearned, habitual patterns of thinking process may become reactivated and, consequently, trigger symptom relapses in vulnerable individuals during times of stress. A ruminative cognitive style and excessive self-focus increase the likelihood that these maladaptive thinking patterns and their corresponding schemas will be reactivated. In addition to traditional cognitive therapy techniques, MBCT incorporates mindfulness training, utilizing techniques drawn from mindfulness-based stress management (Kabat-Zinn, 1994). However, MBCT uses an explicit cognitive framework, and the major goals of therapy are to reactivate adaptive patterns of thinking through nonjudgemental awareness of cognitions, emotions, and bodily sensations, and to develop a decentered stance toward cognitions and feelings, which are viewed as passing events in the mind.

Schema-Based Therapy

Schema-based therapy, or schema therapy, was an outgrowth of Beck's early conceptualization of schema (Beck et al., 1979). Schema therapy was developed to address more specifically the needs of individuals with characterological issues, such as borderline personality disorder, and long-standing or relapsing conditions, such as chronic depression or anxiety, eating disorders, and long-standing relationship or intimacy problems (Young et al., 2003). In schema therapy, a predominant focus is on the occurrence of *early maladaptive schemas*, defined by Young and colleagues as "self-defeating emotional and cognitive patterns that begin early in . . . development and repeat throughout life" (p. 7). Individuals cope with these problematic, painful, or distressing early maladaptive schemas through *schema avoidance*, or rearranging their lives so that problematic schemas are never activated; *schema surrender*, whereby perceptions and behaviors are changed to conform to their schemas; and *schema neutralization/overcompensation*, whereby they act to neutralize the schema by behaving in a manner opposite to what is predicted by the schema. In addition to cognitive techniques, experiential activities, such as guided imagery and role playing, and techniques using the therapeutic alliance, such as reparenting techniques, are utilized both to explore schemas to develop a schema formulation with the client and to provide corrective experiences.

ASSUMPTIONS OF COGNITIVE THERAPY

1. The way individuals construe or interpret events and situations mediates how they subsequently feel and behave. Human functioning is the product of an ongoing interaction between specific, related "person variables" (beliefs and cognitive processes, emotions, and behavior) and environmental variables. These variables influence one another in a reciprocal manner over the course of time.

2. Interpretation of events is active and ongoing. The construal of events allows individuals to derive a sense of meaning from their experiences and permits them to understand events, with the goals of establishing their "personal environment" and forming a response. Behavioral and emotional functioning, as a result, are seen as goal directed and adaptive.

3. Individuals develop idiosyncratic belief systems that guide behavior. Beliefs and assumptions influence perceptions and memories, and memories are activated by specific stimuli or events. The individual is rendered sensitive to specific "stressors," including both external events and internal affective experiences. Beliefs and assumptions contribute to a tendency to attend selectively and to recall information that is consistent with the content of the belief system, and to "overlook" information that is inconsistent with those beliefs.

4. Stressors contribute to a functional impairment of an individual's cognitive processing and activate maladaptive, overlearned coping responses. A feedforward system is established, in which activation of maladaptive coping behaviors contributes to the maintenance of aversive environmental events and consolidation of the belief system. The person who believes, for example, that "the freeway is horribly dangerous" might drive in such a timid manner that he or she causes an accident, thus strengthening the belief in the danger of freeways and the importance of driving even more defensively.

5. The "cognitive specificity hypothesis" states that clinical syndromes and emotional states can be distinguished by the specific content of the belief system and the cognitive processes that are activated.

THE CONCEPT OF PERSONALITY

The foundation of cognitive therapy is the belief or meaning system that forms the identity or "personality" of a given individual. When we speak of "cognitions" we are not limiting ourselves to "automatic thoughts"—that is, to the thoughts and beliefs that comprise a person's moment-to-moment stream of consciousness. Rather, cognitions include our perceptions, memories, expectations, standards, images, attributions, plans, goals, and tacit beliefs. They include multiple factors that have gone into making up the personality of an individual. Cognitive variables, then, include thoughts in our conscious awareness, as well as inferred cognitive structures and cognitive processes.

Although individuals may be born with certain temperaments shaped by genetic heritability, experiences from individuals' earliest years shape how they view the world around them. Beliefs shaped by these experiences are the focus of cognitive therapy. A child who feels secure in the love and attention of his or her primary caregiver will have a belief system that the world is a safe place to explore. Although attachment theory (Bowlby, 1969) is derived from psychodynamic models of thought, cognitive theory has reformulated the original drive-based conceptualization and posits that an individual's characteristic patterns of viewing the world are shaped throughout development and are known as *schemas*.

Schemas play a central role in the formation of an individual's personality. The concept, originally proposed by Kant, has more recently been employed by Piagetian psychologists and associative network theorists to refer to organized, tacit cognitive structures made up of abstractions or general knowledge about the attributes of a stimulus domain, and the relationships among these attributes (Horowitz, 1991). Stored in memory as generalizations from specific experiences and prototypes of specific cases, schemas provide focus and meaning for incoming information. Although not in our conscious awareness, they direct our attention to those elements of our day-to-day experience that are most important for our survival and adaptation. Individuals tend to assimilate their experiences in response to preexisting schemas rather than to accommodate schemas to events that are unexpected or discrepant (Kovacs & Beck, 1978); that is, we tend to make sense of new experiences in terms of what we already believe rather than by changing our preexisting views.

In addition to representations and prototypical exemplars of specific events, schemas also incorporate emotions or "affective valences" related to the events. Events in one's life activate both ideational and emotional content. Cognitive schemas, as a result, might more accurately be described as cognitive–emotional structures (Greenberg & Safran, 1987). They are postulated to account for consistencies in behavior over time and for continuities in one's sense of self throughout one's life. Schemas are often strongly held and are seen as essential for the person's safety, well-being, or existence. Schemas that are consolidated early in life and powerfully reinforced by significant others are often highly valent in the personality style of the individual.

Recent work on schemas has identified certain representative schemas that form the basis of psychopathology for each disorder (Riso, du Toit, Stein, & Young, 2007). For example, highly sociotropic or autonomous personality styles may make an individual more vulnerable to depression. Highly sociotropic individuals have "interpersonal schemas" (Safran, Vallis, Segal, & Shaw, 1986) that are cognitive representations of interactions with others, such as attachment figures that maintain individual relationships. An example is the belief that when I ask for support, others will reject me. On the other hand, highly autonomous individuals focus on achievement and may have schemas about failure or success, such as "If I fail, I will be rejected." In both cases we can see how schemas shape an individual's personality, with a focus on either relatedness or achievement. Schemas are reviewed in greater depth in the subsequent section on psychopathology, but it is essential to note that cognitive schemas form the basis of individual's personality styles according to cognitive theory, and that the growing emphasis on personality in cognitive therapy has led to an surge in the practice of, and the amount of research on, schema-focused therapies. Additionally, books on the treatment of personality disorders now often include a cognitive component that recognizes the importance of schemas to the formation of personality (e.g., Millon, 1999).

PSYCHOLOGICAL HEALTH AND PATHOLOGY

Our "meaning system," our knowledge base, and ways of processing information are organized and coherent. From this perspective, human behavior is both goal directed and generative. It is based on rules and tacit beliefs that are elaborated and consolidated over the course of an individual's life. Cognitive processes, emotional responses, and behavioral skills are adaptive. Cognitive processes are seen as playing a central role in organizing our responses both to daily events and to long-term challenges. Therefore, schemas form the basis of both "healthy" personalities and those of individuals with psychopathology. The standard cognitive therapy model posits that three variables play a central role in the formation and maintenance of common psychological disorders: the cognitive triad, schemas, and cognitive distortions (Beck et al., 1979). These three variables are also present for individuals without psychopathology, and the distinction between adaptive cognitions and cognitions that have become maladaptive for an individual are described in each case.

The Cognitive Triad

The construct of the cognitive triad was first proposed by Beck (1963) as a means of describing the negativistic thoughts of depressed inpatients. He observed that the thoughts of depressed individuals typically include highly negative views of self, the world, and the future. The thoughts of anxious clients, in contrast, tend to differ from those of depressed individuals in each of these domains. They tend to view the world or others as potentially threatening, and to maintain a vigilant and wary orientation toward their future. The concept of the cognitive triad, then, serves as a useful framework for examining the automatic thoughts and tacit assumptions that clients describe. Virtually all client problems can be related to maladaptive or dysfunctional beliefs in one of these three areas. As a result, when beginning therapy, it is often helpful to inquire as to clients' thoughts in each of these areas. Because clients' beliefs and attitudes are quite idiosyncratic, we should anticipate that the specific content of their thoughts regarding the self, the world, and the future will differ. By assessing the degree of contribution of thoughts in each of these areas to clients' distress, the therapist can begin to develop a conceptualization of their concerns.

Schemas

The concept of schemas plays an important role in cognitive models of emotional and behavioral problems. Schemas are maintained, elaborated, and consolidated through processes of assimilation and are changed through accommodation to novel experiences (Rosen, 1989). Schemas are developed over the course of an individual's infancy and childhood. Early maladaptive schemas typically are seen as serving an adaptive function and may represent internalizations of ongoing or repetitious parental behavior. The parent who is unsupportive, punitive, or unpredictable toward his or her infant, for example, will likely behave in a similar manner during later years. The child's nascent beliefs that "my needs won't be met by others," "I am flawed or inadequate," and "I must submit to the control of others to avoid punishment" are initially represented nonverbally as subjective encodings of interactive experiences, and are elaborated and consolidated by later events. They are reified as procedural memories, tacit beliefs, or representations about the self and the world— they become the "givens" of life. Tacit beliefs or schemas are activated by events that are similar to early experiences surrounding their development (Ingram, 1984). These tacit rules, assumptions, and beliefs serve as the wellspring of the various cognitive distortions seen in clients. As the activation of the memory spreads throughout the associative links of the schema's network, other memories, exemplars, expectations, and emotions related to the event are activated. If the schemas are elaborate, individuals become preoccupied with the event. As thoughts about personal weakness, hopelessness, and unremitting disappointment gain predominance, individuals become less active and socially engaged, and their mood becomes increasingly depressed and hopeless. People's observations of themselves in this state only provide further evidence of their inadequacy and contribute to a worsening of their interpersonal problems.

The precise content of schemas is not typically open to introspection or rational disputation. Nonetheless, basic categories for classifying events can be inferred from monitoring the types of information that are most frequently remembered and used (Kovacs & Beck, 1978). In the schema therapy model, *early maladaptive schemas* are presumed to occur in five main domains: (1) disconnection and rejection, in which an individual perceives instability in interpersonal connections; (2) impaired autonomy and performance, in which one has difficulty functioning independently and successfully differentiating self from others; (3) impaired limits in regard to reciprocity and self-discipline; (4) other-directedness that focuses on the needs of others while neglecting one's own needs; and (5) overvigilance and inhibition that involve suppression of one's own impulses and feelings, and an internalization of rigid rules about one's functioning (Young et al., 2003). Highly depressed persons, for example, often maintain the schemas "I'm defective" (impaired autonomy and performance) and "people are unreliable" (disconnection and rejection). Highly angry individuals, in contrast, may or may not believe they are flawed or defective. They do, however, tend to believe that "the world is dangerous" (overvigilance/inhibition), and that "people are malicious" (disconnection and rejection). Although not present in these individuals' daily thoughts, these beliefs strongly influence their behavioral and emotional reactions.

Cognitive Distortions

A potentially infinite amount of information impinges on us in our day-to-day lives. As a result, we must selectively attend to those events or stimuli that are most important to our adaptation and survival. Some events are examined, recalled, and reflected on; others are overlooked, ignored, and forgotten as uninteresting or unimportant. Because our attentional capacities and ability to process information are limited, some distortion of our experiences necessarily *must* occur. An individual's perceptions, memories, and thoughts can become distorted in a variety of adaptive and maladaptive ways. Some individuals may, for example, view life in an unrealistically positive way and perceive that they have control or influence that they may not, in reality, possess. They may take chances that most people would avoid—such as starting a new business or investing in a risky new stock. If successful, the individual is vindicated and may be envied for his or her *chutzpah,* or nerve. Such distortions can, however, be problematic, in that they may lead individuals to take chances that may result in great danger; they might, for example, experience massive chest pains and not consult a physician due to the belief "nothing will happen to me. I'm too young and healthy for a heart attack."

Negative or maladaptive distortions typically become the focus of therapy. One task in treatment is to examine these distortions and assist clients to recognize the impact on functioning. Distortions represent maladaptive ways of processing information and may become emblematic of a particular style of behaving or of certain clinical syndromes. Like many constructs, how we define and understand notions such as "rationality," "distortion," "adaptiveness," "maladaptiveness," and "bias" has important philosophical and practical implications. They should be carefully scrutinized. Typical distortions and examples of the common clinical correlates include the following:

1. *Dichotomous thinking.* "Things are black or white"; "You're with me or against me." This tendency toward "all-or-nothing" thinking is encountered in borderline personality and obsessive–compulsive disorders.
2. *Mind reading.* "They probably think that I'm incompetent"; "I just know that they will disapprove." This processing style is common in avoidant and paranoid personality disorders.
3. *Emotional reasoning.* "I feel inadequate, so I must be inadequate"; "I'm feeling upset, so there must be something wrong." This distortion is common among individuals suffering from anxiety disorders.
4. *Personalization.* "That comment wasn't just random, I know it was directed toward me." At the extreme, this is common in avoidant and paranoid personality disorders.
5. *Overgeneralization.* "Everything I do turns out wrong"; "It doesn't matter what my choices are, they always fall flat." At the extreme, this is common among depressed individuals.
6. *Catastrophizing.* "If I go to the party, there will be terrible consequences"; "It would be devastating if I failed this exam"; "My heart's beating faster, it's got to be a heart attack." This distortion is characteristic of anxiety disorders, especially social anxiety, social phobia, and panic.
7. *"Should" statements.* "I should visit my family every time they want me to"; "They should do what I say because it is right." This is common in obsessive–compulsive disorders and among individuals who feel excessive guilt.
8. *Selective abstraction.* "The rest of the information doesn't matter. This is the salient point"; "I've got to focus on the negative details; the positive things that have happened don't count." At the extreme, this is common in depression.

THE PROCESS OF CLINICAL ASSESSMENT

Identifying specific problems and objectively evaluating the effectiveness of interventions are essential parts of cognitive psychotherapy. Assessment instruments, including self-report questionnaires, behavior rating scales, and clinician rating scales, can be quite useful in this regard. They are frequently administered at the beginning of treatment and at later points.

A large number of well-validated rating scales have been developed in recent years; it is beyond the scope of this chapter to review them. However, we have found several of them to be particularly useful and deserving of note. Among these are the Dysfunctional Attitudes Scale (DAS; Weissman & Beck, 1978; Beck, Brown, Steer, & Weissman, 1991) and the Young Schema Questionnaire (YSQ; Young, 1991). The DAS is used to measure dysfunctional attributions that are thought to make one vulnerable to psychopathology (typically depression). The YSQ is used more generally to assess early maladaptive schemas that could lead to multiple types of psychopathology.

When depression is a primary concern, the Beck Depression Inventory (BDI) is among the most useful tools available to the therapist. The BDI-II (Beck, Steer, & Brown, 1996) is among the most widely used self-report measures for depression in the world and is a well-accepted, reliable, and valid measure of depressed mood. The administration of a self-report depression scale, such as the BDI-II, prior to each session can provide objective data regarding therapeutic progress and can assist in identifying the specific focus of a client's depression. When anxiety is a target symptom, the Beck Anxiety Inventory (BAI), a 21-item self-report symptom checklist designed to measure the severity of anxiety-related symptoms (Beck, Epstein, Brown, & Steer, 1988), the Zung Anxiety Rating Scale (ZARS; Zung, 1971), or the State–Trait Anxiety Inventory (STAI; Spielberger, Gorsuch, Lushene, Vagg, & Jacobs, 1983) may be used. These measures provide a useful, objective measure of the client's general level of anxiety and can be used both quantitatively and qualitatively as a diagnostic aid.

The Beck Hopelessness Scale (BHS) is a brief and highly useful measure of pessimism (Beck, Weissman, Lester, & Trexler, 1974). Because levels of hopelessness are often highly correlated with suicide potential, the BHS can be used in conjunction with a measure of depression as a means of estimating suicide risk (Freeman & Reinecke, 1993).

Assessment of Vulnerability Factors

There are circumstances, situations, or deficits that have the effect of decreasing the client's ability to cope effectively with life's challenges. These factors lower the client's tolerance for stress and may serve to increase suicidal thinking, lower the threshold for anxiety stimuli, or increase vulnerability to depressogenic thoughts and situations (Freeman & Simon, 1989). These include (1) acute or chronic illness, (2) hunger, (3) fatigue, (4) major or minor stressful events, (5) loss of social support or an important relationship, (6) alcohol and substance abuse, (7) chronic pain, and (8) new life circumstances. An essential component of cognitive therapy is to use an unstructured or structured interview to assess for vulnerability factors that may be the diathesis that puts an individual at risk for psychopathology by activating negative schemas and automatic thoughts.

In addition, issues of diversity, such as acknowledging life stressors or circumstances due to an individual's cultural background, expectations for and motivations to pursue therapy, limitations to engage in therapy due to poverty, cultural barriers, linguistic/communication barriers, or exposure to unique stressors (e.g., discrimination or acculturative stress) are important areas for assessment and can aid in conceptualization of the client's problems. Culturally sensitive interventions can include increasing social supports and access to social or community resources, alleviating stressors, and improving coping skills.

THE PRACTICE OF THERAPY

A common element across cognitive-behavioral models is an emphasis on helping clients to examine the manner in which they construe or understand themselves and their world (cognitions), and to experiment with new ways of responding (behavioral). By learning to understand the idiosyncratic ways they perceive themselves, the world, and their prospects for the future, clients can be helped to alter negative emotions and to behave more adaptively. In practice, cognitive therapy sessions are (1) structured, active, and problem oriented; (2) time-limited and strategic; (3) psychoeducational; (4) based on constructivist models of thought and behavior; and (5) collaborative.

Cognitive therapy attempts to identify specific, measurable goals and to move quickly and directly into those areas that create the most difficulty for the client. The approach is similar in this regard to contemporary short-term dynamic and interpersonal psychotherapy. Cognitive therapy does not presume to protect individuals from experiencing distress in the future. Anxiety, depression, and guilt can play an essential and adaptive role in people's lives. Instead, cognitive therapy endeavors not to alleviate these emotions but to provide clients with skills for understanding and managing them.

One reason that individuals experience difficulty coping with internal or external stimuli is a lack of adaptive skills. Cognitive and behavioral skills typically emerge over the course of one's development through structured interactions with supportive caregivers. Developmentally important competencies include the ability to regulate affective arousal, interpersonal, or social skills; the ability to direct and maintain one's attention; and cognitive skills (including executive functions and formal operational thought). An important component of cognitive therapy is to enhance clients' skills and sense of personal competence so that they can more effectively deal with life stressors and have a greater sense of control and self-efficacy.

Cognitive Therapy in Action

Before therapeutic change can occur, a trusting therapeutic collaboration must be established. The first goal in cognitive therapy, then, is to establish rapport through empathic, active listening. Clients need to feel that they are heard, and that their concerns are understood and acknowledged by their therapist. The cognitive therapist encourages and facilitates client speech and promotes the experience of affect in the therapy session. The cognitive therapist also identifies recurrent patterns in the client's behavior and thoughts, points out the use of maladaptive coping strategies or distortions, and draws attention to feelings and thoughts the client may find disturbing. Before specific interventions are made, however, the therapist carefully reviews a client's developmental, familial, social, cultural, occupational, educational, medical, and psychiatric history. These data are useful in helping to turn a client's presenting complaints into a working problem list and a treatment conceptualization (Persons, 2008).

The establishment of a problem list gives both client and therapist an idea of where the therapy is going, a general time frame, and a means of assessing therapeutic progress. The identification of an agenda item leads directly into an examination of the client's emotions and thoughts in a recent situation. Setting an agenda at the beginning of each session allows both client and therapist to bring out issues of concern for discussion. Moreover, it allows for continuity between sessions, so that sessions are not individual events but part of a cohesive whole. The collaborative process may be empowering, because it allows for the co-creation of therapeutic goals. This may be particularly useful for clients from racial/ethnic minorities or disadvantaged backgrounds, because it may help "demystify" the therapy experience for individuals who are unfamiliar with the goals of typical therapy or whose culture may have general prohibitions against obtaining mental health services. A typical agenda might include the following:

1. Discussion of events during the past week and feelings about the prior therapy session.
2. A review of self-report scales filled out by the client prior to the session.
3. A review of agenda items remaining from the previous session.
4. A review of the client's homework. The client's success or problems in doing the homework are discussed, as are the results of the assignment.
5. Current problems that are put on the agenda might involve the development of specific skills (e.g., social skills, relaxation training, or assertiveness skills) or the examination of dysfunctional thoughts.

Each session concludes with a review or summary of the session and gives the client an opportunity to clarify goals, as well as skills, techniques, or insights, that have been discussed. A homework assignment for the next session and factors that may impede its completion are addressed. Finally, the client is asked for his or her response to the session.

Problem Conceptualization and Treatment Planning

After the therapist conducts a comprehensive assessment, the problem conceptualization forms the foundation for a targeted treatment plan. The conceptualization must be (1) useful, (2) parsimonious, and (3) theoretically coherent. It should explain past behavior, make sense of current difficulties, predict future behavior, and yield pragmatic recommendations. The conceptualization process begins with the compilation of a specific, behaviorally based problem list, which is then prioritized. A particular problem may be the primary focus of therapy because of its debilitating effect on the individual. In another case, one may focus on the simplest problem first, thereby giving the client a sense of confidence in the therapy itself, as well as practice in basic problem solving. In a third case, the initial focus might be on a "keystone" problem—that is, a problem whose solution will cause a ripple effect in solving other problems or which is high-risk, such as ongoing suicidal ideation.

The case formulation of the client's problems allows the therapist to develop strategies and interventions individualized to the particular client. As part of this formulation, the therapist develops hypotheses about what reinforces and maintains dysfunctional thinking and behavior, including idiosyncratic thinking patterns and automatic thoughts. A formulation may include a description of beliefs that are either adaptive or maladaptive, and the degree to which these beliefs are held. It is useful to discuss with a client the strength with which he or she believes key automatic thoughts or assumptions. Automatic thoughts containing the phrase "I am _____" can be particularly difficult to change, because they may be statements of a client's actual self-schemas. One young woman, whose frequent and vociferous complaining had led her to be fired at work and to be dropped from the lead role in a theatrical production, stated, "I know I make people defensive, but it's just who I am, and they have to accept me for that. . . . I'm just identifying problems I see for people who are the authorities, so they have to change them. . . . I *can't* change who I am." A formulation should describe the content and structure of maladaptive thinking patterns that are causing the client's distress, impairing functioning, or causing unwanted emotional, behavioral, or cognitive responses. An effective formulation identifies an individual's cognitive distortions, maladaptive beliefs, and the potential schemas that underlie them. Providing an understanding of what may be maintaining the patient's distress may also help to instill a sense of hope and personal efficacy.

Specific Interventions

Interventions should be chosen specifically to address the distortions, maladaptive beliefs, and hypothesized schemas identified in the case formulation that underlie identified problem behaviors. The precise mix of cognitive and behavioral techniques will depend on the client's abilities, the level of pathology, and the specific treatment goals. When working with severely depressed clients, for example, initial treatment goals might center on facilitating behavioral activity, improving self-care, and reducing social isolation.

Pharmacotherapy may be an important adjunct in the therapy program. Cognitive therapy and pharmacotherapy are not mutually exclusive but can be integrated into an effective treatment program. In addition to its value in modifying dysfunctional thoughts or maladaptive behavior that contribute to clients' feelings of dysphoria, anxiety, or anger, cognitive therapy can also be used to improve medication compliance. Maladaptive thoughts, such as "This just proves I'm crazy" and "This means there must be something wrong with my brain," may be quite distressing and undermine treatment compliance. Use of pharmacotherapy alone might not address these beliefs. Antidepressant medications typically take several weeks before improvement is seen. Cognitive therapy, however, can be helpful in a short period and may provide depressed clients with a sense of relief before the medications can be titrated effectively.

Cognitive Techniques

Cognitive techniques may be defined as any intervention or technique that alters a client's perceptions or beliefs. The number of techniques that are potentially available is virtually infinite. Therapists should teach these skills, so that their clients can "become their own therapist." These techniques have been described in detail elsewhere (e.g., Persons, Davidson, & Tompkins, 2001).

IDIOSYNCRATIC MEANING

In many ways, our constructs determine our perceptions. All words carry an idiosyncratic or personal meaning. The exploration of these meanings models the need for active listening skills, increased communication, and the value of examining one's assumptions. The meanings attached to the client's words and thoughts can be explored. The client who believes, for example, that he will be "devastated" by his spouse leaving might be asked, in a supportive manner, what he means by "devastated." He may be asked to reflect on exactly how he would be devastated, and then on the ways he might be spared from "devastation." This may be particularly important for individuals from diverse cultural backgrounds, because the meaning of "common" difficulties such as depression may be experienced and conceptualized differently across cultures. For instance, individuals from Eastern countries sometimes describe "depression" as a feeling of emptiness or loss of a sense of self, whereas, people from Western cultures may describe depression more typically as feeling "down" or "low." Similarly, some clients from non-Western cultures might express psychological distress using idioms that are specific to their culture, such as *nervios*, which encompasses both somatic and psychological components. Exploring these words and terms and what they mean not only for the client but also within the cultural context may help to elucidate specific meaning attached to the construct by the client.

QUESTIONING THE EVIDENCE

This technique involves systematically examining evidence in support of a belief, as well as evidence that is inconsistent with it. The reliability of the sources of the information might be examined, and the individual might come to recognize that he or she has overlooked information that is inconsistent with his or her beliefs. It is important that a clinician question the evidence for the beliefs in a true "spirit of inquiry." The focus should not be on "begging the question" or asking leading questions whose intent is apparent, because this may cause clients to feel that they need to give the "right" answer, or that they are failing, and they may become defensive.

REATTRIBUTION

Clients often take responsibility for events and situations that are only minimally attributable to them. A therapist can help a client distribute responsibility among all relevant parties.

RATIONAL RESPONDING

One of the most powerful techniques in cognitive therapy involves helping the client to challenge dysfunctional thinking. The Dysfunctional Thought Record (DTR) is an ideal format for testing maladaptive beliefs. The process begins with a client identifying the thought, emotion, or situation that causes difficulty. If the client presents with an emotional issue (e.g., "I'm very sad"), the therapist may inquire as to the situations that engender the emotion and the attendant thoughts. If the client presents with a thought (e.g., "I'm a loser"), the therapist ascertains the feelings and the situation. Finally, if the client presents with a situation (e.g., "My husband left me"), the therapist endeavors to determine the thoughts and emotions that precede, accompany, and follow the event. Statements such as "I feel like a loser" are reframed as thoughts, and the accompanying emotions are elicited. After the automatic thought has been identified, a "rational response" can be developed. Rational responding involves four steps: (1) a systematic examination of evidence supporting and refuting the belief; (2) the development of an alternative, more adaptive explanation or belief; (3) decatastrophizing the belief; and (4) identifying specific behavioral steps to cope with the problem.

EXAMINING OPTIONS AND ALTERNATIVES

This involves working with clients to generate additional options. Suicidal clients, for example, often see their alternatives as so limited that death becomes a viable solution. Clients can be assisted to develop, then evaluate, alternative solutions.

DECATASTROPHIZING

Clients are taught to examine whether they are overestimating the severity of a situation or the likelihood of a negative outcome. Through Socratic questioning they are encouraged to "keep the problem in perspective."

FANTASIZED CONSEQUENCES

Clients are asked to describe a fantasy about a feared situation, their images of it, and the attendant concerns. In verbalizing their fantasies, clients can often see the irrationality of their ideas. If the fantasized consequences are realistic, then the therapist can work with a client to assess the danger and develop coping strategies.

ADVANTAGES AND DISADVANTAGES

By asking the client to examine both the advantages and disadvantages of both sides of an issue, the therapist can help the client achieve a broader perspective. This basic problem-solving technique is useful in gaining a perspective, then plotting a reasonable course of action.

TURNING ADVERSITY TO ADVANTAGE

There are times when a seeming disaster can be used to advantage. Having a deadline imposed may be seen as oppressive and unfair, but it may be used as a motivator. Clients are assisted in identifying strengths or competencies they have acquired through overcoming past adversities.

GUIDED ASSOCIATION/DISCOVERY

In contrast to the psychodynamic technique of free association, in guided association or discovery, the therapist works with the client to identify relationships between ideas, thoughts, and images by means of Socratic questioning. Also referred to as the "vertical" or "downward arrow" technique, the therapist encourages the client to identify a series of automatic thoughts. The use of statements such as "And then what?" or "And that means what?" allows the therapist to guide the client toward an understanding of themes within implicit automatic thoughts and to identify possible underlying schemas.

PARADOXICAL INTERVENTIONS

By taking an idea to its extreme, the therapist can help to move the client to a more moderate or adaptive position vis-à-vis a particular belief and, paradoxically, cause the client to develop a sense of control over an "uncontrollable" symptom. For instance, providing homework of "worrying" (for those with generalized anxiety disorder) or "crying" (for those who are depressed) during a given time period may allow clients to see that they have some measure of control over when they choose to engage in a behavior. However, therapists who employ these techniques must do so carefully, flexibly, and in the context of a strong working relationship, because some clients may view such interventions as making light of their problems.

SCALING

The technique of scaling along a continuum can be quite useful to counteract all-or-nothing thinking. Scaling of emotions, for example, can lead a client to gain a sense of distance and perspective. A depressed client who believes that he is "incompetent," for example, might first be asked to rate the strength of his belief in this statement on a 100-point scale. He can then be asked to establish anchor points for his belief—identifying the "most incompetent person in the world" (0) and the "most highly skilled and competent person in the world" (100). When asked to rate himself on the "competence scale" he has developed, he typically would recognize that he is neither entirely incompetent nor the most competent individual, but that, like others, he has strengths and weaknesses, and at least a modicum of competence.

EXTERNALIZATION OF VOICES

Most individuals, when asked to reflect on their thoughts, can "hear" the voice of their thoughts in their head. When clients are asked to externalize these thoughts, they are in a better position to deal with these "voices" and thoughts. By having the therapist take the part of the dysfunctional voice, a client can gain experience in responding adaptively. The therapist might begin, for example, by modeling rational responses to a client's verbalizations of dysfunctional thoughts. With practice, the client comes to recognize the dysfunctional nature of the thoughts and becomes better able to respond adaptively to them.

SELF-INSTRUCTION

Meichenbaum (2009) and Rehm (2009) developed extensive batteries of self-instruction techniques that are useful in working with depressed or impulsive clients. Clients can be taught, for example, to offer direct self-instructions for more adaptive behavior, as well as counterinstructions to avoid dysfunctional behavior.

THOUGHT STOPPING

Given the relationship between thoughts and mood, maladaptive automatic thoughts can have a "snowball effect," in that even mild feelings of dysphoria or anxiety can bias subsequent cognitive processes, leading the individual to feel continually more distraught. Thought stopping is best used when the negative emotional state is first recognized. Anxious clients, for example, can be taught to picture a stop sign or "hear a bell" at the outset of an anxiety attack. This momentary break in the process allows them to reflect on the origin of the anxiety and to introduce more powerful cognitive techniques (e.g., rational responding) before their anxiety escalates.

DISTRACTION

This technique is especially helpful for clients with anxiety problems. Because it is almost impossible to maintain two thoughts simultaneously, anxiogenic thoughts generally preclude more adaptive thinking. Conversely, a focused thought distracts from the anxiogenic thoughts. By focusing on complex counting, addition, or subtraction, clients are rather easily distracted from other thoughts. Having clients count to 200 by 13's, for example, can be effective, as can reading a page of text upside down. When outdoors, counting cars, people wearing the color red, or any other cognitively engaging task will suffice.

DIRECT DISPUTATION

When there is an imminent risk to the client, as in the case of suicide, the therapist might consider direct disputation. Because this approach is in some regard noncollaborative, the therapist risks becoming embroiled in a power struggle or argument with the client. Disputation of core beliefs may, in fact, engender avoidance or a passive–aggressive response. Disputation, argument, or debate must be used carefully, judiciously, and with skill.

LABELING OF DISTORTIONS

Fear of the unknown and "fear of fear" can be important concerns for anxious clients. The more that can be done to identify the nature and content of the dysfunctional thoughts and to help label the types of distortions that clients use, the less frightening the entire process becomes. Clients can be taught to identify and label specific distortions during the therapy session and can be asked to practice the exercise at home. This can be accomplished with the aid of a "thought record" on which clients record their automatic thoughts on an ongoing basis during the day, or with a counter with which they simply record the frequency of the thoughts.

DEVELOPING REPLACEMENT IMAGERY

Many anxious clients experience vivid images during times of stress. Clients can be helped by training in the development of "coping images." For example, rather than imagining failure, defeat, or embarrassment, the therapist assists the client to develop a new, effective coping image. Once well practiced, clients can substitute these images outside the therapy session. ·

BIBLIOTHERAPY

Several excellent books can be assigned as readings for homework. These books can be used to educate clients about the basic cognitive therapy model, emphasize specific points made in the session, introduce new ideas for discussion, or offer alternative ways of thinking about clients' concerns. Some helpful books include *Love Is Never Enough* (Beck, 1989), *Feeling Good* (Burns, 1980), *Mind over Mood* (Greenberger & Padesky, 1995); and *The Anxiety and Phobia Workbook* (Bourne, 2005).

ACT TECHNIQUES

Many techniques used within ACT focus on clients examining and distancing themselves from their cognitions, and encourage examination of problems in the context of client's own experiences. These techniques can include discussing with the client the paradoxical effect of trying to deny or control one's thoughts, which often causes an increase in unwanted thoughts and feelings. ACT also uses several techniques to promote distance from one's thoughts, such as exercises thast encourage the client to view his or her thoughts as if cognitions are "soldiers on parade," so that the client is looking *at* thoughts, not *from* thoughts. In addition, acceptance is promoted through encouraging clients to observe and experience their thoughts and emotions nonjudgmentally as they are (Hayes, 2004).

Behavioral Techniques

Traditional behavioral techniques (see Antony & Roemer, Chapter 4, this volume) are regularly used in CBT. However, the rationale for the use of behavioral techniques differs from that of traditional behavioral therapy. In behavior therapy, adaptive behavior changes are the goal of treatment. In cognitive therapy, adaptive behavioral changes that result from behavioral techniques are indeed viewed as desirable, but behavioral techniques are used primarily to facilitate cognitive changes. Using behavioral techniques, especially at the beginning of stages of therapy, is viewed as important not only to change maladaptive behavior patterns, but also to instill hope and to provide for early success in therapy. For instance, Beck et al. (1979) noted that severely depressed clients might benefit first from behavioral techniques, such as activity scheduling, in order to provide a foundation for eventually challenging their hopelessness about the future and their negative view of self.

Behavioral interventions facilitate cognitive changes by directly challenging a client's faulty assumptions, rules, and ultimately core beliefs. Successful completion of behavioral tasks and skills development, including coping and distress tolerance skills, can enhance an individual's sense of mastery and self-efficacy, and may be particularly beneficial to challenge inaccurate or faulty self-schemas that center on being helpless, ineffectual, powerless, weak, or incompetent. The use of behavioral experiments that encourage a client to engage in a behavior and observe the consequences can help to correct faulty assumptions. For example, catastrophizing can be challenged if the client who engages in the avoided behavior has the opportunity to observe that the extremely severe, feared consequence does not occur. As with cognitive homework assignments, the therapist reviews the thoughts and emotions experienced as clients attempt the behavioral assignments, and uses behavioral assignments strategically and carefully to facilitate clients' success and minimize the chance of failure to perform the task.

Homework

No therapy takes place solely within the confines of the consulting room. Insights and skills gained within the therapeutic milieu, by their nature, may be consolidated and employed in the client's day-to-day life. Practicing cognitive-behavioral skills at home allows for a greater therapeutic focus and more rapid gains.

Homework assignments can be either cognitive or behavioral. They might involve having the client complete an activity schedule (an excellent homework for the first session) or try a new behavior. The homework assignment, when appropriately assigned, should flow directly from the session material. It is an extension of the skills developed during the therapy hour into the client's daily life. It is important to review homework assignments each week, reward progress, and troubleshoot around obstacles or barriers to completion. If homework assignments are not regularly discussed, clients come to see them as unimportant and stop doing them.

Challenges

Noncompliance, sometimes called resistance, often carries the implication that the client does not want to change or "get well" for either conscious or unconscious reasons. Leahy (2001) defines *resistance* as "anything in the client's behavior, thinking, affective response, and interpersonal style that interferes with the ability of that client to utilize the treatment and to acquire the ability to handle problems outside of therapy" (p. 11). Resistance may be manifested directly (e.g., tardiness or missed appointments and failure to complete homework) or more subtly through omissions in the material reported in the sessions. Clinically, we can identify several reasons for noncompliance. They may be due to failure on the therapist's part to validate the client's beliefs and experience, or to a general lack of skill. Noncompliance may also be due to client factors, such as poorly developed coping skills, environmental stressors, or hopelessness. Shared variables, such as lack of a good therapeutic alliance and collaborative relationship, can make progress especially difficult.

When working cross-culturally, it is important to distinguish between psychological reasons for noncompliance and cultural or socioeconomic barriers that directly interfere with one's ability to comply with treatment. Cultural barriers may include linguistic difficulties that contribute to miscommunications or misunderstandings in terms of the rationale of therapeutic interventions or cultural prohibitions against participating in psychotherapy. Socioeconomic barriers may include transportation difficulties and unpredictable or stressful home, work, or school environments that may interfere with the timely completion of homework. For these clients, approaches that focus on a therapeutic relationship may be appropriate, such as schema therapy approaches. Challenges must be identified and collaboratively addressed.

Common Therapist Errors

Mistakes occur during the practice of cognitive therapy, and knowledge of common errors can help us avoid them. These include (1) inadequate socialization of the patient to the model; (2) failure to develop a specific problem list or to share a rationale with the patient; (3) not assigning appropriate homework (and not following up on completed homework assignments); (4) premature emphasis on identifying schemas; (5) therapist impatience and becoming overly directive during therapy in an attempt to resolve the patient's symptoms immediately; (6) premature introduction of rational techniques (before a formulation has been completed); (7) lack of attention to developing a trusting collaborative rapport and inadequate attention to "nonspecific factors" of the therapy relationship; and (8) not attending to the therapist's own emotional reactions, automatic thoughts, and schemas—the countertransference.

Termination

Termination in cognitive therapy begins in the first session. Because the goal of cognitive therapy is not cure per se but more effective coping, the cognitive therapist does not plan for therapy in perpetuity. As a skills acquisition model of psychotherapy, the therapist's goal is to assist clients in acquiring the capacity to deal with internal and external stressors that are a part of life. When objective rating scales, client reports, therapist observations, and feedback from significant others confirm improvement and a higher level of adaptive abilities, the therapy can move toward termination. The final sessions typically include a review of the client's presenting concerns, cognitive and behavioral skills developed over the course of treatment, and a discussion of upcoming events that may precipitate a relapse. Clients are taught to distinguish a lapse from a relapse, and coping strategies for managing difficult life circumstances are reviewed and practiced. Particular attention is paid to cognitive and behavioral factors associated with relapse (e.g., perfectionism, excessive reassurance seeking, negative attributional style, hopelessness, and low personal efficacy). Goals during the final phase of treatment, then, center on consolidating gains and relapse prevention.

Although numerous outcome studies have found that cognitive therapy can be highly effective in 12–15 sessions, there is no typical duration for the treatment. In assisting clients with more severe or chronic difficulties, for example, we have found that meaningful gains can be achieved within several weeks as clients learn cognitive and behavioral techniques for coping with their feelings of depression, anxiety, and anger. However, cognitive therapy can profitably continue for 2–3 years, as the assumptions and schemas underlying clients' difficulties are examined and addressed. With this in mind, we have often found it useful to discuss the expected duration of therapy with clients at the outset, and to negotiate a termination date or a set number of sessions in advance. This process encourages both therapist and client to maintain a problem focus and a sense of urgency in the treatment.

Termination in cognitive therapy is accomplished gradually to allow time for ongoing modifications and corrections. Sessions are tapered off from once weekly to biweekly. From that point, sessions can be set on a monthly basis, with follow-up sessions at 3 and 6 months, until therapy is ended. Clients can, of course, still call for an appointment in the event of an emergency. As the conclusion of treatment nears, the client's thoughts and feelings about the termination are carefully explored, as are schemas and assumptions regarding separation. Termination can afford the therapist an opportunity to explore with clients their thoughts, feelings, and characteristic ways of coping with separations.

THE THERAPEUTIC RELATIONSHIP AND THE STANCE OF THE THERAPIST

As client-centered therapists have observed, therapists who are "nonpossessively warm," empathic, and genuine achieve greater gains than do those who are not. Cognitive therapy recognizes the central importance of these nonspecific relationship variables in facilitating change but views them as "necessary but not sufficient" for therapeutic improvement; that is, the development of a warm, empathic, and genuine relationship is not necessarily accompanied by behavioral or emotional change. That being said, forming an empathic, collaborative therapeutic relationship is an essential first step in cognitive therapy, especially when dealing with clients with personality disorders or psychoses. Without trust and understanding, all of the techniques that follow lack a necessary foundation.

Cultural mistrust, or "healthy cultural paranoia" may occur in cross-cultural dyads, whereby a minority group client may exhibit an initial level of distrust of the therapist or the psychotherapeutic process due to previous experiences with being negatively stereotyped or discriminated against (Sue & Sue, 2007). When relevant, the therapist should demonstrate patience and be prepared openly to acknowledge cross-racial or cross-cultural differences in a nondefensive and open manner in order to facilitate the development of trust. CBT has often been called "collaborative empiricism," and the therapeutic relationship is essential to that collaboration.

The transference relationship also plays an important role in cognitive therapy (Reinecke, 2002). The client's behavior toward the therapist may reflect the activation of schemas (as might the therapist's behavioral and emotional responses to the client). The client's experiences during the therapy hour, as a consequence, can serve as evidence to dispute tacit beliefs. Moreover, schemas activated in the therapeutic relationship can in many ways be similar to those activated in clients' relationships with others. The therapist works, through the use of Socratic questioning, to develop greater awareness in clients of their thoughts, feelings, and perceptions—including those about the therapeutic relationship. Cognitive therapy understands transference and countertransference from a social learning perspective and uses experiences within the therapeutic relationship as a means of clarifying and changing tacit beliefs and maladaptive interpersonal patterns.

The therapist's directiveness can be adjusted over the course of treatment depending on the needs of the client. However, in comparison with psychodynamic or humanistic therapies, CBT is generally considered, like behavioral therapy, to be directive. With a highly depressed client, immobilized by psychomotor retardation and feelings of hopelessness, the therapist may want to adopt a more assertive, directive stance. In contrast, a less directive stance might be employed with a highly passive and dependent client.

EFFICACY AND EFFECTIVENESS

Does cognitive therapy work? The results of empirical outcome studies have generally been both supportive and promising (Butler, Chapman, Forman, & Beck, 2006). In efficacy research, cognitive therapy typically contains behavioral components and is frequently considered to be the same as CBT. Both are distinguished from behavioral therapy by the inclusion of cognitive components (Butler et al., 2006). The efficacy of CBT has been so well established over the years that the focus is no longer on meta-analyses that combine studies into an overall picture of how well CBT works, but on combining the meta-analyses themselves (Butler et al., 2006). CBT is one of the most rigorously investigated empirically supported treatments. A comprehensive review of studies confirming the efficacy of CBT for each disorder is beyond the scope of this chapter, but has been conducted by Butler and colleagues in a rigorous meta-analysis of 16 meta-analyses including 9,995 subjects and 332 studies. These researchers found that by 2006, the number of outcome studies on CBT numbered over 325, and that number has assuredly grown rapidly in the 4 years since publication. They reported that CBT is highly effective in the treatment of depression, generalized anxiety disorder, panic with and without agoraphobia, social phobia, posttraumatic stress disorder, and childhood depression and anxiety disorder. CBT is still effective, although somewhat less so, for the treatment of marital distress, anger management, childhood somatic disorder, and chronic pain. Although CBT was not compared to control treatments, there were significant pre- and posttreatment differences in the symptoms of both bulimia nervosa and schizophrenia, suggesting that CBT is efficacious for these disorders as well. Butler and colleagues also reported that the gains found during treatment with CBT were maintained at follow-up, separating CBT from pharmacotherapy, which usually does not result in long-term gains following termination of treatment. Although there are increasing numbers of research studies investigating the efficacy of CBT for different disorders, the majority by far still focus on CBT for depression.

Depression

A number of randomized controlled trials published during recent years support the utility of cognitive therapy for treating depression among adults (e.g., Hollon, Thase, & Markowitz, 2002; Gloaguen, Cottraux, Cucherat, & Blackburn, 1998; Butler et al., 2006) and youth (Reinecke, Ryan, & DuBois, 1998). Initial findings indicated that relapse and recurrence rates were lower for clients who received cognitive therapy than for those who had received medications. In a meta-analysis of eight studies, Gloaguen and colleagues (1998) reported that CBT was superior to waiting-list or placebo controls, although it was equivalent to behavior therapy in effect size. They also reported that at 1-year minimum follow-up, 29.5% of the CBT clients relapsed, compared to 60% of clients treated with antidepressants. Moreover, providing CBT booster sessions or maintenance therapy after initial remission can reduce the risk of relapse (Jarrett et al., 2001). Additional research on the ways in which psychotherapy may serve to prevent relapse and recurrence of depression is sorely needed.

Not all studies, however, have been entirely supportive of cognitive therapy as the most efficacious treatment for depression. Although cognitive therapy typically has been found to be as effective as medications for the acute treatment of clinical depression, this was not found to be the case in the National Institute of Mental Health (NIMH) Treatment of Depression Collaborative Research Program (Elkin et al., 1989), a multisite clinical trial comparing cognitive therapy, interpersonal therapy, the antidepressant medication imipramine, and a placebo control (pill with adjunctive clinical management). Although the initial results of the NIMH study are inconsistent with those of other controlled outcome studies, further findings suggest that the efficacy of cognitive therapy may vary based on therapist skill and expertise (at least for more severely depressed individuals) (Hollon et al., 2002).

CBT is also useful in treating atypical depression (Mercier, Stewart, & Quitkin, 1992), chronic depression (in conjunction with medications) (Keller et al., 2000), and depression in adolescents (Reinecke et al., 1998). Controlled trials, however, tend to use highly selected samples and typically are carried out in university research clinics. The question arises: Is cognitive therapy effective in community settings? Is it useful in treating the broader and more complex range of clinical problems encountered in general clinical practice? Although research is limited, preliminary findings have been positive (e.g., Persons, Burns, & Perloff, 1988).

Although the outcomes of cognitive therapy have been found to be equal to those of behavioral therapy, and superior to placebo or no-treatment controls, comparison of the outcomes of cognitive therapy with those of other forms of psychotherapy in the treatment of depression has yielded less consistent results (Butler et al., 2006). Gloauguen and his colleagues (1998) reported in their meta-analysis that cognitive therapy is more efficacious than "other therapies" for depression. Wampold, Takuya, Baskin, and Tierney (2002) redid the metanalysis by Gloaguen et al. (1998) and claimed that cognitive therapy is superior only to "non-bona fide" treatments for depression, meaning therapies that did not contain common therapeutic factors such as therapeutic relationship, belief in the treatment by the therapist, and a clear case formulation. However, others have noted that common factors are not necessarily more important than specific factors (e.g., factors unique to cognitive therapy) when evaluating therapy efficacy. DeRubeis, Brotman, and Gibbons (2005) argued that evidence exists for the superiority of some therapy approaches, including cognitive therapy, when examining specific disorders, and that research examining the relationship between therapeutic alliance, the most "potent" common factor, and symptom improvement has been inconsistent, implying that specific factors are also important.

In additional research on the topic, the NIMH project reported that CBT and interpersonal therapy resulted in roughly equivalent gains for depressed individuals (Elkin et al., 1989). Shapiro et al. (1994) also reported that CBT and psychodynamic–interpersonal therapy were roughly equivalent in outcome, although long-term gains were worse for short-term treatment with psychodynamic–interpersonal therapy when compared with longer therapy of this kind and short- or long-term CBT. Rigorous meta-analyses comparing the efficacy of CBT with other treatments, and the relative importance of common and specific factors, are needed.

Generalized Anxiety Disorder

Controlled outcome studies suggest that cognitive-behavioral interventions may be helpful in alleviating anxiety for clients with generalized anxiety disorder, and that gains are maintained over time (Borkovec & Costello, 1993).

Panic Disorder with and without Agoraphobia

A number of CBT protocols have been developed to treat panic disorder (e.g., Craske, Brown, & Barlow, 1991; Craske & Barlow, 2008). Controlled outcome studies indicate that these approaches are superior to wait-list, medication, pill placebo, and relaxation training controls (Beck, Sokol, Clark, Berchick, & Wright, 1992). Gould, Otto, and Pollack (1995) concluded in their meta-analysis that cognitive-behavioral techniques combining cognitive restructuring with interoceptive exposure were the most efficacious. They also reported that CBT techniques were effective at 1-year follow-up.

Posttraumatic Stress Disorder

Cognitive-behavioral models based on information-processing and emotion-processing paradigms (Resick & Schnicke, 1992) have proven quite useful in providing an understanding of the ways traumatic experiences can disrupt core cognitive processes or schemas and may result in the activation of "pathological fear structures" (Hembree & Foa, 2003). The results of controlled outcome studies suggest that "trauma-focused" cognitive-behavioral approaches can be quite helpful in treating individuals with posttraumatic stress disorder, and are superior to waitlist or no treatment controls (Powers, Halpern, Ferenschak, Gillihan, & Foa, 2010; Bisson et al., 2007).

Social Phobia

Cognitive-behavioral interventions for social anxiety, including psychoeducation, relaxation training, identification of maladaptive thoughts and expectations, rational disputation, social skills training, and *in vivo* exposure, have been developed (e.g., Chambless & Hope, 1996; Wells, 1997). Outcome studies indicate that these approaches are superior to wait-list and supportive therapy controls, and that gains tend to be maintained over time (Wilson & Rapee, 2003).

Cognitive-behavioral models and treatments have also been shown to be efficacious forms of treatment for diverse problems such as body dysmorphic disorder (e.g., Veale et al., 1996), obsessive–compulsive disorder (e.g., Clark & Purdon, 2003), anger management (e.g., Dahlen & Deffenbacher, 2001), marital problems (e.g., Epstein & Schlesinger, 2003), and eating disorders (e.g., LeGrange, 2003).

TREATMENT APPLICABILITY

Cognitive Specificity Hypothesis

Of particular importance for the clinician is the *cognitive specificity hypothesis*—the postulate that emotional states (and clinical disorders) can be distinguished in terms of their specific cognitive contents and processes. Cognitive specificity directs our attention toward cognitive and behavioral processes that mediate specific disorders, and that may serve as a focus of treatment. Depressed individuals' views of themselves and their world are filtered through the dark prism of negativistic attributions and expectations. The schemas of depressed persons encompass associations related to themes of deprivation, loss, and personal inadequacy (Guidano & Liotti, 1983). Anxiety disorders, in contrast, stem from a generalized perception of threat in conjunction with a belief that one is unable to cope with the impending danger. Each of the specific anxiety disorders (obsessive–compulsive disorder, panic disorder, simple phobia, generalized anxiety disorder, and social anxiety) can be distinguished by the nature of the perceived threat (Freeman, Pretzer, Fleming, & Simon, 1990). Other emotions (including anger, guilt, relief, disappointment, despair, hope, resentment, jealousy, joy, pity, and pride) and clinical disorders (including personality disorders) also can be distinguished in terms of their specific cognitive contents and processes (Beck, Freeman, & Associates, 1990). The cognitive specificity hypothesis is of central importance in the clinical practice of cognitive therapy, in that it allows us to provide clients with a rationale for understanding emotional reactions that might otherwise be seen as inscrutable, and to target our interventions toward specific central beliefs and attitudes that mediate their distress. Our interventions vary, as such, depending on the specific constellation of beliefs, expectations, attributions, and skills deficits that clients demonstrate.

Recent findings have been consistent with predictions of the cognitive model regarding cognitive mediation of depression. This research generally supports the ideas that (1) cognitive therapy causes changes in negative cognitions; (2) these cognitive changes in cognitions covary with symptom improvement; and (3) cognitive mediation variables can distinguish responders from nonresponders in cognitive therapy (Garratt, Ingram, Rand, & Sawalani, 2008). Thus, the bulk of research supports the idea that cognitive changes predict improvement in depressive symptomatology.

When comparing cognitive therapy to other therapies that might cause cognitive changes, it is unclear whether cognitive therapy predicts substantially larger changes in cognitions. However, studies that have found nonsignificant differences between cognitive therapy groups and other groups often had directional but nonsignificant trends for greater cognitive changes in the cognitive therapy conditions compared to other forms of therapy. Studies that did not find statistically significant effects had smaller mean sample sizes compared to those studies that did find significant effects, suggesting that nonsupportive studies were underpowered. Current research does suggest, however, that cognitive therapy leads to more changes in maladaptive cognitions when compared to pharmacotherapy. Generally, these findings are all consistent with what would be predicted from the cognitive therapy model (Garratt et al., 2008).

Anxiety

As anxious individuals confront a problematic situation (e.g., an upcoming exam), their perceptions of that event are influenced by their existing beliefs, memories, schemas, and assumptions. In evaluating the situation, they make two judgments—an assessment of the degree of risk or threat (which incorporates assessments of the severity of the outcome and the probability that it will occur) and an assessment of their ability to cope with that risk. Treatment of anxiety disorders, then, involves reexamining beliefs, assumptions, and schemas; developing appropriate coping skills; enhancing perceptions of personal efficacy; decatastrophizing perceived threats; and discouraging avoidance or withdrawal.

Anxious individuals appear to share a number of beliefs and may demonstrate attentional biases toward threat-relevant stimuli. Research suggests that anxious clients tend to believe that if a risk exists, then it is adaptive to worry about it (anxious overconcern), it is necessary to be competent and in control of situations (personal control/perfection), and it is adaptive to avoid problems or challenges (problem avoidance). Moreover, they tend to demonstrate heightened levels of anxiety sensitivity, self-focused attention, and deficits in emotion regulation. As noted, common themes shared by the anxiety disorders are a perception of a threat and a belief that the threat cannot be managed or avoided. The threats may be real or imagined, internal (somatic sensations, emotions, and thoughts) or external (job loss), and are most often directed toward the person or the personal domain. All, however, are similar in that they are perceived as endangering physical, psychological, emotional, or social well-being.

The cognitive model of anxiety involves several elements. Anxiety, which is an adaptive response to one's environment, begins with the perception of threat in a specific situation.

As noted, the meaning that an individual attaches to the situation is determined by his or her schemas and memories of similar situations in the past. The individual then assesses the seriousness of the threat and evaluates his or her ability to cope with it. If the situation is viewed as threatening, a sense of danger ensues. If a mild threat is perceived, the individual responds to it as a challenge and feels excitement and enthusiasm. Cognitive and perceptual processes can be affected by an individual's current mood. In this case, when an individual begins feeling anxious, he or she is likely to become even more vigilant to perceived threats and begin to recall threatening experiences in his or her past. The individual, as a consequence, may come to perceive threat where none existed before.

The course of cognitive therapy for anxiety disorders follows from the foregoing discussion of general principles. In conceptualizing an individual's anxiety, we begin by assessing his or her *anxiety threshold,* or ability to tolerate anxiety. Each person has a general anxiety threshold as well as an ability to tolerate anxiety in specific situations. These thresholds may shift in response to stresses in the individual's day-to-day life and available supports. The therapist begins, then, by asking what specific events, situations, or interactions trigger the individual to become anxious.

Next, an assessment is made of automatic thoughts accompanying the feelings of anxiety. Although the thoughts of anxious individuals often incorporate themes of threat and vulnerability, their specific content can be quite personal or idiosyncratic and may be related to a specific syndrome. As the cognitive specificity hypothesis suggests, each of the anxiety disorders can be distinguished on the basis of its accompanying cognitive contents and processes. *Panic disorder,* for example, is characterized by a sensitivity or vigilance to physical sensations and a tendency to make catastrophic interpretations of these somatic feelings. *Agoraphobia* typically involves a fear of being unable to reach a "safety zone" rapidly, such as one's house—leading the individual to avoid cars, planes, crowded rooms, bridges, and other places where ready escape might be blocked. *Phobias,* in contrast, stem from a fear of specific objects (e.g., a large dog) or a situation (e.g., speaking in public). *Obsessive–compulsive disorder* is characterized by a fear of specific thoughts or behaviors, whereas *generalized anxiety disorder* involves a more pervasive sense of vulnerability and a fear of physical or psychological danger.

Not all anxiety reactions are the same. Rather, symptom patterns vary from person to person. One individual may experience predominantly physical symptoms (e.g., tachycardia, difficulty breathing, dizziness, indigestion, wobbliness, or hot flashes), necessitating the development of an individualized treatment program. Another individual's anxiety, however, might be characterized by "fears of the worst" happening and thoughts of losing control. This treatment program would be somewhat different. When treating anxiety disorders, it is helpful to keep this variability in mind and to address each of the component symptoms individually.

As with other clinically important problems, treatment of anxiety begins with the development of a parsimonious case conceptualization. By adopting a phenomenological stance, we attempt to understand individuals' thoughts, feelings, and behavioral responses as they confront anxiety-provoking situations. Questions to be addressed include the following: Is the client in real danger, or is his or her response out of proportion to the threat? What are the client's coping skills? What is the client's anxiety threshold? What are the clients attributions–automatic thoughts–schemas? What behavioral skills are needed? Consideration of these questions guides the therapist toward a more systematic and effective treatment program. Interventions are directed toward addressing the identified specific beliefs and coping deficits.

Personality Disorders

Personality disorders refer to enduring patterns of thought, perception, and interpersonal relatedness that are inflexible and maladaptive. They tend to occur in a range of settings and are often accompanied by significant distress. More often than not, they greatly impair individuals' social or occupational functioning. They are both chronic and pernicious. Personality disorders differ from other clinically important problems (e.g., major depression or anxiety disorders) in that they tend not to fluctuate over time and are not characterized by discrete periods of distress.

Like other problems we have discussed, each personality disorder can be described in terms of a specific constellation of cognitive contents and processes (Freeman, 2002). The schemas of a dependent individual, for example, tend to be characterized by beliefs of the form, "I am a flawed or incapable person" (self) and "The world is a dangerous place" (world), and by the assumption, "If I can maintain a close relationship with a supportive person, then I can feel secure." As a consequence, the individual with a dependent personality disorder continually seeks relationships with others, fears the loss of relationships, and feels despondent and anxious when deprived of the support of others.

A schizoid individual, in contrast, may not only hold the belief that "the world is a dangerous place" (world) but also maintain the schema, "Others are dangerous or malevolent" (world), and the assumption, "If I can avoid intimate relationships with others, then I can feel secure." As a consequence, the behavioral and emotional responses of such an individual are quite different. Such an individual tends to be indifferent to the praise or criticism of others, to maintain few close friendships, and to be emotionally aloof from others. As one client succinctly stated, "My dream is to get through law school so I can get a lot of money . . . then I'd buy an island . . . I'd never have to deal with anyone, that would be ideal."

Personality disorders reflect the activity of maladaptive schemas and assumptions (Freeman, 2002; Riso, Maddux, & Santorelli, 2007). Although these schemas may have been adaptive in the context in which they were developed, they have lost their functional value. Clients tend (at least initially) not to view their perceptions, thoughts, or behavior as problematic. They believe that the problems reside in others.

Individuals with personality disorders typically seek treatment due to other concerns—most often, feelings of depression, anxiety, anger, or difficulties maintaining jobs or relationships. It is important to remember that the client's goals in seeking treatment may not be shared with others (including the therapist). If a client is not willing to work on "core" issues, then therapy may still prove useful, providing the client with techniques for controlling his or her feelings of depression or anxiety, and assisting the client to develop trusting relationships. Although more time-consuming, the gradual uncovering of schemas through guided discovery, and the demonstration that they are maladaptive through Socratic questioning, can be far more fruitful than direct confrontation.

Cognitive therapy of personality disorders differs from short-term cognitive therapy in that it incorporates a more comprehensive exploration of the developmental origins of the schemas (a "developmental analysis") and examines the ways in which the schemas are expressed in the therapeutic relationship. Unlike the psychodynamic psychotherapist, however, the cognitive therapist does not focus on the transference relationship as a means of permitting interpretation of underlying drives, defenses, or ego functioning. As in other approaches, the development of an angry or depressive relationship with the therapist may undermine therapeutic collaboration. Such negative perceptions, attributions, or expectations are challenged directly, and the therapeutic relationship serves as evidence that the tacit belief is not true.

The therapeutic relationship plays a central role in the treatment of personality disorders and serves as a microcosm of the client's responses to others. The sensitive nature of the relationship means that the therapist must exercise great care. Being even 2 minutes late for a session with a client with a dependent personality may elicit anxiety about abandonment. The same 2 minutes of lateness may raise in clients with paranoid personalities the specter of being taken advantage of.

It is often valuable to discuss the time frame for treatment with clients at the outset of therapy. Many clients, for example, may have read about cognitive therapy and expect that they will be "cured" in 12–20 sessions. Given the greater severity and chronicity of their difficulties, however, a longer time frame might be anticipated. Although clients may expect some symptomatic improvement within a relatively short period, a longer time is necessary to identify and change tacit beliefs (12–20 months is a far more reasonable time frame).

Cognitive therapy of personality disorders is a rapidly evolving area for clinical theory and research (see the section on schema-based therapy). Although few controlled outcome studies (e.g., Giesen-Bloo, van Dyck, Spinhouen, van Tilburg, Dirksen, et al., 2006) have yet been completed, our clinical experience suggests that the model provides a parsimonious means of understanding a range of persistent and self-defeating patterns of thought, emotion, and behavior. The potential value of cognitive therapy for treating these most challenging clients, though not yet realized, is great.

Psychotic Disorders

One of the more recent emphases in cognitive therapy has been the treatment of psychotic disorders. This advancement of treatment to a complex and difficult group is an indication of cognitive therapy's growing sophistication, integrative capacity, and complexity. The treatment of psychotic disorders historically lay in the realm of psychotropic medication, social skills training, and crisis management. Individual psychotherapy was often regarded as futile for individuals suffering from delusions and hallucinations by many in the medical community. CBT for psychotic disorders (CBTp; e.g., Beck, Stolar, Rector, & Grant, 2009) has changed both the understanding and the treatment of these disorders, and is now frequently used as an adjunct to medication or as the sole treatment in cases that involve problems with medication management and resistance. An increasing number of empirical investigations in recent years has examined the efficacy of CBTp. More recently, there has also been an increased focus on the use of preventive and early intervention cognitive treatments with individuals and groups at high risk for the development of psychosis.

The Cognitive Theory of Psychotic Disorders

Overall, cognitive therapy views schizophrenia and other psychotic disorders as the result of neurobiological vulnerabilities that make such patients highly sensitive to environmental stressors, with fewer psychological resources to cope with this stress. Additionally, the cognitive theory of schizophrenia and psychotic disorders differentiates the mechanisms behind the positive symptoms of these disorders, such as delusions and hallucinations, and the negative symptoms, such as restricted emotional expression, diminished fluency of thought and speech (*alogia*), and decreased motivation to engage in goal-directed behavior (*avolition*).

Positive Symptoms

Historically, the positive symptoms of psychotic disorders have been understood as neurobiological and not amenable to psychological intervention. Cognitive-behavioral therapists agree with the neurobiological underpinnings of such disorders, but they also see such symptoms as being the result of identifiable cognitive biases and distortions that maintain symptoms and can be understood within the context of the patient's life (Beck et al., 2009). They are exaggerated manifestations on a continuum of normal perceptions, thoughts, or beliefs that can be understood and treated in a manner similar to other disorders. The main difference between more normative beliefs and psychotic hallucinations or delusions is that they are not as amenable to corrective feedback and the content is taken at face value, without examining contradictory evidence or alternative explanations. Within this framework, for example, auditory hallucinations or voices can be understood as thoughts generated by the patient that have been externalized and are perceived as emanating from outside of the self. The content of these hallucinations varies and is consistent with the patient's pre-existing beliefs and expectations about the self, others, or the world. Like other automatic thoughts, such hallucinations tend to be triggered by stressful situations or in response to difficult or negative internal or external cues. Similarly, delusions are seen as distorted beliefs, imaginings, or hypotheses that are taken as fact or reality, and that may function to protect the patient from feelings of vulnerability or low self-esteem. Such beliefs often have their roots in the patient's predelusional beliefs; therefore, understanding these earlier beliefs can help in discerning the meaning of the current belief system. Furthermore, these beliefs may reflect particular cognitive biases, such as egocentrism, externalization, and intentional attribution, which can be identified, understood, and challenged (Rector & Beck, 2002). Such distorted beliefs or cognitions are then open to cognitive restructuring through the use of Socratic questioning, examination of the evidence for and against such beliefs, reality testing, and adoption of alternative hypotheses or explanations.

Negative Symptoms

Initially seen by cognitive therapists as symptoms of comorbid depression or responses to positive symptoms, today cognitive theory views negative symptoms as the result of a combination of neurobiological, environmental, and psychological processes. Following a diathesis–stress model, neurobiological influences may predispose some individuals to experience negative symptoms, which may result from and/or contribute to adverse responses to environmental stresses. These individual responses to stress may be further mediated by psychological variables, which can be a focus of intervention. In particular, individuals with schizoid personality traits may be particularly vulnerable to negative symptoms because such symptoms may represent an intensification of preexisting negative beliefs about the self and others. These cognitions may include negative beliefs about social engagement, personal adequacy, and performance, and may be activated in response to the occurrence of positive symptoms as compensatory strategies. Such negative symptoms may serve to protect individuals from painful positive symptoms and perceived external pressure or threats. Furthermore, many patients with schizophrenia display a specific negative cognitive set "characterized by low expectancies for pleasure, success and acceptance, as well as the perception of limited resources" (Rector et al., 2005, p. 252), that contribute to the negative symptoms in a circular manner.

Cognitive Treatment of Psychotic Disorders

CBTp follows closely the practice of cognitive therapy with depression, anxiety, and other nonpsychotic disorders. The overall goal, as noted earlier, is to identify patients' distorted beliefs or cognitions, examine the evidence for and against such beliefs, and develop alternative hypotheses or explanations. The treatment is typically active, structured, and time-limited. Early sessions focus on development of the collaborative therapeutic relationship, a thorough assessment, and mutually agreed upon treatment goals. Psychoeducation about the interaction among thoughts, feelings and behavior, the role of cognitive biases and distortions, and the cognitive model of schizophrenia or other psychotic disorders also takes place, allowing for normalization of symptoms. This phase of treatment may take longer than with nonpsychotic patients, because the therapist must work to establish trust and rapport. Similarly, therapists must be flexible in their approach, take frequent breaks, alter session length, and modify goals from session to session as needed by the patient.

The context of individual sessions follows a standard cognitive therapy model of checking the patient's mood and medication use. The work of the previous session is reviewed, and a structured agenda for the current session is developed. Cognitive and behavioral strategies addressing the session goals are practiced within the session, and the patient is assigned homework to monitor and test beliefs experimentally *in vivo*.

Specific strategies used in cognitive therapy for people with delusions and hallucinations include identification of the antecedents of the delusions, beliefs, or hallucinations, and current triggers to the occurrence of the delusions or hallucinations. This is followed by Socratic questioning of the interpretation of these occurrences and examination of the evidence for this interpretation. When working with psychotic patients, it is important that such questioning be gentle and nonjudgmental, and occur in the context of a trusting therapeutic relationship. Questions should not be experienced as a direct challenge to the patient's beliefs. Confrontation or collusion with the patient's dysfunctional belief system should be avoided. By questioning the interpretation of the event, the patient is able to consider alternative hypotheses. Repeated questioning and testing of alternative explanations for events, with behavioral experiments to test these hypotheses assigned as homework, are thought to lead eventually to changes in the patient's belief system or perceptions. The patient is able to see the delusions and hallucinations as one interpretation of the meaning of events rather than as absolute truth, and the certainty with which the patient holds the beliefs begins to weaken.

In addition to working with patients in challenging the interpretation and content of the delusions and hallucinations, cognitive therapy also helps patients to cope with the distress caused by their positive symptoms and potential comorbid conditions, such as depression and anxiety, often reflected in the negative symptoms. Cognitive-behavioral approaches to these symptoms parallel the cognitive approach to depression and anxiety in other disorders. Behaviorally, this can include self-monitoring; activity scheduling; ratings of pleasure and mastery; graded task assignments; and training in assertiveness, social skills, or coping and relaxation methods. Cognitively, therapy focuses on eliciting the patient's thoughts about activity, performance, or socializing, gently questions the veracity of those cognitions, and tests those beliefs with behavioral experiments as homework assignments.

Empirical Findings on CBT and Psychotic Disorders

Cognitive-behavioral treatment of psychosis is used either as an adjunct to pharmacotherapy or alone, as an alternative to pharmacotherapy in cases of treatment resistance or reluctance to take medication. This is particularly true for patients with schizophrenic disorders, with less robust results for other forms of psychosis.

Several meta-analyses of CBTp for schizophrenia that have appeared in the last few years have examined the efficacy of from seven to 34 randomized controlled trials of CBTp versus control conditions, routine mental health care, supportive psychotherapy, and other common adjunctive interventions (e.g., Gould, Mueser, Bolton, Mays, & Goff, 2001; Rector & Beck, 2001; Wykes, Steel, Everitt, & Terrier, 2008; Zimmerman, Favrod, Trieu, & Pomini, 2005). Aggregatively, these many controlled studies have included patients with both acute and chronic conditions and 6- to 18-month follow-up periods. In addition to findings that demonstrate lower treatment dropout rates for CBTp, these reviews show improvements in such clinically meaningful domains as patients' negative and positive symptoms, general life functioning, and social anxiety.

As in any area of research on the outcomes of psychotherapy, the findings from these important clinical trials have not gone uncriticized on methodological grounds (e.g., Gaudiano, 2005; Lynch, Laws, & McKenna, 2010), and some critics who have examined findings from many of the same controlled trials included in the meta-analyses reached less positive conclusions about the efficacy of CBTp for psychotic conditions (e.g., Jones, Cormac, Silvera de Mota Neto, & Campbell, 2004).

Moreover, outcomes for CBTp appear to be less positive with increased patient comorbidity, chronicity of the condition, and level of denial or rigidity. Many important patient questions remain to be investigated by research in this area (e.g., whether the results seen to date reflect the effect of CBTp on the central mechanisms responsible for the psychosis itself or on the secondary consequences of the illness). Similarly, the mechanisms of change in these clinical methods are not clear and require further exploration.

Despite these cautionary notes, expert groups of clinicians and researchers (e.g., Kreyenbuhl, Buchanan, Dickerson, & Dixon, 2010; National Institute for Clinical Excellence [NICE], 2009) have independently concluded that CBTp should be included as a recommended treatment for schizophrenia. For example, in the United Kingdom, where the bulk of the treatment and research on CBTp has been conducted, NICE (2002) published its recommendations advocating the inclusion of cognitive-behavioral approaches in the treatment of schizophrenia in its clinical guidelines, as the standard of care for psychological treatment of the illness. This recommendation was reaffirmed in the 2009 update of the NICE recommendations.

CASE ILLUSTRATION

Presenting Problems

Bob, 20 years of age, was living with his parents at the time of his referral for cognitive therapy. He was working part-time as a box boy at a local parts warehouse and had recently taken a leave of absence from a prestigious university. Bob was mildly obese and, although appropriately attired, had an unkempt, disheveled look—as if he had not showered in several days. He walked with a heavy, plodding gait and mumbled, making his speech difficult to understand. His eye contact was poor, and his speech was driven and rambling. His diagnoses at the time of his referral were bipolar disorder and depressed and avoidant personality disorder.

Bob's presenting concerns included a history of severe depression, suicidality, feelings of worthlessness, social anxiety, manic episodes (characterized by decreased sleep, agitation, constant talking, irrational spending, grandiose delusions, and motoric overactivity), and poor social skills. He had participated in psychoanalysis four times a week for several years and had received trials of a number of medications—all to no avail. Although his episodes of mania were reasonably well controlled by lithium (which he took regularly), his feelings of depression continued to worsen. Bob had been hospitalized twice due to suicidal ideations, and his psychiatrist had recommended that he be placed in a residential treatment program due to his deteriorating condition. His parents were interested in a second opinion before placing their son in a long-term treatment facility and felt that cognitive therapy was their "last hope."

Initial Assessment

Complete developmental, social, and medical histories were obtained, and a battery of objective rating scales was administered to gain a clearer idea of Bob's problems. His scores on the BDI, BAI, and BHS were 28, 51, and 19, respectively. These scores are indicative of clinically severe depression, anxiety, and pessimism. His responses on the Minnesota Multiphasic Personality Inventory (MMPI) yielded a 2-8-7 profile, with concomitant elevations of scales 3, 4, and 10. His responses on the MMPI were similar to those of persons who are highly anxious, depressed, agitated, and tense. Bob was dependent and unassertive in his relationships with others and felt unable to meet the challenges of day-to-day life. His responses on a series of automatic thought questionnaires revealed that he was highly concerned that others like him, that he experienced difficulty being alone, and that he could not avoid thinking about his past mistakes.

Background

Bob was the younger of two children and had grown up in an affluent suburb and attended exclusive schools. Although he had done quite well academically during his elementary and high school years, his interpersonal and emotional functioning were quite poor. He was plagued by feelings of self-doubt and worthlessness, and made self-critical comparisons with others on an almost continual basis. He believed that others were of "stellar quality" and that he was "stupid and a fraud." When asked to elaborate, Bob noted that although he had graduated near the top of his high school class, his father had written many of his papers. While away at college, Bob began to withdraw. He rarely attended class, and during one fire drill remained in his room, "hoping to be killed in the flames." After several weeks of desperate calls to his parents and increasing suicidal ideations, Bob returned home. His father, concerned by possible repercussions of leaving the university, devised an elaborate story that Bob needed to return home because his mother was having brain surgery. When Bob returned home, his father was disappointed and could not tell anyone in the family or community about it. To protect his secret, whenever they left the house, Bob was required to lie on the floor of the car, covered by a blanket.

Although Bob had done well academically and had attempted to be a "perfect child," he struggled internally with feelings of anger, depression, and inadequacy. He reported experiencing sadistic fantasies of attacking children in the neighborhood and recalled having made obscene phone calls to an 8-year-old boy while in high school.

Cognitive Formulation

Bob's depression and anxiety were superimposed on a self-critical and perfectionistic personality style. He maintained high, even grandiose, standards for his own performance (e.g., believing that he needed to earn the Nobel Prize in literature) and anticipated rejection from anyone who would come to know him. Bob's beliefs and actions were characteristic of many depressed individuals and fit well with cognitive models of depression. Negative views of self, world, and future, for example, were readily apparent in his thoughts. His social skills were poor, and he tended to behave in ways that led others to withdraw from him. Bob's social problem-solving capacities were poorly developed, and he engaged in few activities that would provide a sense of accomplishment or pleasure. When he did do well on a task, he would minimize the significance of his accomplishment and begin recounting past failures. He tended to respond to feelings of depression and anxiety though rumination and withdrawal rather than through adaptive coping. Given the information available to this point, one might conceptualize Bob's difficulties as follows:

- *Behavioral coping strategies.* Avoidance or withdrawal. Seeking reassurance from others.
- *Cognitive distortions.* Dichotomizing (e.g.,"If I'm not right,I must be wrong . . . I can't even think right"). Selective abstraction (e.g., "I wasn't comfortable in class that first day; it didn't feel right. I knew it; that just tells you I'll never make it in college"). Personalization (e.g.,"Everybody was sitting at other tables in the cafeteria . . . it shows nobody likes me"). "Should" statements (e.g., "I should be smarter and do more . . . I have to"). Magnification/minification (e.g., "I know he sent me a letter about how much he liked my paper, but it doesn't mean anything . . . it doesn't count"). Catastrophizing (e.g., "I'm incompetent at life . . . I have no abilities"). Self-critical comparison (e.g., "Everyone is better than me; I can't even blow a bubble").
- *Automatic thoughts.* "I'm so stupid . . . I'm an unintelligent jerk." "People will discover I'm a fake." "I'll never be a success." "My life is meaningless . . . I have no one to share it with." "I'm really disturbed . . . I have a hollow head."
- *Assumptions.* "If I can avoid others, then I can feel secure." "If I'm successful, then I can feel good about myself."
- *Schemas.* "I'm fundamentally defective" (self). "The world is a dangerous place" (world). "People are unreliable and unsupportive" (social relations).

Course of Therapy

The first goals in treatment were to establish trust and rapport, develop a problem list, and educate Bob about the process of cognitive therapy. During the initial sessions, Bob invariably appeared sad and anxious. He maintained a pessimistic outlook and continually sought reassurance from the therapist that he was "ok." Bob expressed a great deal of anger about his limited progress in psychoanalysis and was skeptical about cognitive therapy. We began, then, with a discussion of his feelings about therapy, what he had learned in his analysis, and his goals for the future. He conceded that he had developed a number of important insights during his analysis, and that he "really didn't know much" about cognitive therapy.

Bob remarked that he just wanted "to be an average person in college," a reasonable and appropriate goal, and he agreed to read a short book on cognitive therapy before our next session. His first formal homework assignment was to "write down his thoughts when he was feeling upset during the week"—an initial step toward completing a DTR (Beck et al., 1979).

Bob's feelings of dysphoria and anxiety became more severe as he became adept at identifying his automatic thoughts. This is not uncommon and appears to reflect clients' increasing sensitivity to thoughts they have been attempting to avoid. Rational responding, a countering technique (McMullin, 1986), was introduced to alleviate these feelings. Bob was asked to write down his thoughts when he was feeling particularly depressed or anxious. He then systematically examined evidence for and against each of the distressing thoughts (*rational disputation*), listed alternative ways of thinking about the evidence (*reattribution*), and developed more adaptive ways of coping with the concerns (*decatastrophizing* and searching for alternative solutions). For example, Bob felt he was "an unintelligent jerk." A brief review of Bob's recent past revealed that although he had left several schools, he had graduated near the top of his high school class, had received a score of 1580 (out of a maximum of 1600) on his college entrance exams, and had been admitted to the honors program at an Ivy League university. Taken together, the evidence suggested that Bob was not unintelligent. In fact, he was quite bright. A more parsimonious (and reasonable) interpretation of his experiences was that he lacked confidence in his abilities given events during his junior and senior years in high school, and he was unprepared to cope with the anxiety of moving away from his home and parents. A goal of therapy would be to help Bob develop skills to accomplish this goal.

Given his low motivation and social isolation, Bob was encouraged to begin completing daily activity schedules (Beck et al., 1979). He wrote down his activities on an hour-by-hour basis, then rated them as to their degree of "mastery/sense of accomplishment" and "pleasure/fun." As might be expected, Bob engaged in few activities that provided him with a sense of worth, accomplishment, or enjoyment. Depressed clients such as Bob often avoid challenging tasks and experience difficulty completing tasks they had accomplished with ease before the onset of their depression. Thoughts such as "I can't do it" and "What's the point?" inhibit them from engaging in activities that might provide them with a sense of competence or pleasure. Moreover, their avoidance of tasks and impaired performance serves as further evidence that "there's something wrong with me . . . I can't do it." Activity scheduling served to directly counteract these processes. Bob and his therapist developed a list of simple activities he would attempt each day. He was encouraged, for example, to get out of bed at 10:00 A.M. and take a shower (rather than lounging in bed until midafternoon), to call a friend on the phone, to accept an invitation from a friend to play cards, and to go to the local gym for a swim. As Bob began to employ these techniques, his feelings of anxiety and dysphoria began to decline. These gains were reflected in Bob's improving scores on several objective rating scales. His scores on the BDI, for example, declined from a 28 (*severe depression*) at week 2 of treatment to a 9 (*mild depression*) at week 23. His scores on the BAI declined from a 51 (*severe anxiety*) to a 3 (*negligible anxiety*) during this same period.

In addition to symptom reductions in dysphoria and anxiety, an important focus of therapy was addressing long-term life goals, specifically, Bob's inability to develop close relationships with others and to live independently from his parents. Behavioral interventions (e.g., modeling appropriate eye contact and role playing basic conversational skills) were introduced to develop Bob's social skills, and a hierarchy of social activities (beginning with playing cards with his friends, concluding with going on a date with a woman) was established. Bob was able to progress through the hierarchy over several months, but he encountered a great deal of anxiety with each new step. Relaxation training, rational responding, guided imagery, and role playing of the activities were useful in helping Bob to develop these skills.

At the same time, Bob was encouraged to consider ways of returning to college. Because he was highly anxious about leaving home (his last two attempts to live on his own had ended in psychiatric hospitalizations), Bob began by taking night classes at a local university. Not surprisingly, he did quite well. His tendency to minimize these accomplishments was addressed directly in therapy, as was the effect of these accomplishments on his mood and self-esteem. After approximately 6 months, Bob began to discuss the possibility of applying to college once again. His fears of another "breakdown," as well as his uncertainty about possible majors and careers, became the focus of therapy. Once again, he began seeking reassurance from the therapist that he would "be ok." This provided an opportunity for examining experiences that had contributed to the consolidation of his schemas and the ways they were reflected in the therapy relationship. For example, Bob frequently sought reassurance and assistance from his mother during his childhood, and his father's attempts to assist him with his homework during high school had maintained his belief that he was "incompetent" and "stupid." Bob acknowledged that reassurance (whether from his therapist or his parents) did little to alleviate these feelings, and that his search for support precluded him from solving problems on his own. Experiences during his childhood that were inconsistent with these beliefs were examined, and Bob was encouraged to test the current validity of the beliefs by completing tasks without seeking support or reassurance.

Bob was subsequently accepted at a major university several hundred miles from home. Before leaving for college, however, we felt it would be beneficial for him to have an experience that would give him confidence that he could live alone. To this end, Bob applied for a position as a relief worker in a small South American village. During his 6 weeks away from home, Bob was confronted with numerous challenges that previously he would have felt he could not handle. He returned home with a new (longer) hairstyle, an earring, and a developing sense of identity as an individual who might be able to help others. Bob left for college several weeks later. After a difficult first year, Bob became a residence hall counselor and his grades began to stabilize. Booster sessions were held approximately once a month. Therapy was concluded after approximately 3 years. Bob graduated from college, began teaching inner-city children in another state, and was accepted to graduate school. Although he remained somewhat anxious and self-critical, he became able to function autonomously. The gains made over the course of treatment are reflected not only in his improved scores on objective rating scales but also in the quality of his life. The goals of therapy were not limited to the alleviation of depression and anxiety but included a focus on latent beliefs and the establishment of an adult identity. Individuation from his parents, a return to school, the development of career goals, and the acquisition of social skills were all important objectives.

This case illustrates how strategic interventions can be employed in treating severe and long-standing psychological difficulties. The treatment of this individual was multifaceted and incorporated traditional cognitive and behavioral approaches, as well as interpersonal interventions focusing on the ways in which unstated beliefs or schemas are expressed in the therapeutic relationship (Safran & McMain, 1992; Safran & Segal, 1990). Social problem solving, rational responding, attributional retraining, behavioral skill training, and developmental analysis of underlying schemas and assumptions all played a role. With the exception of three family sessions, Bob's parents were not included in his treatment. This was explicitly discussed with Bob—a goal of therapy was to encourage him to accept responsibility for the course of his treatment and to function more autonomously.

CONCLUSION

The usefulness of cognitive therapy for treating a range of behavioral and emotional difficulties has been well established. Refined models of depression and the anxiety disorders have been proposed and have generated a great deal of empirical interest. Controlled studies of cognitive therapy's effectiveness in the treatment of other clinically important problems, however, remain to be completed. Moreover, the processes underlying change over the course of therapy are not well understood. What specific cognitive and behavioral techniques, for example, are most closely associated with clinical improvement? Do rationalistic and constructivist variants of cognitive therapy differ with regard to their effectiveness in treating specific disorders? What changes in clients over the course of their treatment? Cognitive models of psychopathology will continue to evolve in response to the needs of our clients and the results of empirical research. Although important practical and conceptual problems remain, cognitive therapy stands as a useful paradigm for understanding human adaptation and improving the quality of our clients' lives.

SUGGESTIONS FOR FURTHER STUDY

Recommended Reading

Beck, A. T., Rush, A. J., Shaw, B. F., & Emery, G. (1979). *Cognitive therapy of depression*. New York: Guilford Press.—The original manual for cognitive therapy of depression and suicide.

Dobson, K. S. (Ed.). (2010). *Handbook of cognitive-behavioral therapies* (3rd ed.). New York: Guilford Press.—More than a compendium of techniques, the authors offer critical reviews of recent research and suggest areas of inquiry.

Leahy, R. (2003). *Cognitive therapy techniques: A practitioner's guide*. New York: Guilford Press.—This book provides a comprehensive, detailed overview of basic cognitive assessment and intervention techniques.

Persons, J. (2008). *The case formulation approach to cognitive-behavior therapy*. New York: Guilford Press.— This book provides a useful framework for integrating cognitive behavioral therapy models and techniques into the conceptualization and treatment of individual clients.

Riso, L. P., du Toit, P. L., Stein, D. J., & Young, J. E. (2007). *Cognitive schemas and core beliefs in psychological problems: A scientist-practitioner guide*. Washington, DC: American Psychological Association.— An excellent overview of schema-based therapy approaches for a range of psychological disorders.

Hayes, S. C., Follette, V. M., & Linehan, M. M. (2004). *Mindfulness and acceptance: Expanding the cognitive-behavioral tradition*. New York: Guilford Press.—A comprehensive overview of the theoretical underpinnings and therapeutic methods of "third-wave" cognitive-behavioral therapies.

DVDs

Beck, J. (2006). *Cognitive therapy* (Systems of Psychotherapy Video Series). Washington, DC: American Psychological Association.

Meichenbaum, D. (2007). *Cognitive behavior therapy with Donald Meichenbaum* (Systems of Psychotherapy Video Series). Washington, DC: American Psychological Association.

Wright, J. H., Ramirez Basco, R., & Thase, M. E. (2006). *Learning Cognitive Behavior Therapy: An illustrated guide*. Washington, DC: American Psychiatric Press.—This accessible resource includes a book and companion DVD containing multiple examples of cognitive and behavioral assessment and intervention techniques.

Young, J. E. (2007). *Schema therapy* (Systems of Psychotherapy Video Series). Washington, DC: American Psychological Association

REFERENCES

Abramson, L., Metalsky, G., & Alloy, L. (1989). Hopelessness depression: A theory-based subtype of depression. *Psychological Review, 96,* 358–372.

Abramson, L., Seligman, M., & Teasdale, J. (1978). Learned helplessness in humans: Critique and reformulation. *Journal of Abnormal Psychology, 87,* 49–74.

Adler, A. (1968). *The practice and theory of individual psychology*. New York: Humanities Press.

Arch, J. J., & Craske, M. G. (2008). Acceptance and commitment therapy and cognitive behavioral therapy for anxiety disorders: Different treatments, similar mechanisms? *Clinical Psychology: Science and Practice, 15,* 263–279.

Beck, A. (1989). *Love is never enough*. New York: HarperCollins.

Beck, A. T. (1963). Thinking and depression: I. Idiosyncratic content and cognitive distortions. *Archives of General Psychiatry, 9,* 324–333.

Beck, A. T. (1972). *Depression: Causes and treatment*. Philadelphia: University of Pennsylvania Press.

Beck, A. T., Brown, G., Steer, R. A., & Weissman, A. (1991). Factor analysis of the Dysfunctional Attitudes Scale in a clinical population. *Psychological Assessment: A Journal of Consulting and Clinical Psychology, 3,* 478–483.

Beck, A. T., Epstein, N., Brown, G., & Steer, R. (1988). An inventory for measuring clinical anxiety. *Journal of Consulting and Clinical Psychology, 56,* 893–897.

Beck, A. T., Freeman, A., & Associates. (1990). *Cognitive therapy of personality disorders*. New York: Guilford Press.

Beck, A. T., Rector, N. A., Stolar, N., & Grant, P. (2009). *Schizophrenia: Cognitive theory, research, and therapy*. New York: Guilford Press.

Beck, A. T., Rush, A. J., Shaw, B. F., & Emery, G. (1979). *Cognitive therapy of depression*. New York: Guilford Press.

Beck, A. T., Sokol, L., Clark, D., Berchick, R., & Wright, F. (1992). A crossover study of focused cognitive therapy for panic disorder. *American Journal of Psychiatry, 149*(6), 778–783.

Beck, A. T., Steer, R. A., & Brown, G. K. (1996). *Manual for Beck Depression Inventory–II*. San Antonio, TX: Psychological Corporation.

Beck, A. T., Weissman, S., Lester, D., & Trexler, L. (1974). The measurement of pessimism: The Hopelessness Scale. *Journal of Consulting and Clinical Psychology, 42,* 861–865.

Bergin, A. E., & Garfield, S. L. (2003). *Handbook of psychotherapy and behavior change*. New York: Wiley.

Bisson, J. I., Ehlers, A., Matthews, R., Pilling, S., Richards, D., & Turner, S. (2007). Psychological treatments for chronic post-traumatic stress disorder: Systematic review and meta-analysis. *British Journal of Psychiatry, 190,* 97–104.

Borkovec, T., & Costello, E. (1993). Efficacy of applied relaxation and cognitive-behavioral therapy in the treatment of generalized anxiety disorder. *Journal of Consulting and Clinical Psychology, 61,* 611–619.

Bourne, E. J. (2005). *The anxiety and phobia workbook* (4th ed.). Oakland, CA: New Harbinger.

Bowlby, J. (1969). *Attachment and loss: Vol. 1. Attachment*. New York: Basic Books.

Bowlby, J. (1985). The role of childhood experience in cognitive disturbance. In M. Mahoney & A. Freeman (Eds.), *Cognition and psychotherapy* (pp. 181–200). New York: Plenum Press.

Burns, D. (1980). *Feeling good*. New York: Morrow.

Butler, A. C., Chapman, J. E., Forman, E. M., & Beck, A. T. (2006). The empirical status of cognitive-behavioral therapy: A review of meta-analyses. *Clinical Psychology Review, 26,* 17–31.

Chambless, D. L., & Hope, D. A. (1996). Cognitive approaches to the psychopathology and treatment of social phobia. In P. Salkovskis (Ed.), *Frontiers of cognitive therapy* (pp. 345–382). New York: Guilford Press.

Clark, D. A., & Purdon, C. (2003). Cognitive theory and therapy of obsessions and compulsions: A critical re-examination. In M. Reinecke & D. Clark (Eds.), *Cognitive therapy across the lifespan* (pp. 90–116). Cambridge, UK: Cambridge University Press.

Craske, M. G., & Barlow, D. H. (2008). Panic disorder and agoraphobia. In D. H. Barlow (Ed.), *Clinical handbook of psychological disorders: A step-by-step treatment manual* (4th ed., pp. 1–64). New York: Guilford Press.

Craske, M. G., Brown, T. A., & Barlow, D. H. (1991). Behavioral treatment of panic disorder: A two-year follow-up. *Behavior Therapy, 22*(3), 289–304.

Dahlen, E., & Deffenbacher, J. (2001). Anger management. In W. Lyddon & J. Jones (Eds.), *Empirically supported cognitive therapies: Current and future applications* (pp. 163–181). New York: Springer.

DeRubeis, R., Brotman, M. A., & Gibbons, C. J. (2005). A conceptual and methodological analysis of the nonspecifics argument. *Clinical Psychology: Science and Practice, 12,* 174–181.

Elkin, I., Shea, M., Watkins, J., Imber, S., Sotsky, S., Collins, J., et al. (1989). National Institute of Mental Health Treatment of Depression Collaborative Research Program: General effectiveness of treatments. *Archives of General Psychiatry, 46,* 971–982.

Ellis, A. (1962). *Reason and emotion in psychotherapy.* New York: Lyle Stuart.

Ellis, A., & Harper, R. (1961). *New guide to rational living.* New York: Crown.

Epictetus. (1983). *The handbook of Epictetus* (N. White, Trans.). Indianapolis, IN: Hackett.

Epstein, N., & Schlesinger, S. (2003). Treatment of family problems. In M. A. Reinecke, F. M. Dattilio, & A. Freeman (Eds.), *Cognitive therapy with children and adolescents: A casebook for clinical practice* (pp. 304–337). New York: Guilford Press.

Freeman, A. (2002). Cognitive-behavioral therapy for severe personality disorders. In S. G. Hofmann & M. C. Tompson (Eds.), *Treating chronic and severe mental disorders: A handbook of empirically supported interventions* (pp. 382–402). New York: Guilford Press.

Freeman, A., Pretzer, J., Fleming, B., & Simon, K. (1990). *Clinical applications of cognitive therapy.* New York: Plenum Press.

Freeman, A., & Reinecke, M. A. (1993). *Cognitive therapy of suicidal behavior: Manual for treatment.* New York: Springer.

Freeman, A., & Simon, K. (1989). Cognitive therapy of anxiety. In A. Freeman, K. Simon, L. Beutler, & H. Arkowitz (Eds.), *Comprehensive handbook of cognitive therapy* (pp. 347–366). New York: Plenum Press.

Freud, S. (1923). The ego and the id. *Standard Edition, 19,* 1–66. London: Hogarth Press.

Garratt, G., Ingram, R. E., Rand, K. L., & Sawalani, G. (2007). Cognitive processes in cognitive therapy: Evaluation of the mechanisms of change in the treatment of depression. *Clinical Psychology: Science and Practice, 14,* 224–239.

Gaudiano, B. A. (2005). Cognitive behavior therapies for psychotic disorders: Current empirical status and future directions. *Clinical Psychology: Science and Practice, 12,* 33–50.

Giesen-Bloo, J., van Dyck, R., Spinhoven, P., van Tilburg, W., Dirksen, C., Van Asselt, T., et al. (2006). Outpatient psychotherapy for borderline personality disorder: Randomized trial of schema-focused therapy versus transference-focused psychotherapy. *Archives of General Psychiatry, 63,* 649–658.

Gloaguen, V., Cottraux, J., Cucherat, M., & Blackburn, I. M. (1998). A meta-analysis of the effects of cognitive therapy in depressed patients. *Journal of Affective Disorders, 49,* 59–72.

Goldfried, M. R. (2003). Cognitive-behavior therapy: Reflections on the evolution of a therapeutic orientation. *Cognitive Therapy and Research, 27,* 53–69.

Goldfried, M. R., & Merbaum, M. (Eds.). (1973). *Behavior change through self-control.* New York: Holt, Rinehart & Winston.

Gould, R. A., Mueser, K. T., Bolton, D., Mays, V., & Goff, D. (2001). Cognitive therapy for psychosis in schizophrenia: An effect size analysis. *Schizophrenia Research, 48,* 335–342.

Gould, R. A., Otto, M. W., & Pollack, M. H. (1995). A meta-analysis of treatment outcome for panic disorder. *Clinical Psychology Review, 15,* 819–844.

Greenberg, L. S., & Safran, J. D. (1987). *Emotion in psychotherapy.* New York: Guilford Press.

Greenberger, D., & Padesky, C. A. (1995). *Mind over mood: A cognitive therapy treatment manual for clients.* New York: Guilford Press.

Guidano, V. F., & Liotti, G. (1983). *Cognitive processes and emotional disorders: A structural approach to psychotherapy.* New York: Guilford Press.

Hays, P. (2009). Integrating evidence-based practice, cognitive-behavior therapy, and multicultural therapy: Ten steps for culturally competent practice. *Professional Psychology: Research and Practice, 40,* 354–360.

Hayes, S. C. (2004). Acceptance and commitment therapy and the new behavior therapies: Mindfulness, acceptance, and relationship. In S. C. Hayes, V. M. Follette, & M. M. Linehan (Eds.), *Mindfulness and acceptance: Expanding the cognitive-behavioral tradition* (pp. 1–29). New York: Guilford Press.

Hembree, E., & Foa, E. (2003). Promoting cognitive change in posttraumatic stress disorder. In M. Reinecke & D. Clark (Eds.), *Cognitive therapy across the lifespan* (pp. 231–257). Cambridge, UK: Cambridge University Press.

Hollon, S., Thase, M., & Markowitz, J. (2002). Treatment and prevention of depression. *Psychological Science in the Public Interest, 3,* 39–77.

Horowitz, M. (Ed.). (1991). *Person schemas and maladaptive interpersonal patterns.* Chicago: University of Chicago Press.

Ingram, R. (1984). Toward an information processing analysis of depression. *Cognitive Therapy and Research, 8,* 443–478.

Jarrett, R., Kraft, D., Doyle, J., Foster, B., Eaves, G., & Silver, P. (2001). Preventing recurrent depression using cognitive therapy with and without a continuation phase: A randomized clinical trial. *Archives of General Psychiatry, 58,* 381–388.

Jones, C., Cormac, I., Silveira de Mota Neto, J., & Campbell, C. (2004). Cognitive behavior therapy for schizophrenia. *Cochrane Database of Systematic Reviews, 4,* 1–57.

Kabat-Zinn, J. (1994). *Wherever you go there you are: Mindfulness meditation in everyday life.* New York: Hyperion.

Keller, M. B., McCullough, J. P., Klein, D. N., Arnow, B., Dunner, D. L., Gelenberg, A. J., et al. (2000). A comparison of nefazodone, the cognitive behavioral-analysis system of psychotherapy, and their combination for the treatment of chronic depression. *New England Journal of Medicine, 342,* 1462–1470.

Kovacs, M., & Beck, A. (1978). Maladaptive cognitive structures in depression. *American Journal of Psychiatry, 135,* 525–533.

Kreyenbuhl, J., Buchanan, R. W., Dickerson, F. B., & Dixon, L. B. (2010). The Schizophrenia Patient Outcomes Research Team (PORT): Updated treatment recommendations 2009. *Schizophrenia Bulletin, 36,* 94–103.

Leahy, R. L. (2001). *Overcoming resistance in cognitive therapy.* New York: Guilford Press.

LeGrange, D. (2003). The cognitive model of bulimia nervosa. In M. A. Reinecke & D. Clark (Eds.), *Cognitive therapy across the lifespan* (pp. 293–314). Cambridge, UK: Cambridge University Press.

Lynch, D., Laws, K. R., & McKenna, P. J. (2010). Cognitive behavioural therapy for major psychiatric disorder: Does it really work? A meta-analytical review of welll-controlled trials. *Psychological Medicine, 40,* 9–24.

Mahoney, M. (1977). Reflections on the cognitive-learning trend in psychotherapy. *American Psychologist, 32,* 5–13.

McMullin, R. E. (1986). *Handbook of cognitive therapy techniques.* New York: Norton.

Meichenbaum, D. (1977). *Cognitive behavior modification.* New York: Plenum Press.

Meichenbaum, D. (2009). Self inoculation training. In W. T. O'Donohue & J. E. Fisher (Eds.), *General principles and empirically supported techniques of cognitive behavior therapy* (pp. 627–630). Hoboken, NJ: Wiley.

Mercier, M., Stewart, J., & Quitkin, F. (1992). A pilot sequential study of cognitive therapy and pharmacotherapy of atypical depression. *Journal of Clinical Psychiatry, 53,* 166–170.

Millon, T. (1999). *Personality-guided therapy.* New York: Wiley.

Morrison, A. P., French, P., Parker, S., Roberts, M., Stevens, H., Bentall, R. P., & Lewis, S. W. (2007). Three-year follow-up of a randomized controlled trial of cognitive therapy for the prevention of psychosis in people at ultrahigh risk. *Schizophrenia Bulletin, 33*(3),682–687.

National Institute for Clinical Excellence (NICE). (2002). *Schizophrenia: Core interventions in the treatment and management of schizophrenia in primary and secondary care* (Clinical Guideline 1). London: Author.

National Institute for Clinical Excellence (NICE). (2009). *Schizophrenia: Core interventions in the treatment and management of schizophrenia in adults in primary and secondary care* (Update of NICE Clinical Guideline 1). London: Author.

Organista, K. C., & Munoz, R. F. (1996). Cognitive behavioral therapy with Latinos. *Cognitive and Behavioral Practice, 3*, 255–270.

Persons, J. (2008). *The case formulation approach to cognitive therapy.* New York: Guilford Press.

Persons, J., Burns, D., & Perloff, J. (1988). Predictors of dropout and outcome in private practice patients treated with cognitive therapy for depression. *Cognitive Therapy and Research, 12*, 557–575.

Persons, J., Davidson, J., & Tompkins, M. (2001). *Essential components of cognitive-behavior therapy for depression.* Washington, DC: American Psychological Association.

Powers, M. B., Halpern, J. M., Ferenschak, M. P., Gillihan, S. J., & Foa, E. B. (2010). A meta-analytic review of prolonged exposure for posttraumatic stress disorder. *Clinical Psychology Review, 30*, 635–641.

Rector, N. A., & Beck, A. T. (2001). Cognitive behavioral therapy for schizophrenia: An empirical review. *Journal of Nervous and Mental Disease, 189*, 278–287.

Rector, N. A., & Beck, A. T. (2002). Cognitive therapy for schizophrenia: From conceptualization to intervention. *Canadian Journal of Psychiatry, 47*, 39–48.

Rector, N. A., Beck, A. T., & Stolar, N. (2005). The negative symptoms of schizophrenia: A cognitive perspective. *Canadian Journal of Psychiatry, 50*, 247–257.

Rehm, L. (2009). Self-management. In W. T. O'Donohue & J. E. Fisher (Eds.), *General principles and empirically supported techniques of cognitive behavior therapy* (pp. 627–630). Hoboken, NJ: Wiley.

Reinecke, M. (2002). Cognitive therapies of depression: A modularized treatment approach. In M. Reinecke & M. Davison (Eds.), *Comparative treatments of depression* (pp. 249–290). New York: Springer.

Reinecke, M. A., Ryan, N. E., & DuBois, D. L. (1998). Cognitive-behavioral therapy of depression and depressive symptoms during adolescence: A review and meta-analysis. *Journal of the American Academy of Child and Adolescent Psychiatry, 37*(1), 26–34.

Resick, P. A., & Schnicke, M. K. (1992). Cognitive processing therapy for sexual assault victims. *Journal of Consulting and Clinical Psychology, 60*, 748–756.

Riso, L. P., du Toit, P. L., Stein, D. J., & Young, J. E. (2007). *Cognitive schemas and core beliefs in psychological problems: A scientist-practitioner guide.* Washington, DC: American Psychological Association.

Riso, L. P., Maddux, R. L., & Santorelli, N. T. (2007). Early maladaptive schemas in chronic depression. In L. P. Riso, P. L. du Toit, D. J. Stein, & J. E. Young (Eds.), *Cognitive schemas and core beliefs in psychological problems: A scientist-practitioner guide* (pp. 41–58). Washington, DC: American Psychological Association.

Rosen, H. (1989). Piagetian theory and cognitive therapy. In A. Freeman, K. Simon, L. Beutler, & H. Arkowitz (Eds.), *Comprehensive handbook of cognitive therapy* (pp. 189–212). New York: Plenum Press.

Safran, J., & McMain, S. (1992). A cognitive-interpersonal approach to the treatment of personality disorders. *Journal of Cognitive Psychotherapy: An International Quarterly, 6*, 59–67.

Safran, J. D., & Segal, Z. V. (1990). *Interpersonal process in cognitive therapy.* New York: Basic Books.

Safran, J., Vallis, T., Segal, Z., & Shaw, B. (1986). Assessment of core cognitive processes in cognitive therapy. *Cognitive Therapy and Research, 10*, 509–526.

Scott, J., & Freeman, A. (2010). Beck's cognitive therapy. In N. Kazantis, M. A. Reinecke, & A. Freeman (Eds.), *Cognitive and behavioral theories in clinical practice* (pp. 28–75). New York: Guilford Press.

Segal, Z. V., Teasdale, J. D., & Williams, J. M. G. (2004). Mindfulness-based cognitive therapy: Theoretical rationale and empirical status. In S. C. Hayes, V. M. Follette, & M. M. Linehan (Eds.), *Mindfulness and acceptance: Expanding the cognitive-behavioral tradition* (pp. 45–65). New York: Guilford Press.

Seligman, M. (1975). *Helplessness: On depression, development, and death.* San Francisco: Freeman.

Shapiro, D. A., Barkham, M., Rees, A., Hardy, G. A., Reynolds, S., & Startup, M. (1994). Effects of treatment duration and severity of depression on the effectiveness of cognitive-behavioral and psychodynamic-interpersonal psychotherapy. *Journal of Consulting and Clinical Psychology, 62*, 522–534.

Spielberger, C. D., Gorsuch, R. L., Lushene, R. E., Vagg, P. R., & Jacobs, G. A. (1983). *Manual for the State–Trait Anxiety Inventory*. Palo Alto, CA: Consulting Psychologists Press.

Sue, D. W., & Sue, D. (2007). *Counseling the culturally diverse*. New York: Wiley.

Tolman, E. (1949). *Purposive behavior in animals and men*. Berkeley: University of California Press.

Veale, D., Gournay, K., Dryden,W., Boocock, A., Shah, F., Willson, R., et al.. (1996). Body dysmorphic disorder: A cognitive-behavioural models and a pilot randomized controlled trial. *Behaviour Research and Therapy, 34*, 717–729.

Voss Horrell, S. C. (2008). Effectiveness of cognitive-behavioral therapy with adult ethnic minority clients: A review. *Professional Psychology: Research and Practice, 39*, 160–168.

Wampold, B. E., Takuya, M., Baskin, T. W., & Tierney, S. C. (2002). A meta-(re)analysis of the effects of cognitive therapy versus 'other therapies' for depression. *Journal of Affective Disorders, 68*, 159–165.

Weissman, A. N., & Beck, A. T. (1978, March). *Development and validation of the Dysfunctional Attitudes Scale: A preliminary investigation*. Paper presented at the meeting of the American Educational Research Association, Toronto, ON.

Wells, A. (1997). *Cognitive therapy of anxiety disorders*. Chichester, UK: Wiley.

Wilson, J., & Rapee, R. (2003). Social phobia. In M. A. Reinecke & D. Clark (Eds.), *Cognitive therapy across the lifespan* (pp. 258–292). Cambridge, UK: Cambridge University Press.

Wykes, T., Steel, C., Everitt, B., & Tarrier, N. (2008). Cognitive behavior therapy for schizophrenia: Effect sizes, clinical models, and methodological rigor. *Schizophrenia Bulletin, 34*(3), 523–537.

Young, J. (1991). *Cognitive therapy for personality disorders: A schema-focused approach*. Sarasota, FL: Professional Resource Exchange.

Young, J. E., Klosko, J. S., & Weishaar, M. E. (2003). *Schema therapy: A practitioner's guide*. New York: Guilford Press.

Zimmerman, G., Favrod, J., Trieu, V. H., & Pomini, V. (2005). The effect of cognitive behavioral treatment on the positive symptoms of schizophrenia spectrum disorders: A meta-analysis. *Schizophrenia Research, 77*, 1–9.

Zung, W. W. K. (1971). A rating instrument for anxiety disorders. *Psychosomatics, 12*, 371–379.

CHAPTER 6

Behavior Therapy
Functional–Contextual Approaches

William C. Follette
Glenn M. Callaghan

HISTORICAL BACKGROUND

One way of understanding the history of behavior therapy is to distinguish among three waves or generations of behavior therapies. The first wave of behavior therapy was a reaction to clinical practices of the day that were not based on well-established basic principles of behavior and behavior change. Those practices included psychoanalysis and humanistic therapies, among others. Behavior therapies well-rooted in behavior analytic learning principles were increasingly important and included practices such as desensitization, token economies, behavioral treatment for autism, exposure therapies; and other applications of applied behavior analysis. With some exceptions, the initial wave of behavior therapy largely eschewed intrapersonal and relationship concerns.

Though there was earlier evidence, by the late 1960s, the role of cognitive processes in human behavior and the explosion in mechanistic computer analogies to cognition gave rise to the second wave of behavior therapy. This generation of behavior therapy came on the heels of Albert Bandura's (1977) extension of behavior theory to include cognitive models and processes of change, learning by observation, and a theory of self-efficacy. By the end of the 1970s, cognitive therapy was made mainstream with the publication of Beck's (Beck, Rush, Shaw, & Emery, 1979) famous treatment manual for depression and Albert Ellis's (1977) work on rational emotive therapy. Part of the reason for the ascension of cognitive processes was the perceived unwillingness of behaviorism to address language and private events, including thoughts and emotion. While this criticism was only partially valid, as we discuss shortly, it did provide the opportunity for the second wave to gather momentum. It is worth noting that the cognitive-behavioral therapies emerging at the time were not closely tied to basic cognitive research going on in laboratories. It is this departure from the close ties between clinical interventions and basic research that also differentiated the first and second waves of behavior therapies.

The origins of the third wave of behavior therapy are more difficult to describe. More recent studies of the posited mechanisms of change for cognitive therapy have called into question the actual role and process of changing cognitions, and a seminal component analysis of cognitive therapy for depression suggested that that the behavioral rather than the cognitive components of cognitive therapy were responsible for observed changes in depression (Jacobson et al., 1996). The methodology of a somewhat mechanistic view of human behavior that was utilized by cognitive-behavioral therapy (CBT) researchers began to look as if it had not paid the dividends anticipated. A philosophical shift characterized the third generation of behavior therapy.

The philosophy of behavioral psychotherapy and behavioral clinical psychology has generally followed one of two traditions. The first, mechanism, can be understood using a machine metaphor. This worldview (ontology) presumes that there are realities to be discovered; that these realities are composed of parts, forces and relationships; and that there are lawful relations governing these realities to be identified. To understand the machine, in our case behavior, one must understand the components and the lawful relationships among them. To "repair" dysfunctional behavior one would need to identify the part or the process that was not working properly and repair it. One example of mechanism is the stimulus–response (S-R) psychology of John B. Watson, who argued the reductionistic position that all activities can be defined as muscle movement and glandular activity. Though it might not seem so, CBT is also mechanistic, in that it presumes elaborated cognitive processes that mediate outcomes. Distress was proposed to result from dysfunctional beliefs about the meaning of antecedent stimuli. If one learned to dispute or correct those erroneous beliefs, psychological distress would be ameliorated.

The second philosophical position is that of pragmatism or contextualism. Pragmatism argues that distinctions matter only when they make a difference. Statements, scientific or otherwise, are true to the extent that they produce an outcome that makes a practical difference. While there are a variety of contextualist perspectives (Hayes, Hayes, Reese, & Sarbin, 1993), this chapter focuses on *functional contextualism* (for a more complete discussion of functional contextualism as a philosophy for behavioral science see Gifford & Hayes, 1999). The link with pragmatism is that the activities of the scientist or, in our case, the therapist, are not directly concerned with formal statements of cause and effect, but rather the identification of useful functional relations, about which we say more later.

Perhaps surprisingly, it is the radical behaviorism of B. F. Skinner (1953) that characterizes contemporary functional contextualism. Though Skinner did not overly concern himself with philosophy, he did reject the simple notion of local (temporally ordered) cause and effect in favor of function. Skinner viewed the acquisition of behavior to occur over time as the organism's behaviors are selected based on an accumulated history (Chiesa, 1992). *Radical behaviorism* directed the scientist to consider behavior in a context of which the scientist was also an inextricable part. The exact scale over time of that context depended on the intended goals of a particular analysis.

Gifford and Hayes (1999) have characterized contemporary functional contextualism as follows:

> Functional contextualism seeks analyses that achieve prediction and influence with *precision* (a restricted set of constructs apply to any particular event), *scope* (a wide number of events can be analyzed with these constructs), and *depth* (analytic constructs at the psychological level cohere with those at other levels). The goal of prediction and influence provides a specific kind of utility or "successful working." Specifically, prediction and influ-

ence is accomplished when an analysis (a) identifies contextual features that permit the prediction of the behavior of interest, and (b) demonstrates that the manipulation of these contextual features affects the probability of occurrence of this behavior. (pp. 307–308; emphasis in original)

Nowhere in the description is a notion of strict causality. The criterion by which an analysis is judged is whether or not it allows one to accomplish the goals set forth at the beginning of the analysis.

Though perhaps not obvious, the notion that function was the key to assessing a useful analysis allowed Skinner a methodology to explore both verbal behavior and private events, including thoughts and feelings. In his analysis, the meaning of psychological terms was derived from the contingencies that surrounded the use of such terms. One could not operationally define such terms for someone, but one could identify the history and function of the use of descriptions of private events. This assertion opened the subject matter of CBT to a different kind of analysis than had previously occurred. Private events, such as relationships, thoughts, feelings, and emotions, became legitimate objects of study. However, from a functional perspective, private events are considered dependent variables (i.e., things to be explained) rather than independent (i.e., causal) variables that exist without reference to the context in which they occur.

The third wave of therapies is difficult to characterize. However, they share an interest in pragmatic goals, rely less on strict cause–effect explanations of behavior, but instead tend to understand behavior as acts-in-context. In addition, they tend to concern themselves with the interpersonal and language stimulus functions that can produce unnecessary suffering. What are these therapies? Often included in such lists are functional analytic psychotherapy (FAP; Kanter, Tsai, & Kohlenberg, 2010; Kohlenberg & Tsai, 1991; Tsai et al., 2009), acceptance and commitment therapy (ACT; Hayes, Strosahl, & Wilson, 1999), and dialectical behavior therapy (DBT; Linehan, 1993). Other candidates include behavioral activation and mindfulness-based cognitive therapy.

THE CONCEPT OF PERSONALITY

Functional contextualism does not find the concept of personality to be a very useful heuristic. As classically discussed, personality is generally a structuralist notion that behavior is the result of covert internal intrapsychic structures. Functionally, the construct of personality does not particularly help the clinician do anything differently with respect to changing behavior. Attributing behavioral tendencies or perceived rigidity to some personality feature of the client generally restricts the likelihood that the therapist will look for controllable environmental factors that may produce change if properly arranged.

Having minimized the importance of the concept of personality, now let us backtrack to discuss how radical behaviorally oriented contextualists would discuss the issues of response variability or invariability. For more detailed discussion of the issues described here the reader is referred to Baum's (2005) *Understanding Behaviorism* and Nelson-Gray and Farmer's (2005) *Personality-Guided Behavior Therapy*.

From our perspective, behavior is selected over time because of environmental consequences. Problematic and adaptive behaviors arise through the same processes. What may look like maladaptive behavior from one perspective has likely been, on average, more frequently reinforced than alternative behaviors in the same situation. Giving either a com-

The positive psychology movement has classified six virtues and 24 character strengths in the process (Peterson & Seligman, 2004). Between DSM and positive psychology the field has tied anchors at suffering and happiness. However, there is not yet a coherent linkage between the extremes that seems clinically useful.

In 1993 we put forward some initial ideas about a behavior analytic conceptualization of psychological health and later positive psychology (Follette, Bach, & Follette, 1993; Follette, Linnerooth, & Ruckstuhl, 2001). In the article on psychological health, we offered the following hypothetical scenario for a discussion between a therapist and two clients. Both had been treated for depression, and both currently had depression scores of 0, indicating no depression. Consider these different responses the clients might have given as therapy ended:

> CLIENT A: I have worked through the pain and I can now live with it. As much as it hurt, I know I can survive, and sharing my life with someone else again is very important to me.
>
> CLIENT B: I have worked through the pain and now I can live with it and get on with my life. But I am never going to get involved like that again or permit myself to be so vulnerable and hurt. (Follette et al., 1993, p. 304)

Without some notion of psychological health these two outcomes would be indistinguishable, because the initial depressive symptoms had resolved according to whatever depression scale was used. Yet, as therapists, we readily appreciate a significant difference in outcomes between these two clients. Client A is more likely to engage a richer variety of social reinforcers than Client B, even if entails some risk of future pain. Client B alludes to a future in which relationships are much more tightly managed and limited and that in turn will limit opportunities for both hurt and fulfillment. Avoidance of future pain is more important than intimacy to Client B. It is important to be able to differentiate these outcomes.

In offering some ideas about psychological health we realized that no conceptualization of psychological health or pathology is made that does not somehow involve the values and goals behind asserting such a conceptual scheme. One advantage of the way a functional contextualist approaches the issue is that the principles that produce distress are the same as those that can be used to increase satisfaction. Notice we did not use the term *happiness,* because constantly being happy is not our definition of psychological health. Interestingly, not all contemporary functional contextualists would agree on all aspects of psychological health. We have more to say on this later. What is presented here comes from the following values.

Some behavioral accounts describe a well-adjusted person as having a learning history that includes a wide range of positive reinforcement for healthy behaviors. We presume that the influence of broad and deep sources of reinforcement that do not impinge on the rights of others produce a more satisfying life experience. Another element of psychological health is *behavioral flexibility*, which has been defined as "the ability to contact the present moment more fully as a conscious human being, and to change or persist in behavior when doing so serves a valued goal" (Hayes, Luoma, Bond, Masuda, & Lillis, 2006, p. 7). This implies that an individual behaves under the contingent control of the environment in which he or she functions rather than according to strict rule-governed behavior that he has been taught or constructed for oneself. Inflexibility results from weak or counterproductive contextual control over language processes.

At many points in our lives it is adaptive to learn by following *rules* (descriptions of the relationship between setting, behavior, and consequences). "Don't touch a strange dog" might be a behavior better learned by rule than by experience. However, a rule such as "Join in a conversation when you are sure what to say" limits social opportunities and should be tested occasionally. Other rules are probably enduring ("Don't leave the house without wearing pants"). The psychologically healthy individual finds a reasonable balance and the ability to recognize when conditions of reinforcement might have changed, and how to relate to language and cognitions effectively so they do not restrict opportunities to behave in valued ways.

Maximizing the conditions in which one functions under positively reinforcing conditions implies that one can construct a reasonable balance between short-term and long-term reinforcers. This requires that one have social networks that support the achievement of long-term reinforcers by supplying short-term and intermediate reinforcement for the effort. For example, building up to run a marathon is more likely to be successful if one runs with a partner or has friends who provide reinforcement each time one runs a longer distance than before. The fact that we argue that these repertoires are valuable would not mean very much if we had no technology for establishing such behaviors, but in fact we do.

Perhaps the most significant change that has occurred as part of the third wave of behavior therapy is the special attention paid to the role of language and cognition in psychopathology and therapy. Skinner attempted to account for verbal behavior and in so doing provided some useful, functional language. However, among other limitations, his account of verbal behavior did not adequately address how stimuli could come to have discriminative functions without a direct learning history. In nonverbal organisms (all organisms other than humans), this only occurs via stimulus generalization, when some formal property of a new stimulus resembles the originally learned stimulus. A pigeon may learn to peck a green key when reinforced for doing so and may then also peck a blue-green key without a direct history of receiving reinforcement. The formal property of "greenness" has sufficiently shared physical characteristic so that the key pecking occurs. However, nonverbal organisms cannot then be presumed to peck when presented with the sound of the word *green* without additional conditioning. Humans do so starting at very early ages. Language allows many complex relations among stimuli to emerge. This line of research has been called relational frame theory (RFT; Hayes, Barnes-Holmes, & Roche, 2001) and represents the scientific basis for therapies such as ACT to alter the context under which cognition and language function.

Two features of language and cognition that are of particular interest are *bidirectionality* and *relational networks*. Nonverbal organisms can learn to discriminate previously neutral stimuli that predict events. A dog learns to respond to "Go for a walk?" if the phrase precedes the walk. That same dog will not learn this relationship if the "Go for a walk?" follows the walking. Bidirectionality in humans is demonstrated when learning occurs, although the neutral stimulus follows the event. For example, if one takes a child to the circus and buys her caramel popcorn, which she readily devours, and later you tell the child what they had was "caramel popcorn," she will likely agree if you subsequently offer to buy her caramel popcorn, even though the label followed the stimulus. This bidirectionality of stimulus relations is important, because in therapy it is an account of why talking about a traumatic event after it has already occurred can still evoke distress. When the talk and the event become one and the same, a client will avoid the conversation, because the conversation acquires the aversive properties of the events. If one learns to equate the words with the event itself, unnecessary distress can occur when talking about an aversive event is the same as the event itself.

The second important feature of RFT is the notion of *relational responding*. There are many kinds of relational responding. For example, *stimulus equivalence* is demonstrated when one is shown that $A = B$ and $B = C$. One then easily determines that $A = C$ without ever directly contacting either B or C. Once these relations are established, a relational network has formed. Many kinds of relational networks can be formed in addition to "equal to or same as," including "greater than," "better than," "more than," "less than," "sooner than," and so on.

The last concept we present is what RFT calls the *transformation of function*, the basis for derived relational responding. If one has learned that A is more than B, and then B is reinforced at some level, it is likely that A, in the absence of any other contingencies, will serve greater reinforcing functions because of its "more than" relationship with B. It is through this process that one could transfer an aversive conditioned response from one member of an equivalence class to another, without ever directly contacting the aversive contingency for each member of the class. In terms of psychological health and psychopathology, transfer of stimulus function can lead to efficiencies in learning as well as unexpected avoidance of stimuli (people or experiences) that occur as a result of inappropriate transfer of stimulus function. A disappointing experience with one person can lead to avoidance of others who might be members of an equivalance class. While a more detailed explanation of RFT is not possible here, it provides an experimental basis for studying complex verbal processes, something that is consistent with the initial appeal of the first wave of behavior therapies but was not available until RFT.

Whether we consider the clinical behavior analysis portion or the RFT portion of the third wave, both share the notion that the underlying processes that can lead to psychological health can also lead to psychopathology. Healthy behavior or pathological behavior stems from the person acting in a context. Change occurs by altering that context. It is the history of the person within his or her environment that produces the outcome, not some internal defect or disease. Intervention builds on one's history rather than trying to eliminate symptoms. A recent statement by Dahl, Plumb, Stewart, and Lundgren (2009) places the ACT/RFT scientists and practitioners in the contextualist camp:

> Behavior analysis, as a broad field subsuming both ACT and RFT, represents the application of functional contextualism in psychology. The fundamental behavior analytic unit is the operant, or three-term, contingency involving antecedents, . . . behavior, and consequences. . . . This relates to ACT and RFT because we are not interested in analyzing a behavioral event . . . by breaking it down into its component parts. Rather, we are interested in seeing how behaviors occur within the context of a person's unique personal history and influences of the present environment. How we change behavior in ACT is related to understanding context, as opposed to changing the content of thought or the form of feelings. We work to change not a person's thoughts about her painful history, but rather a relationship to those very thoughts, so that she might live in a meaningful life guided by her values, as opposed to her past or current private experiences. (p. 4)

The focus of ACT is not to eliminate or even necessarily to alter the frequency of thoughts but to change the way in which one relates to those thoughts by altering the context in which the functions of those thoughts occur, so as to not interfere with behaving in a manner consistent with living a valued life.

Third-wave therapies that attempt to alter the context of one's cognitive behaviors so that they are noticed as just being behaviors ("I'm noticing the thought that I might fail") rather than being a cause ("I'm incompetent") are addressing this issue in some fashion. These approaches are quite different from any that might directly attempt to eliminate those thoughts.

THE PROCESS OF CLINICAL ASSESSMENT

Psychological assessment by a contemporary behavioral researcher or practitioner is fundamental to the process of treatment and is collaborative and openly shared with clients. In order to determine which behaviors to address in treatment, the clinician uses a *functional analysis*. This is a process of determining the variables that give rise to and support everything a client does.

Functional Analysis in Brief

Ultimately, the goal of a functional analysis of client behavior is to understand the ABCs of behaviorism—the antecedents, the behaviors, and the consequences. More technically, one would say, the *discriminative stimuli* (S^D), the *response repertoire* (R), and the *contingencies of reinforcement* (S^R). In any event, the therapist must understand what occurs before a behavior that signals it or sets the occasion for it to occur, and what follows the behavior that makes it more or less likely to occur in the future. The analysis also includes an assessment of the quality (successful functioning) of the behavior in the context in which it occurs. The conditions that would signal reinforcement (S^D) may be present, but the behavior itself may not be "good enough" to get reinforced. The behavior analysis of the response is rich and somewhat complex. We seek to understand the behavior not by how it may appear more superficially, but by its function (hence the term *functional analysis*). The superficial appearance of behavior, also known as its *topography*, is what is most readily visible to us and often is quite salient. For example, stating that a client cries, self-injures, or repeatedly washes her hands is to describe the topography of that response. These are likely very important behaviors to notice and may even be shorthand terms to help describe targets for clinical intervention, but identifying behaviors does not constitute a functional analysis.

The therapist's goal here is to understand the function of these behaviors or how they come about and are sustained for the client. While self-injury, for example, is important to note, it is more important to understand what purpose that behavior serves. A functional-analytic question may be, "What does it cost or benefit the client in the short and long term to engage in such a response?" If, for example, the client engages in self-injury to "help feel calmer afterward," then we may have part of a functional analysis, namely, the behavior may be negatively reinforced by removing some aversive state. If the self-injury occurs during times of distress that include cognitive and affective states and is followed by the reduction in distress, we may have begun to define a type of functional response for the client. In fact, the client may engage in a variety of problematic coping strategies when experiencing distress that all serve temporarily to reduce this distress but may have longer-term, less desirable consequences. If all of these behaviors result in reducing that distress as a consequence (contingencies of *negative reinforcement*), then we have defined a functional class of behaviors for the client. A *functional class* is a group of behaviors with similar antecedents and consequences for a client, despite their difference in appearance. These topographical dissimilarities can be striking. For example, a client may make jokes, cry out, miss sessions, or quickly acquiesce, all in the service of escaping or avoiding difficult emotional experiences in a clinical session.

At its broadest conceptual level, a functional analysis attempts to make clear the function of *important* (explain a significant amount of outcome if altered), *causal* (reliably precedes and covaries), and *alterable* (can be changed in therapy) variables (Haynes & O'Brien, 1990). Specifically, a therapist tries to identify those variables that seem pertinent or essential to what the client and therapist have identified as targets for an intervention. These are, then, important to the case. The challenge is that some variables that "look" or "feel" important may simply be more salient or interesting based on the therapist's underlying epistemic assumptions about what causes suffering. A client's childhood may or may not be important. Furthermore, events in the past may seem "important" when, in fact, they are no longer causally related to why the client engages in the behavior in the present. This is called *functional autonomy* and refers to the difference between variables that may have been important at one time and those that maintain the behaviors seen in the present. The bottom and most elemental line here is that the variables identified in any functional analysis are causal; that is, there is a demonstrable relationship between the variables described in a functional analysis and those that are used to alter the behaviors of interest. This is what is meant by *alterable*.

In this way, then, a functional analysis in the assessment of client behavior is an iterative or a step-by-step process that is recursive. We state what we believe is a useful analysis. If we attempt to alter some client behavior to help alleviate suffering, perhaps by teaching a different repertoire to the client, then we must determine whether this actually had any real change or impact on that suffering. If the client does not improve, then we are required to go back to revisit and modify the analysis until it helps the therapist produce clinical improvement.

The Concept of Resistance

To the behavioral therapist, *resistance* simply refers to a behavioral repertoire of the client when he or she is not yet able to engage in the targeted response; that is, when treating someone who is constantly washing his or her hands, and who still cannot seem to really decrease this responding, the client is not "resisting" treatment. There is not a deeper cause of the lack of treatment gain. One simply has either asked the client to engage in a response that has not been sufficiently learned, or one has failed to understand all of the variables in the functional analysis that need to be in place for the client to engage in another response. In any case, the behavior therapist goes back to the drawing board.

The Role of Psychiatric Diagnoses and the Selection of Interventions

It may be evident to the reader that a good deal of precision and accuracy is necessary during the assessment process of therapy. The precise description of client behaviors is essential in creating these working hypotheses of the variables that control client behaviors. It does not serve the therapist's analysis, and hence the client in treatment, if the therapist prematurely stops his or her description of client behaviors or uses descriptors that are imprecise. As convenient as it may be to describe a client's behavior as "panicked" or "dysthymic," it tells us very little in the way of what these behaviors are, and it tell us nothing about where they came from and why they continue. This is more generally true with diagnostic labels and standard psychiatric nosology. The important question is highlighted in the famous quote by Gordon Paul: "What treatment, by whom, is most effective for this individual with that specific problem, and under which set of circumstances?" (1967, p. 111).

One challenge a contemporary behavior therapist may face lies with personal preferences for different behavior therapies. Some therapies (e.g., ACT) focus on intrapersonal events, such as intolerance of emotional experience and subsequent escape and avoidance behaviors, while others (e.g., FAP) may have a personal focus on interpersonal processes, including the therapeutic relationship. Personal interests are perfectly fine. They speak to our own reinforcement histories and even to our values or identified salient reinforcers for which we work. The challenge lies with deciding to use one of these therapies before a functional analysis or behavioral assessment has taken place. This a priori-driven conceptualization is, in fact, not a behavioral conceptualization at all.

The Client Repertoire: Strengths and Weaknesses

An effective functional analysis attempts to identify the contingencies responsible for not only ineffective client problem behaviors but also those that effectively move clients toward their goals. The behavioral therapist tries to specify those behaviors, typically referred to as strengths or weaknesses, in the repertoire that may be excessive or deficient and contribute to human suffering, while also identifying behaviors that actually do serve the client's goals or help to alleviate suffering. The behavior therapist's goal is to build a more effective client repertoire, not to eliminate problems directly. By identifying aspects of the client's repertoire that are already in place, the therapist can more efficiently and effectively help the client improve. Typically referred to as a constructivist approach to therapy, this approach is at the heart of much of what we do (see Goldiamond, 1974).

Values: Identifying Salient Reinforcers

Values are essentially the client's identification of salient reinforcers toward which he or she works, or would like to move. It is important to notice that verbal behavior related to identification of reinforcers may not always correspond to the reality of the client's current behavior. In FAP, clients may be asked to write a mission statement that can help to influence behavioral choices when other environmental contingencies are not present. ACT makes use of similar exercises, such as having clients write their own eulogy, imagining what they would like others to say about their lives.

Cultural Factors: Contextual Variables

Contextual variables also include the client's race, ethnicity, spirituality, and experience of social class. Often gender roles, sociopolitical values, and other deeply personal behaviors may be related to verbal behaviors in the form of rules for which the client has a history of reinforcement for following. In this way, a behavior therapist often finds it helpful to assess for a client's own description of what was or is expected of him or her in a given role. For example, we may ask of a female client who considers leaving her partner in search of a more independent life, "What were the expectations of women when you grew up? What expectations do you feel now? Are these reasonable or understandable to you? How might you try to do that differently? What might that gain for you? Could it also have its costs? What would it be like not to be in a relationship?" These types of variables frequently present as unspoken conflicts between what is expected and what is preferred. We have more to say about cultural factors later.

Those trained in functional analysis might believe that the technique will identify the important variables to consider in treatment planning regardless of any differences in ethnicity, culture, spirituality, sexual preference, and the like. One might believe this is the case, because a functional analysis is iterative and self-correcting. This is not the case. While clients may be patient during the assessment phase of therapy, their patience is not without limits. It is presumptuous to believe that a variety of circumstances do not apply when it is appropriate to seek outside consultation on how to evaluate probable strengths and reinforcers when cultural differences are significantly large.

Unit and Level of Analysis

We hope we have made clear that behavior is understood as an act in context and is evaluated by the effectiveness of the behavior in achieving a goal. Behavior is situated action and is only understood in the context in which it occurs. It is important to note that the context in which to appreciate the function of a behavioral class is dynamic. It is rarely meaningful to consider only a single ABC analysis in therapy. Although sometimes an immediate exchange between the client and therapist is significant in isolation, it is often useful to consider whether a particular behavior is part of a larger pattern that may emerge over time. As we mentioned earlier, the topography of a behavior may vary across sessions, but the more salient function may better be understood by examining the impact of the client's behavior on the therapist to determine whether different topographies elicit the same response from the therapist (and others). Assessing whether one has chosen the correct level of analysis depends on whether it leads the therapist to engage the client in developing a more successful behavioral repertoire.

THE PRACTICE OF THERAPY

The basic structure of most contemporary contextual behavior therapies is similar to most traditional therapies. Most commonly, individual sessions are held weekly for the proverbial 50-minute hour. In research settings, treatment protocols generally range from 16 to 22 weeks (see later discussion regarding the scalability of ACT). In more natural environments, therapy can and does last much longer. The reason for long-term treatment is that the scope of the problems addressed by contemporary behavior therapies is much broader than that in first- or second-wave therapies.

It is important to remember that FAP and ACT are not designed to be eliminative therapies; that is, the goal of each of these therapies is not to eliminate symptoms that fit into some diagnostic category, but to establish a context (history and skills) that allows clients to develop behaviors consistent with attaining their personal goals and values. This process is more open-ended because the scope is broader and clients often continue to expand their goals and values as they progress. To the extent that clients meet criteria for a diagnostic category, we generally presume that it is because important areas of functioning do not provide the quality and quantity of reinforcement needed, and contextual factors that are in place impede the necessary learning to achieve these goals.

We use FAP to illustrate some of these clinical principles. Often ACT techniques are used within FAP (Callaghan, Gregg, Marx, Kohlenberg, & Gifford, 2004) and will be briefly described. As noted earlier, assessment and treatment are intertwined. While some assessment is being conducted, the therapist is also shaping therapy engagement. The therapist needs to be aware that therapy is difficult for the client. Those who have not been in therapy before often do not know exactly what to expect and how to behave. Some clients may ask halfway facetiously whether they should lie on a couch. Those more familiar with therapy may be looking for similarities or differences between this therapy and other experiences. The first three to four sessions are usually introduced in ways familiar to most therapists.

THERAPIST: In this first part of therapy I am going to get to know you and your view of why therapy makes sense for you. That might take as little as one session but more commonly takes two to four sessions. I'll listen and ask questions, and answer those you may have. At some point during this phase I'll develop some idea of what I think might be the important issues for us to address. Much of that information will come from you, but I will also be paying attention to what is happening in sessions and suggest some additional ideas that occur to me as well. I'll share those ideas with you to see if they make sense to you, and I'll describe how therapy works. During that same time I'm going to try to make an honest assessment of whether I believe I can be helpful working with you. During that same time, you have a job as well.

CLIENT: What is that?

THERAPIST: Your job is to decide whether you want to work with me. You are the consumer here. It is important that we be able to work well together. While I believe I can most often be helpful, it is important that you feel comfortable with that decision as well. So at the time I am able to share my ideas about how to proceed with you, I will ask you if you would like to work with me. I believe therapy can be very helpful for almost everyone, and I want you to have a good experience, even if some of the sessions are difficult. That is more likely to happen if you feel comfortable with your therapist. I will be honest with you and tell you if I think I can be helpful, and I want you to be honest with me about whether you feel comfortable working with me. If you don't feel comfortable I will be happy to help refer you to another therapist with whom you might feel more comfortable. That choice is strictly up to you.

CLIENT: That sounds fair. I'm sure we can work together.

THERAPIST: I suspect so as well, but we will make the choice together when the time comes.

During these initial sessions the therapist does two things. One is that he or she begins a functional analysis of the presenting problems. The information for that analysis comes from the client and the therapist's reactions to what the client says, how effective or aversive the client's behavior might be, and how effectively the therapist responds to the client. Some clients have overly high expectations about how quickly therapy proceeds, while others are quite reticent. These could be clinical issues. In these early sessions it is important to reinforce effort, attendance, and any data gathering that may be required. The interactions between the client and therapist are a rich source of information about the interpersonal functioning of the client. The second task for the therapist is to have the client identify the values for which he or she genuinely strives. Following this initial assessment, the following conversation might take place that marks a transition into deeper levels of work.

THERAPIST: I think I have a pretty good idea what some of your primary concerns are. Let me summarize what I understand the issues to be, and then you can correct or elaborate on anything I've said. Your first concern is that you are unhappy in your current relationship with Beth. You said, "I'm unhappy and I don't know why." Additionally, you said that your life seemed "boring." What you wanted out of therapy is to improve your relationship with Beth and find some meaning in life. Does that sound about right?

CLIENT: Yes, those seem to be the things that are most weighing on my mind.

THERAPIST: I also noticed some other things you didn't mention that might be important for us to consider. During the last couple of sessions, it seemed as if you wanted to ask some questions of me but decided not to. There was also one occasion when I had to take an emergency phone call and you looked slightly annoyed. But when I asked if the call was annoying or distracting, you said, "No." So in addition to what you said about Beth and finding more meaning in life, I have this loosely held hypothesis that you have a hard time either labeling some of your emotions or figuring out how to express them effectively. I'm not sure where that comes from, but I think it could be relevant to why you initially came in to treatment. Does that make any sense?

CLIENT: It kind of does. Sometimes during conversations I have some sense that things aren't going well, but I don't know what to say, and by the time I figure it out the opportunity has passed.

THERAPIST: So it sounds like what I said makes sense to you. Did anything I said sound wrong, exaggerated, or as if I missed something that is important to you?

CLIENT: No, I think you did a good job. What next?

THERAPIST: Well, I'm pretty confident that I can be useful for you. I very much enjoy our interactions and look forward to working with you. In a moment I'll ask whether you would like to work with me, but first, I want to explain how therapy would proceed. You've done a great job so far, but the harder work is ahead of us. In the kind of therapy I do, I believe that the problems you have in your relationship with Beth will actually show up between you and me during sessions. In fact, I think some of that has already happened. I suspect you were annoyed when our session was interrupted but were unwilling or unable to express your displeasure. I had some sense of that at the time, but when I asked you about it, you said there was no problem. I believe there are many opportunities between you and Beth to better express what makes you happy, sad, annoyed or joyful that gets missed. I'm not sure why quite yet, but I'm certainly wondering if that happens. When it happens between us, you and I will both try to notice when it happens and behave more effectively in the moment. So therapy will be a time during the course of our relationship when we keep an eye out for things you do well and things you can do better. When either of those happens I'm going to point it out, and we can experiment with different ways of responding. In some ways our relationship is just like any other close, confiding relationship you have, except that you can try different ways of expressing yourself and I'll hang in there with you, no matter how difficult the struggle. There may be some homework, but the main work will be done in the context of a close relationship between the two of us. What do you think?

CLIENT: That sounds fine.

THERAPIST: Would you tell me if it didn't?

CLIENT: I'm not sure.

THERAPIST: (*smiling*) Perfect! I think we can work together.

CLIENT: (*smiling*) I do, too.

The nature of FAP is that therapy is tailored to the concerns and functioning of a particular client. Still, common functional classes can be observed. Callaghan (2006) has provided an assessment instrument called the Functional Idiographic Assessment Template (FIAT) that can help conceptualize problems fairly efficiently. The FIAT suggests five classes of interpersonal functioning to assess. These classes are described in Table 6.1. Note that examples given for problems recognize contextual cues or discriminative stimuli in the environment in which the class of behaviors could be emitted and reinforced. Examples are also provided for problems with the quality, function, or timing of the client's responses. In most of the behavior classes in which there are problems with responses, those responses are not likely to serve as effective reinforcers or discriminative stimuli for another person's interpersonal responses. These five classes of behaviors are certainly not unrelated and overlap each other.

The purpose of the FIAT is to help organize more technical aspects of behavior the therapist may use to conceptualize a case in language a client can readily understand. The FIAT was not developed to be exhaustive or the only way to conceptualize client problem areas. It is an example of some ways in which one might begin thinking functionally about a client's problems. Though we have not listed examples here, the therapist should also be noting client strengths on which to build as therapy progresses.

Earlier we mentioned that we helped clients identify important values (reinforcers) toward which to organize their behavior. In the case presented earlier, the client is behaving as if he values the avoidance of conflict more than developing an intimate, egalitarian relationship. This short-term avoidance is likely contributing to his relationship dissatisfaction and his failing sense of purpose. Identifying more distal, fundamental values will be useful. FAP and ACT both spend time with clients in various values clarification exercises (Dahl et al., 2009). Helping the client prioritize values may help to establish greater motivation to attempt new behaviors even at the cost of some short-term distress. During the course of therapy, the client will have many opportunities to refine how effectively he expresses his feelings and negotiates change with his partner. At many points during therapy, the client will be asked, "Is what you are doing consistent with what you want to be about?" This longer-term motivating question is coupled with immediate support for constructive change during each session.

Clinically Relevant Behaviors and the Five Rules for FAP

In forming the case conceptualization based on the functional analysis, the therapist identifies functional classes of behavior called *clinically relevant behaviors* (CRBs). CRBs fall into one of two categories, either behavioral excesses or deficits that are problematic for the client. Those that appear in session are called CRB1s. Client improvements that appear in session are termed CRB2s. In principle delivering FAP is straightforward. The ordering of how treatment is done depends on the presenting problems of the client, how the client actually behaves in a particular session, the evolving nature of the case conceptualization, and an evaluation of whether behavioral improvements can be shaped or whether some behaviors interfere sufficiently with therapy that they have to be addressed before a more effective repertoire can be established.

TABLE 6.1. FIAT Classes of Problematic Interpersonal Functioning

Contextual cues/discriminative stimulus functions	Response repertoire
Class A: Assertion of needs	

• Problems with identification or specification
  ○ Unable to identify or specify needs or values
    as they occur
    or
  ○ Cannot identify that a request could be made
    to meet his or her own need
• Problems with appropriate contextual control
• Problems with undergeneralizing features of
  relationships
• Problems with overgeneralizing features of
  relationships
	• Escape or avoidance repertoire
	  ○ Escape repertoire
	  ○ Avoidance repertoire
	    —Rejecting that a need is present
	    —Ineffective or unclear assertion of needs
	    —Disguised request
	    —Excessive requests or demands for needs to be met
	    —Aversive response style

Class B: Bidirectional Communication	

• Problems with identification or specification
  ○ Identifying or describing his or her impact
    on others
  ○ Identifying that feedback is being given by
    another person
  ○ Discriminating whether feedback is accurate
  ○ Discriminating that feedback can be given
	• Escape or avoidance repertoire
	  ○ Escape Repertoire
	    —Hypersensitivity to observed impact and feedback
	     from others on others
	  ○ Avoidance repertoire
	    —Failure to solicit feedback from others
	    —Lack of response to observed impact or feedback
	     from others
	    —Insensitivity to feedback
	    —Rejection of feedback by others
	    —Providing feedback to others
	    —Failure to provide feedback
	    —Ineffective/overelaborated/unclear feedback
	    —Negativistic feedback
	    —Overly detailed feedback to others
	    —Perseveration of feedback

Class C: Conflict	

• Problems with identification or specification
• Problems with appropriate contextual control
	• Escape or avoidance repertoire
	  ○ Excessive acquiescence
	  ○ Social withdrawal
	  ○ Excessive appeasing or conciliatory responses
	  ○ Indirect/ineffective attempts to resolve conflict
	  ○ Unwillingness to compromise in conflict
	  ○ Conflict—facilitating or escalating repertoire

Class D: Disclosure and interpersonal closeness	

• Problems with identification or specification
• Problems with appropriate contextual control
  ○ Overdisclosing
  ○ Underdisclosing
	• Escape or avoidance repertoire
	  ○ Infrequent seeking of interpersonally close
	    interaction
	  ○ Low desire for closeness
	  ○ Failure to solicit other's disclosure
	  ○ Problems with general prosocial repertoire
	  ○ Unclear or inaccurate self-disclosure
	  ○ Excessive self-disclosure or seeking closeness
	  ○ Failure to respond to another's disclosure or
	    requests and/or reciprocate with social support

(cont.)

TABLE 11.1. *(cont.)*

Contextual cues/discriminative stimulus functions	Response repertoire
Class E: Emotional experience and expression	

• Problems with identification or specification
• Problems with appropriate contextual control
   ○ Inability to recognize that an emotional experience would be expected in that context
   ○ Cannot discriminate when to report or express a feeling
	• Escape or avoidance repertoire (infrequent experience)
	   ○ Escape repertoire
	   ○ Avoidance repertoire
	     —Inaccurate label of emotional experience/ restricted range of expression
	     —Ineffective or unclear description of emotional experience
	     —Excessive affective expression

Note. Data from Callaghan (2006).

• *Rule 1: Notice the presence of CRBs when they occur in a session.* In many ways this is the simplest of the rules, yet it requires considerable skill. First one must have a solid case conceptualization to know what to notice. Some behaviors may appear to be clinically important, but whether they are depends on the case conceptualization. If a client asks for a change in fees or time, that may be a CRB1, if the client has a history of seeming uncooperative with others; a CRB2, if the client has a clinically important difficulty with assertion; or nothing at all, if the requests do not appear relevant to the case. Whether an in-session behavior is determined to be a CRB requires that the therapist be very attuned to his or her own reactions. Therapists should ask themselves several questions when assessing their ability to notice CRBs. What client behaviors have a negative impact on you? Is the client keeping your attention? What does the client do to deflect or gain your attention? These and other questions help therapists develop their own noticing repertoire.

• *Rule 2: Evoke CRBs.* Often in therapy clients emit a CRB1 in response to an event being discussed or, ideally, in response to something the therapist does (evokes a CRB). Initially, this is an opportunity for the therapist to strengthen his or her interpersonal relationship by developing trust and understanding, and to take risks with clients to create opportunities for change. What a therapists evoke also depends on the case conceptualization. A therapist expression of genuine caring can evoke a CRB1, CRB2, or nothing (in the sense that responses to intimacy are not a problem for a particular client). Rules 1 and 2 are made important by virtue of Rule 3.

• *Rule 3: Naturally reinforce CRB2s.* When a CRB1 occurs, it is an opportunity to shape alternative, more useful responses. While there may be times when punishing the occurrence of CRB1s is necessary, such as with extremely high rates of behavior that interfere with therapy, most of the time the therapist notes the occurrence of a CRB1 and prompts a CRB2 and reinforces it, or an approximation of it. The absolutely important word in this rule is *naturally,* which means that the nature of the reinforcement resembles and functions similarly to caring relationships in the client's world. To do FAP, the therapist must have a personal repertoire to care deeply for and about clients. Without any intention to infantilize the client, one aspect of this kind of caring is like that of a parent or sibling who is supportive and invested in the success of one's child or sibling as he or she tries to master life. Interest, appreciation and compassion are important components of the relationship necessary to reinforce change naturally. Simply uttering words such as "That's great" is arbitrary (and perhaps rule-governed) and unlikely to sustain change and change efforts, whereas the genuine expression of caring and excitement can.

- *Rule 4: Observe the potentially reinforcing effects of therapist behavior in relation to client CRBs.* Being aware of one's impact on a client is important, because reinforcement is defined by the actual consequences it has on client behavior and *not* by the intended impact. Sometimes one can ask a client directly, "What was it like to hear me say that I'm sad?" At other times such direct inquiries can seem arbitrary. The ability to determine one's impact on the client is another important clinical skill.

- *Rule 5: Provide functional analytically informed interpretations and implement generalization strategies.* It can be useful to teach and support a client in recognizing the context in which his or her behaviors occur. This can help the client becomes a better observer of what maintains or inhibits his or her own behavior and that of valued others. The function of this, just like any other behavior, is crucial. The intention of this rule is to help clients understand important controlling variables in their lives so they can alter and control them, thereby making it easier to generalize the understanding gained in therapy to support behavior change in other contexts. One must be sure that when clients understand the "reasons" for their behavior that these do not become reasons to explain not changing in valued directions.

Intrapersonal and Interpersonal Functions

At the risk of presenting a false dichotomy between intrapersonal and interpersonal functions, we do so hoping it is a useful heuristic rather than actual distinction, because, in the end, behavior is behavior. The term *intrapersonal* for our purposes in this chapter is intended to highlight those aspects of assessment and intervention that focus on how a client relates to his or her cognitions and affective experiences in ways that permit or restrict flexibly pursuing life goals. For example, if one were to act as if the thought "I'll never be in a good relationship" is anything more than a thought, but instead an accurate predictor of all relationships, it would diminish the likelihood that one would actively seek new, meaningful relationships or fully engage in existing ones. Therapy would create a context in which the client relates to that thought as if it were just that—a thought—and not an actual predictive rule. One might think of such experiences as an intrapersonal focus. Notice that *intrapersonal* here does not refer to an implicit personality structure. Instead, therapy would focus on creating a context, or adding to one's history, such that having a thought does not prevent actively behaving constructively.

ACT uses a variety of principle-based techniques to address how a client can learn to behave with more psychological flexibility by changing the context in which thoughts and affective experiences occur. Detailing these processes is beyond the scope of this chapter, but they are briefly described in Table 6.2. The application of these techniques might be used to address our hypothetical client's reluctance to express displeasure or annoyance with his wife and the therapist. This behavior prevents the client from enjoying all the potential richness that marriage might hold for him. His reluctance might be because he avoids any conversations that might involve conflict. The therapist might raise this issue as session progress as follows:

THERAPIST: Just now when I said that I found it painful to watch you struggle with telling me that, once again, you couldn't tell me that you were unable to disagree with your wife. You started to tear up.

CLIENT: (*Says nothing, but blinks to fight back tears.*)

TABLE 6.2. Core ACT Processes

Process	Type of process	Description
Acceptance[a]	Mindfulness and acceptance	Active and aware embrace of private events arising from one's history without attempts to alter frequency or form (e.g. teaching anxious client to feel anxiety)
Defusion[a]	Mindfulness and acceptance	Alter the undesirable functions of thoughts in order to change the way client interacts with or relates to thoughts
Being present[a]	Mindfulness and acceptance/commitment and behavior change	Promoting ongoing nonjudgmental contact with psychological and environmental events using language to note and describe events, not predict and judge them
Self as context[a]	Mindfulness and acceptance/commitment and behavior change	Being aware of one's flow of experiences without attachment to them—developed from a sense of self as a locus or perspective
Values	Commitment and behavior change	Chose qualities of purposive action that cannot be obtained as an object but can be used to support behaviors in the moment
Committed action	Commitment and behavior change	Development of larger patterns of effective action in the service of chosen values

Note. Based on Hayes, Luoma, Bond, Masuda, and Lillis (2006, pp. 7–10).
[a]These constructs comprise how ACT conceptualizes "mindfulness."

THERAPIST: I can see that this is hard for you . . . that you aren't wanting to have the thought that you could be upset and still act to make your feelings known. I'm going to just take a moment and sit with my sadness. (*A minute passes.*) I'm sad. And I had the thought that I wasn't being a good therapist. I noticed that I had that thought, and then I let it pass on its own. I think we're doing important work and this is an important moment. I can think all of those thoughts and still be here with you—watching and caring.

CLIENT: I could never do that.

THERAPIST: Hold that thought—the thought you could never let yourself feel afraid. Watch yourself having that thought. Play with that thought. (*Some moments pass.*) Now see if you can make it go away. Don't think of being afraid. (*More time passes.*) Do you notice that the only way to see whether you were successful at keeping the thought away was to have the thought "Am I feeling afraid?"

Whatever the history that makes it difficult for the client to engage fully, his marriage needs to be addressed. At this point in therapy the client is behaving as if his thought is a valid rule to which he should adhere. ACT processes can be very useful, and the therapeutic relationship is a part of the context that can make experimenting with new ways of behaving with respect to having thoughts that are not in the service of enriching his relationship easier to explore.

ACT has several techniques that function to change the context in which the client responds to his cognitions. Many are accomplished with experiential exercises and metaphors. Metaphors are useful, because they can move cognitions into other relational frames.

By talking about controlling thoughts or emotion as struggling against quicksand, clients may begin to see the struggle as counterproductive. Let us briefly describe some strategies and techniques that might be applicable to this client who does not express his displeasure, and who wants to distance from his wife to avoid conflict and the negative emotions he experiences.

- *Creative hopelessness.* Are clients willing to consider that there might be another way to proceed that does not require knowing [what to do]? In order for clients to move forward, it is necessary to give up the struggle not to have negative feelings. Asking clients what they have tried and how it has worked can be useful. As clients recite all of the (unsuccessful) things they have tried, it may become apparent that they have no way out of the dilemma. Metaphors, such as "the only way to win a tug of war with a monster is to drop the rope," or "when you find yourself in a hole, quit digging," or likening the struggle to a Chinese finger puzzle ("the more one pulls, the tighter the trap") all help the client to see the hopelessness of trying not to experience negative emotions.

- *Identifying values and goals.* As we discussed with FAP, having clients define life goal-directed behavior is an important component of treatment. In many instances, avoidance of emotion directly interferes with other larger goals, such as enjoyment of a fulfilling relationship or being a good partner.

- *Acceptance.* Among many notions of acceptance is that of willingness to experience thoughts and feelings for what they are rather than reacting to them in ways that have limited how one engages life. The techniques used include mindfulness and acceptance exercises, such as attending to one's breathing while learning to "watch" and have anxiety-related feelings and sensations come and go.

- *Cognitive defusion.* Cognitive fusion can lead clients to become caught up in the content of what they are thinking and feeling. *Fusion* implies that a thought is not just a thought but actually entails the real events the word implies. Thoughts of discomfort become a story of how discomfort is horrible. Defusion is a fundamental ACT process in which clients learn to observe thoughts as just thoughts rather than literal truths on which they must act. Defusion exercises are intended to alter the stimulus function of anxiety from "Anxiety is horrible and I must escape it" to "I am noticing that my heart rate is high" or even "I am anxious," without the need to act upon the observations.

These and other processes (see Table 6.2) all support taking value-guided action, while still having thoughts and feelings (but nothing more). ACT processes are intended to change the context in which thought and actions occur.

If adding to history so that having thoughts and emotions is no longer a barrier to the client expressing feelings to his partner, there are still interpersonal processes that must be continually assessed and addressed in treatment. Though the client may be willing to express his needs, that also does not mean he has the repertoire to do so. If he can express his needs, that does not mean he can recognize the optimal circumstances in which he can express them. Expressing his needs does not necessarily mean that he does a thoughtful job of expressing his appreciation when they are met. As therapy progresses, the therapist watches for opportunities for the client to express both pleasure and displeasure at whatever is happening in the therapeutic relationship, and creates the conditions in which the client may make successive approximations of affective expressions that are effective and likely to work well outside of therapy as well. When the approximations represent some noticeable improvement in effort or function, the therapist naturally supports the client. When they do not, the therapist can be "in the moment" with the difficulty of the task and encourage the client's continued effort.

Common Mistakes

Assuming that the therapist has learned the appropriate science behind the techniques utilized in therapy, several mistakes are common. The most significant mistake an FAP therapist can make is to fail to recognize the importance of establishing him- or herself as an important source of social reinforcement for change. This sounds technical, but it is intensely interpersonal. Supervision sessions often involve addressing the differences between therapists' natural caring responses to their closest friends in whose welfare they are truly invested and those topographically similar but functionally inadequate expressions in therapy.

Another understandable mistake is that therapists can do too much work for a client. It is common for improvements to be incremental. As any good behavior therapist knows, it is important to discriminate small improvements and (naturally) reinforce them. When a noticeable improvement has occurred, therapists sometimes fail to continue to raise the bar for even more effective client responding. Therapists are genuinely happy for the change that has occurred and lose sight of change that is still needed. After a period of time, the client–therapist relationship can resemble that of others with whom the therapist is close. The therapist "knows" what the client means and accepts an expression of feeling from the client that would not be effective in a different relationship. Though therapy can become comfortable for the dyad, eventually the client recognizes that therapy has stagnated and loses motivation for change. It can be difficult to require more effort from the client after such periods, though the client's reaction to new therapist efforts to promote change can be grist for the therapeutic mill.

Therapists all have individual and cultural histories that can help or hinder appreciating unique features of their clients' behaviors that, although different from what the therapist is used to or expects, still work. In a therapy like FAP it is crucial to look for a variety of behaviors that work in the service of the client even if these are very different from how the therapist might accomplish the same goal. Therapists have to learn to recognize effective responses that may differ from their own. While we train therapists to recognize that they each can accomplish certain goals in a variety of ways, it is not always easy to remind them that the same is true for clients.

The last mistake we mention here is for the therapist to be oblivious to his or her own strengths and weaknesses as a person that also show up in an intense therapeutic relationship. In supervision, we spend considerable time asking ourselves and noticing in others what our own strengths and liabilities are in particular situations. For example, it is not uncommon for either of us to use humor both effectively and ineffectively (though we think we are funny). Sometimes humor can make difficult contingent responding seem more gentle while still being effective. At other times, humor used inappropriately can be an escape or avoidance response that allows either therapist or client to avoid an intense reaction or keeps one from persisting to identify important functional relations that hinder interpersonal functioning. It can be a useful exercise before a session to remind oneself of the case conceptualization, what characteristics of the client are most problematic for the therapist, and what would be the most useful thing to do in that situation.

Termination

Because of the intense nature of the relationship between client and therapist in FAP, termination is particularly important to process. Termination can be an opportunity for clients to develop a repertoire for having intense relationships even those defined as time-limited. A willingness to immerse oneself in such relationships is a demonstration of acceptance. It is also an opportunity to express loss and even grief, while reviewing the behaviors that initially interfered with closeness, and those that ultimately produced it. Termination is also an opportunity for therapists to experience both satisfaction and loss. If neither occurs, it is likely the therapist has not fully engaged with the client in the relationship.

THE THERAPEUTIC RELATIONSHIP AND THE STANCE OF THE THERAPIST

In FAP, the intense, important therapeutic relationship is essential to producing change. The goal of the therapist is to establish him- or herself as a salient provider of accurate verbal descriptors and social reinforcers. Such relationships are established when the client understands that he or she sets the goals of therapy in the service of living a valued life. This happens collaboratively. As shown earlier, the therapist shares with the client the mutual nature of assessing what each person views as the issues for therapy, whether the therapist believes he or she can be helpful, and whether the client agrees and wishes to work with the therapist. There are no coercive elements in the collaboration. The choices of how to respond to clients are determined by assessing what is in the client's best interests at the moment and naturally reinforcing clinically relevant behaviors. The close, genuine relationship with the therapist should be experienced by the client as one without guile or any hidden agenda.

Contextual behavior therapists presume that clients are behaving "as they should given the context" and unconditionally support their experience. Thus, there is no blame or guilt to be assigned to clients. Lack of progress in therapy is attributed to the therapist having an incomplete functional analysis or inadequate reinforcing properties to produce change.

Therapy is guided by the goals stated by the client, but therapy is principle-based. Therapist and client have created a treatment approach collaboratively, and it is often the therapist's job to keep the two on task. This means that the agendas for the session often are set depending on what is required at a given point in therapy. Exactly how directive any session is depends on the case conceptualization. If seeking control of important aspects of a client's life is a clinically relevant behavior, sessions may be more guided by the client's preferences, or the converse may be true if giving up control is a valued goal for the client. If a client is at a point in therapy where contacting real-world contingencies would be useful, behavioral activation components of therapy might be quite directive.

The importance of self-disclosure has received considerable attention (Farber, 2006). The importance of therapist self-disclosure about personal history is determined by the function it has in a particular instance. Disclosure of the therapist's immediate responses to CRBs is essential. The degree to which personal self-disclosure is useful depends on the relevance of the history of the therapist and the stimulus properties of the therapist to the client. On many occasions, self-disclosure of relevant personal history is the appropriate social reinforcer for a CRB. On such occasions, self-disclosure can deepen the therapeutic relationship and make it more likely to facilitate client behavior change. The therapist has to be careful that such disclosures do not change the focus of therapy rather than reinforce the client's behavior.

In ACT, the essential feature of the relationship is unconditional acceptance of the client's experience. By therapist modeling and sharing of how he or she is experiencing an interaction with the client, such disclosure can also create a close relationship in which the client can disclose freely. When the therapist him- or herself can fully experience the client without avoidance of discomfort, the therapist is freer both to enquire and to disclose.

The concept of countertransference is often invoked in discussions about therapists responding to clients. While the traditional construct is not useful to contemporary behavior therapists, certainly it is the case that therapists, like clients, respond to the stimulus properties of a client or the verbal process that occurs in-session. Because this is the case, the therapist may respond to the client based on the his or her history with people who have similar stimulus functions as the client. Here, the therapist does not respond to the client "as if" he or she were a person in the therapist's past; instead, the therapist may simply respond to the client as he or she would given a history of reinforcement for those responses.

These therapist behaviors, then, may be effective in session or they may be ineffective—just like a client's. To the extent they are ineffective, they should be the focus of supervision and additional training. In FAP, care is taken during training to make sure ethical boundaries are strictly maintained. Given the degree of disclosure and caring that occur during therapy, the characteristics of the relationship may be confused by client and therapist with those of a romantic or sexual relationship. While training, great care is taken to make sure FAP therapists can discriminate their own feelings and identify such feeling in clients so as to not reinforce such behaviors or exploit client vulnerabilities.

Essential Therapist Skills

There is only one essential therapist skill for functional contextualists: Act effectively in the best interests of the client. To do so requires a sophisticated *noticing repertoire*. Therapists in training often ask some version of "What should I do when X happens?" While those learning a new therapy find concrete answers soothing, the answer is, "What do you think is going on?" By asking that question we suggest that what to do should be evident if one considers the situation in the context of the case conceptualization. Is the client making an awkward attempt at establishing closeness? Is the client trying to make the therapist uncomfortable and divert the conversation? Once the therapist makes this assessment (which is admittedly difficult to do in the moment during a session), what to do becomes clearer.

The other is issue is *how* does the therapist respond to accomplish a particular goal? The principle we emphasize is that of equifinality; there are many ways to attain the same function and it is the function that matters, not the form. What is perceived as supportive from one person may function as disingenuousness from another. Something complimentary from one person may be seen as sexualized from another. A smile may be a potent reinforcer in one instance and a punisher in another. Thus, the essential noticing repertoire extends to being able to assess the impact the therapist is having on the client.

None of the essential qualities requires perfection—only awareness. It can be therapeutic to make mistakes in a session and analyze with the client what went wrong and how to do things more effectively. It is often the case that the client's interactions outside the room encompass mistakes as well, so the therapist working through his or her own mistakes is a useful exercise in which the client can participate.

It is essential that FAP therapists be fully aware of what controls their behavior in therapy, as well as what functions as reinforcers for them in the therapy room. Events in one's personal life may, for example, change one's focus during therapy if intimacy is suddenly lacking in one's own life. In such an instance the therapist would be acting unethically, because the session is serving the therapist's interests rather than the client's. Every client presents different stimulus properties that interact with the therapist's own history. It is essential that the therapist constantly assesses whether the interaction produces positive or potentially problematic therapist behavior.

CURATIVE FACTORS OR MECHANISMS OF CHANGE

Change is produced by adding to a client's history so that the context for new, more adaptive, goal-directed behavior is learned. For FAP the mechanism is therapist-contingent responding to clinically relevant behaviors to shape more effective, valued behavioral repertoires that will be maintained by natural consequences. For ACT the mechanism is to alter the relationship between thoughts and actions, so that one's feelings, thoughts, and cognitions are without unnecessary encumbrances and one still moves effectively toward a valued goal.

Insight

Learning without awareness is probably the modal occurrence for much of human behavior. Therapy can proceed quite readily without the client fully noticing how change is taking place. From the client's perspective the sessions may be moving to new topics, or outside changes may be occurring, though the client cannot say precisely why. The initial problems for which the client sought therapy may be resolving without the client necessarily knowing the exact process that is occurring.

We have found it useful to add some structure to therapy to prompt clients to track the goals and effectiveness of interactions. We ask clients to consider what they want to have happen in any particular conversation with the therapist or individuals outside of therapy. At opportune times or after an interaction we might ask, "What do you want to have happen? Is this the right time for that to happen? Is that happening? Should you do something different? Did you do anything to make it more likely to happen in the future?" We are developing a noticing repertoire in the client. In essence, we would like our clients to become functional analysts of their own behavior.

We should also offer some caveats about a client's need to have insight. If the client has organized his or her suffering around a core of "I just need to know why I do this," then a discussion of the role of insight (or lack thereof) in therapy may be important. Likely, the therapist will want to help the client differentiate the importance of understanding how to make things different from how things have come to be. Clients often believe that if they can find the reasons for their behavior, change can ensue. One of the problems with this endeavor is that we end up with long lists of reasons that are not actually causal variables, and reason giving itself becomes an impediment to change. One can tell a convincing story that still does not actually point to variables that need to be addressed. For these reasons, contemporary behavior therapists tend to be leery of the role of insight in favor of alterable, controllable, causal variables. These terms are not always as seductive as the term *insight*, but they may be effective in getting the job done.

In cases where interventions make use of experiential exercises, defusion, metaphors, or related techniques, it is likely that some kind of insight is necessary. For example, if one is asked to defuse (decouple) words from the events to which they refer, the whole point of such exercises is to provide people with knowledge they did not previously have about the nonliterality of words. The simple defusion exercise of saying, "milk, milk, . . . milk," until the word and sound no longer entail the beverage, imparts an intended insight that seems necessary for that technical process to be successful. The same is likely true for mindfulness exercises in which clients are taught to notice themselves having thoughts rather than giving the thoughts content during the exercises.

Interpretations

Interpretations are verbal accounts of how behavior came to be or what maintains it. The degree to which a therapist supplies an interpretation depends on how much a client benefits rather than gets stuck in constructing a narrative of his or current state. In FAP these "reasons" are intended to help clients assess their environment in order to makes changes that will be supported. When a therapist presents a case conceptualization or describes a functional class, he or she is providing some kind of reason (function) to the client. In order for reasons not to become obstacles to change, therapy can point to how a better understanding of (no longer relevant) reasons can make new efforts at behavior change less risky.

The Therapist's Repertoire

To be an effective FAP therapist, one must become a meaningful source of social reinforcement to a wide variety of clients. If behavior change does not happen readily in a FAP case, the therapist begins to wonder why he or she does not matter enough to the client. There are two responses to that concern when it inevitably arises in supervision. The first is that there has not been enough time to establish a new and potent history with the client. There is certainly individual variability in this regard. The second answer is more difficult to hear. Indeed, the therapist may not be bringing the salient part of his or her repertoire into the room when doing therapy. It is easy for therapists to provide arbitrary reinforcement but harder to supply deep, meaningful natural reinforcement. We often spend considerable time in supervision asking therapists to bring out that part of their repertoire they would show to their partner or to a child they are helping through a difficult time. That level of caring and vulnerability is recognized as something much more important to the change process than saying in a monotone, "I'm feeling really close to you right now." That intense relationship, when coupled with a strong functional analysis, can produce striking change.

It is not clear how well developed a therapist's own interpersonal repertoire must be in order to shape it in the client. At a metaphoric level, does the therapist need to be able to play Rachmaninov to teach something as basic as "chopsticks"? It is difficult to see how a therapist would teach acceptance skills (a repertoire of experiencing rather than escaping emotions) if that therapist dominantly engaged in experiential avoidance. How much of the repertoire must be intact? This is an empirical question. Perhaps there is comfort to be found by recognizing that many pupils exceed the skills of their teachers. Unfortunately, some do not.

Commonalities

Functional contextual behavior therapies share a great deal in common with other psychotherapies. Consistent with person-centered therapies (Rogers, 1961), behavioral interventions begin with clients' attempts to understand the world from their own experience in order to conduct a meaningful functional analysis. Like a person-centered approach, the behavior therapist holds empathy and unconditional regard as central to good therapy. Empathy may be operationalized as understanding the client's unique history the way that history was experienced. If the therapist had that same history, he or she (as the product of the contingencies of that history) might feel and behave very similarly. Unconditional regard may be understood as genuine respect for the client. The genuineness or authenticity Rogers (1957) wrote about is essential in some applications of behavior therapy, particular FAP, but it may not always be fundamental. Indeed, though genuineness, unconditional regard, and empathy were seen as the necessary and sufficient elements of clinical change from a person-centered perspective, they are likely seen by the contemporary behavior therapist as neither always necessary nor by themselves sufficient. It may be better to understand those components as part of doing good therapy than to understand essential aspects of functional contextualistic behavior therapy.

Contemporary behavior therapy also shares much in common with CBT, in which the mechanism of change is both cognitive (changing thoughts to produce behavior change) and behavioral (altering contextual contingencies to produce behavior change). These different philosophical mechanisms are, in fact, at odds with each other and may represent an untenable philosophical eclecticism. However, inherent in both contemporary behavioral therapies and CBT, the intervention is seen as collaborative. The problem list is developed cooperatively by therapist and client. Both therapies are very active and directive, and often involve outside-of-session "homework" activities. Both can involve a playful and inquisitive therapist approach with the client, with a focus on what is working for the client and what is not. Although the mechanism of action is different than that in a cognitive approach, contemporary behavior therapies are deeply interested in cognition as it relates to human suffering. However, cognition is not seen as causal; it is seen as one of the contingencies that can give rise to and maintain suffering.

TREATMENT APPLICABILITY AND ETHICAL CONSIDERATIONS

Functional contextual therapies are broadly applicable and have been shown to be effective with a range of diagnostic categories. In the course of contemporary functional contextualistic therapies, clients develop new, more effective repertoires that successfully displace less useful behaviors.

There are some broadly held beliefs that can initially interfere with a client fully engaging in therapy. Most clients who seek therapy hold two assumptions. The first is that thoughts cause feelings, and the second is that painful thoughts should be eliminated. Both of these assumptions are not supported by either FAP or ACT as exemplars of functional contextualistic therapies. Both therapies, but more explicitly ACT, address the reduction of unnecessary suffering (i.e., suffering that results from the struggle to not feel any kinds of painful emotions). Not only is that struggle futile, but efforts to limit negative feelings also inevitably limit richer positive feelings. To the degree that the underpinning goals of therapy are ultimately incommensurate with those of the client, therapy may be rejected. A referral might be appropriate, but the contextualist therapist would clearly see the client's unwillingness to let go of these assumptions as a key sign that this would be an appropriate therapy.

The ethical issues that can arise from these interventions are not unique. For FAP it is essential for the therapist to have a repertoire to establish an intense interpersonal relationship with a variety of clients. If one cannot establish such a relationship, the effectiveness of the treatment is significantly diminished, because much behavior change that occurs in therapy is mediated by the social reinforcing contingencies supplied by the therapist. One would reasonably expect that potential clients who do not find intense interpersonal relationships reinforcing would do less well in FAP than in other, more directive therapies focusing on more specific problem-solving strategies.

Transcultural Issues

Since a client's behavior is understood functionally within the context in which it occurs, any analysis of the relevant antecedents and consequences of problem behaviors or improvements is incomplete until the analysis includes an assessment of the culture-specific antecedents and consequences that may be asserting influence (Vandenberghe et al., 2010). In any particular therapy session, the history of the therapist and client, both in the past and in the moment, interact with all the prior history, culture, and biology of both members of the dyad. It is often important to consider the multiple operating factors that may contribute to the client's apparent resistance or compliance, as well as subtle influences on how the therapist may endorse some goals and values over others (Hays, 2001).

The selection of goals and values can be particularly difficult to understand in clients who have quite dissimilar backgrounds from the therapist and his or her available consultants. Therapists should assess the level of acculturation that clients demonstrate, as well as the goals they endorse. The goal of therapy is not necessarily to have clients adapt their behavior to that of the mainstream culture; rather, it is how to optimize their access to reinforcement in all cultures in which they participate. On occasion, such choices may be at odds with the cultural norms of the therapist. For instance, the child of an immigrant family may be struggling about whether to maintain a deferential relationship with her parents or seek more independence. The choice is the client's. However, in many circumstances there are opportunities for the client to gain reinforcement from both cultures if she can discriminate the circumstances in which each kind of behavior will be reinforced.

Among other consequences of adopting new behavioral repertoires when adjusting to a new set of cultural influences is the likelihood that new behaviors will lead to novel emotional responses for the client. For instance, if a normative cultural practice is to avoid direct expression of affect, clients may have difficulty contacting new contingencies available in current culture. Clients may feel embarrassed or aggressive and cease behaving before they experience any reinforcement for expressing wants and desires. The therapist can help clients discriminate between the actual consequences provided. Therapy may also address how clients can learn usefully to label new emotions that are not typically discussed in the culture of origin. An emerging sense of self may result from these activities, but even the notion of self may be very different between cultures.

The nature of intimacy can be very different between cultures as well. FAP is an intimate form of therapy in which therapists are effective when clients are aware that they very much matter to the therapist. Just as can occur between clients and therapists in a Western culture, intense and confusing feelings that result in transcultural therapy situations must become legitimate learning moments for clients and therapists alike.

Certainly, when doing therapy with a client who has obvious cultural differences with the therapist, it is sometimes (wrongly) expedient to attribute therapy difficulties to the cultural differences. It is often said that there is more behavioral variance within cultures than between cultures. Whether this is true in any particular case, it is useful to conceptualize culture as part of the context in which behavior occurs, but more proximal (i.e., therapy) factors are likely to be important, causal, and changeable.

RESEARCH SUPPORT AND EVIDENCE-BASED PRACTICE

One of the appeals of contextualistic therapies is that the practices themselves are built on well-researched principles of learning. FAP is easily understood as the application of operant principles to shaping behavior change. The importance of the therapeutic relationship as a mediator of social reinforcement has been articulated for several decades, and the importance of the therapeutic alliance is supported by a robust literature. While the principles of FAP are simple to disseminate, the training of therapist skills in applying these principles has been less simple. The history of clinical behavior analysis has been more in the single-subject or idiographic tradition and has not been as influential as group design studies since the beginning of the empirically supported treatment movement. New methodologies for combining single-subject studies that are being developed may significantly extend the influence of such designs (Shadish, Rindskopf, & Hedges, 2008).

Case study data supporting the effectiveness of FAP address a variety of clinical problems, including several categories of anxiety disorders, depressive disorders, personality disorders, as well as interpersonal relationship difficulties (Baruch et al., 2009). FAP has also been successfully combined with ACT, cognitive therapy, and DBT. The primary stumbling block to more FAP research using group designs lies in demonstrating contingent responding has occurred and has impacted behavior. This process is very labor-intensive. It generally involves using a lag-sequential approach of continuously coded exchanges between the therapist and client. The benefit of having such a strongly principle-based therapy is that if the therapist is adhering to the FAP principles described earlier, there is likely to be corresponding change is the client's clinically relevant behaviors, because of the direct relationship between CRBs and the clinician's immediate contingent response. So far, a more expedient method for documenting FAP adherence and effectiveness has not yet been fully developed.

ACT has undergone much more extensive outcome research and has been shown to be effective in a wide variety of situations, ranging from reduction of the suffering associated with mental disorders, including psychosis, chronic diseases, pain and stigma, to enhancment of job performance (Hayes et al., 2006). Several lines of research provide support for the efficacy and effectiveness of ACT. Correlational studies have shown a relationship between self-report processes targeted by ACT and a variety of quality-of-life and psychopathology measures. Results show a relationship between psychological flexibility (acceptance and valued action) and better outcomes.

A number of outcomes testing the relative strength of ACT versus structured interventions show a weighted effect size in favor of ACT, about 0.44 (Cohen's d) at posttest and 0.63 at follow-up. When ACT is compared to treatment as usual, wait list, or placebo control, the posttest and follow-up effect sizes are 0.99 and 0.71, in favor of ACT. In a small number of direct comparisons between ACT and cognitive therapy or CBT. ACT has shown a similar size advantage in effect size.

In the last several years, psychotherapy outcome researchers have begun to appreciate the importance of testing whether the change observed in outcome studies is the result of a theory-specific mechanism of action. The processes targeted by ACT are imperfectly measured, as is the case for most theory-based interventions. However, the available data support the notion that ACT produces its clinical effects by change processes in ways that are theoretically consistent with the ACT model (see processes in Table 6.2). While it is premature to conclude that ACT researchers understand all the elements that produce change as a result of ACT, it is impressive that ACT brings about change not by trying to eliminate symptoms, but by changing how clients relate to thoughts about the symptoms, so that they can freely engage life in a manner consistent with their valued goals.

Last, ACT seems to be very scalable. By that we mean that ACT has shown useful effects when given as fairly intensive psychotherapy over a long period of time, all the way down to 3 hours of intervention to clients adjusting to positive psychotic symptoms. It is not likely that such widely variable "doses" of ACT produce salutary effects to the same degree or via the same mechanism, but there are multiple sources of evidence that varieties of ACT can be flexibly applied to a broad spectrum of issues using many different formats.

CASE ILLUSTRATION

Kim, a 32-year-old white female, presents for therapy complaining of sad mood, social isolation, and general feelings of distress. She has tried two courses of antidepressants without benefit. While Kim does meet criteria for dysthymic disorder and evidences some of the criteria of major depressive disorder, she is not currently suicidal. Her physician has suggested that she try psychotherapy.

Kim works at a large corporation and describes her role there as "very middle management." She feels somewhat challenged in her job intellectually, but her largest challenge is interacting with both her employers and her associates. More than this, though, Kim reports being unable to have friends and feel "connected" to others. She feels unsupported in life, and she genuinely marvels at the way her colleagues seem to be able to talk to others and stay emotionally connected. Kim is currently single, and describes a heterosexual orientation and a desire to date men. She also describes a "normal" childhood with age-appropriate relationships throughout her development, and a relationship with her parents that was "strict but loving." In this description, her parents were both physical in their discipline, but there is no evidence of any abuse either sexually or physically. Her description of a "loving" relationship with her parents appears accurate but severely limited in terms of expression of affect, either verbally or nonverbally, among Kim, her parents, and her younger sister.

From a contemporary behavioral framework, the goal of the therapist is to identify those operant behaviors that function both to allow social interactions that result in reinforcers and those that do not. In Kim's case, her values are to live a "connected" life with others, which we further understand through questions with Kim as meaning one that is richer with social reinforcement. Given that she has the value of engaging others, the therapist must determine what aspects of an operant analysis prevent this from occurring. Is it the conditions under which she seeks social interactions that do not produce this reinforcement? That is, does she know when, with whom, or how often to engage in social interaction?

This is the discriminative stimuli side of the equation. In addition, other discriminative stimuli need to be assessed. Does Kim know when *she* wants or needs social engagement? While this appears to be a very simple task, clinicians likely recognize the essential nature of this early step in seeking support or "connection" with others. Does Kim know what she wants, when she wants it, and can she *then* seek it out in appropriate contexts?

Next in a behavioral analysis is the *response repertoire*, and this term is by far the most complex and richest contextually. For Kim, we want to know what happens when others engage her. Does she respond appropriately, or does she not really know what to do? Does she return a person's inquiry with too little disclosure, so that others do not seek her out again? Conversely, does she overdisclose, creating an aversive context for others? Does she begin to feel affect during a social interaction, then quickly attempt to escape her own emotional experience, resulting in a rather odd or "disconnecting" interaction with others? The variety of questions in the assessment phase of a contemporary behavioral interview ranges from assessing a repertoire that is insufficiently developed to one that is excessive in nature.

The final term in the behavioral analysis is the *contingencies of reinforcement*. In this case, we want to assess the client's sensitivity to discriminating social reinforcement and its actual impact. In addition, and as is the case with assessing discriminative stimuli or antecedent functions, we want to know whether the client even is putting herself in a context to receive social reinforcement when her behaviors are more effective.

In Kim's case, she has a reasonably complex repertoire problem, along with a challenge in discriminating when to engage with others in activities she could find reinforcing or "connecting." Kim has trouble knowing when others are making efforts to connect with her and tends to attribute those efforts to things that do not suggest she should try to engage others in return. Consider the following interaction during the assessment phase:

KIM: It's just, I don't know, they don't really include me, I guess. It makes me really sad.

THERAPIST: That's gotta be tough, feeling like that. That you're sad, and not included. I can't help thinking, though, you just said earlier today that your friend Shelly called and asked you to go bowling with everyone.

KIM: I know, but she probably just felt like she had to do that.

THERAPIST: Really? Was it work-related?

KIM: No.

THERAPIST: That's what I thought. I think this was Shelly asking to do something with you.

KIM: Yeah? Maybe you're right. I don't know how to even tell that in the moment.

Part of Kim's difficulty here is discriminating when to connect with others. Another key aspect of her social difficulties in her repertoire can be seen in the rest of that interaction.

THERAPIST: Yeah, I think that's right. I think that's one of the problems here, that you don't actually know when others are kind of inviting you to connect with them.

KIM: But why? I mean, why don't I?

THERAPIST: I don't know. I guess that's the big million dollar question, isn't it? Maybe it's that the way you were raised makes it harder to see this in others, but in a lot of ways, that doesn't really matter does it?

KIM: No?

THERAPIST: Well, I don't know that it totally does. I mean it makes this all make sense, doesn't it? If it were related to the way you were raised. But still, here we are, and here you are, and we need to figure out how to get you connected. I think the big "why" question may take us down another path altogether, and then, really who knows if that's right?

KIM: Yeah, you're right.

THERAPIST: Maybe. So let me ask you this, though. Let's say that you did know another person was asking you to come do something, let's say you could tell that. Would that fix it?

KIM: I don't think so.

THERAPIST: Me neither. Or at least I am worried that it wouldn't.

KIM: What do you think I would do?

THERAPIST: You tell me.

KIM: I wouldn't go.

THERAPIST: 'Cause . . .

KIM: It would freak me out. I wouldn't know what to do.

THERAPIST: Yeah. And if you didn't go, you'd feel better?

KIM: I guess. Better than going or trying to go. But really, just more sad. This makes me really sad. I can't stand this feeling of being alone. I can't stand that feeling of deciding not to go either. This is so hard.

This last interaction helps provide evidence that one of Kim's key operant behaviors in addition to her difficulties is to know when and with whom to engage to "feel connected" or have access to social reinforcers. She has a very difficult time engaging others when she feels sad. Here, the operant analysis can show that under conditions when Kim feels something, "sad affect," she engages in some escape response that then immediately has the negative reinforcing consequence of not feeling anxious or troubled, but with the longer-term consequence of being more isolated.

It is important to remember that Kim's feelings, and her thoughts, come from some history. Her feelings do not make her stay home. She feels something in response to an environmental event (here an offer for social engagement), then engages in some response that is contingently reinforced (escape behaviors that serve to reduce aversive affect). Ultimately, her thoughts and feelings are understood as a product of contingent reinforcement, too; that is, Kim feels worry in response to an offer to go out and have fun with others. This is a particular response based on an individual learning history.

In this case, Kim's operant response of not going out with others is in part due to her inability (1) to discriminate opportunities for social reinforcement, and (2) to experience difficult feelings, such as sadness or anxiety, that come with these opportunities. While her immediate repertoire is negatively reinforced through escape and avoidance behaviors, ultimately she is isolated and feels lonely and sad. One challenge that lies before Kim is the ability to express her feelings with others once she is able to notice and experience them. It is the belief of the therapist that developing these behaviors will allow Kim to move closer to her values, her identified salient reinforcers.

We jump forward in Kim's treatment to an interaction working on Kim's experience of difficult affect:

THERAPIST: So, how did the trip out with the gang from work go?

KIM: Oh, you know. Hard, I guess.

THERAPIST: Yeah.

KIM: Yeah. I tried some of the things we worked on. I just don't know about feeling stuff I don't want to feel. I am so tired of this sadness stuff.

THERAPIST: I don't blame you for feeling tired. It looks really exhausting, what you have described to me. Getting the call. Deciding to go. Getting ready. Going there. Being there. All the time *feeling* this *stuff.* Yikes! It is hard.

KIM: I know. I mean, why can't I just not feel it.

THERAPIST: Totally. Why not?

KIM: 'Cause it's mine?

THERAPIST: 'Cause it's yours. Because from what you have described, when you try not feel it, to get rid of it, to do everything but have it, what happens?

KIM: It gets worse.

THERAPIST: Yeah. Well, I think maybe in the short run it doesn't, right? But in the long run, you feel really alone.

KIM: I gotta feel it?

THERAPIST: I don't know, you know, it's your stuff. This is really hard for us. What will work better for you?

KIM: To feel it.

THERAPIST: To feel it. I think so, and then move in the direction you want your life. Get connected, be part of this big thing called "life with other people."

KIM: It's just hard.

THERAPIST: It is. And . . .

KIM: And I keep moving.

THERAPIST: And . . . for you, I mean . . .

KIM: And I keep feeling.

THERAPIST: I think so. Is it working?

KIM: I think so. I mean, I had a really nice time. Shelly is so nice. And there was this guy there . . .

In this exchange, Kim describes the challenges inherent in experiencing difficult affect, then doing what she wants to do, go out with her friends. The goal of the therapist here is to help her develop an alternative repertoire that might be differentially reinforced, one that requires Kim to feel her feelings rather than continue to escape those opportunities. It is essential, as described elsewhere in this chapter, that the therapist remember to approach this type of work with compassion. This is very hard for us to do, to feel what we do not want to feel. In fact, as therapists, we avoid our own difficult affect. We ask clients to feel what they need to feel to continue to work toward their own salient reinforcers or values. (We should ask the same of ourselves as therapists.) We also want to remember that when we talk to clients, we focus on their response to their own discriminative stimuli, their own contextual antecedents. Feelings do not make us do one thing or another, nor do thoughts. Feelings and thoughts are behaviors that come from somewhere, and our job is to understand that. When they come from some environmental context, they may be reinforced. When they are, they can then serve as discriminative stimuli for other responses, such as escape and avoidance behaviors, that in turn are negatively reinforced.

Kim is learning that to feel what she feels is still only part of her therapeutic work. She also needs to develop a repertoire for expressing those feelings. She may have a fairly limited ability to do this given her relationship history and her isolation. Developing her repertoire for expressing her feelings requires some ability to experience them, but it does not assume that her ability to experience her affect will translate into a vocabulary for that expression. In fact, her inability to express these feelings successfully may create more opportunities for Kim to try to escape and avoid her feelings when interacting with others. This cyclical or recursive pattern may feed on itself, creating more social isolation. Consider the following excerpt:

KIM: I think the date was a total disaster. I am an idiot.

THERAPIST: I am sorry to hear that. What happened?

KIM: I just got really flustered. I like him. He knows that. He likes me, and I know that.

THERAPIST: But . . . ?

KIM: I don't know. I felt so nervous at one point. Like I didn't know what to say. Like I didn't know how to say what I felt.

THERAPIST: And you felt something?

KIM: Oh, I felt it all right. I am not sure what it was. I just started off all "touchy-feely" and he seemed fine, then I got lost in what I was saying, like I don't know the words.

THERAPIST: What are you feeling right now, Kim, as we are talking about this?

KIM: Huh? Well, I don't know.

THERAPIST: Right now. What do you feel here telling *me* this? Sharing this with me?

KIM: Sheesh, I don't know. This is hard enough.

THERAPIST: And here we are having an interaction, and you don't know your feelings.

KIM: Duh.

THERAPIST: OK, so what do you want to do?

KIM: About what?

THERAPIST: Not knowing what you feel.

KIM: I don't know, you tell me.

THERAPIST: I can't, can I? But here we are having this difficult interaction where you feel something, right?

KIM: Oh, I feel it. I don't want to, but I feel it. I think I want to talk about something else now. Maybe you could just back off a bit.

THERAPIST: OK, I want to respect your wishes here, but I think we've stumbled into your way of disconnecting from others. Here with me. So I want you to try something. I want you to stay connected to me, 'cause I really want to know about this, about this part of you that is so important to what we work on in here.

KIM: My feelings?

THERAPIST: Yeah, and more importantly, how you feel in here with me, as we interact here.

KIM: It matters.

THERAPIST: It matters immensely. This is how I really know you. I want you to feel what you feel, for sure. Then I want you to be able to share that with me, with others. This is how we connect, really. Right?

KIM: I am just confused.

THERAPIST: And . . . ?

KIM: And I need help?

THERAPIST: With . . . ?

KIM: With you understanding me. And I don't have the words for this. I don't have the way to tell you how hard this is, but I so need you to understand. Can you help?

THERAPIST: This is it, Kim. I am all ears, I think I really get how much this matters. I so appreciate you asking me for help. I think I can help, too, but let's see.

KIM: What can I do?

THERAPIST: Let's start at the beginning. When we are talking, when do you start to get confused? I think this may be a lot like what happens with Todd, what happened with him on your last date. I think that when you get confused, it spirals a bit, but I think there is a real way to slow this down and have you really feel what you feel, and have others like me, like Todd, or whoever, really lean in and help out. That's our job as the people who care about you. What we do here, well, that will work for me, but remember, you gotta try connecting lots of different ways with different people. Wanna try?

In this interaction, the therapist is attempting to use an in-session opportunity to help contingently shape a more effective interpersonal repertoire for Kim to express her emotions, even when they are confusing or hard to pinpoint. The therapist attempts to notice the conditions that give rise to an ineffective repertoire, then bring that into the therapy interaction to create a chance to work on that very skill set. Here the therapist quickly recognized the repertoire of disengagement, when Kim was flustered or confused about her feelings (that occurred on her date), show up in the context of the two of them. The therapist then allowed the client to show that repertoire in an effort to prompt a more effective behavior, one that he could reinforce, then suggest she try outside with others.

Overall, in functional–contextual behavior therapy, the clinician attempts to create a case conceptualization based on the principles of operant conditioning. This case conceptualization will evolve over the course of therapy and guide the therapist with respect to when and how he or she should intervene with any client. The choice of strategies, ACT or FAP, DBT, or behavioral activation, all depend on this particular client with his or her particular behaviors. The therapist continues to focus on the function of those behaviors, not their appearance, and attempt to alter either the contingencies of reinforcement or the discriminative stimulus conditions that give rise to the responses. Or, as is often the case, the therapist addresses the complex repertoire itself, which will then likely create different consequences.

This form of intervention, as a balance of science and service delivery, is one of the most thoughtful, idiosyncratic, and vital interventions among the different principle-based approaches. When the behavioral clinician is in the role as therapist, he or she is a vital part of the client's context in which behavior is observed, understood, and changed. When Skinner introduced the term *radical behaviorism*, he was referring to the fact that the behavioral scientist is an integral and inextricable part of what he or she studies. In FAP, the same is true of the therapist. The therapist is both fallible and helpful, and is always an active ingredient in the process of clinical change.

SUGGESTIONS FOR FURTHER STUDY

In addition to the resources listed below, both the FAP and ACT communities are active online. For more information and resources related to FAP, go to *www.functionalanalyticpsychotherapy.com*. For extensive resources related to ACT, but also contextual behavioral science in general, go to *www.contextualpsychology.org*.

Recommended Reading: Clinical Case Studies

Eifert, G. H., Forsyth, J. P., Arch, J., Espejo, E., Keller, M., & Langer, D. (2009). Acceptance and commitment therapy for anxiety disorders: Three case studies exemplifying a unified treatment protocol. *Cognitive and Behavioral Practice, 16*, 368–385.—An excellent overview of the principles used in ACT, as applied to three different cases with an anxiety disorder.

Tsai, M., Kohlenberg, R. J., Kanter, J. W., & Waltz, J. (2009). Therapeutic technique: The five rules. In M. Tsai, R. J. Kohlenberg, J. W. Kanter, B. Kohlenberg, W. C. Follette, & G. M. Callaghan (Eds.), *A guide to functional analytic psychotherapy: Awareness, courage, love and behaviorism* (pp. 61–102). New York: Springer.—Outlines the basic processes in FAP and contains transcripts to illustrate how one might apply them.

Twohig, M., & Hayes, S. C. (2008). *ACT verbatim: Depression and anxiety*. Oakland, CA: New Harbinger.—The title says it all.

Recommended Reading: Research

Hayes, S. C., Luoma, J. B., Bond, F. W., Masuda, A., & Lillis, J. (2006). Acceptance and commitment therapy: Model, processes and outcomes. *Behaviour Research and Therapy, 44*, 1–25.—An accessible overview of current views of the ACT model and a solid presentation of empirical data about ACT.

Baruch, D. E., Kanter, J. W., Busch, A., Plummer, M. D., Tsai, M., Rusch, L. C., et al. (2009). Lines of evidence in support of FAP. In M. Tsai, R. J. Kohlenberg, J. W. Kanter, B. Kohlenberg, W. C. Follette, & G. M. Callaghan (Eds.), *A guide to functional analytic psychotherapy: Awareness, courage, love, and behaviorism* (pp. 21–36). New York: Springer.—A summary of the evidence related to the effectiveness of FAP in an easy-to-read form.

DVDs

Hayes, S. C. (2008). *Acceptance and commitment therapy* (Systems of Psychotherapy Video Series). Washington, DC: American Psychological Association.—ACT is used to address anger and guilt issues. The case is particularly interesting, demonstrating the role of value-guided behavior in ACT.

There are no formally distributed videos of FAP currently available. The Association for Behavioral and Cognitive Therapies (*www.abct.org*) has a video entitled *Doing Psychotherapy: Session 3—Clinical Grand Rounds,* in which Robert J. Kohlenberg discusses integrating a variety of methods of treatments for a role-played anxiety and depression client with other prominent CBT therapists. This video does not demonstrate FAP but does show Kohlenberg uniting therapy and the underlying behavioral principles that might guide intervention choices.

REFERENCES

Bandura, A. (1977). *Social learning theory.* Englewood Cliffs, NJ: Prentice-Hall.

Baruch, D. E., Kanter, J. W., Busch, A., Plummer, M. D., Tsai, M., Rusch, L. C., et al. (2009). Lines of evidence in support of FAP. In M. Tsai, R. J. Kohlenberg, J. W. Kanter, B. Kohlenberg, W. C. Follette, & G. M. Callaghan (Eds.), *A guide to functional analytic psychotherapy: Awareness, courage, love, and behaviorism* (pp. 21–36). New York: Springer.

Baum, W. M. (2005). *Understanding behaviorism: Behavior, culture, and evolution* (2nd ed.). Malden, MA: Blackwell.

Beck, A. T., Rush, A. J., Shaw, B. F., & Emery, G. (1979). *Cognitive therapy of depression.* New York: Guilford Press.

Callaghan, G. M. (2006). The Functional Idiographic Assessment Template (FIAT) system. *Behavior Analyst Today, 7,* 357–398.

Callaghan, G. M., Gregg, J. A., Marx, B. P., Kohlenberg, B. S., & Gifford, E. (2004). FACT: The utility of an integration of functional analytic psychotherapy and acceptance and commitment therapy to alleviate human suffering. *Psychotherapy: Theory, Research, Practice and Training, 41,* 195–207.

Chiesa, M. (1992). Radical behaviorism and scientific frameworks: From mechanistic to relational accounts. *American Psychologist, 47,* 1287–1299.

Dahl, J., Plumb, J., Stewart, I., & Lundgren, T. (2009). *The art and science of valuing in psychotherapy: Helping clients discover, explore, and commit to valued action using acceptance and commitment therapy.* Oakland, CA: New Harbinger Press.

Ellis, A. (1977). The basic clinical theory of rational-emotive therapy. In A. Ellis & R. Grieger (Eds.), *Handbook of rational-emotive therapy* (pp. 3–34). New York: Springer.

Farber, B. A. (2006). *Self-disclosure in psychotherapy.* New York: Guilford Press.

Follette, W. C. (1997). A behavior analytic conceptualization of personality disorders: A response to Clark, Livesley, and Morey. *Journal of Personality Disorders, 11,* 232–241.

Follette, W. C., Bach, P. A., & Follette, V. M. (1993). A behavior analytic view of psychological health. *Behavior Analyst, 16,* 303–316.

Follette, W. C., Linnerooth, P. N., & Ruckstuhl, L. E. (2001). Positive psychology: A clinical behavior analytic perspective. *Journal of Humanistic Psychology, 41,* 102–134.

Gifford, E. V., & Hayes, S. C. (1999). Functional contexualism: A pragmatic philosophy for behavioral science. In W. O'Donohue & R. Kitchener (Eds.), *Handbook of behaviorism* (pp. 285–327). San Diego: Academic Press.

Goldiamond, I. (1974). Toward a constructional approach to social problems: Ethical and constitutional issues raised by applied behavior analysis. *Behaviorism, 2,* 1–85.

Hayes, S. C., Barnes-Holmes, D., & Roche, B. (Eds.). (2001). *Relational frame theory: A post-Skinnerian account of human language and cognition.* New York: Kluwer Academic/Plenum Press.

Hayes, S. C., Hayes, L. J., Reese, H. W., & Sarbin, T. R. (Eds.). (1993). *Varieties of scientific contextualism.* Reno, NV: Context Press.

Hayes, S. C., Luoma, J. B., Bond, F. W., Masuda, A., & Lillis, J. (2006). Acceptance and commitment therapy: Model, processes and outcomes. *Behaviour Research and Therapy, 44,* 1–25.

Hayes, S. C., Strosahl, K., & Wilson, K. G. (1999). *Acceptance and commitment therapy: Emotion, cognition, and human suffering.* New York: Guilford Press.

Haynes, S. N., & O'Brien, W. H. (1990). Functional analysis in behavior therapy. *Clinical Psychology Review, 10,* 649–668.

Hays, P. (2001). *Addressing culural complexities in practice: A framework for clinicians and counselors.* Washington, DC: American Psychological Association.

Jacobson, N. S., Dobson, K. S., Truax, P. A., Addis, M. E., Koerner, K., Gollan, J. K., et al. (1996). A component analysis of cognitive-behavioral treatment for depression. *Journal of Consulting and Clinical Psychology, 64*, 295–304.

Kanter, J. W., Tsai, M., & Kohlenberg, R. J. (Eds.). (2010). *The practice of functional analytic psychotherapy*. New York: Springer.

Kohlenberg, R. J., & Tsai, M. (1991). *Functional analytic psychotherapy*. New York: Plenum Press.

Linehan, M. M. (1993). *Cognitive-behavioral treatment of borderline personality disorder*. New York: Guilford Press.

Nelson-Gray, R. O., & Farmer, R. F. (2005). *Personality-guided behavior therapy*. Washington, DC: American Psychological Association.

Paul, G. (1967). Strategy of outcome research in psychotherapy. *Journal of Consulting and Clinical Psychology, 31*, 109–118.

Peterson, C., & Seligman, M. E. P. (2004). *Character strengths and virtues: A handbook and classification*. Washington, DC: American Psychological Association.

Rogers, C. R. (1957). The necessary and sufficient conditions of therapeutic personality change. *Journal of Consulting Psychology, 21*, 95–103.

Rogers, C. R. (1961). *On becoming a person*. Boston: Houghton Mifflin.

Shadish, W. R., Rindskopf, D. M., & Hedges, L. V. (2008). The state of the science in the meta-analysis of single-case experimental designs. *Evidence-Based Communication Assessment and Intervention, 2*, 188–196.

Skinner, B. F. (1953). *Science and human behavior*. New York: Free Press.

Tsai, M., Kohlenberg, R. J., Kanter, J. W., Kohlenberg, B., Follette, W. C., & Callaghan, G. M. (2009). *A guide to functional analytic psychotherapy: Awareness, courage, love and behaviorism*. New York: Springer.

Vandenberghe, L., Tsai, M., Varlero, L., Ferro, R., Kerbauy, R. R., Wielensha, R. C., et al. (2010). Transcultural functional analytic psychotherapy. In J. W. Kanter, M. Tsai, & R. J. Kohlenberg (Eds.), *The practice of functional analytic psychotherapy* (pp. 173–185). New York: Springer.

PART IV

EXPERIENTIAL AND HUMANISTIC APPROACHES

Person-Centered Psychotherapy and Related Experiential Approaches

Arthur C. Bohart
Jeanne C. Watson

T he focus of this chapter is person-centered psychotherapy and two experiential psycho-therapies related to it: focusing-oriented psychotherapy (Gendlin, 1996) and emotion-focused therapy, the process–experiential approach (PE-EFT; Greenberg, Rice, & Elliott, 1993). We also briefly address Gestalt psychotherapy in our "Historical Background" section, because PE-EFT is partially based upon it.

Person-centered therapy refers to a theoretical view of the nature of human beings and their interactions, originally developed by Carl Rogers in the 1940s and 1950s, and to a philosophy of how to relate to human beings in growth-producing ways, both inside and outside psychotherapy. Rogers first developed his ideas in the form of *client-centered therapy* and later changed the name to "person-centered" when he expanded the practice of his ideas to other realms of human interaction, such as education and international conflict resolution. Both focusing-oriented psychotherapy and PE-EFT evolved out of the person-centered approach. We consider them to be part of a larger "family" of person-centered experiential psychotherapies (PCEP).

HISTORICAL BACKGROUND

Carl Rogers

Several influences led Carl Rogers to develop the person-centered view of psychotherapy and of human beings. As a youth, Rogers spent much of his time on a farm, where he was particularly interested in the processes of facilitating growth. He also studied scientific experimentation with respect to agriculture. Facilitating growth and testing hypotheses characterized Rogers's experimental attitude toward both life and understanding human interaction. This attitude guided the development of his theoretical constructs.

Rogers was raised in a religiously conservative family and initially planned to be a minister. However, over the course of his college years his views gradually liberalized. A trip to China at the end of his senior year of college had a particularly significant impact on him; for example, he became aware that there were many different ways to look at the world. He also witnessed extensive human suffering, and his goal became to help people. He then attended graduate school at the Union Theological Seminary, which furthered the liberalization process in which Rogers was already engaged. These experiences contributed to Rogers's emphasis on accepting people and on looking for the best in them. During his time at Union Theological Seminary, he finally realized that he could help people just as well as a psychologist, and he changed over to Columbia University, where he pursued his PhD.

Later, when Rogers was working as a child guidance counselor, he was exposed to the ideas of Otto Rank. Rankian ideas that influenced Rogers included an emphasis on individuals' creativity and potential, with the aim of therapy being acceptance of the self as unique, and on individuals' self-reliance. Rogers saw the client as the central figure in the therapeutic process, emphasizing that the client is his or her own therapist, and focused on clients' present experience in therapy (Raskin & Rogers, 1989).

Another influence was the *Zeitgest* of the 1930s (Barrett-Lennard, 1998), the "Roosevelt years." Some of the features of those times that influenced Rogers, Barrett-Lennard speculates, included a focus on empowering people, on learning through trial and error, and on openness to new thought and solutions. Roosevelt also emphasized participation in appraisal and decision making by those affected. He encouraged and accepted divergent thinking and pressed for the integration of opposites. His managerial style was a supportive one, in which he tried to release the creativity of his subordinates. Roosevelt held an optimistic view of human nature, in that people were to be treated as basically trustworthy and reasonable, even if their behavior was not always rational.

For Rogers, however, the most formative influences came from his experience with clients. This is how he recalled their impact:

> I had been working with a highly intelligent mother whose boy was something of a hellion. The problem was clearly her early rejection of the boy, but over many interviews I could not help her to this insight. . . . Finally I gave up. I told her that it seemed we had both tried, but we had failed, and that we might as well give up our contacts. She agreed . . . and she walked to the door of the office. Then she turned and asked, "Do you ever take adults for counseling here?" When I replied in the affirmative, she said, "Well then, I would like some help." She came to the chair she had left, and began to pour out her despair about her marriage, her troubled relationship with her husband, her sense of failure and confusion. . . . Real therapy began then, and ultimately it was very successful. This incident was one of a number which helped me to experience the fact . . . that it is the *client* who knows what hurts, what directions to go in, what problems are crucial. (Rogers, 1961a, pp. 11–12)

In the 1940s Rogers formulated an early version of person-centered therapy, also known as "nondirective therapy." This stage was characterized by a fundamental emphasis on the therapist's nondirectiveness: The goal was to create a permissive, open atmosphere that was not driven by therapists' techniques or agendas but rather was designed to facilitate clients' self-diclosure and openness to their own experience. The major therapeutic "interventions" were acceptance of the client and clarification of what the client was saying. By the 1950s, empathic understanding of the client was increasingly emphasized, along with the therapist's receptivity to the client's feelings. Later, in the 1960s, this shifted to an emphasis on the congruence or genuineness of the therapist.

Subsequently, Rogers's interests expanded beyond the field of psychotherapy. He began to work increasingly in group settings to facilitate growth in nonpatient populations and, in his last years, focused his energy on using the group format to foster world peace. He studied the potential of bringing together warring political factions to promote open, constructive dialogue. Groups were conducted, for instance, with blacks and whites from South Africa, and with Protestants and Catholics from Northern Ireland. The person-centered perspective was also extended to education and medicine.There have been many other innovations and derivations that have flowed from the person-centered philosophy, including communication skills training, as well as programs for training parents, leaders, and teachers, and for enhancing relationships (see Larson, 1984).

Carl Rogers's impact on the field of psychotherapy has been profound. Smith (1982) conducted a poll of members of the Clinical and Counseling Psychology divisions of the American Psychological Association, as well as of members of the American Counseling Assocation. Rogers was rated the most influential of all therapists, even more so than Freud. A more recent survey (Cook & Biyanova, 2009) also found that Rogers is rated by psychotherapists as the person who had most influenced their work.

Eugene Gendlin

Another important figure in the person-centered and experiential psychotherapy approach was Eugene Gendlin, born in Vienna, Austria, in 1926. As Jews, forced to flee the rise of the Nazis, his family emigrated to the United States in 1939. In getting his family out of Austria safely, Gendlin's father had to meet with various sources and leads. In one case, after meeting with a man who supposedly was going to help them, he decided he could not trust the man to ensure his family's safe passage out of Germany. His father explained his decision by saying that his feeling had said "No." It subsequently turned out that his father had been correct about the man: "I was surprised then and often asked myself later what kind of feeling it is which tells you something. Sometimes I tried to find such a feeling within myself, but I could not. But that I started to look for it had its effect in the end. Forty years later when I was asked how I could discover focusing, I remembered these circumstances" (Korbei, 1994, page number unavailable). Later, when his father ran into someone else whom he felt he could trust, they followed that person's guidance and escaped successfully.

Gendlin (personal communication, April 2, 2007) has also said that his parents did not get along well, and from this he learned to see things from different points of view. He could understand each of their points of view, but they could not understand each other's. He found that he became bored with that with which he agreed, and so would read other points of view. As a college undergraduate he developed a method whereby he could communicate with people on both sides of various issues (e.g., religious people and atheists, Marxists and McCarthyites, Behaviorists and Freudians). The method was to accept their entire system, then try to formulate whatever point was being made in terms of the ideas and symbols from within that system. This became one of Gendlin's primary interests: the symbolization of experience.

In 1958, Gendlin received his PhD in Philosophy from the University of Chicago. There he became interested in psychotherapy, because he recognized that it was the process of *symbolizing experience* freshly. Consequently, he approached Carl Rogers and asked to be included in his clinical practicum. Rogers (personal communication, August, 1985) was at first ambivalent about accepting a philosopher into his practicum, but he eventually relented. Gendlin became one of his best students; he became involved in Rogers's research projects and was later Research Director of the Wisconsin Schizophrenia Project (Rogers, Gendlin, Kiesla, & Traux, 1967).

Laura Rice and Leslie Greenberg

Another important figure in the PCEP approach was Laura Rice, who worked to understand and promote clients' experiencing in the session. Rice had studied with Rogers at the University of Chicago in the 1950s (Rice, 1992). Born in 1920 in New England to parents of Puritan descent, Rice was home schooled; she was in her early teens before she went to a public school with her peers, an experience that had a lasting impact on her as she struggled to fit in (Watson & Wiseman, 2010). After graduating, Rice worked in the Counseling Center at the University of Chicago before moving to a faculty position in the newly formed Department of Psychology at York University in Toronto, Canada. There she established a strong research tradition in psychotherapy process, while mentoring a number of students who later became prominent, including Leslie Greenberg, Jeanne Watson, William Pinsoff, and Robert Elliott, all of whom continue her work today.

Leslie Greenberg was one of Rice's graduate students and later a colleague; together they established a research paradigm called task analysis to help illuminate different client processes in therapy. Out of this work they developed the process–experiential approach to psychotherapy (Greenberg et al., 1993). While Rice was a firm adherent of Rogers's client-centered therapy, Greenberg was integrating her influence with that of Gestalt therapists (see below). They each developed models of specific in-session change processes, including *systematic evocative unfolding* for *problematic reactions, two-chair dialogues* at *conflict splits,* and *empty chair dialogues* for *unfinished business,* which they subjected to empirical testing and verification and that would later become the basis for PE-EFT (PE-EFT) (Greenberg, 1979, 1980, 1983; Greenberg & Webster, 1982; Rice & Greenberg, 1984; Rice & Saperia, 1984).

Gestalt Psychotherapy

We briefly review Gestalt psychotherapy because process–experiential psychotherapy is an integration of it and person-centered therapy. Gestalt therapy is an important humanistic–experiential approach in its own right (Strümpfel & Goldman, 2002; Yontef, 1995). Although it developed independently of person-centered therapy, philosophically they share much in common (C. Rogers, personal communication, April 1971). However, at the level of practice they are considerably different.

Gestalt psychotherapy was codeveloped by Fritz Perls, Laura Perls, and Paul Goodman, although Fritz Perls, because of his charismatic persona, has popularly gotten most of the credit for being its "founder," or "finder," as he often referred to it. Gestalt therapy emphasizes awareness and contact. A person who is in full contact with his or her environment and self on an ongoing basis is able to make effective choices. If there is awareness and contact, then the organism has the capacity to organize and reorganize itself spontaneously for effective functioning. Gestalt therapy is a field theory. It holds that the organism is a system and exists in a systemic relationship with its environment. The person *is* an interaction: There is a fluidity between self and world, such that the person is in continuous dialogue or contact with his or her world. Therefore, he or she has the capability to organize and reorganize him- or herself so that the "self" is appropriately functional at given moments.

As with person-centered therapy, Gestalt therapy emphasizes growth. It does not focus on specific symptom removal. The process of Gestalt therapy is based on developing the client's capacities for maintaining ongoing direct contact and awareness. This leads the individual to be able to make effective choices and to be "response-able" (responsible). The Gestalt therapist facilitates this by providing an empathic and responsive here-and-now relationship, and by suggesting various experiments designed to help clients explore their capacities for contact and awareness. For instance, clients may be asked to track what they are aware of in the moment, by saying "Now I am aware of. . . . " Clients may be asked to exaggerate gestures to see what they become aware of. Instead of talking about a dream, a client may be asked to role-play the various parts of the dream.

The most well-known experiments are those that involve "chair work." Following from the goal of helping clients learn how to stay in contact, Gestalt therapists believe that sometimes "just talking" about a problem can allow the person to stay *out* of contact. To bring clients into contact with the immediacy of experience, they have them enact role plays. For instance, the client may be talking about a problem with "the other person." With the empty chair procedure, the Gestalt therapist has the client imagine that the person is sitting in an empty chair across from him or her, then speak directly to that person, thus bringing the client into fuller contact with the immediacy of experiencing that other person. Then the client is asked to switch chairs and to role-play the other person's side, and to continue switching chairs to continue the dialogue. Different forms of chair work have become integral parts of PE-EFT.

Types of Clients with Whom the Approach Was Originally Developed

Person-centered therapy was developed from work with a wide range of clients in a number of different settings. Carl Rogers's first clinical work was at a psychoanalytically oriented child guidance clinic in Rochester, New York, where he worked with underprivileged children and their families. Later, at the University of Chicago Counseling Center, he and his colleagues saw clients from both the community and the college campus. Person-centered therapists worked with problems of all types, including depression, anxiety, personality disorders, and psychosis. During the late 1950s, a major research project with people with schizophrenia resulted in additions to both theory and practice.

THE CONCEPT OF PERSONALITY

Personality as Process

Person-centered therapy has not had a theory of personality *structure* so much as of personality *functioning and change*. The core of the person-centered concept of personality is that humans are growing, changing organisms. It is therefore important to understand the processes involved in personality functioning. Personality structures are not fixed in early childhood—they evolve. Personality characteristics are "structures in process." Even when a personality trait such as dependency continues throughout a lifetime, it can grow and change such that the way a person is dependent as an adult may be different from, and more adaptive than, the way the person was dependent as a child. Support for this idea is provided by a study that found that immature dependency evolved into a mature form of maintaining dependent relationships, with people becoming effective and caring partners with significant others (Caspi, Elder, & Herbener, 1990).

According to the person-centered view, persons have a capacity for continual *growth*. This capacity manifests itself in moment-by-moment adaptation. Behavior in any given situation is an application of stored knowledge or personality predispositions to act in accordance with the specific circumstances of a particular situation. The blend of preexisting knowledge and current circumstances always results in slightly new and different behavior than before. As behaviorist Robert Epstein (1991) has said, "The behavior of organisms has many firsts, so many, in fact, that it's not clear that there are any seconds. We continually do new things, some profound, some trivial. . . . When you look closely enough, behavior that appears to have been repeated proves to be novel in some fashion. . . . You never brush your teeth exactly the same way twice" (p. 362). This implies that the most important characteristics of the human being are the capacity for learning and creativity. Learning results in constantly fleshing out and modifying beliefs, concepts, schemas, constructs, and personality traits. On occasion, it leads to major, significant shifts in personality or belief.

In order for this process to operate most effectively, persons have to be able to be *present in the moment*. This means they have to be open to information within themselves and to information in the environment. For Rogers, the essence of effective functioning can be expressed in one word: *openness*. It is important to understand that being "present-centered" does not mean "eat, drink, and be merry for tomorrow you shall die," or any such endorsement of an impulsive hedonistic approach to life. Rather, it means that in making effective and responsible long-range choices for both self and society, people do it best if they are open to all the information available in the moment and realize that they can do now only what they can do now, while keeping the future in mind.

Carl Rogers originally discussed this capacity for growth in terms of an *actualizing tendency* in living things. He later expanded this idea by suggesting that it was an individual form of a broader, formative tendency found in the universe. This formative tendency is for things (such as crystals, as well as living creatures) to move toward greater order, complexity, and interrelatedness. On the level of the individual person, the *actualizing tendency* is the inherent tendency of individuals to develop by forming more differentiated and integrated personal life structures.

It is because of this tendency that persons have a built-in potential for resilience. Based on their research on children who grow up and survive in adverse circumstances, Masten, Best, and Garmezy (1990) suggested that "studies of psychosocial resilience support the view that human psychological development is highly buffered and self-righting" (p. 438). Following Carl Rogers, Bohart and Tallman (1999) have argued that it is people's capacities for self-righting that are the primary force that makes psychotherapy work.

The view of persons as ongoing, evolving processes implies that they are inherently interactional. They are in continual dialogue with themselves and their environments. Their behavior arises both from their personalities and from relationships in their "ecological niches." It is meaningless to talk about individuals as if they are completely free of contexts. In this respect person-centered theory has been called a "field" theory, meaning that behavior arises from the person's perception of the field of relationships or environment within which he or she is embedded.

The concept of *self* is key for person-centered theory. However, the self is not a "homunculus" or thing inside the person. It is a concept, or a "map," that the person develops to help navigate the world. This map must be held tentatively, because no map is itself the territory. One may continually discover new aspects of the self and need to change one's map.

Holding the map of the self rigidly can lead to psychological dysfunction. *Self-actualization* is the tendency of the organism to enhance its own self-development. It can go in either positive or negative directions depending on whether the person holds his or her self-concept tentatively (which promotes productive learning) or rigidly (which promotes defensive and maladaptive development).

In spite of the emphasis on context, Rogers posited individual autonomy as a major goal of human development, similar to most theories of personality developed in the West. Rogers saw the fully functioning person as having an internal locus of control and operating on the basis of personally chosen values rather than by rigidly conforming to the dictates of society. However, the emphasis on a separate, bounded, autonomous self that "self-actualizes" has been criticized as reflecting largely Western, white male values. In other cultures the boundary of the self does not stop at the skin of the person but is extended to the family or the group. Within these other cultures the determinants of behavior are seen as located in a field of forces, which includes the self, in contrast to Western psychology, in which causes are located inside the individual.

Rather than focus on autonomy, we suggest that the operative ingredient in Rogers's theory is a sense of *agency:* a sense that one can confront challenge. A sense of ableness or effectance may be more important than a sense of self-sufficiency. Because challenge is an inherent part of doing most things that are worthwhile in life (careers, relationships, childrearing), having a sense of ableness that one can confront and cope with challenges is fundamental to effective functioning (Dweck & Leggett, 1988).

The recognition that different cultures have different concepts of self is part of a larger recognition that personal and social realities are fundamentally multiple. Individuals and cultures find different viable but workable ways of constructing personal realities. Therefore, PCEP therapists respect the growth potential available within each person's personal reality rather than try to impose an objectively "correct" way of being on them. This belief makes PCEP theory particularly compatible with belief in the importance of respecting cultural diversity.

Because person-centered therapists assume that there is some "sense" in each individual's perceptual universe, facilitating communication among different people's personal realities, including those between therapist and client, is more important than judging who has the correct view. PCEP therapists believe that open sharing of feelings and perspectives in a mutually respecting and accepting atmosphere will facilitate movement toward mutual understanding among the parties involved, and mobilize both individual wisdom and the "wisdom of the group" (O'Hara & Wood, 1983).

An open *internal* process of communication in which all aspects of the self are respected and listened to is equally important. Open, "friendly" listening to all aspects of thoughts, feelings, and experiences, including internalized "voices" from parents and society, allows one's "community within" to move toward creative synthesis. All internal voices may have something to contribute. This is what person-centered therapists call *congruence.*

Experiencing and Feelings

Person-centered and experiential therapists value both intellectual, rational thinking and feelings and experience as important sources of information about how to deal with the world creatively. However, being open to internal experience is particularly important for effective functioning. Rogers originally talked about an "organismic valuing process." He argued that the organism "knows" what it needs for survival and growth. Persons function most effectively when they are aware of and take into account the "wisdom of their organisms."

Later, Gendlin developed his theory of *experiencing*, which Rogers adopted. Experiencing is a different, more fundamental way of knowing self and world than can be acquired from rational, conceptual thinking. Experiencing is also different from emotion; it is the immediate, nonverbal sensing of patterns and relationships in the world and within the self. It includes what is often called "intuitive knowing." However, there is nothing mysterious about it. We can sense or perceive relationships that we cannot easily describe in words. People can, for instance, sense or "feel" when a human face is drawn out of proportion, long before they can cognitively and intellectually identify what is wrong with it (Lewicki, 1986).

The meanings that are acquired through direct experiencing are much more powerful than meanings acquired through conceptual thought. The *experience* of feeling loved in a relationship is a complex, whole-bodied sense of interaction that has much more to it than any intellectual or conceptual description can convey. Infants can tell from their interactions with their mothers whether the latter are empathically attuned to them, before they can put that knowing into words. Gendlin (1970) believes that experiencing is more complex than conscious verbal–conceptual thought and is the source of creativity. Einstein, for instance, had a nonverbal "felt sense" of relativity theory before he had spelled it out in concepts. Internally we have a "felt sense" of how our lives are going and how each specific situation presents itself to us. It is at the level of felt sense that therapeutic change must take place, according to Gendlin. Therapy must lead to a directly felt shift in how we relate to the world, rather than merely to intellectual change. Gendlin's (1996) focusing-oriented psychotherapy is based on this idea.

Person-centered therapists are well-known for advocating "getting in touch with" and "trusting" feelings. Feelings, from a person-centered view, are not synonymous with emotions. Although we can feel anger and sadness, we also feel or sense complex meaning patterns. To be aware of feelings, therefore, is to be aware of both emotions and of sensed patterns of relationships between self and world at a given moment. One can "feel that something is wrong in a relationship" and "feel that one's life is out of balance." To "trust one's feelings" means to listen to them as a source of information. It does not mean to do what they say.

For example, a client came to one of us (ACB) after seeing another therapist. His problem was that he was *feeling* that his wife did not love him. Yet intellectually, when he thought about it, he could identify no logical reason for that feeling. His wife claimed she loved him, and the other therapist had concluded that he was misperceiving the situation based on childhood problems with his mother. A month or two after he had started to see Art, his wife suddenly announced that she was leaving him. She admitted that she had been having an affair for months and was in love with someone else. Clearly, the client's feeling had been based on his apprehension of a set of subtle changes in his wife's manner of relating that were so subtle that his intellectual, rational side could not identify them. If he had been able to trust his feelings, he would have explored his experience more carefully and might have been able to identify the subtle cues involved.

Feelings may not always be an accurate guide, especially if they are based on misperceptions or erroneous interpretations. Thus, sometimes we are misled because something "feels right" when it is not. It could have been that the client's feelings about his wife were wrong—that perhaps it was not that she did not love him, but that she was distracted because of problems at work but did not want to talk about it. If, in that case, he had been able to trust his feelings, he would have been able to check them continuously against his ongoing experience with his wife and would have discovered that his interpretation of those subtle cues to mean she did not love him was not accurate. The legacy from his childhood was not so much that he projected lack of love onto his wife but that he had learned to distrust his feelings.

Person-centered theorists believe that fully functioning people use *all* their faculties. They use their ability both to think rationally and to problem-solve, and to experientially sense what is personally meaningful to the self. Either source of information can be mistaken: Full functioning takes both into account.

Emotion

Theorists of PE-EFT, while agreeing with the importance of experiencing, have particularly emphasized the role of emotion in both human functioning and psychotherapy, and have incorporated emotion theory and dialectical constructivism into their view of human functioning and change. These theorists emphasize the role of emotion, which they see as fundamentally adaptive and as providing information quickly and efficiently to individuals about the impact of their environments, so that they can respond to meet their needs and goals. For example, seek solace when sad, or set limits when violated. According to recent developments in PE-EFT theory, emotion alerts individuals to what is important and significant in their environment and provides a sense of the personal meaning of events. It is regarded as coordinating experience and providing a sense of unifying wholeness (Elliott, Watson, Goldman, & Greenberg, 2004). Process–experiential theorists suggest that emotion schemes are a fundamental way in which experiences are organized. Emotion schemes provide a higher-order organization of experience consisting of four elements, including perceptual–situational, bodily–expressive, motivational–behavioral, and symbolic–conceptual aspects.

The perceptual–situational aspect consists of the person's awareness of the external situation, as perceived and often accessed through episodic memories. The bodily–expressive aspect consists of the bodily reaction and felt sense (e.g., experiencing a sense of helplessness when ridiculed). The symbolic–conceptual aspect refers to the verbal and visual representations of experience; or the labels we apply to differentiate states (e.g., irritation, anger, rage). Often these are metaphorical articulations or imagistic representations of one's felt sense of being in the world. The motivational–behavioral aspect consists of the actions and behavioral responses that accompany different emotional states (e.g., crying when sad and running away when scared) (Greenberg, Rice, & Elliott, 1993).

Another aspect of emotion theory that informs recent variants of PE-EFT is the role of affect regulation. These theorists (Elliott, Watson, et al., 2004; Greenberg et al., 1993; Kennedy-Moore & Watson, 1999) identify a number of processes and activities that facilitate affect regulation, including awareness, acceptance, labeling, reflection, and modulation of distress and expression. They see these activities as key to the therapeutic process and to person-centered and experiential psychotherapies in particular (Elliott, Watson, et al., 2004; Kennedy-Moore & Watson, 1999; Watson, 2007). An important component of person-centered theory is the focus on clients' inner experience. Rogers observed that one of the processes in person-centered therapy is that clients become more aware of their experience and work to symbolize or represent that experience in words. This process is akin to becoming aware of feelings and labeling them in conscious awareness (Wexler &

Rice, 1974). In addition, process–experiential theorists are concerned with helping clients to accept and tolerate their emotional experience and learn to soothe themselves when it is intolerable, as well as develop ways of expressing it that help them to realize their goals and meet their needs in ways that are appropriate to their current context (Greenberg et al., 1993).

Dialectical Constructivism

The other important influence incorporated into PE-EFT theorists' accounts of personality is *dialectical constructivism* (Greenberg & Pascuel-Leone, 2001). According to this view, the self is a constantly evolving but organized multiplicity of selves (Elliott, Watson, et al., 2004; Greenberg et al., 1993). Thus, people are seen as being made up of different voices, or aspects of the self. Other experiential theorists describe them as *experiencing potentials* (Mahrer, 1983). These experiencing potentials or voices emanate from different emotion schemes that are triggered by interactions with the environment. According to this view, no single way of construing the world is dominant; rather, there are an infinite number of ways a person can construe and interact with the world given the multiplicity of voices and ways of perceiving experience.

Theory of Development

Person-centered theory has implied but not emphasized a view of development. First, the infant at birth is an active, curious, exploratory organism, interested in learning about the world and intrinsically interested in developing its own capacities. The child listens to and learns from all sources of his or her experiences: parents, peers, relatives, teachers, neighbors, cultural stories, and so on. The child is particularly interested in learning what results from his or her own efforts and exploratory activity.

The child is seen as a growing organism whose development will continue across the lifespan. In contrast to psychoanalytic theory, in which early experience is seen as "foundational," and as the primary shaping influence on all later constructions of personal reality, PCEP approaches hold that as people develop, they incorporate what was learned earlier into broader and more inclusive frameworks for understanding themselves and their world. This view is more compatible with the theory of Jean Piaget than with that of Freud. In Piaget's (Cowan, 1978) view, development is an expanding process in which later stages involve transcending and reorganizing what has come before. Earlier ideas and experience are retained but are incorporated in newer, more sophisticated constructions of reality in such a way that the form in which they were originally learned is altered. Freudian models view development as being like a pyramid, with early learning forming a broad base for what comes later. Person-centered theory sees development more like a series of Chinese boxes, one within the others. Early childhood is like the smallest box, which gets incorporated into the next largest box, and so on. Each new developmental experience forms a broader and more coherent framework for personal integration than the previous one.

Furthermore, humans are oriented more toward exploring and confronting challenge than toward avoiding pain and frustration. Psychodynamic theorists assume that humans have a "ubiquitous tendency to avoid pain" (Strupp & Binder, 1984, p. 32), and that children commonly avoid, deny, and repress painful experiences or emotions. In contrast, we are frequently amazed by our clients' courage and persistence in confronting pain and challenge, and their attempts to master them. Children also repeatedly face up to painful events and frustrating experiences in attempts at mastery. Consider, for instance, a child as she learns to walk. She repeatedly falls, yet gets up and keeps trying. Humans do avoid pain and frustration but primarily when they feel incompetent to deal with them (Bandura, 1986), as might occur with overwhelming experiences such as early childhood abuse.

PSYCHOLOGICAL HEALTH AND PATHOLOGY

From a PCEP perspective, abnormal behavior is likely to arise if a person is unable to operate in an evolving, growing way. Psychological problems are not faulty beliefs or perceptions, dysfunctional emotional reactions, nor are they inadequate or inappropriate behavior per se. As humans confront challenges in life they periodically misperceive, operate on mistaken beliefs, experience anxiety or depression, and behave inadequately. Dysfunctionality occurs if we *fail to be open to information so that we can learn* from feedback. As a result, we remain stuck in misperceptions, dysfunctional emotions, or inadequate behavior. Dysfunctionality is the result of blocks to learning.

According to Rogers, a primary cause of dysfunction is incongruence between aspects of the self-concept and experience. For example, Janet was a premed student one of us (ACB) knew in college. Part of her self-image was that she was going be a doctor, yet she experienced classes in biology and chemistry as alien and unfulfilling. The incongruence between her self-concept and experience troubled her.

However, it is not incongruence per se that creates dysfunctionality but how the person responds to and tries to resolve the incongruence. All people experience incongruence periodically. If constructs are held tentatively, one will be able to work toward integrating disparate aspects of the self, and it is from such integration that creativity arises. However, if aspects of the self-concept are held rigidly, integration and synthesis are blocked.

People learn to hold parts of their self-concept rigidly when parents, teachers, or culture impose *conditions of worth* on them. They are made to feel that they are worthwhile only when they conform to others' standards and values. This leads to the adoption of rigid "shoulds" about how they are supposed to be. When incongruence between rigid "shoulds" and experience occurs, people are unable to challenge their "shoulds" and so may respond by trying to ignore their experience or by misinterpreting it. Being unable to listen to their own experience, they disempower themselves. They then must rely exclusively on the rigid "shoulds" to guide their choices. When that does not resolve anxiety and incongruence, they feel helpless and may develop dysfunctional behavior. Janet had been "programmed" for years by parents and teachers to become a doctor. To follow this program she had to ignore inconsistent feelings, such as those toward her chemistry and biology classes. This appeared to affect her personality as well: She came across as a distant and guarded person. One day, however, she came to class and was open, warm, and friendly. She told the author (ACB) that she had made a major decision and had changed her major to literature. She disclosed that she had finally begun to listen to her experience and had realized that she did not want to be a doctor. Trusting that part of her experience allowed her to "open up" in other ways.

Janet's problem was that she was holding her belief that she was to be a doctor rigidly. When she was able to hold it tentatively and evaluate it against her experience, she chose to change her major. However, she could have gone in the opposite direction. As she began to trust her feelings, she might have found that she deeply valued helping people. She might then have chosen to become a doctor, even if it meant overcoming her dislike of chemistry and biology. Only the choice would then have been based on a deep personal value rather than on a rigid "should" imposed on her by others. What was important was that Janet be open to her experience, so that she could question and challenge her constructs.

In general, it is when individuals are not open to experience, particularly internal experience, that problems arise. Gendlin held that psychological problems result from a failure to listen empathically to the flow of internal experience (to "focus") in a manner that promotes creatively working on problems. In cases of major disruptions in personal functioning, such as schizophrenia (Gendlin, 1967), individuals come to feel that their own inner life is so chaotic and "sick" that they turn away from it altogether, assuming that there is nothing there to be trusted.

PE-EFT theorists have a related but slightly different view. These authors particularly emphasize the importance of emotional reactions in human functioning. Emotions reflect action tendencies, which inform people how they need to react in a given moment. Therefore, the failure to be aware of or to access emotional information interferes particularly with adaptive capabilities. This failure may lead to a persistence in dysfunctional reactions and an inability to choose new behaviors flexibly to meet the demands of a situation.

Recent variants of PE-EFT theory distinguish between primary adaptive emotion and three types of dysfunctional emotional responses (Elliott, Watson, et al., 2004; Greenberg et al., 1993). *Primary adaptive emotion* is regarded as a direct emotional response that is consistent with the situation and enables the person to take appropriate action in response to it. Examples include expressing happiness at seeing a significant other or taking a rest when tired. These types of automatic responses are essential for survival. In contrast, dysfunctional responses include maladaptive emotional responses, secondary reactive emotions, and instrumental emotions. These theorists see *maladaptive emotions* as emanating from overlearned responses to difficult and traumatic experiences. They are viewed as not adaptive to the current life situation and as interfering with current functioning. *Secondary emotions* are those that occur in response to adaptive emotions so as to transform them (e.g., becoming angry when hurt in order to hide vulnerability; or being disgusted by fear when forcing oneself to be brave in the face of danger). *Instrumental emotions* are deliberate attempts to use emotional reactions as a way of manipulating or controlling others. When using instrumental emotions, a person is being deliberately and consciously incongruent in order to try to influence another's behavior (e.g., appearing sad to receive a reward, or acting hostile in an attempt to intimidate the other). Emotion schemes enable a person to synthesize experience, and they provide both a holistic sense of the person in a given situation and specific emotional reactions, which organize the person for action. Psychological problems occur because individuals either fail to attend to and symbolize their own internal reactions or because their reactions come out of rigid "emotion schemes."

When One Is Functioning Fully

For Rogers, people are able to function most fully when they are open to information. Rogers and his colleagues (e.g., Rogers, 1961b) developed a Process Scale to measure change in therapy from "dysfunctional" to more "fully functional" ways of being. Rogers described the scale thus: "It commences at one end with a rigid, static, undifferentiated, unfeeling, impersonal type of psychologic functioning. It evolves through various stages to, at the other end, a level of functioning marked by changingness, fluidity, richly differentiated reactions, by immediate experiencing of personal feelings, which are felt as deeply owned and accepted" (p. 33). When people are functioning fully, they are therefore fluid and flexible: holding constructs tentatively, testing them against experience, open to and accepting of feelings, listening to and learning from feedback, dialoguing with themselves and their surroundings, and experiencing themselves as able to direct their own lives.

Full functioning refers to a mode of being, namely, that of operating as an evolving process. This does not mean the person necessarily feels fulfilled, content, or even happy (Rogers, 1961a). Nor is there such a thing as a "fully functioning *person*" who is always operating optimally. Even when functioning fully, people may periodically feel blocked, incompetent, inadequate, or frustrated. However, by being in touch with the inner flow of experience and processing it, they are able to struggle with problems, try to learn, and continue to develop.

THE PROCESS OF CLINICAL ASSESSMENT

Person-centered therapists generally do not find traditional diagnostic or assessment procedures useful. Such procedures encourage an "outside" expert perspective on the client, as if the client were being put under a microscope and dissected. This is antithetical to the person-centered, empathic stance in which the therapist tries to feel him- or herself into the client's unique experience. Diagnosis tips the power balance in favor of the therapist. Categorizing people tends to bias the therapist toward treating the individual as a member of a *class* rather than as a unique being. A person-centered therapist would be interested in understanding and relating to Jack or Carolyn, not Jack-the-borderline-personality-disorder or Carolyn-the-narcissist. Moreover, the nature of the PCEP relationship encourages greater sharing of power, because the client is seen as the expert on his or her experience and the therapist, as a companion or guide. However, because the mental health field uses diagnostic labels, person-centered therapists employ them for communication purposes. Rather than assess and diagnose, the PCEP therapist's focus is on the client's moment-to-moment experience, with the goal of facilitating that process as it emerges and progresses. Thus, PCEP therapists are careful to provide the therapeutic conditions of empathy, respect, congruence, and acceptance to support clients as they attend to and formulate their experiencing.

In contrast to other PCEP therapists, process–experiential therapists (Greenberg et al., 1993) make *process diagnoses* in therapy, which is an assessment of the presence of a dysfunctional emotion scheme the client might want to change, and of the client's readiness to work on it at any given moment in therapy. It is important to note that the therapist focuses not on the *content* of this emotion scheme (e.g., anger toward one's father) but merely on evidence that the client is experiencing some block in the process of resolving a personal problem. Process–experiential therapists look for "markers," which are specific verbal, behavioral, or emotional signs that a client is struggling with a particular kind of emotional processing problem. For instance, a marker for a *problematic reaction point* (PRP) is that clients are puzzled by their reaction to a situation or person, which may consist of feeling that their reactions were unreasonable, dysfunctional, exaggerated, or unexpected.

The identification of a specific kind of marker suggests to the therapist what type of intervention could be used at that moment to foster and deepen the client's exploration. Process diagnoses and the corresponding interventions have been developed by therapists trying to make explicit their implicit knowledge of what happens in therapy, as well as intensive study of clients' successful performances and resolution of specific blocks such as problematic reactions. Thus, at a marker for a PRP, a PE-EFT therapist might suggest that clients engage in systematic evocative unfolding to access their episodic memory of a situation and the emotion evoked to identify the trigger for the reaction and to help clients gain a better understanding of it. If clients agree that focusing on the PRP would be useful, their PE-EFT therapist gently suggests ways of representing their experience to help them gain a better sense of their experiencing in the moment when the reaction occurred.

THE PRACTICE OF THERAPY

The core of PCEP practice is for therapists to focus on what is happening between themselves and the client in the moment. This includes focusing on both the client's moment-by-moment experience and their own moment-by-moment experience with the client. Working with what is most "alive," present, or central for the client is thought to be the best way to support clients' processes for change. Therapists therefore focus on understanding and working as clients' ongoing attempts to change, stabilize, understand, or reorganize themselves emerge in the moment. Although most PCEP therapists would agree with this, there are differences in *how* they work with the moment-by-moment process. Traditional person-centered therapists (e.g., Brodley, 1993) operate in a "nondirective" way. The therapist's goal is primarily to be a companion on the client's journey of self-discovery. By being warm, empathic, accepting, and genuine, the therapist provides an atmosphere in which the client's own thrust toward growth can operate. Therapists largely stay within the client's frame of reference, focusing their efforts on understanding and reflecting the client's communication and experience. Rarely would a traditional person-centered therapist suggest a technique or engage in self-disclosure.

A trend in the 1960s among some person-centered therapists was to treat person-centered therapy more as a philosophy of therapy than as a specific way of doing it. It was argued that if therapists were warm and accepting, empathic, and genuine, while respecting the client's growth process, they could go beyond the traditional nondirective mode, share their own thoughts and reactions, and even suggest techniques from other therapies (Holdstock & Rogers, 1983). For many therapists, person-centered therapy became a philosophy in whose context they could practice in eclectic ways. As a result, some person-centered therapists have incorporated behavioral, hypnotic, and Gestalt techniques into their practice. Natalie Rogers (1997) includes art and dance in her "person-centered expressive therapy." Similarly, Gendlin's (1996) focusing-oriented therapy and Greenberg et al.'s (1993) process–experiential therapy hold that therapists can systematically facilitate clients' experiencing in the moment to help them resolve problematic issues and grow.

Currently there is controversy among the various "tribes" of the PCEP approach over whether it is appropriate for the therapist to self-disclose, suggest techniques, or try systematically to facilitate experiencing. Traditional person-centered therapists (Brodley, 1993) particularly disagree with experiential approaches that attempt to facilitate clients' experiencing in the session. They believe that to use any technique, such as the "empty chair," systematically is to violate the basic "nondirective attitude" of following the client, and letting the client find his or her own pathway to growth.

Philosophy of Therapy

Person-centered and experiential therapies are based on the belief that it is clients who ultimately "heal" themselves and create their own self-growth (Bohart & Tallman, 1999). Growth and healing is generated from within the person, though external processes can either facilitate or retard that process. As analogies to the person-centered view, plants and children grow naturally, though farmers and parents contribute to fostering or retarding that growth.

Person-centered and experiential therapies are unique in how much they emphasize the self-righting, self-healing tendencies of the person. Although therapists with other approaches agree that humans have positive potential within, they believe people might not use this potential unless guided to do so by the therapist, presumably because clients are so motivated by their desires to avoid pain and to gain security that they avoid dealing with issues that unlock that potential, or because they are trapped in faulty thinking from which they must be freed by the therapist. The therapist becomes the "expert guide" on what issues the client needs to face in order to grow.

In contrast, the job of person-centered and experiential therapists is to provide optimal conditions under which the intrinsic self-organizing and self-transcending capabilities of the person can operate. Under supportive conditions, the client's thrust toward growth overrides any tendencies toward avoidance of pain. Given proper conditions, clients naturally move towards wholeness and psychological health.

Therapists do not have to make clients face up to even extremely repressed, painful experiences, such as those of early childhood abuse. If conditions are provided under which clients can begin to begin to develop a sense of self-efficacy in their own capacity for self-righting and growth, they will come to want to face up to such experiences when necessary for their continued development. At that point, such experiences begin to emerge slowly as a part of the process of self-healing.

Person-centered and experiential psychotherapists accept clients where they are when they come into therapy. If the client's problem is feeling chronically tense, the PCEP therapist works on what the client chooses to focus on and does not assess whether there are "deeper issues" to confront. This is due to the belief that clients' development of their capacities for self-direction and self-regulation are the most important aspect of therapy, and that clients delve deeper when necessary, and when they are ready. This is also true for experiential psychotherapists who may try to facilitate and augment clients' experiencing by suggesting different ways of working in therapy. However, they remain respectful of their clients' sense of self-direction and what is important to them at different times.

Basic Structure of Person-Centered and Experiential Therapies

Person-centered and experiential therapists are flexible in how they structure the therapy interaction. Although they typically meet with the client for a 1-hour session on a once-a-week basis, person-centered therapists modify this format to conform to the needs of a particular client. A client might be seen more or less than once a week, sessions might last either longer or shorter than 1 hour, and meetings might or might not be held in the therapist's office. For example, Gendlin (1967) worked with hospitalized patients by taking them for a walk down to the hospital cafeteria. One of us (ACB) worked with a young hospitalized client with paranoid schizophrenia by meeting with him on the hospital lawn. The other (JCW) worked with a severely developmentally challenged and autistic young man by accompanying him in an exploration of a garden reflecting his interests and actions, in a manner that is known and formulated as pretherapy (Prouty, 1990). PCEP therapists do not dictate the number of sessions that may be required for each person. Although usually several sessions are necessary, person-centered and experiential therapists believe that it is possible for important change to occur in a single session. At the other end of the continuum, some people may need to be in therapy for a number of years to address adequately the issues they seek to resolve. Thus, no meaningful "average length" can be prescribed for person-centered therapy.

Person-centered and experiential therapists might use any or all of individual, couple, family, or group therapy formats. However, the choice is jointly decided by the therapist and all the participants.

Goal Setting

Person-centered and experiential therapists believe that it is the client who, at some level, knows what hurts and what needs to be changed, although it may take the therapy process to access this knowledge. Therefore, these therapists do not set goals for what changes clients need to undergo in order to improve (e.g., "become more assertive," "stop thinking irrationally," or "get out of your dysfunctional relationship"). Rather, the goal is to provide conditions under which the client's own intrinsic capacity for confronting and exploring problematic experiences, extracting new and important meanings, and creatively reorganizing experience in more productive ways can operate.

Why can the therapist not simply tell the client "the answer"? We stated earlier that people live in different personal realities of which therapists can know only little bits. In a famous film of Carl Rogers working with Gloria (Shostrom, 1965), Gloria's problem was that she had lied to her daughter Pammy about the fact that she was having sexual relationships although she was not married. She wanted Rogers to tell her whether to tell her daughter the truth. Rogers refused to do so and helped Gloria arrive at her own answer. In watching the film, students have often expressed frustration: Why can Rogers not just tell her to be honest?

One reason is that only Gloria knows the true subtleties and complexities of her life and of her relationship with her daughter. Only Gloria knows the intricate "web" of relationships that constitutes her "ecological niche." What might seem wise from an outside perspective might not be wise from inside Gloria's life. Therefore, only Gloria knows how, ultimately, to reorganize and synthesize all the factors to provide a solution that is personally wise, that takes care of both herself and her daughter, and that honors other relationships and values in her life. If Rogers were to give generalized advice ("Yes. It's better to be honest"), it might work. However, it also is possible that if Gloria simply followed this advice, without working out its wisdom, it might backfire. For instance, if Gloria still felt conflict, she might convey that conflict and spread her own anxiety to her daughter.

Although all person-centered and experiential therapists agree on not setting goals for *what* the client needs to change, they differ on whether to have goals regarding *how* best to help the client find his or her own answers. Traditional person-centered therapists set no goals for their clients or for the therapy process at all. Although traditional person-centered therapists believe that therapy leads to outcomes such as people being more open to experience, more fluid, and more differentiated, they believe that these changes are most likely to occur if they do not try to make them happen but focus instead on how they can best be present with their clients. Traditional person-centered therapists' goals are ones they set for *themselves:* to be empathic, accepting, respectful, and congruent. The therapist, in some sense, works on *him- or herself* in therapy in order to be more effectively present. The therapist who feels that he or she is not understanding the client struggles to do so. If the therapist feels incongruent, he or she struggles to be effectively congruent.

In contrast, while focusing-oriented and process–experiential therapists, like their person-centered counterparts, agree that there are no clearly defined outcomes other than the ones set by their clients, they nonetheless may suggest specific process goals to clients. This is an attempt to help clients who are stuck to resolve certain cognitive–affective problems, such as lack of awareness of, or representation of, experiencing, or conflicts about two different courses of action.

Techniques and Strategies

Person-Centered Psychotherapy

For person-centered therapy, the establishment of a facilitative therapeutic relationship is itself the therapeutic technique and strategy. The process of "being with" the client in the sense of accepting the client as he or she is, entering imaginatively into the client's world of perception and feelings, and being authentic, is sufficient for the facilitation of a process of change.

What the therapist primarily does is express his or her struggles to understand the client's experience. This often comes out in the form of *reflection,* which is a way of responding in which the therapist tries to communicate his or her understanding of what the client is experiencing and trying to say. Therapists can reflect feelings, meanings, experiences, emotions, or any combination thereof. They often go beyond what the client has explicitly *said* to try to grasp what the client is experiencing but has been left unsaid. However, the therapist tries to grasp only what is within the client's current range of awareness of experiencing. The therapist does not try to grasp possible unconscious aspects of the client's experience, which is the main theoretical difference between a reflection and a psychodynamic interpretation. The following example compares a reflection and an interpretation:

> *Client:* "I'm feeling so lost in my career. Every time I seem to be getting close to doing something creative, which would lead to a promotion, I somehow manage to screw it up. I never feel like I am using my potential. There is a block there."
>
> *Reflection:* "You're feeling really frustrated and you don't know what's happening. You get in your own way every time you have a chance to use your potential."
>
> *Psychodynamic interpretation:* "It sounds like every time you get close to success you unconsciously sabotage yourself. Perhaps success means something to you that is troubling or uncomfortable, and you are not aware of what that is."

Notice that this interpretation may, in fact, be accurate, but it is an attempt to make the client think about his or her behavior as opposed to mirroring and adequately representing his experiencing. Thus, it works to bring to the client's attention something that is not *currently* in the client's awareness. This is the key difference between reflections and interpretations.

For person-centered therapists it is important to react in a therapeutically spontaneous manner to whatever is happening in the moment between themselves and their clients. Although reflection has been the traditional form for expressing empathy, spontaneous expressions of empathy may take many other forms (Bozarth, 1997) such as self-disclosure of the therapist's own experience in "resonance" with that of the client. At a given moment, the sense of sharing between therapist and client might also lead the therapist spontaneously to suggest a technique. Person-centered therapists are not banned from suggesting techniques. It is *how* they suggest techniques that is important. A technique is only suggested when to do so furthers the process of client and therapist being together in a real, empathic relationship. It is not an attempt to "do anything" to the client or "make anything happen." The client is always free to reject the technique. However, techniques are suggested relatively infrequently by person-centered therapists. Whereas the experiential therapists also emphasize the client-centered nature of the relationship and prize the therapeutic conditions emphasized by Rogers, they, more than their person-centered colleagues, tentatively introduce other techniques or ways of working to facilitate clients' process in the session more frequently.

Focusing-Oriented Psychotherapy

Gendlin's (1996) focusing-oriented psychotherapy is based on the idea that change arises from tuning into and working with a "bodily felt sense." Research has shown that clients grow when they actively refer inwardly to their experience and feelings, and articulate that experience (Hendricks, 2002). They are less likely to grow if they talk about their problems in distanced, intellectual ways or focus externally on the situations in their lives. Based on this premise, focusing-oriented psychotherapists try to facilitate this experiencing process in psychotherapy in three basic ways. First, they use a variant of empathic responding—"experiential" responding. Experiential responses specifically focus on the felt aspects of the client's present experience and often rely on metaphors. An experiential response to our aforementioned client might be as follows: "It sounds like you're feeling really up against it, like up against a big wall, which you're trying to push aside, and you don't know how to."

A second technique used by experiential therapists is the sharing of their own immediate experience in the therapy relationship with their clients (Gendlin, 1967). The therapist attends to his or her own immediate experience in the situation and tries to explicate it in words. This helps therapist and client clarify the nature of what is going on between them, and provides for clients a model of how to relate inwardly to their own experience. For instance, the therapist might say to a silent, sad client who has just suffered a loss: "Part of me wants to reach out and contact you and talk about the loss, and part of me feels like I just want to sit in silence with you and keep you company in your pain. I'm not sure what you want, but I want you to know that I'm here if you want to talk, and I'm here even if I just stay silent with you for a while."

The third technique is *focusing* (Gendlin, 1996). A client is asked to focus inwardly and to "clear a space" by imagining that he or she has set all problems aside for the moment. Then the client takes one problem and tries to focus on how the problem feels inside. Although a person can think about only parts of a problem at any given moment, he or she can feel all those parts together. The client waits and listens to see whether some words or concepts come from the feeling. This process often leads to a *felt shift* in which the sense of the problem reorganizes, so that the person can get a better "handle" on the crux of it.

Any concept or technique from other therapies might be used by a focusing-oriented therapist if it helps to facilitate contacting, exploring, and articulating inner experiencing. Experiential therapists have used Gestalt role playing, body techniques, cognitive techniques, and relaxation. They may talk about psychoanalytic ideas if these concepts help clients directly refer to their immediate felt experience. Thus, Gendlin's theory of experiencing has provided a theoretical rationale for eclectic therapeutic practice (Gendlin, 1996).

Process–Experiential/Emotion-Focused Psychotherapy

PE-EFT (Greenberg et al., 1993), an integrative psychotherapy based in a person-centered view of the nature of the human being, also draws on ideas from both cognitive theory and Gestalt psychotherapy. It is a member of a larger class of integrative, emotion-focused psychotherapies that also includes "emotion-focused therapy for couples" (Greenberg & Johnson, 1988; Johnson & Boisvert, 2002).

Carrying forward work by Wexler and Rice (1974) and others, process–experiential therapists (Greenberg et al., 1993) view clients' problems as resulting from the failure to explore productively certain classes of cognitive–affective information. The goal of the PE-EFT therapist is to facilitate different types of cognitive–affective operations in the client at different times to best enhance deeper exploration. The job of the therapist is (1) to identify the problem the client is struggling with and select the intervention that best facilitates work on the specific problem at any given moment, and (2) to guide the client systematically, if agreeable, through the operations involved in the chosen intervention. Different client behaviors serve as therapeutic markers to guide the therapist in choosing which intervention to use.

Greenberg and colleagues (1993) have modeled five basic therapeutic markers, two of which we briefly describe. The first client marker is that of a conflict split, with the client in conflict about something. Usually there is a "should" side saying "do this," and a "want" side saying "I don't want to." With this marker, the Gestalt two-chair exercise is used. A clients role-plays both sides, speaking from the "should" side, then switching chairs to speak from the "want" side. The client goes back and forth until some integration is reached, which occurs as the client clearly articulates each side of his or her experience, with its concomitant needs, wishes, hopes, and fears. There is a shift in the power balance as the client's "should" side moves from talking in oppressive, controlling language to expressing concerns, hopes, and fears. Instead of "You should study harder," it says, "I'm worried that if you don't study harder, you won't achieve your goals, and that makes me scared, because how will we support ourselves?"

A second marker occurs when the client has "unfinished business" with another person. For this problem, a version of the Gestalt empty-chair exercise is used. The client role-plays dialogues between him- or herself and the other person, taking both roles. This role-play allows the client to arrive at a personal resolution of the emotional pain experienced in the relationship with the other person. For instance, a sexually abused daughter might role-play a dialogue between herself and her father. In her chair she expresses her rage, guilt, and sadness over what her father has done to her. She may play her father as someone whom she can ultimately forgive, or she may play him as an "unrepentant bastard." In either case, she becomes able to let go of her guilt and her experience of the past, and to reclaim a sense of her own worth and potency (Elliott et al., 2005; Greenberg & Paivio, 1997).

Process of Therapy

For each of the previously described therapies, the therapeutic process is one of staying closely with the "flow" of what is happening in the session. Therapists focus on what clients bring up to talk about and do not try to guide the conversation toward topics they think are important. For instance, Gloria shifted topics several times over the course of her half-hour session with Rogers. He stayed with her shifts, and it is clear that there was a kind of intuitive wisdom to these shifts that led Gloria to deepen her exploration.

What is talked about is not nearly as important as the moment-by-moment process: For example, are clients relating to themselves in a productive, self-evolutionary way no matter what the content? The process of therapy, therefore has its own intrinsically structured flow, and clients often recycle topics several times before they are resolved.

From person-centered and experiential perspectives, "resistance" is not a useful concept. What other therapists call *resistance* may be defined as occurring when the *therapist* thinks the client should be talking about something, feeling something, or doing something other than what the *client* is doing. When clients are "resisting," they are trying to follow what they feel will best help them maintain or grow at that time. As with anything else the client is doing, person-centered and experiential therapists "respect the resistance" and try to empathize with "where the client is coming from" at that moment. Moreover, if there is resistance, then PCEP therapists use this as an indicator that they are not fully in tune with a client's experience and need to work harder at being more empathic and congruent in the session. Were an experiential therapist to use a technique at that point, it would be used in an experimental way to see whether it helps the client move forward. It would not be used to "break through" the resistance. This is the best way to facilitate the process of moving forward. Clients may grow out of resistance if the therapist remains in empathic and genuine contact but may get stuck in resistance if the therapist (or anyone else) relates to them in a "superior" manner—correcting them or imparting "truth" to them.

Because person-centered and experiential therapists invest so much trust in clients' ability to direct their process of growth, termination of therapy is rarely a problem. In our experience, clients are motivated to move away from being dependent on the therapist to "trying their wings" when they are ready. They do not need to be "fully healed," with all problems resolved, to try to live on their own. Problems are a part of life, and clients sometimes leave because they now feel they can manage the problems on their own. Sometimes clients ease themselves into termination by deciding to come every other week for a time instead of every week, before they decide to stop altogether. In other instances, clients just decide they are ready to stop.

When a client decides to stop therapy, therapist and client talk over the decision. If the therapist has reservations about the client's termination, he or she may express them, especially if the client asks for the therapist's opinion. But contrary to the "expert therapist" model, in which clients are sometimes told that they are avoiding or resisting because they want to stop therapy, a person-centered therapist confines him- or herself to a *personal* self-disclosure (e.g., "I worry that we didn't quite work through that issue, and I wonder if it might bother you again, but you know I'm here if you ever do feel a need for further work").

Virtually all the errors a person-centered or an experiential therapist may commit arise from failing to be warm, empathic, and genuine; imposing an agenda upon the client; or failing to be in touch with the unfolding moment-by-moment process.

THE THERAPEUTIC RELATIONSHIP AND THE STANCE OF THE THERAPIST

The therapeutic relationship is the single most important factor in both person-centered and experiential approaches. According to Rogers (1957), the three primary conditions of a good therapeutic relationship are *unconditional positive regard* or *warmth, empathic understanding*, and *genuineness* or *congruence*. Rogers postulated that these basic relationship conditions are "necessary and sufficient" for therapeutic growth to occur, although Bozarth (1993) has suggested that these conditions are sufficient but not absolutely necessary, because the self-actualizing tendency may sometimes facilitate growth even without a therapeutic relationship.

The implications of Rogers's (1957) statement were (and are) radical: It is the relationship that is the "healing" element in therapy. Techniques, theoretical points of view, and even professional training have little to do with making therapy work. Strupp and Hadley (1979), for instance, found that untrained college professors, chosen for their sensitivity, were on average as therapeutic as professional therapists.

Although experiential therapists would agree that the relationship is healing, they believe that the use of additional techniques and strategies can facilitate the growth process in therapy. In a sense, while they might agree that the relationship conditions are necessary and sufficient for most clients much of the time, sometimes they are insufficient for clients who may be blocked; that is, the use of exercises, such as the empty-chair and focusing, can enhance the effectiveness of the process.

Warmth or unconditional positive regard has also been called "acceptance," "respect," "liking," "prizing," or even "nonpossessive love." The quality is a basic attitude of liking, respecting, or prizing directed at the client as a whole person. It rests on a distinction between the client as a person and the client's behavior. Just as good parents continue to like and prize their children even while disliking specific behaviors (e.g., writing on the walls with crayons), the person-centered therapist continues to prize the client as a person even when the client's behavior is dysfunctional. Unconditional regard does not mean the person-centered therapist conveys support or approval for dysfunctional behavior.

Feeling liked and prized as people, clients begin to feel safe to explore their experience and to take a more objective look at their behavior. Clients are able to distinguish between their intrinsic worth as persons and the dysfunctionality of current ways of experiencing and behaving. Bozarth (1997) has held that unconditional positive regard is the core healing element in therapy.

Empathic understanding is based on the ability to intuit oneself inside the client's personal reality, to come as close as one can to seeing and feeling as the client sees and feels. From an "outside" perspective, client behavior often seems irrational, self-destructive, manipulative, narcissistic, rigid, infantile, or egocentric. However, from an "inside" perspective, behaviors that seemed dysfunctional and irrational from the outside usually make "sense" in terms of how the client is experiencing the world. This does not mitigate the behavior's dysfunctionality. Rather, it suggests that from within the client's skin, there is some sense underlying it.

One client was arrested for exposing himself to his neighbor's 12-year-old daughter. As the therapist struggled to understand from the viewpoint of the client's personal reality, it became clear that the client felt totally helpless and impotent in his dealings with this girl whom he experienced as consistently making fun of him and treating him with disrespect. Exposing himself was an extreme (albeit dysfunctional) reaction to one particularly hurtful show of disrespect, and his way of expressing helplessness, anger, and rage. We later describe what happened in this case.

There are a number of different positive therapeutic effects of empathic understanding. First, the experience of being known seems to be intrinsically therapeutic. When a person feels fully known by another, it is as if the person comes into focus to him- or herself. The person feels better able to sort things out and to make choices. Second, finding that there is some sense in his or her experience, even when he or she has acted dysfunctionally, makes the person feel generally less crazy or dysfunctional. The person begins to have some confidence in his or her own inner experience, which allows him or her to look at things more carefully and to confront painful experience.

Third, therapist empathic understanding provides a model of a "friendly" way for clients to listen to their own experience. This friendly listening lets clients accept and hear meanings that they previously feared because they seemed "unfriendly" to the self, thus allowing them to begin to find more productive ways of dealing with those feelings and meanings. As the aforementioned client began to listen to his own experience in a friendly manner, he began to realize there was some "sense" in his impulsive act of exposing himself to his neighbor's daughter. He was trying to assert himself. He decided that he wanted to develop more proactive and less harmful ways of asserting himself and dealing with his anger, which is what he and the therapist worked on.

Fourth, therapist empathic understanding helps to soothe the client and modulate emotions. As the client begins to put experience into words and feels heard and understood, he or she feels calmer and less anxious, and more able to confront difficult and painful experiences. Fifth therapist empathic understanding facilitates the clients' deconstruction of his or her experiencing and worldviews (Watson, 2002).

Genuineness or *congruence* refers to the degree to which a therapist is in touch with and aware of him- or herself in therapy. This does not mean that the therapist acts out feelings or says whatever is on his or her mind. Rather, genuineness and congruence are matters of *inner* connection. They have to do with the degree to which therapists are in touch with the flow of their inner experience, and the extent to which their outward behavior reflects some truly felt aspect of their inner experience.

Lietaer (1991) has distinguished between congruence and *transparency*. *Congruence* is attending inwardly to one's experience and working to sort out its meanings. *Transparency* is the open self-disclosure of what is within the therapist. Although person-centered therapists value self-disclosure in therapy, it should be "sensitively relevant" to what promotes the therapeutic process. Rogers has argued that therapists should only disclose their reactions when (1) they are persistent and (2) are getting in the way of the therapeutic relationship itself.

Gendlin (1967) cautions that therapists must self-disclose in more effective and productive ways than the person in the street. The way people in the street are "honest" is often to label, criticize, and judge (e.g., "You're boring"). If the therapist has a reaction to a client (e.g., anger), which she concludes she should share, she first must work with it herself before self-disclosing. She tunes inward and tries to sort out the degree to which her reaction reflects her own issues from the degree to which it reflects something useful in the relationship to be shared. She then shares it as her reaction, not as the "truth."

Genuineness as a Basis for Therapeutic Eclecticism

From the 1960s on, many person-centered therapists increasingly have emphasized genuineness as the most important of the therapeutic conditions, although only in the context of warmth and empathy, and with a belief in the client's intrinsic self-directive capacities. The emphasis on genuineness fueled the shift by some person-centered therapists toward a more integrative way of practicing. First, it encouraged therapists to find their own styles for expressing empathy instead of expressing it primarily in the form of reflection. Genuinely expressed empathy became a matter of tuning in and timing rather than a specific kind of response. One client, for instance, did not experience reflections as empathic, and the therapist soon gave up sharing understanding in that way. The client felt more comfortable with the therapist expressing his own reactions. He experienced the therapist as "really understanding him" when the therapist responded in that manner. With another client, empathy sometimes was expressed in a light, humorous, almost bantering way of interacting.

Second, the emphasis on genuineness provided a philosophical basis for therapists to disclose their opinions or suggest techniques. It was argued that if the therapist had an opinion or a thought, or knew of a technique and deliberately withheld it in order to "play the role of a nondirective therapist," then the therapist was not being genuine. The issue was not *whether* a technique was suggested but *how*. Was it suggested by the expert trying to fix the client, or by one human being sharing his or her own experience with another? In the latter case, the implicit message was "This is something from my experience that you may find useful; however, it is up to you to evaluate its usefulness and to use it if you wish." With this modification, as we have noted, many person-centered therapists have incorporated hypnosis, dream work, Gestalt techniques, and behavioral techniques into their practices.

Third, the emphasis on genuineness contributed to idea of the therapist working at *relational depth* with the client (Mearns & Cooper, 2005), which has to do with the sense of closeness and connectedness that develops between therapist and client. These experiences of "deep meeting" are not only highly meaningful for clients and therapists alike but also therapeutic.

Transference and Countertransference

Many person-centered therapists, including the authors, do not find the concepts of transference and countertransference to be either meaningful or therapeutically helpful. These terms originate in traditional or Freudian psychoanalytic theory. *Transference* refers to the tendency of the client to read things into the therapist's behavior based on the client's past experience, primarily those with caretakers. *Countertransference* refers to the tendency of the therapist to read things into the client's behavior based on the therapist's past experience and unresolved problems.

These concepts are not helpful, because they do not make meaningful distinctions between different kinds of experiences. To understand the present we *always* "transfer" past experience onto it. We are "transferring" right now when we interpret these words as being in "English" based on past experience. Whenever we use past experience to interpret the present, there is the possibility of error. For instance, in some other cultures, people stand much closer to one another when they talk than they do in Northern European American culture. Based on our past experience, we might misinterpret the behavior of people from such a culture as being intrusive or overly familiar. We might continue to feel uneasy around them, even when we know intellectually that we are just dealing with a cultural difference. We might also make dysfunctional decisions about the persons based on our erroneous interpretation.

The key is not whether we use our past experience to understand the present—we always do that. It is whether we attend to the *discrepancies* between what is new and different in the present and our past experience, and use that to learn and to adjust our perceptions. Clients often appear to persist in their "misreadings" of the therapist, but, from a PCEP point of view, that is not because they are "transferring." Rather, their ability to listen openly to corrective information, both from others and from their own inner experiencing, has been compromised by a lack of self-trust. As they come to trust themselves and the therapist, and as they learn how to listen to their feelings, they become better and better at correcting misreadings of situations.

It is interesting to note that person-centered and experiential psychotherapists do not often speak of transference issues with their clients. One reason for this might be that it does not manifest as readily, if at all, in relationships where the objective is to remain within clients' frame of reference. While it is possible that PCEP therapists, like all therapists, might inadvertently trigger a response from their clients by their behavior (e.g., a misunderstanding of what a client is trying to communicate might make a client feel invisible, which might resonate with extremely painful feelings of not being seen and cared for as a child), as long as therapists are able to respond with empathy, acceptance, and understanding of those feelings, as well as to validate how the client might have experienced the interaction, it is likely that the feelings will be modulated and the relationship repaired. It is as if by trying to remain within their clients' frame of reference and being accepting of their reactions and perceptions, PCEP therapists fly under the radar and seldom activate painful feelings from the past within the therapeutic relationship.

With respect to countertransference, it might be argued that therapists always see clients at least partially through the lens of their own past experience. This includes experience from their personal past, with previous clients, and from what they have been taught in school and their professional training, It includes cultural norms and expectations. Some therapists tend to see clients through the eyes of either psychiatric diagnoses or pet theories.

As we have already noted, therapists' personal reactions can be productively used in therapy if they are expressed therapeutically and owned as therapists' own reactions rather than presented as objective truth about the client. Therapists need to listen to clients to see whether their perceptions and reactions are fitting with clients' experience. In other words, therapists need to notice discrepancies between their own perceptions of their clients and clients' actual reactions, whether these perceptions are based on theory, cultural background, or therapists' personal experience.

What is important is that both therapists and clients engage in a process of getting to know what is unique and different about this person and this situation compared to the past. The question is: Is the individual exploring preconceptions in order to modify them over time and truly getting to know him- or herself in relation to other people and different situations? This process is crucial for effective coping in life. This is the process the therapist must develop for him- or herself and the process that person-centered therapy models for the client through its emphasis on acceptance and open exploration.

CURATIVE FACTORS OR MECHANISMS OF CHANGE

From a person-centered point of view, the major "mechanism" of change is the client's capacity for productive and creative self-organization and growth, or what Bohart (in press) has called "self-organizing wisdom." Therapists foster this capacity through how they relate to clients. Provision by person-centered and experiential therapists of an engaged, experientially supportive, and empathic relationship, including the use of empathically attuned techniques and procedures, provides a "conflict-free zone" that mobilizes clients' "critical and creative intelligence." As clients feel understood, supported, and "met" by the therapist, their creative intelligence begins to overcome self-criticism, defense, and emotional blocks. Clients become curious about their own experience and perceptions, and begin to explore them. This exploratory process leads to the creative synthesis of incongruities between different thoughts and perspectives, or thoughts and experiences. It leads clients to learn to incorporate and include all their experience. Clients feel free to try out new behaviors, and to fail with them, before they refine them so that they become truly effective. They also experiment with developing more effective, satisfying, and responsible relationships with others.

As part of that process, clients relate to old traumatic experiences in new ways, allowing them to be worked through and more productively incorporated into personal functioning. A person who was abused as a child may come to appreciate and value the processes whereby she managed to preserve herself and survive. She may mine that for a sense of strength rather than one of weakness. She may find ways of using her experience to develop her own sensitivity and capacity for caring. Therefore, working through past trauma is not really repairing damage as much as it is learning how to assimilate and reorganize traumatic experience to mobilize potential.

Because the therapy process is creative, therapists often have no idea how new but adaptive solutions will emerge. Mahoney (1991) and others have talked about Ilya Prigogine's research in chemistry and physics, which found that systems confronted with disorganization sometimes spontaneously jump to entirely new, more sophisticated levels of organization. Person-centered therapists believe this is what often happens in therapy. Therefore, the therapist does not have to be the expert who knows the answer. Rather, the therapist must be a "process expert" who can facilitate the creative process.

Through clients' own self-experimentation, they begin to build a sense of *efficacy*: I can learn and change and move my life forward. Clients learn that they can struggle with something they are up against and make some productive accommodation with it, no matter how awful the problem. For instance, a client may learn to live productively even if paralyzed. One learns that life is a process of continual confrontation of problems and challenges, and of moving onward.

In addition to mobilizing clients' cognitive processing skills so that they can begin to solve their problems in living, another active ingredient is internalization of the therapeutic relationship. Barrett-Lennard (1997) speaks of the self-empathy that develops out of the therapeutic relationship. With the development of self-empathy, clients come to learn to accept and view as legitimate their experience, and to represent it accurately, so that they can modify harsh conditions of worth and develop other guidelines for living that are less annihilating or neglectful of self. In addition, as clients come to attend to, accept, and try to represent accurately their inner experiences, they learn to regulate their affect. In the process of exploring their experience with their therapists, clients learn to become aware of their feelings and to label them, more able to tolerate negative affect and to modulate both levels of arousal and expression of feelings and emotions (Elliott et al., 2003; Watson, Goldman, & Greenberg, 2007).

Focusing-oriented and process–experiential psychotherapists particularly emphasize the role of feelings and emotions in the change process. However, unlike their more client-centered counterparts, experiential and process–experiential therapists believe that it can be helpful to provide clients with active guidance in processing different kinds of emotional experiences that may be getting in the way of their capacity for productive self-reorganization. Focusing-oriented therapy stresses the importance of clients tuning into the bodily felt sense of their problems and turning that felt sense into words. This leads to a creative unfolding process that produces a bodily shift in how the problem is experienced, accompanied by a bodily felt reorganization of the problem in a new, more productive way. Similarly, process–experiential therapy stresses a process of accessing emotions so as to facilitate the restructuring of emotion schemes in terms of seeing a situation differently, accessing different feelings in response to a situation, identifying new needs and goals, or symbolizing experience in new ways.

Person-centered therapists do not explicitly teach life skills, as do some behavioral therapists. Nevertheless, the process is one in which skills such as learning to explore and to listen to one's experience, as well as good communication skills, are modeled and experienced. The client learns that there is something valuable and trustworthy in everyone's experience, and that it is better to listen to others than to impose one's will and values upon them. Dialoguing in an open, cooperative way about mutual problems is the best way to find a solution and mobilizes the "wisdom of the group." Respecting different ways not only is interpersonally important, but it also fosters the creativity that comes from openness to difference. Experiential therapists, however, may include some teaching of life skills. The focusing exercise, for instance, can be taught, then utilized as a self-help skill outside of psychotherapy.

Insight

Acquiring insight is not a primary change mechanism in person-centered or experiential therapy, although clients often may attain it. Change often occurs without insight. It is the direct experience of the therapy relationship itself that has the most impact. *What* one learns about oneself is less important than *the changes that come about in how* one relates to oneself, to others, and to problematic experience. These are complex, lived, whole-bodied changes that occur in an experiential manner rather than being guided "from above" by insight.

The Role of the Therapist's Personality

We have previously described how the therapist's ability to be congruent and to be a real person in therapy is crucial to the change process. Good therapists seek out their own therapy whenever it appears that their problems or personalities are getting in the way of providing a therapeutic environment for the client.

Factors That Limit the Success of Person-Centered and Experiential Therapies

Practically all the factors that limit the success of person-centered and experiential therapists have to do with whether the client and therapist create a good enough working relationship so that the client engages actively in the tasks of therapy. Although person-centered and experiential therapists have developed ways of working with unmotivated clients (e.g., Gendlin, 1967), effectiveness is limited by low client motivation. To work with clients who are in therapy against their will, such as court-referred clients or adolescents brought by their parents, is challenging. The establishment of a good relationship becomes even more central with such populations.

Clients with whom it is difficult to establish a relationship can likewise limit the effectiveness of person-centered and experiential therapy. Working with clients labeled with "borderline personality disorder," for instance, is difficult not because their personality structure is primitive but because some have difficulty staying with the frustrations that are a normal part of the working environment of therapy. We believe that if a strong therapeutic alliance can be formed, then these clients can be worked with effectively.

It has been asserted at times that person-centered therapy is not useful with "nonverbal" clients. However, person-centered therapists have had success with nonverbal clients with schizophrenia (Gendlin, 1967), and Prouty (1990) developed pre-therapy for working with people both severely regressed schizophrenia and with mental retardation.

Curative Factors Shared with Other Approaches

There are features of person-centered and experiential therapies shared by other approaches. One example is the emphasis on the relationship and on empathy (e.g., Bohart & Greenberg, 1997). The importance of accessing emotion and experiencing is becoming more and more emphasized in cognitive therapy.

Motivational interviewing (Miller & Rollnick, 2002), an approach developed for the treatment of alcoholism and other addiction problems, it is based on the same fundamental premise as PCEP therapies: that humans have considerable potential for self-righting and self-healing. The core therapeutic strategy is the use of empathic listening. Miller (2000) reports research that shows that empathic listening works better than confrontation with people who have alcohol problems. In addition to empathic listening, motivational interviewing adds other strategies that encourage clients to think out for themselves why it is to their benefit to modify their drinking.

PCEP therapies place a heavy emphasis on acceptance. The empathic, accepting therapeutic environment allows clients to access and to accept their experience. Rogers often noted that clients need to accept themselves and their experience in order to change. This idea of acceptance is now a key part of many modern cognitive-behavioral therapies, such as Linehan's dialectical behavior therapy (Linehan, 1993), and acceptance and commitment therapy (Hayes, Strosahl, & Wilson, 1999).

TREATMENT APPLICABILITY AND ETHICAL CONSIDERATIONS

Person-centered and experiential therapies have been used with a wide range of client problems, including alcoholism, schizophrenia, anxiety disorders, and personality disorders. They have also been used with individuals with a mental handicap and older adults (cf. Lietaer, Rombauts, & Van Balen, 1990). Process–experiential therapy has been successfully applied to the treatment of depression (Greenberg & Watson, 2006). Focusing-oriented therapy has been used with a variety of problems, including borderline personality disorders and cancer (Greenberg, Elliott, & Lietaer, 1994). A number of person-centered therapists have developed models for working with families and couples (Levant & Shlien, 1984; Lietaer et al., 1990). Emotionally focused therapy (Johnson & Boisvert, 2002), a variant of process–experiential therapy, is an empirically supported approach for couples (see Gurman, Chapter 10, this volume). Person-centered therapy was originally developed in a child guidance clinic, and person-centered play therapy has been used successfully with children (Bratton & Ray, 2002).

A good relationship in which the child learns that he or she is valuable, understandable, and acceptable through the therapist's empathy, congruence, and acceptance, is even more of a primary change agent than that found in adult psychotherapy. The therapy format is one in which the child and the therapist play, and feelings are talked about in that context. Similarly, establishing a good therapeutic bond is the primary treatment goal with adolescents. Many adolescents are in therapy against their will and do not trust adults. Establishing a trustful empathic relationship in which the therapist is willing to be open is already therapeutic, regardless of talked-about issues. Santen (1990) has also used focusing with traumatized children and adolescents.

Their philosophy makes person-centered and experiential therapies particularly appropriate for work with women, minorities, people of different cultural backgrounds, or people of alternative sexual orientations. This is because the therapist is not an "expert" who is going to impose the "right way of being" on the client; rather, the therapist is a "fellow explorer" who tries to enter the life world of the client in a curious, interested, accepting, and open way. The therapist tries to work from the frame of reference that the client thinks is important. Paradoxically, this might lead the therapist to become somewhat more directive with a client who might want directiveness based on his or her cultural background, at least until the client become comfortable taking the "reins" into his or her own hands.

Working with people who come from different experiential backgrounds than the therapist, however, imposes a particular responsibility on the therapist to check continually to make sure his or her perceptions of clients' experience are not being colored by his or her own background and preconceptions. Despite the fact that PCEP theory dictates an openness to different ways of experiencing and construing reality, PCEP therapists, like all therapists, must be careful that their implicit cultural assumptions do not color what they do. O'Hara (1996) analyzed a film of Carl Rogers working with a woman and pointed out how Rogers's implicit cultural assumptions, particularly about autonomy, interfered with his hearing her.

None of the person-centered therapies discussed in this chapter would be the treatment of choice for problems in which the teaching and learning of specific skills is important, as is the case in sex therapy. Such problems may best be treated by behavioral methods. We would not require a client to obtain medication but, with certain kinds of problems (e.g., major affective disorders), would make the client aware of the availability of medication and tell the client that there is a good possibility that his or her problem could be alleviated by it.

There are no particular ethical issues unique to person-centered or experiential therapy. However, the egalitarian, democratic stance of the therapist, along with the belief in clients' self-healing potential, can sometimes create a disparity with the perspectives of other professionals. The problem is that person-centered and experiential therapists do not adopt an "expert" stance vis-à-vis the client. Although they may have expertise, they share it with their clients in a collaborative, nonauthoritarian way and do not prescribe treatment for the client. The field of psychotherapy is currently increasingly adopting a "medical" view in which the therapist is the "expert/professional" who decides on the course of treatment. For instance, for a client who has been sexually abused as a child, some abuse therapists hold that the number-one priority of therapy must be working with the abuse. Because a crucial part of person-centered and experiential therapy is to trust the client's judgment, if a client chose not to explore his or her childhood abuse, the therapist would go along with that decision. This might bother therapists who believe it is largely the expert/professional's role to decide what focus is best.

This does not mean a person-centered or experiential therapist would go along with any decision a client made. There are cases when a person-centered or experiential therapist chooses to impose his or her judgment upon the client, though this is avoided as often as possible. Person-centered and experiential therapists have loyalties to society, as well as to their clients, and would take action to protect others from a client's choices if necessary. As members of society we might make a personal choice to hospitalized an acutely suicidal client, even against our client's judgment. However, we would take the responsibility for the decision—we did it because we wanted to save the client's life—rather than because we, as the experts, know what is "best" for the client.

Generally a person-centered or experiential therapist might look for a number of different indicators as signs that therapy is effective, including greater client access to and acceptance of feelings and experiencing; a greater sense of client self-acceptance and self-trust; signs of the client showing more initiative in making personal choices; signs that the client is beginning to relate more as an equal to the therapist; more client comfort with personal self-disclosure; and signs that the client can better tolerate, face up to, and continue to try to master adversity. Ultimately, because client-centered and experiential therapists place their trust in clients' increasing capacities to know their own experience, the single most important criterion of effectiveness is the client's own judgment that he or she is making progress.

RESEARCH SUPPORT

The PCEP approach has had a long and distinguished history of exploring its effectiveness through empirical research. Carl Rogers, often called the "father of psychotherapy research," was the first to record psychotherapy interviews for research study. Other person-centered and experiential researchers, such as Leslie Greenberg, Laura Rice, Eugene Gendlin, Robert Elliott, and William Stiles, have become internationally known for their work (e.g., Castonguay, Muran, Angus, Hayes, Ladany, & Anderson, in press). Below we consider findings on PCEP.

Research on Therapy Outcome

A recent research review (Elliott & Friere, 2008) has concluded that there is considerable evidence for the effectiveness of person-centered and experiential psychotherapies. The review consisted of a meta-analysis of 178 studies in which changes were measured before and after therapy in 13,032 clients. In 59 of these studies, employing 2,023 clients, person-centered or experiential therapy was compared to a control group, and in 109 studies, employing 10,352 clients, person-centered or experiential therapy was compared to another form of therapy. Effect sizes (ESs: a measure of impact) were as follows (0.8 is considered a large ES; 0.2 or less is a small ES): on pre–post treatment studies; that is, comparing changes within the client group, the ES at the end of treatment was 1.03, and at 12-month follow-up was 1.14. The ES compared to untreated controls was 0.81. The ES versus other forms of therapy was –0.01 (a small, nonsignificant difference suggesting equivalence between these and other forms of therapy).

In particular, the two most researched therapies from this group, person-centered therapy and PE-EFT, both appear to be as effective as cognitive-behavioral therapy (CBT). Person-centered therapy is virtually equivalent in effectiveness to CBT (ES = −0.09), with even that small difference disappearing when analysts statistically control for the allegiance of the researcher. PE-EFT appears to be somewhat superior in effectiveness to CBT (ES = 0.35), although that difference could in part be due to researcher allegiance.

As concrete examples of these findings, Stiles, Barkham, Mellor-Clark, and Connell (2008) studied 5,613 clients who received either person-centered therapy, CBT, or psychodynamic therapy in the United Kingdom for various disorders. They found that the average client showed significant improvement, but there was no difference in effectiveness among the three approaches. Watson, Gordon, Stermac, Steckley, and Kalogerakos (2003) compared PE-EFT with CBT in the treatment of major depression in a researcher-allegiance-balanced randomized clinical trial. Client levels of depression, self-esteem, general symptom distress, and dysfunctional attitudes significantly improved in both therapy groups. Although the outcomes for clients in both treatment groups were generally equivalent, there was a significantly greater decrease in clients' self-reports of their interpersonal problems in PE-EFT than in CBT. Additional support for the effectiveness of client-centered therapy and PE-EFT in the treatment of depression was provided in a study by Goldman, Greenberg, and Angus (2007).

The conclusion is that there is substantial evidence for the effectiveness of these psychotherapies. Although there is less evidence supporting focusing-oriented psychotherapy, it can be effective in coping with cancer, in dealing with weight problems, and in helping with public speaking anxiety (Greenberg et al., 1994). Studies have also found that focusing is effective with prison inmates, older adults, health-related concerns, and stress management (Hendricks, 2002).

Other evidence (Elliott, 2002; Elliott, Greenberg, & Lietaer, 2004) indicates that person-centered and experiential therapies are ameliorative for problems of depression, anxiety, "mixed neurotic" problems, schizophrenia and personality disorders, health-related problems, problems of minor adjustment, and relationship problems. Bratton and Ray (2002) have concluded that humanistic play therapy, particularly person-centered therapy, is empirically supported. In most of these areas the evidence is strong enough to meet formal criteria for what is considered "empirically supported therapy."

Research on Therapy Process

Rogers emphasized two qualities of importance to successful therapy: the active self-healing agency of the client and the therapeutic relationship. Rogers hypothesized that clients have the capacity to heal themselves if they have a warm, empathic, and supportive relationship within which they can engage in the kind of self-exploration/self-examination process that leads to personal evolution. What is the evidence for this proposition?

Bohart and Tallman (1999, 2010) concluded after reviewing the literature that therapy is primarily a process of mobilizing clients' capacities for change. First, there is now considerable evidence for humans' capacities for resilience and self-righting. Second, client involvement is one of the best predictors of change in therapy. Third, clients creatively utilize and transform what they gain from therapy and actively work outside therapy to facilitate change. Finally, Rennie (2002) has found that clients are highly active and agentic in how they pursue their aims in therapy, picking and choosing what they want to use from therapists' communications, subtly trying to influence the therapist if they feel the therapist is off track, and so on. In summary, Rogers's faith that clients have considerable capacities for self-healing, and that it is they who make therapy work, has received research support.

Second, research has generally shown that the most important factor that therapists provide is the therapeutic relationship (e.g., Norcross, in press). In keeping with Rogers's hypothesis, the quality of the relationship seems to be a stronger predictor of outcome than the use of therapeutic techniques. Rogers (1957) hypothesized that the necessary and sufficient conditions for psychotherapy to work are the therapist's levels of warmth, empathy, and genuineness. It has not been shown that these conditions are necessary and sufficient. However, there is evidence linking them to psychotherapy outcome. A meta-analysis of studies relating empathy to therapy outcome, found an ES of 0.30, suggesting a moderate relationship between therapist empathy and outcome (Elliott, Watson, & Greenberg, in press). Similarly, after a review of the research on positive regard, Farber and Doolin (in press) concluded that it also bore a positive but moderate relationship to therapeutic outcome. The research on congruence/genuineness found a small to moderately positive relationship between therapist genuineness and therapeutic outcome (Kolden, Klein, Wang, & Austin, in press). Similar evidence found a weak but positive link between self-disclosure and outcome (Hill & Knox, 2002).

Another hypothesis about therapy process concerns the role of experiencing and emotion in facilitating change. Hendricks (2002) concluded that 50 studies found that the client's level of "focusing" (the degree to which the client is tuning into his or her experience) is correlated with therapy outcome. With regard to emotion, there is evidence that emotional activation is also important in facilitating change in many therapeutic conditions (Elliott et al., in press). Ratings of clients' depth of experiencing have been related to good outcome consistently in person-centered/experiential psychotherapy (Elliott, Greenberg, et al., 2004; Hendricks, 2002; Klein et al., 1986; Orlinsky & Howard, 1978; Pos, Greenberg, Goldman, & Korman, 2003; Watson & Bedard, 2006). Moreover clients' emotional processing in the session has been found to be beneficial across a range of therapeutic approaches other than person-centered and experiential therapy, including CBT and psychodynamic therapy (Castonguay, Goldfried, Wiser, & Raue, 1996; Giyaur, Sharf, & Hilsenroth, 2005; Godfrey, Chaider, Risdale, Seed, & Ogden, 2007; Leahy, 2002; Stanton et al., 2000). In conclusion, Rogers's two major hypotheses concerning the importance of the client's self-healing capacities and the relationship have both received research support. In addition there is growing support that focusing and emotional activation are also important factors in the change process.

CASE ILLUSTRATION

Kevin, age 35, came to therapy suffering from severe depression. He felt unable to carry on and was seriously thinking of ending his life. He was not sure that psychotherapy could help, but he was desperate to try to overcome his intense pain. Kevin, who was married with three children, described his family life as difficult. His wife was an invalid who required a lot of care. Since she had become ill, her moods were unpredictable and she was given to angry outbursts. After her illness, Kevin gave up many of the activities he had enjoyed, including playing the piano, swimming, and tennis, as he spent his time trying to care for his wife and three children. Initially in therapy he focused on the demands of his present situation. However, as he began exploring it and realized how much his wife's moods affected him, he began to recall his experiences growing up.

Kevin was the eldest of three children and had always tried to be responsible and grown up. He recalled that when he was 3, his mother had become severely ill and was hospitalized for a number of months. He had gone to live with his paternal grandmother, an arrangement that ended when his mother returned home. Kevin was uncertain what his mother had been hospitalized for when he was 3, but he thought it might have been depression, because she had been hospitalized for depression when he was 12 and again when he was 16. During the final hospitalization, Kevin recalled that his mother had become almost catatonic, and that he was unable to communicate with her when he visited in the hospital. Growing up, he recalled that he lived in fear that his mother would disappear. He was especially careful to suppress his own needs as he tried to assist his mother and ensure that she did not leave again. His other two siblings were more difficult than he and required special care. One had a learning disability and the other was given to emotional outbursts that dominated the household. His mother seemed unable to cope with his youngest brother and instead catered to his tantrums, leaving Kevin feeling invisible and forgotten.

In an effort to escape the difficulties at home, Kevin formed a band with some friends and took solace in playing his piano. At the age of 18 he left home to go to university, where he studied to become a social worker. There he met his wife, who was also studying social work. After they married, both worked until they had children, at which time Kevin continued working while his wife stayed home to raise their three sons. When Kevin's sons were teenagers his wife took ill, and Kevin began cutting back on his own activities, spending more time at home to care for his family, and gradually becoming more and more depressed.

When one of us (JCW) first saw Kevin, she worked to establish a person-centered relationship, one in which he felt prized, accepted, safe, and respected. Her focus was on understanding his experience of himself and his world. Kevin became aware that he had never had the opportunity to put his experience into words, which was difficult but comforting for him in therapy. He valued the experience of being listened to, as well as the opportunity to share his experiences and view them differently for the first time. At first he and the therapist worked together to understand the source of his depression. He began to realize that it stemmed from the conditions of worth that he internalized as a boy, that he had to be good and not make any trouble in order to ensure that his mother not become depressed again and forsake the family. As Kevin began to explore his experience, it became apparent that he was very rational and intellectual, because he constantly tried to understand his problems and find solutions. But it was difficult for him to know what he was feeling and experiencing. It was very frustrating for Kevin when his therapist would ask how he was feeling, and he began to realize how out of touch he was with his inner experience.

At this point his therapist suggested that perhaps he might be interested in learning *focusing* to help him get in touch with his inner experiencing. He realized that in order to cope, he had shut away his own experiencing, and that he was also very scared of opening it up. He worried that it might be so overwhelming that he would not know how to cope. His therapist explored his fears with him in a person-centered way; as he continued to vacillate between trying to access his inner experience in the session and maintaining distance, his therapist asked if he would like to work with his conflict using *two-chair work*. Hesitantly, Kevin agreed. In spite of his reservations he found the two-chair work very useful and was able to become aware of his fears and the worry that he might end up like his mother and have to be hospitalized to get in touch with his pain. He was also able to access a strong and resilient part of himself that wanted to heal. By accessing the part that felt strong enough to heal, Kevin was able to move further into accessing and representing his inner experience. To assist him with this, the therapist once again offered to teach him focusing. Kevin accepted, and he and the therapist began to work together to listen to his inner experience, to give it words and try to represent it symbolically, so that he could become more aware of it and see what it meant.

As he explored memories of his childhood and inner experience, Kevin became aware of how scared he had been as a child and how much he had lived in fear that his mother would leave. He also recalled how sad he had felt when he left his grandmother to return home. His grandmother had died when he was 11, and Kevin missed her greatly but tended to push his sadness away, out of fear that it would be overwhelming. At this point his thera-pist asked whether Kevin would perhaps like to speak with his grandmother and express his sense of loss, in the hope that he might be able to overcome some of his pain. Kevin agreed and his therapist initiated an empty chair task by asking him to imagine his grandmother sitting in front of him. Kevin was able to recall his grandmother from pictures. His sense was of an older woman with kind blue eyes, smiling at him in encouragement.

Kevin was able to express how sad he had been when he went home after his mother returned from the hospital. He recalled that his time with his grandmother had been happy and fun. He had memories of working in the garden with her and helping to prune her peonies. He recalled how she had cuddled him and that somehow he felt safe around her. He expressed his sadness after she died, noting that there was no one there for him to play with or to soothe him when things were rough at home. After expressing his sadness, Kevin was able to assume the role of his grandmother. In this role, he told Kevin what a special child he had been and that he was dearly loved. His grandmother affirmed that they had had a lot of fun together when his mother was in the hospital and that she had missed him, too, when he returned home. She said it made her sad to see him hurting and asked him to hold on to the happy memories, and to know that she loved him very much.

Kevin seemed stronger after this empty chair work. His depression lifted somewhat, and he began to focus on how he could best cope with his wife's illness. The worst was her moodiness. He realized that this triggered an extreme reaction he did not understand. His therapist suggested that this sounded like a *problematic reaction*; the client agreed and was willing to try *systematic evocative unfolding* to try to understand it better. As Kevin vividly described one of the incidents with his wife that led him to become severely anxious and depressed, he realized that her tantrums reminded him of his sibling. He recalled how awful it was at home when his sibling was upset, and how everything began to revolve around him. Kevin felt that he not only became invisible but also very scared that his brother's behavior would be too much, and that his mother would go back to hospital.

Once he realized what his feelings and reactions were about, Kevin began to explore the impact of his mother's repeated hospitalizations more fully. He processed how scary it was for him and realized how much he suppressed his own feelings for fear of triggering thoughts of his mother. He had carried this style of being into his adult relationships, con-tinually monitoring and accommodating himself to the wishes of his wife and colleagues, so that by the time he entered therapy he felt almost annihilated. Kevin continued in therapy for the next 2 years, slowly reprocessing his experiences as a child and seeing how they affected him in the present. He engaged in more empty chair work with his mother to come to terms with the pain he had experienced as a result of her treatment of him and her illness, as well as with his sibling to free himself of resentment and grief over his sibling's needs always seeming to take precedence when he was a child. Kevin grieved the loss of adequate nurturing, allowing his childhood wounds to heal, and he gradually assumed greater care for himself, so that rather than ignore his experience, he tried to meet his needs in ways that were balanced with those of his family. As he continued in therapy, Kevin slowly learned to be more aware of his own feelings and needs, and to find ways to meet and express his needs in his relationship with his wife.

Interestingly, as Kevin began to hear himself better, he was also better able to be with his wife and her pain, so that he listened to her in such a way that she stopped needing to lash out at him to feel heard and understood. His therapist was primarily client-centered in her approach, while offering other types of experiential interventions if she thought they might be useful. However, it was very much at her client's discretion whether they were implemented. Much of the work was to help the client give voice to his organismic experience in therapy, experience that he had previously silenced and kept from awareness because it was contrary to maintaining his sense of safety as a child.

SUGGESTIONS FOR FURTHER STUDY

Recommended Reading

Burry, P. J. (2008). *Living with the Gloria films: A daughter's memory.* Ross-on-Wye, Wales: PCCS Books.— A fascinating look at the most famous series of films on psychotherapy ever made, and on the woman who worked with both Carl Rogers and the Gestalt therapist Fritz Perls.

Cain, D. J., & Seeman, J. (Eds.). (2002). *Humanistic psychotherapies: Handbook of research and practice.* Washington, DC: American Psychological Association.—This comprehensive volume summarizes research on each of the approaches covered in this chapter, as well as humanistic therapy with children, group therapy, relationship variables, the self, and emotion.

Farber, B. A., Brink, D. C., & Raskin, P. M. (Eds.). (1996). *The psychotherapy of Carl Rogers: Cases and commentary.* New York: Guilford Press.—Cases of Carl Rogers with commentaries by eminent psychotherapists from person-centered and other psychotherapeutic traditions.

Gendlin, E. T. (1996). *Focusing-oriented psychotherapy: A manual of the experiential method.* New York: Guilford Press.—This book gives details on practicing focusing-oriented psychotherapy and gives extensive case history material.

Greenberg, L. S., Rice, L. N., & Elliott, R. (1993). *Facilitating emotional change: The moment-by-moment process.* New York: Guilford Press.—This book on process–experiential psychotherapy has detailed case histories at the end.

Kirschenbaum, H. (2008). *Life and work of Carl Rogers.* Alexandria, VA: American Counseling Association.

DVDs

Gendlin, E. T. *Focusing with Eugene T. Gendlin.* Available at *www.focusing.org.*

Greenberg, L. S. (2006). *Emotion-focused therapy over time* (Psychotherapy in Sizx Sessions Video Series). Washington, DC: American Psychological Association.

Greenberg, L. S. (2007). *Emotion-focused therapy for depression* (Specific Treatments for Specific Populations Video Series). Washington, DC: American Psychological Association.

Shostrom, E. L. (Producer). (1965). *Three approaches to psychotherapy: Carl Rogers.* Orange, CA: Psychological Films.—The most famous film of Carl Rogers working with Gloria.

REFERENCES

Bandura, A. (1986). *Social foundations of thought and action: A social-cognitive analysis.* Englewood Cliffs, NJ: Prentice-Hall.

Barrett-Lennard, G. T. (1997). The recovery of empathy: Toward others and self. In A. C. Bohart & L. S. Greenberg (Eds.), *Empathy reconsidered: New directions in psychotherapy* (pp. 103–121). Washington, DC: American Psychological Association Press.

Barrett-Lennard, G.T. (1998). *Carl Rogers' helping system: Journey and substance.* Thousand Oaks, CA: Sage.

Bohart, A. C. (in press). Person-centered psychotherapy: Working with self-organizing wisdom. In *International Conference Person-Centered Counseling and Psychotherapy Today: Evolution and Challenges,* June 24–28, 2009, Conference Proceedings. Athens: Aspri Lexi.

Bohart, A.C., & Greenberg, L.S. (1997). Empathy and psychotherapy: An introductory overview. In A. C. Bohart & L. S. Greenberg (Eds.), *Empathy reconsidered: New directions in psychotherapy* (pp. 3–32). Washington, DC: American Psychological Association Press.

Bohart, A. C., & Tallman, K. (1999). *How clients make therapy work: The process of active self-healing.* Washington, DC: American Psychological Association Press.

Bohart, A. C., & Tallman, K. (2010). Clients as active self-healers: Implications for the person-centered approach. In M. Cooper, J. Watson, & D. Höelldampf (Eds.), *Person-centred experiential therapies work* (pp. 91–131). Ross-on-Wye, Wales: PCCS Books.

Bozarth, J. (1997). Empathy from the framework of client-centered theory and the Rogerian hypothesis. In A. C. Bohart & L. S. Greenberg (Eds.), *Empathy reconsidered: New directions in psychotherapy* (pp. 81–102). Washington, DC: American Psychological Association Press.

Bozarth, J. D. (1993). Not necessarily necessary but always sufficient. In D. Brazier (Ed.), *Beyond Carl Rogers: Toward a psychotherapy for the 21st century* (pp. 287–310). London: Constable.

Bratton, S. C., & Ray, D. (2002). Humanistic play therapy. In D. J. Cain & J. Seeman (Eds.), *Humanistic psychotherapies: Handbook of research and practice* (pp. 369–402). Washington, DC: American Psychological Association Press.

Brodley, B. T. (1993). Response to Patterson's "Winds of change for client-centered counseling." *Journal of Humanistic Education and Development, 31,* 139–143.

Caspi, A., Elder, G.H., & Herbener, E.S. (1990). Childhood personality and the prediction of life-course patterns. In L. E. Robins & M. Rutter (Eds.), *Straight and devious pathways from childhood to adulthood* (pp. 13–35). New York: Cambridge University Press.

Castonguay, L. G., Goldfried, M. R., Wiser, S., & Raue, P. J. (1996). Predicting the effect of cognitive therapy for depression: A study of unique and common factors. *Journal of Consulting and Clinical Psychology, 64*(3), 497–504.

Cook, J. M., & Biyanova, T. (2009). Influential psychotherapy figures, authors, and books: An Internet survey. *Psychotherapy: Theory, Research, Practice and Training, 46*(1), 42–51.

Cowan, P. A. (1978). *Piaget: With feeling.* New York: Harcourt.

Dweck, C. S., & Leggett, E. L. (1988). A social-cognitive approach to motivation and personality. *Psychological Review, 95,* 256–273.

Elliott, R. (2002). The effectiveness of humanistic therapies: A meta-analysis. In D. J. Cain & J. Seeman (Eds.), *Humanistic psychotherapies: Handbook of research and practice* (pp. 57–82). Washington, DC: American Psychological Association Press.

Elliott, R., Bohart, A. C., Watson, J. C., & Greenberg, L. S. (in press). Empathy. In J. C. Norcross (Ed.), *Psychotherapy relationships that work* (2nd ed.). New York: Oxford University Press.

Elliott, R., & Friere, E. (2008, July). *Empirical support for person-centred/experiential psychotherapies: Meta-analysis update 2008.* Paper presented at the Conference of the World Association of Person-Centered and Experiential Psychotherapy and Counseling, Norwich, UK.

Elliott, R., Greenberg, L. S., & Lietaer, G. (2004). Research on experiential psychotherapies. In M. Lambert (Ed.), *Bergin and Garfield's handbook of psychotherapy and behavior change* (5th ed., pp. 493–540). New York: Wiley.

Elliott, R., Watson, J. C., Goldman, R. N., & Greenberg, L. S. (2004). *Learning emotion-focused therapy: The process–experiential approach to change.* Washington, DC: American Psychological Association Press.

Epstein, R. (1991). Skinner, creativity, and the problem of spontaneous behavior. *Psychological Science, 2,* 362–370.

Farber, B. A., & Doolin, E. (in press). Positive regard and affirmation. In J. C. Norcross (Ed.), *Psychotherapy relationships that work* (2nd ed.). New York: Oxford University Press.

Gendlin, E. T. (1967). Therapeutic procedures in dealing with schizophrenics. In C. R. Rogers, E. T. Gendlin, D. J. Kiesler, & C. B. Truax (Eds.), *The therapeutic relationship and its impact* (pp. 369–400). Madison: University of Wisconsin Press.

Gendlin, E. T. (1970). A theory of personality change. In J. T. Hart & T. M. Tomlinson (Eds.), *New directions in client-centered therapy* (pp. 129–174). Boston: Houghton Mifflin.

Gendlin, E. T. (1996). *Focusing-oriented psychotherapy: A manual of the experiential method.* New York: Guilford Press.

Giyaur, K., Sharf, J., & Hilsenroth, M. J. (2005). The capacity for dynamic process scale (CDPS) and patient engagement in opiate addiction treatment. *Journal of Nervous and Mental Disease, 193*(12), 833–838.

Godfrey, E., Chaider, T., Ridsdale, L., Seed, P., & Ogden, J. (2007). Investigating the "active ingredients" of cognitive behaviour therapy and counselling for patients with chronic fatigue in primary care: Developing a new process measure to assess treatment fidelity and predict outcome. *British Journal of Clinical Psychology, 46*(3), 253–272.

Goldman, R. N., Greenberg, L. S., & Angus, L. (2005). The effects of adding specific emotion-focused interventions to the therapeutic relationship in the treatment of depression. *Psychotherapy Research, 15*, 248–260.

Greenberg, L. S. (1979). Resolving splits: Use of the two chair technique. *Psychotherapy: Theory, Research and Practice, 16*(3), 316–324.

Greenberg, L. S. (1980). An intensive analysis of recurring events from the practice of Gestalt therapy. *Psychotherapy: Theory, Research and Practice, 17*, 143–152.

Greenberg, L. S. (1983). Toward a task analysis of conflict resolution. *Psychotherapy: Theory, Research and Practice, 20*, 190–201.

Greenberg, L. S., Elliott, R., & Lietaer, G. (1994). Research on humanistic and experiential psychotherapies. In A. Bergin & S. Garfield (Eds.), *Handbook of psychotherapy and behavior change* (4th ed., pp. 509–542). New York: Wiley.

Greenberg, L. S., & Johnson, S. M. (1988). *Emotionally focused therapy for couples.* New York: Guilford Press.

Greenberg, L. S., & Pascual-Leone, J. (2001). A dialectical constructivist view of the construction of personal meaning. *Journal of Constructivist Psychology, 14*, 165–186.

Greenberg, L. S., Rice, L. N., & Elliott, R. (1993). *Facilitating emotional change: The moment-by-moment process.* New York: Guilford Press.

Greenberg, L. S., & Watson, J. (1998). Experiential therapy of depression: Differential effects of client-centered relationship conditions and process–experiential interventions. *Psychotherapy Research, 8*, 210–224.

Greenberg, L. S., & Watson, J. C. (2006). *Emotion-focused therapy for depression.* Washington, DC: American Psychological Association Press.

Greenberg, L. S., & Webster, M. (1982). Resolving decisional conflict by means of two-chair dialogue and empathic reflection at a split in counseling. *Journal of Cognitive Psychology, 29*, 468–477.

Hayes, S. C., Strosahl, K. D., & Wilson, K. G. (1999). *Acceptance and Commitment Therapy: An experiential approach to behavior change.* New York: Guilford Press.

Hendricks, M. N. (2002). Focusing-oriented/experiential psychotherapy. In D. J. Cain & J. Seeman (Eds.), *Humanistic psychotherapies: Handbook of research and practice* (pp. 221–252). Washington, DC: American Psychological Association Press.

Hill, C. E., & Knox, S. (2002). Self-disclosure. In J. C. Norcross (Ed.), *Psychotherapy relationships that work: Therapist contributions and responsiveness to patients* (pp. 255–265). New York: Oxford University Press.

Holdstock, T. L., & Rogers, C. R. (1983). Person-centered theory. In R. J. Corsini & A. J. Marsella (Eds.), *Personality theories, research, and assessment* (pp. 189–228). Itasca, IL: Peacock.

Johnson, S., & Boisvert, C. (2002). Treating couples and families from the humanistic perspective: More than the symptom, more than solutions. In D. J. Cain & J. Seeman (Eds.), *Humanistic psychotherapies: Handbook of research and practice* (pp. 309–338). Washington, DC: American Psychological Association Press.

Kennedy-Moore, E., & Watson, J. C. (1999). *Expressing emotion: Myths, realities and therapeutic strategies.* New York: Guilford Press.

Kolden, G. G., Klein, M. H., Wang, C., & Austin, S. B. (in press). Congruence/genuineness. In J. C. Norcross (Ed.), *Psychotherapy relationships that work* (2nd ed.). New York: Oxford University Press.

Korbei, L. (1994). Eugene Gendlin. In O. Frischenschlager (Ed.), *Wien, Wo Sonst. Die Entstehung der Psychoanalyse und ihrer Schulen* [*Vienna, where else. The emergence of psychoanalysis and their schools*] (pp. 174–181). Weimar: Böhlau Verlag.

Larson, D. (Ed.). (1984). *Teaching psychological skills: Models for giving psychology away.* Monterey, CA: Brooks/Cole.

Levant, R. F., & Shlien, J. M. (Eds.). (1984). *Client-centered therapy and the person-centered approach: New directions in theory, research, and practice.* New York: Praeger.

Lewicki, P. (1986). *Nonconscious social information processing.* New York: Academic Press.

Lietaer, G. (1991, July). *The authenticity of the therapist: Congruence and transparency.* Paper presented at the international Conference on Client-Centered and Experiential Psychotherapy, Stirling, Scotland.

Lietaer, G., Rombauts, J., & Van Balen, R. (Eds.). (1990). *Client-centered and experiential psychotherapy in the nineties.* Leuven, Belgium: Leuven University Press.

Linehan, M. (1993). *Cognitive-behavioral treatment of borderline personality disorder.* New York: Guilford Press.

Mahoney, M. (1991). *Human change processes.* New York: Basic Books.

Mahrer, A. R. (1983). *Experiential psychotherapy: Basic practices.* Ottawa, Canada: University of Ottawa Press.

Masten, A. S., Best, K. M., & Garmezy, N. (1990). Resilience and development: Contributions from the study of children who overcome adversity. *Development and Psychopathology, 2,* 425–444.

Mearns, D. (2002). Theoretical propositions in regard to self theory within the person-centered approach. *Person-Centered and Experiential Psychotherapies, 1*(1–2), 14–27.

Mearns, D., & Cooper, M. (2005). *Working at relational depth.* London: Sage.

Miller, W. R. (2000). Rediscovering fire: Small interventions, large effects. *Psychology of Addictive Behaviors, 14,* 6–18. (Internet version, pp. 1–15)

Miller, W. R., & Rollnick, S. (2002). *Motivational interviewing: Preparing people to change* (2nd ed.). New York: Guilford Press.

Norcross, J. C. (Ed.). (in press). *Psychotherapy relationships that work* (2nd ed.). New York: Oxford University Press.

O'Hara, M. M. (1996). Rogers and Sylvia: A feminist analysis. In B. A. Farber, D. C. Brink, & P. M. Raskin (Eds.), *The psychotherapy of Carl Rogers: Cases and commentary* (pp. 284–300). New York: Guilford Press.

O'Hara, M. M., & Wood, J. K. (1983). Patterns of awareness: Consciousness and the group mind. *Gestalt Journal, 6,* 103–116.

Pos, A. E., Greenberg, L. S., Goldman, R. N., & Korman, L. M. (2003). Emotional processing during experiential treatment of depression. *Journal of Consulting and Clinical Psychology, 71*(6), 1007-1016.

Prouty, G. F. (1990). Pre-therapy: A theoretical evolution in the person-centered/experiential psychotherapy of schizophrenia and retardation. In G. Lietaer, J. Rombauts, & R.Van Balen (Eds.), *Client-centered and experiential psychotherapy in the nineties* (pp. 645–658). Leuven, Belgium: Leuven University Press.

Raskin, N. J., & Rogers, C. R. (1989). Person-centered therapy. In R. J. Corsini & D. J. Wedding (Eds.), *Current psychotherapies* (4th ed., pp. 155–194). Itasca, IL: Peacock.

Rennie, D. L. (2002). Experiencing psychotherapy: Grounded theory studies. In D. J. Cain & J. Seeman (Eds.), *Humanistic psychotherapies: Handbook of research and practice* (pp. 117–144). Washington, DC: American Psychological Association Press.

Rice, L. N. (1974). The evocative function of the therapist. In D. A. Wexler & L. N. Rice (Eds.), *Innovations in client-centered therapy* (pp. 282–302). New York: Wiley.

Rice, L. N. (1992). From naturalistic observation of psychotherapy process to micro theories of change. In S. Toukmanian & D. Rennie (Eds.), *Psychotherapy process research: Paradigmatic and narrative approaches* (pp. 1–21). Newbury Park, CA: Sage.

Rice, L. N., & Greenberg, L. S.(Eds.). (1984). *Patterns of change: Intensive analysis of psychotherapy process.* New York: Guilford Press,

Rice, L. N., & Greenberg, L. S. (1992). Humanistic approaches to psychotherapy. In D. K. Freedheim (Ed.), *History of psychotherapy: A century of change* (pp. 197–224). Washington, DC: American Psychological Association.

Rice, L. N., & Saperia, E. (1984). Task analysis of the resolution of problematic reactions. In L. N. Rice & L. S. Greenberg (Eds.), *Patterns of change: Intensive analysis of psychotherapy process* (pp. 29–66). New York: Guilford Press.

Rogers, C. R. (1957). The necessary and sufficient conditions of therapeutic personality change. *Journal of Consulting Psychology, 21,* 95–103.

Rogers, C. R. (1961a). *On becoming a person.* Boston: Houghton Mifflin.

Rogers, C. R. (1961b). The process equation of psychotherapy. *American Journal of Psychotherapy, 15,* 27–45.

Rogers, C. R., Gendlin, E. T., Kiesler, D. J., & Traux, C. B. (Eds.), (1967). *The therapeutic relationship and its impact.* Madison: University of Wisconsin Press.

Rogers, N. (1997). *The creative connection: Expressive arts as healing.* Palo Alto, CA: Science and Behavior Books.

Santen, B. (1990). Beyond good and evil: Focusing with early traumatized children and adolescents. In G. Lietaer, J. Rombauts, & R. Van Balen (Eds.), *Client-centered and experiential psychotherapy in the nineties* (pp. 779–796). Leuven, Belgium: Leuven University Press.

Shostrom, E. L. (Producer). (1965). *Three approaches to psychotherapy* [Film]. Orange, CA: Psychological Films.

Smith, D. (1982). Trends in counseling and psychotherapy. *American Psychologist, 37,* 802–809.

Stiles, W. B., Barkham, M., Mellor-Clark, J., & Connell, J. (2008). Effectiveness of cognitive-behavioural, person-centred, and psychodynamic therapies in UK primary-care routine practice: Replication in a larger sample. *Psychological Medicine, 38*(5), 677–688.

Strümpfel, U., & Goldman, R. (2002). Contacting Gestalt therapy. In D. J. Cain & J. Seeman (Eds.), *Humanistic psychotherapies: Handbook of research and practice* (pp. 189–220). Washington, DC: American Psychological Association Press.

Strupp, H. H., & Binder, J. L. (1984). *Psychotherapy in a new key: A guide to time-limited dynamic psychotherapy.* New York: Basic Books.

Strupp, H. H., & Hadley, S. W. (1979). Specific versus nonspecific factors in psychotherapy: A controlled study of outcome. *Archives of General Psychiatry, 36,* 1125–1136.

Watson, J. C. (2002). Revisioning empathy: Theory, research and practice . In D. Cain & J. Seeman (Eds.). *Handbook of research and practice in humanistic psychotherapies* (pp. 445–473). Washington, DC: American Psychological Association Press.

Watson, J. C. (2007). Reassessing Rogers' necessary and sufficient conditions of change. *Psychotherapy: Theory, Research, Practice and Training, 44*(3), 268–273.

Watson, J. C., & Bedard, D. (2006). Clients' emotional processing in psychotherapy: A comparison between cognitive-behavioral and process-experiential psychotherapy. *Journal of Consulting and Clinical Psychology, 74*(1), 152–159.

Watson, J. C., Goldman, R. N., & Greenberg, L. S. (2007). *Case studies in emotion-focused treatment of depression: A comparison of good and poor outcome.* Washington, DC: American Psychological Association Press.

Watson, J. C., Gordon, L. B., Stermac, L., Steckley, P., & Kalogerakos, F. (2003). Comparing the effectiveness of process–experiential with cognitive-behavioral psychotherapy in the treatment of depression. *Journal of Consulting and Clinical Psychology, 71*(4), 773–781.

Watson, J. C., & Wiseman, H. (2010). Laura Rice: Natural observer of psychotherapy process. In L. Castonguay, C. Muran, L.Angus, J. Hayes, N. Ladany, & T. Anderson (Eds.), *Bringing psychotherapy research to life: Understanding change through the work of leading clinical researchers* (pp. 174–184). Washington, DC: American Psychological Association Press.

Wexler, D. A., & Rice, L. N. (Eds.). (1974). *Innovations in client-centered therapy.* New York: Wiley.

Yontef, G. (1995). Gestalt therapy. In A. S. Gurman & S. B. Messer (Eds.), *Essential psychotherapies* (pp. 261–303). New York: Guilford Press.

CHAPTER 8

Existential–Humanistic Psychotherapies

Kirk J. Schneider

HISTORICAL BACKGROUND

There is one ongoing and implicit question in existential–humanistic (E-H) therapy: "How is one *willing* to live—in this remarkable moment, in the care of this inimitable relationship, in the face of these unrepeatable opportunities?" This is the foundation stone—the well-spring—for generations of healers and seekers, as they broach the E-H challenge. Accompany me now, as we plumb this challenge—and the treasures it harbors. I think you will find, as many have, that today's E-H therapy is at the forefront of a professional, philosophical, and even cultural renaissance.

Existential humanism is rooted in the deepest recesses of recorded time. All who addressed the question "What does it mean to be fully and subjectively alive?" have partaken in the E-H quest. Existentialism derives from the Latin root *ex-sistere*, which literally means to "stand forth" or to "become" (May, 1958, p. 12), whereas humanism originates in the ancient Greek tradition of "knowing thyself" (Grondin, 1995, p. 112). Together, existential humanism embraces the following three values: (1) freedom (e.g., to know oneself), (2) experiential reflection (e.g., to discover what one is becoming), and (3) responsibility (e.g., to act on or respond to what one is becoming).

Although existential humanism has its roots in Socratic, Renaissance, Romantic, and even Asiatic sources (Moss, 1999; Schneider, 1998b; Taylor, 1999), not until the mid-19th century was existential philosophy, as such, formalized. With the advent of Søren Kierkegaard's (1844/1944) *The Concept of Dread,* a new era had dawned in which freedom, experiential reflection, and responsibility played an increasingly pivotal philosophical and therapeutic role. In Kierkegaard's thesis, freedom emerges from crisis, and crisis from intellectual, emotional, or physical imprisonment. In Kierkegaard's time, this imprisonment often took the form of acquiescence to the Catholic Church or to objectifying trends in science. In one of the most damning oppositions to social objectification (and doctrinaire living) ever waged, Kierkegaard called for a complete transformation of values. We must move, Kierkegaard exclaimed, from a mechanized or externalized life to one that is centered in the subject, and that struggles for the truth of the subject. It is only through facing and grappling with our selves, Kierkegaard elaborated, that consciousness can expand, deepen, and seek its vibrant potential.

Writing at about the same period, but with an even feistier style, Friedrich Nietzsche (1844–1900) traced the devitalization of conventional culture to the dominance of Apollonian (or rationalist–linear living) over Dionysian (or nonrationalist–spontaneous) living. Although these strains were in tension—in Nietzsche's time, as in the time of the ancient Greeks who formulated them—Nietzsche foresaw the era when Apollonian technocracy would overshadow and level all in its path. To remedy this situation, and to restore the Dionysian spirit, Nietzsche (1889/1982) called for a Dionysian–Apollonian rapprochement. This rapprochement would "afford" people "the whole range and wealth of being natural" but also, and in concert with the latter, the capacity for being "strong, highly educated," and "self-controlled" (p. 554).

The next major revolution in E-H psychology occurred in the early 20th century, with the advent of behaviorism and psychoanalysis. Behaviorism, championed by advocates such as John Watson, stressed the mechanistic and overt aspects of human functioning, whereas psychoanalysis, spearheaded by Freud and his followers, promoted a covert intapsychic determinism. In neither case, existential humanists contended, was the human psyche illuminated in its radiant and enigmatic fullness—its liberating and yet vulnerable starkness—and so they rebelled. Among these rebellions were the rich and far-ranging meditations of William James (1902/1936), Otto Rank (1936), C. G. Jung (1966), and Henry Murray (1938). But while this group drew tangentially from E-H philosophy, another group of mainly former Freudians drew directly on the E-H lineage. Ludwig Binswanger (1958) and Medard Boss (1963), for example, based their psychiatric practices on the existential and phenomenological philosophies of Martin Heidegger (1962) and Edmund Husserl (1913/1962). Expanding on Kierkegaard's emphasis on the subjective, Heidegger developed a philosophy of being. By *being*, Heidegger meant neither self-enclosed individualism nor deterministic realism, but a "lived" amalgam of the two that he termed "being-in-the-world." Being-in-the-world" is Heidegger's attempt to illustrate that our Western tradition of separating inner from outer, or subjective from objective, is misleading and that, from the standpoint of experience, there is no clear way to separate them. In a phrase, we are both separate subjective selves *and* related to the external world, according to Heidegger. To develop his thesis, Heidegger drew on the method and practices of phenomenology, originated by his mentor, Edmund Husserl. According to Husserl (1913/1962), the chief task of phenomenology is to apprehend human experience in its living reality, that is, in its full subjective and intersubjective context (see also Churchill & Wertz, 2001; Giorgi, 1970).

By the 1960s, E-H psychotherapy had evolved into a mature and recognized movement, but it was also a diverse movement. Whereas most E-H practitioners stressed freedom, experiential reflection, and responsibility, they did so with varying degrees of intensity. There were times, for example, such as in the aftermath of World War II and during the flowering of the human potential movement of the 1960s, when existential freedom may have been stressed to the neglect of responsibility (e.g., see May, 1981; Merleau-Ponty, 1962; Yalom, 1980), or other times when responsibility was accented to the detriment of freedom (Rowan, 2001) or experiential reflection to the neglect of responsibility (Spinelli, 2001), and so on. These controversies persist today (see Cooper, 2003, on differences between European and U.S. approaches).

However, today's E-H practitioners have an advantage over those of their predecessors—hindsight. With such hindsight, many contemporary E-H therapists are wary of one-sided formulations, be they of the E-H variety or those with which E-H practitioners traditionally differ. Contemporary E-H practitioners, moreover, tend to value holism, integration, and complementarity. They tend to see the intrapsychic aspects of therapy on a par with those of intersubjectivity (i.e., Schneider & Krug, 2010); the social and cultural implications of their work on a level with individual transformation; and the intellectual and philosophical bases of practice on a plane with those of emotion and spirit. Finally, the contemporary E-H practitioner does not shy away from behavioral or even biological interventions, as those may be appropriate (i.e., Schneider, 1995, 2008).

This breadth of outlook has widened the E-H client base. Less and less is E-H practice confined to the rarified environs of its psychoanalytic forebears, or to upper-class elites; rather, it is opening out to the world within which most of us dwell (O'Hara, 2001; Schneider, 2008; Schneider & Krug, 2010). Put another way, the E-H *attitude* can be seen in a variety of practice settings, from drug counseling (Ballinger, Matano, & Amantea, 2008) to therapy with war veterans (Decker, 2007), to therapy with minorities (Alsup, 2008; Rice, 2008; Vontress & Epp, 2001) to gay and lesbian counseling (Brown, 2008; Monheit, 2008), to therapy with psychotic clientele (Dorman, 2008; Thompson, 1995; Mosher, 2001), to emancipatory practices with groups (E. Bugental, 2008; Montuori & Purser, 2001; O'Hara, 2001), and from cognitive-behavioral interventions with anxious and phobic clients (Bunting & Hayes, 2008; Wolfe, 2008) to psychodynamic mediations with spiritually and religiously distressed clients (Hoffman, 2008), to neurobiological and experiential interventions with sufferers of attachment disorder (Fosha, 2008) .

Yet in spite of their expanded vision, contemporary E-H practitioners still share a core value with their predecessors: the personal or intimate search process that is at the crux of depth practice. As we shall see, this process entails four basic stances or conditions—the cultivation of therapeutic presence, the activation of presence through struggle, the working through of resistance or "protections," and the rediscovery of meaning and awe.

In the next section I describe the theory of personality that underlies this core value and the practical consequences that follow.

THE CONCEPT OF PERSONALITY, PSYCHOLOGICAL HEALTH, AND PATHOLOGY

The concept of personality is useful but, for our purposes, limited. From the standpoint of E-H psychology, one does not experience a personality; one lives an experience. Similarly, the notions of psychological health and pathology can have static, culturally normative qualities that may not reflect the lived experience of distinctive individuals (see Becker, 1973). Nevertheless, there are *patterns* within these lived experiences—characterological structures—which existential humanists have carefully described phenomenologically. Let us consider a sampling of these.

As suggested earlier, the E-H understanding of *functionality* (i.e., psychological health) rests on three interdependent dimensions—freedom, experiential reflection, and responsibility. Although E-H theorists almost invariably highlight all three of these dimensions, they do so in diverse ways. For example, Rollo May (1981) gives primary attention to freedom and that which he terms "destiny." By *freedom*, May means the capacity to choose within the natural and self-imposed (e.g., cultural) limits of living. Freedom also implies responsibility, for, as he suggests, if we are conferred the power to choose, is it not incumbent upon us to exercise that power?

May defines *destiny* in terms of the consciousness of our limits. He then goes on to define four basic limits or forms of destiny—the cosmic, the genetic, the cultural, and the circumstantial. *Cosmic destiny* embraces the limitations of nature (e.g., earthquakes and storms), *genetic destiny* addresses the limits of physiology (e.g., lifespan and temperament), *cultural destiny* entails preset social patterns (e.g., language and class), and *circumstantial destiny* pertains to sudden situational developments (e.g., war and recession).

How, then, do we deal with these contending forces according to May, and what happens when we do not? Let us consider the latter first. The failure to acknowledge our freedom, according to May (1981) leads to a dysfunctional identification with destiny or limits (e.g., depression, obsessive–compulsiveness, and hyperanxiety), whereas the failure to acknowledge our limits leads to a dysfunctional identification with our possibilities (e.g., narcissism, impulsivity, and psychopathy). Hence, the failure to acknowledge freedom can be seen in the forfeit of the capacity for wonder, experimentation, and boldness. Among those who embody those imbalances are the shy and retiring wallflower, the rigid bureaucrat, and the robotic conformist. The failure to acknowledge limits, on the other hand, can be detected in the sacrifice of the ability to discern, discipline, and prioritize one's life. Among those who illustrate this polarity are the aimless dabbler, the impulsive philanderer, and the arrogant abuser.

The great question, of course, is how to help people redress these imprisoning dispositions—how to help them broaden and thereby mobilize their range of behavioral, cognitive, and affective resources. Although there is no simple answer to this query, May finds that intra- and interpersonal struggles (or encounters) are key ameliorative dimensions. It is only through struggle, according to May (1981), that freedom and destiny—capabilities and limits—can be illuminated in their fullness, substantively explored, and meaningfully transformed.

The polarities of freedom and destiny or limitation, and the challenge to respond to these polarities, are central to leading E-H conceptions of psychological health. James Bugental (Bugental & Sterling, 1995), for example, draws on a similar dialectic with his emphasis on the self as embodied yet changing; choiceful yet finite; isolated yet related. We are ever in the process of change according to Bugental, no matter how we choose to conceive it. Our challenge, Bugental elaborates, is to face that change, sort through its manifold features, and etch out of it a meaningful and action-oriented response.

Irvin Yalom (1980) conceives of four "givens" of human existence—death, freedom, isolation, and meaninglessness. Depending on how we confront these givens, Yalom elaborates, we confront the design and quality of our lives. To the extent that we confront death, for example, we also encounter the urgency, intensity, and seriousness that death arouses. To the extent that we confront isolation, we also contact and become aware of our need for relation, or its opposite, solitude. For Yalom, the composition of a life is directly proportional to the composition and array of one's relationship to givens, and the priorities one sets to integrate, explore, or coexist with those givens.

I have elaborated a constrictive–expansive continuum of conscious and subconscious personality functioning (Schneider, 1995, 1999, 2008). This continuum is identified as a capacity that is both freeing and yet limited. We have a vast capacity to "draw back" and constrict thoughts, feelings, and sensations, as well as an equivalent capacity to "burst forth" and expand thoughts, feelings, and sensations. At the same time, each of these capacities is delimited. We can only constrict (e.g., focus and accommodate) and expand (e.g., enlarge and assimilate) so far, before the givens of existence (e.g., death, genes, and culture) deter and curtail us. For me, it is the interplay among constrictive and expansive capacities, and the ability to respond to those capacities and the ability to integrate those responses into a meaningful whole that constitute optimal personal and interpersonal dynamics.

In more recent years, I (Schneider, 1995, 2008) have developed an "existential–integrative" (E-I) approach to therapy. This approach holds that levels of "liberation" (e.g., the physiological, the environmental, and the interpersonal) are interwoven into the constrictive–expansive continuum noted earlier. E-I therapy is now at the forefront of a broadened—and steadily growing—E-H practice philosophy (Bradford, 2007; Schneider & Krug, 2010; Wampold, 2008; Watson & Bohart, 2001). This practice philosophy draws from conventional E-H principles but also differs in one major respect—scope of practice. While the conventional E-H model emphasizes only the experiential level of client contact, and thus restricts its practice base, the E-I model explicitly embraces diverse levels of client contact and thus expands its capacity to serve. Put another way, the E-I approach arose out of the need to address today's ethnically and diagnostically diverse clinical populations, whereas the older E-H modality arose out of a narrower set of priorities (May, 1958; Schneider, 2008). Within that context, E-I interventions are viewed as "liberation conditions," and client dysfunctions as (often restricted) "levels of freedom" or choice (Schneider, 2008, p. 35). Liberation conditions can represent a wide range of interventions (e.g., from the relatively "nonexperiential" medical and behavioral strategies to the "semiexperiential" psychoanalytic and intersubjective modalities, to the relatively "experiential" existential and transpersonal approaches). Depending on the client's desire and capacity for therapeutic change, E-I therapy proceeds holistically toward an experiential level of contact. By *holistically*, I mean that even when E-I therapy is engaged non- or semiexperientially, it is still engaged within an ever-varying, ever-available experiential context.

Maurice Friedman (1995, 2001) echoes the philosophy of Martin Buber with his "dialogical" approach to psychological functioning. The dialogical approach, based on Buber's philosophy of "I–thou" relationships, emphasizes the interpersonal and interdependent dimension of personality. For Friedman, psychological growth and development proceed not merely or mainly through the encounter with self but through the encounter with another. This "healing through meeting," as Friedman puts it, is characterized by the ability to be present to and confirming of oneself, at the same time being open to and confirming of another. The freedom and limits of such a relationship then become transferred to the freedom and limits experienced within oneself, and the trust developed to risk affirmation of the self.

THE PROCESS OF CLINICAL ASSESSMENT

The question of assessment is essentially the question of understanding: On what basis do E-H therapists understand an individual's pattern of interaction, symptomatology, and adaptive resources? E-H therapists employ a variety of means to understand lives. Among these means can be paper-and-pencil tests, ratings of symptomatology, and history taking. However, these modalities tend to be implemented sparingly rather than as a staple of practice. The reason for this caveat is that, as a rule, assessment—like therapy—is an ongoing process for E-H practitioners and not a linear or mechanistic procedure. Appraisal is holistic, in other words, and should not be mistaken for a global or rigid declaration (Bugental & Sterling, 1995). Client *X* may be a "depressive" for an E-H practitioner, but he is also a living, dynamic human being, and this is pivotal information—both for client and therapist.

E-H practitioners are concerned as much or more with depth and breadth of context as with specific overt behaviors. Ideally, nothing is spared in E-H therapeutic assessment. The unfolding moment, the client's explicit and implicit intentions in the moment, the horizons of the past, and the full person-to-person field that is evoked each moment are of equal and abiding import (Fischer, 1994; Schneider, 1985/1995, 2009).

Generally speaking, contemporary E-H practice is an integrative practice (Schneider & Krug, 2010; Yalom, 1980). E-H practitioners value the whole human being—conscious and nonconscious, past, present, and evolving—in the therapeutic encounter. Cultural background, too, is integral for E-H practitioners. Although E-H therapy does not proclaim to be a "one size fits all model," increasingly it urges practitioners to learn as much as possible about cultural—as well as political—influences on practice, and it draws on therapeutic presence to deepen and refine those sensibilities (Brown, 2008; Comas-Diaz, 2008; Schneider & Krug, 2010) As such, E-H practitioners are concerned with how best to understand clients in their moment-to-moment unfolding, and their given level of relation and experience. *Presence* is the chief tool of E-H assessment. Through presence, the holding and illuminating of clients' moment-to-moment experience, E-H therapists are able to attune to the subtlest nuances of clients' concerns, from the cognitive and behavioral to the affective and spiritual. Physiological (e.g., nutritional) and even medical support are not ruled out by the contemporary E-H practitioner; the question is, are these approaches understood within an overarching context of how a person is willing to live his or her life?

Although E-H therapists value the *content* (or explicit features) of clients' experiences, they are acutely and simultaneously sensitized to the *process* or implicit aspects of those experiences. For example, whereas the content of a client's report (e.g., binge eating) may be physiological in nature, the process or implicit aspects may be intensely spiritual, ontological, or interpersonal in nature. E-H assessment, therefore, is predicated on not only a client's presenting problem (or complaint) but also the entire atmosphere of a client's predicament. Everything and anything is open to investigation within the E-H framework, from the initial manner in which the client greets the therapist to the position of the client's hands while elaborating her concern. Put another way, every E-H assessment is holographic. Every moment is believed to be a microcosm and in some sense dovetails with every other moment, and no moment stands in isolation.

For example, one of the first areas of focus within E-H therapy—even before any words are exchanged—is "What is my client expressing in his body?" The E-H therapist is particularly attuned to the manner in which these expressions resonate within him- or herself—their shape, texture, and future intimations. In effect, the E-H therapist uses his or her body as a barometer or register of clients' tacit and overt struggles. Here is a sample of my own thoughts upon greeting a given client:

> What kind of world is this man trying to hold together? What kind of life-design do his muscles, gestures, and breathing betray? Is he stiff and waxy or limber and fluid? Is he caved in and hunched over or stout and thrust forward? Does he curl up in a remote corner of the room or does he "plant himself in my face"? What does he bring up in *my* body? Does he make me feel light and buoyant or heavy and stuck? Do my stomach muscles tighten, or do my legs become jumpy? Do my eyes relax, or do they become "hard," or guarded? What can I sense from what he wears? Is he frumpy and inconspicuous or loud and outrageous? What can be gleaned from his face? Is it tense and weather-beaten or soft and innocent? (Schneider, 1995, p. 154).

Each of these observations begins to coalesce with others, cumulatively, to disclose a world. Each oscillates with others to form a shape, sense, and overarching Gestalt of this particular man's strife.

Presence, then is the sine qua non of E-H assessment. Through the illumination of presence, E-H therapists open to and begin to discover clients' overt and covert scripts, ostensible and tacit agendas, and unfolding rivalries within the battleground of self. Furthermore, they begin to sense the shape of their own responses to these revelations and how best to "meet" or facilitate them. For example, an E-H therapist might ask (silently to herself), what are the resources, difficulties, and potential tools necessitated to address an acutely fragile client? What about a combative client, or a client who resists exploration? These issues challenge any serious-minded therapist but are especially trying to E-H practitioners, who prize depth of connection over symptom relief. The question for the E-H therapist is, How can I best meet this client "where he lives," within the abilities and constraints of where he or she lives, and yet hold out the possibility for a fuller and deeper connection? This holding out of the possibility for an enlarged and deepened contact is one of the primary distinctions between prevailing and E-H visions of healing. Whereas conventional practitioners may tend to calibrate their actions to given parts of the therapeutic concern (e.g., those that pertain to behavior or cognition or childhood), E-H practitioners endeavor to be available to clients across the range of their difficulties, from the measurable and overt to the felt and unformed. It is in this sense that diagnosis is a part of the ongoing contact in E-H therapy, and that formulations must fit people and not the other way around (Fischer, 1984/1994; May, 1983).

Given its evolving and holistic approach, then, E-H assessment must be artfully and mindfully engaged. While psychiatric diagnoses may be useful to E-H practitioners at given stages of therapy, the assessment overall is based on therapist attunement, experience, and clinical judgment. As a rule, the client's desire and capacity for change and the therapist's mindful and sensitive alertness to these criteria guide the ensuing work.

THE PRACTICE OF THERAPY AND THE STANCE OF THE THERAPIST

The aim of E-H therapy is to "set clients free" (May, 1981, p. 19). By freedom, E-H therapists do not at all mean caprice or licentiousness, or even truth in the unqualified sense. What they do mean, however, is the cultivation of the capacity for choice; and choice, as is well established in the existential literature, implies limits, ambiguities, and risk (May, 1981; Tillich, 1952).

Freedom is limited because it arises in a sociobiological–spiritual context, only degrees of which are accessible, changeable, and clear. It is ambiguous because for every choice there is a choice not taken, and for every gain there is a commensurate relinquishment. If I devote myself to sports, for example, my ability to perform intellectually is likely to suffer. If I affirm social visibility, I relinquish my capacity to withdraw, and so on. Finally, freedom is risk because it is ever set against uncertainty and the potential for collapse. But freedom is also vibrant, poignant, and energizing; and for many, it is the point of being alive, in spite of and perhaps even in light of its many challenges.

As suggested earlier, contemporary E-H therapy is both integrative and incremental in its approach to freedom. The client's desire and capacity for change (Schneider, 2008), the alliance and context of the therapy (Bugental, 1987), and practical elements (Yalom, 1989) all figure in. Hence, for some E-H clients, at some stages of therapy, choice can mean drug-induced stability or nutrition-based evenness of mood or reasoned-based empowerment, and so on. However, that which distinguishes E-H facilitation is its ability to address, not merely programmatic (i.e., externally based) adjustments but also internally sparked commitments. Commitment, for E-H therapists, refers to a sense "I-ness," agency, or profound caring about a given direction. It implies a sense that the life one chooses really matters to oneself and is worth one's whole (embodied) investment. This ontological or experiential level of commitment manifests clinically as a sense of immediacy (aliveness), affectivity (passion), and kinesthesia (embodiment) and is typified in the deepest and most pivotal stages of therapy. In short, E-H therapists endeavor not only to meet clients "where they are at" but also to be available to the fullest potential of those clients to "own" or claim the life that is presented to them.

In light of this background, E-H therapy can vary in both length and intensity. It can proceed, on rare occasions, within one or two sessions (e.g., see Galvin, 2008; Laing, 1985) or it can occur in a limited way within a short-term, focused format (e.g., Bugental, 2008; Schneider & Krug, 2010). Typically, however, E-H engagements are intimate (e.g., trust building), long term (e.g., 2–5 years), and intensive (e.g., weekly to twice weekly). Furthermore, E-H therapy can be of benefit to a more diverse range of clientele than is generally presumed (e.g., see May, 1972; Rice, 2008; Vontress & Epp, 2001), although those who tend to be introspective, emotionally tolerant, and exploratory are likely to derive maximal benefits. Put another way, E-H therapists try not to preconceive the contexts within which clients operate. Although they are mindful of the general influence of those contexts, be it religious, cultural, or political, it is still the living, breathing human being that takes primacy.

To summarize then, the chief question for the E-H therapist is how does one help this person (client) find choice—direction, meaning, and depth—in his or her life, *in spite of* (and sometimes in light of) all the threats to these possibilities? Clearly, there are no easy answers to this question, yet it is precisely its difficulty, its *struggle,* that for E-H therapists is key to its unfolding. In other words, E-H therapists challenge clients to grapple with their concerns, and not just intellectually, behaviorally, or programmatically, but experientially, in order to maximize their capacities to transform themselves.

Existential Stances or Conditions

To achieve the aforementioned aims, E-H therapists use a variety of means. These means, however, are not techniques in the classical sense; they are stances or conditions through which experiential liberation, or profound experiential transformation, can take root. Among the core (intertwining and overlapping) E-H stances are the following: *the cultivation of therapeutic presence (presence as ground); the activation of therapeutic presence through struggle (presence as goal); the encounter with the resistance to (or protections from) therapeutic struggle; and the coalescence of the meaning, intentionality, and awe that can result from the struggle.* I now proceed to elaborate on these dimensions.

The Cultivation of Therapeutic Presence: Presence as Ground

The gravity of presence is illustrated by Rollo May's (2007) incisive declaration that in dedicated E-H therapy, it is "the client's life that is at stake," and that is how the therapist should view it. There is a vivid distinction, in my view, between a therapist who approaches a client as a problem-solving "doctor" and a healer who is available for inter- and intrapersonal connection. The former offers a specific set of remedies for an isolated and definable malady; the latter offers a relationship, an invitation, and an accompaniment on a journey. And although the former is likely to appeal to a client's immediate needs for relief, the latter is likely to appeal to a client's underlying urges for discovery, self-sustainment, and vitality.

To be sure, *both* modalities are often relevant over the course of a given therapy, and both are useful. But in today's market-driven, standardizing atmosphere, rarely are both made available.

Through the dimension of presence, however (including a willingness to negotiate fees!), both the problem-solving and journey-accompanying modalities can be made available to clients. And clients, in turn, can substantively benefit from these resources. Without the latter (journey-accompanying) mode, however, clients are likely to feel shortchanged, and, arguably, short-circuited.

Presence is the "soup," the seedbed of substantive E-H work (e.g., see also the growing mainstream support for this conception by investigators such as Wampold [2008]). In this light, Yalom (1980) draws an intriguing parallel between the masterful preparation of a meal and E-H therapy.

Whereas the average cook prepares a meal in accordance with a standardized menu, the masterful cook, while not ignoring the latter guidelines, attunes to the evolving, emerging, and subjectively engaging in her preparation. The masterful cook, in other words, has a good sense of how to prepare a basic meal but can also throw in spices, seasonings, and flavorful mixtures that can radically enhance and transform it. For Yalom (1980), it is precisely these nonprescriptions, these "throw-ins" (p. 3), as he puts it, that matter most.

Analogously, it is precisely the present and attuned therapist who is prepared to help his or her client most, according to E-H practice philosophy. Such a therapist is optimally prepared to provide the atmosphere, personality, and moment-to-moment adjustments that can mobilize client change (Bugental, 1987). Interestingly, even standardized psychotherapy research upholds the latter postulate: Wampold (2001), for example, found that "common factors," such as therapist–client alliance and personality variables, account for about nine times the variance in outcomes over specific therapeutic techniques. Yalom (1989) puts it this way:

> The capacity to tolerate uncertainty is a prerequisite for the profession. Though the public may believe that therapists guide patients systematically and sure-handedly through predictable stages of therapy to a foreknown goal, such is rarely the case. . . . The powerful temptation to achieve certainty through embracing an ideological school . . . is treacherous: such belief may block the uncertain and spontaneous encounter necessary for effective therapy. (p. 13)

"This encounter," Yalom concludes, is "the heart of psychotherapy, ... a caring, deeply human meeting between two people, one (generally, but not always, the patient) more troubled than the other" (p. 13).

Finally, the value of being present as a vulnerable and yet distinctive *person* is illustrated by Friedman (1995) in the following client-authored vignette. Following a 4-year therapy with Friedman, his client, "Dawn," reports the following:

> When I think about our therapeutic relationship, it is the *process* that stands out in my memory, not the content.
>
> Up until the time I met Maurice, I had always "picked out" a male authority figure (usually a teacher or psychologist), put him on a pedestal, and obsessed about him a lot—not usually in a romantic or sexual way, although there was an erotic element. I just wanted him to like me and approve of me and to think I was smart and interesting. A real relationship, though, was terrifying to me—I kept my distance and rarely ever talked to them. The greater the attraction, the greater the fear.

When I first met Maurice, I could feel myself wanting to fall into this same pattern with him. However, I could never quite feel intimidated by him—although I think I really wanted to. He was too human for that. I never felt that I had to be interesting or smart, good, bad, happy, or sad—it just wasn't something I had to be concerned with. If the therapist can be human and fallible, that gives me permission to be human and fallible, too. (p. 313)

For Friedman, as with most E-H therapists, then, presence is the foundation that both holds and illuminates. It holds by supporting, embracing, and opening to clients' travails, and it illuminates by witnessing, disclosing, and engaging with those travails. In short, presence holds and illuminates that which is palpably (immediately, affectively, and kinesthetically) signicant within the client and between the client and therapist, and it is the ground and goal of substantive E-H transformation.

The Activation of Therapeutic Presence through Inner Struggle: Presence as Goal

As suggested earlier, presence not only forms the ground for E-H encounter, but it also culminates in its goal. To the extent that clients can attune, at the most embodied levels, to their severest conflicts, healing in the E-H framework is likely to ensue. This healing is a kind of reoccupation of oneself—an immersion in the parts of oneself that one has designed a lifetime to avoid, and it is an integration thereby of the potential or openings that become manifest through that reoccupation. The question for this particular phase of the therapeutic process is: What are the ways and means to activate presence in the client? Or, how can therapists help to *mobilize* clients' presence? (Bugental, 1987).

As we shall see, the activation of client presence within E-H therapy is characterized by two basic modes or access points— the intrapsychic and the interpersonal. Although these modalities overlap, and indeed intertwine (Merleau-Ponty, 1962), they nevertheless reflect two basic E-H practice styles that are gradually, and for many, refreshingly, beginning to merge (Fosha, 2008; Krug, 2009; Portnoy, 2008).

Bugental (1987), for example, is more representative of the intrapsychic or individualist tradition, although this characterization is far from discrete, and much about his approach can be considered interpersonal as well (Krug, 2009). Within the former tradition, then, Bugental (1987) outlines four basic practice strategies, or what he terms "octaves" for activating clients' presence. These are listening, guiding, instructing, and requiring.

The first octave, *listening*, draws clients out, encourages them to keep talking, and obtains their story without "contamination" by the therapist. Examples of listening include "getting the details" of clients' experiences, "listening to emotional catharsis, learning [clients' views of their] own life or . . . projected objectives" (Bugental, 1987, p. 71). The second octave, *guiding*, gives direction and support to clients' speech, keeps it on track, and brings out other aspects. Examples of guiding include exploration of clients' "understanding of a situation, relation, or problem; developing readiness to learn new aspects or get feedback" (p. 71).

The third octave, *instructing*, transmits "information or directions having rational and/ or objective support. Examples include "assignments, advising, coaching, describing a scenario of changed living," or reframing (Bugental, 1987, p. 71). Finally, the fourth octave, *requiring*, brings a "therapist's personal and emotional resources to bear" to cause clients to change in some way. Examples of requiring include "subjective feedback, praising, punishing [e.g., admonishing], rewarding," and "strong selling of [a] therapist's views" (p. 71).

Listening and guiding comprise the lion's share of E-H activation of presence. Whereas instructing and requiring can certainly be useful from the E-H point of view, they are implemented in highly selective circumstances. For example, instructing may be helpful to clients at early stages of therapy, or for those who have fragile emotional constitutions, such as victims of chronic abuse, or for clients from authority-dependent cultures. Requiring, similarly, may be useful not only in the foregoing situations but also in the case of therapeutic impasses or entrenched client patterns, as we shall see. For the majority of E-H practice situations, however, listening and guiding are pivotal to the deepening, expanding, and consolidating of substantive client transformation.

May (1981) illustrates the value of listening with his notion of the pause:

> It is in the pause that people learn to listen to silence. We can hear the infinite number of sounds that we normally never hear at all—the unending hum and buzz of insects in a quiet summer field, a breeze blowing lightly through the golden hay. . . . And suddenly we realize that this is *something*—the world of 'silence' is populated by a myriad of creatures and a myriad of sounds. (p. 165)

The client, similarly, is almost invariably enlivened in the pause. As Bugental (1987, p. 70) suggests, it is in the therapist's silence at given junctures, that abiding change can take root.

The provision of a working "space," a therapeutic pause, not only helps the therapist to understand, but most importantly, also assists the client to vivify him- or herself. Vivification of a client's world is one of the cardinal tasks of E-H therapy. To the extent that clients can "see" the worlds in which they have lived, the obstacles they have created, and the strengths or resources they possess to overcome those obstacles, they can proceed to a foundational healing. Listening promotes one of the most crucial realizations of that vivification—the contours of a client's battle.

The client's battle—and virtually every client has one—becomes evident at the earliest stages of therapy. For some this battle takes the form of an interpersonal conflict, for others an intrapsychic split; for some it may encompass the compulsion for and rejection of binge eating; for others it may relate to a conflict with one's boss; for still others it may be a struggle between squelched vocational potential and evolving aspirations, and so on. Regardless of the content of clients' battles, however, their form can be understood in terms of two basic valences—the part of themselves that endeavors to emerge, and the part of themselves that endeavors to resist, oppose, or block themselves from emerging (Schneider, 1998a).

Whereas therapeutic listening acquaints and sometimes immerses clients in their battle, therapeutic guiding intensifies that contact. Therapeutic guiding can be further illustrated by encouragements to clients to personalize their dialogue (e.g., to give concrete examples of their difficulties, to speak in the first person, and to "own" or take responsibility for their remarks about others). Guiding is also illustrated by invitations to expand or embellish on given topics, such as in the suggestion "Can you say more?" or "How does it feel to make that statement?" or "What really matters about what you've conveyed?" Finally, guiding is exemplified by the notation of content–process discrepancies, such as "You smile as you vent your anger at him," or "Notice how shallow your breathing is right now" (Bugental, 1987; Schneider, 1995).

I have formulated a mode of guiding that I call *embodied meditation* (Schneider, 1995, 1998a, 2008), which in essence is client-guided and begins with a simple grounding exercise, such as breathing awareness or progressive relaxation (usually assisted by the closing of the eyes). From there, it proceeds to an invitation to the client to become aware of his or her body. The therapist may then ask what, if any, tension areas are evident in the client's body. If the client identifies such an area, which often occurs, the therapist asks the client to describe, as richly and fully as possible, where the tension area is and what it feels like. Following this, and assuming the client is able to proceed with the immersion, he or she is invited to place his or her hand on the affected area (I find that this somatic element can often although not necessarily, be experientially critical). Next, the client is encouraged to associate experientially to this contact. Prompts such as "What, if any, feelings, sensations, or images emerge as you make contact with this area?" can be of notable therapeutic value. I have seen other clients open emotional "floodgates" through this work, but I have also seen clients who feel overpowered by it. It is of utmost importance, again, for the therapist to be acutely attuned while practicing this and other awareness-intensive modes.

Guidance is also illustrated by a variety of experimental formats that can be offered in E-H therapy. These experiments, including role play, rehearsal, visualization, and experiential enactment (e.g., pillow hitting and kinesthetic exercises), serve to liven emergent material and vivify or deepen the understanding of that material (Mahrer, 1996; May, 1972; Schneider, 2008; Serlin, 1996). The phrase "truth exists only as it is produced in action" (Kierkegaard, cited in May, 1958, p. 12), has much cachet in this context. When clients can enact (as appropriate) their anxieties, engage their aspirations, and simulate their encounters, they bring their battles "out on the table," so to speak—in "living color"—for close and personal inspection.

While experimentation within the therapeutic setting is invaluable, experimentation outside the setting can be of equivalent or even superior benefit. After all, it is the life outside therapy that counts most for clients, and it is in the service of this life that therapy proceeds. Experimentation outside therapy, then, has two basic aims: (1) It reinforces intratherapy work, and (2) it implements that work in the most relevant setting possible—the lived experience. Accordingly, E-H therapists encourage clients to practice being aware and present in their outside lives. They may gently challenge clients to reflect on or write about problematic events, or they may propose an activity or therapeutic commitment (e.g., Alcoholics Anonymous or assigned readings). They may also challenge clients to do *without* a given activity or pattern. For example, Yalom (1980) challenged his promiscuous client Bruce to try living without a sexual partner for an extended period. This was a highly demanding exercise for Bruce, whose sexual compulsions were formidable and afforded no pause. Yet after the exercise, Bruce reported rich therapeutic realizations, such as the degree to which he felt empty in his life, and the blind and compulsive measures he took to fill that emptiness. Emptiness, Yalom reported, subsequently became the next productive focus.

Prompts to clients to "slow down," or "stay with" charged or disturbing experience can also facilitate intensified self-awareness. I have known many a supervisee (and even seasoned colleague) who has had difficulties with this latter facilitation. They are superb at helping clients to reconnect with the parts of themselves they have shunted away, and they inspire deep somatic immersion in expressiveness, but they are left with one gaping question: "What do I do after the client is immersed?" The exasperation in this puzzlement is understandable. E-H work can seem tormenting. It can instigate profound moments of unalloyed pain. The last thing a therapist wishes to do in such a situation is to enable increased suffering, or to hover in continued despair. Yet given the client's desire and capacity for change, these are precisely the allowances that E-H therapists must provide; precisely the groundworks they must pursue. They must develop trust, and a sense that the work will unfold (Welwood, 2001). Hence, what do I advise my supervisees and colleagues? I suggest that it is in their interest to trust; in particular, to trust that gentle prompts to "stay with" or "allow" intensive material will almost invariably lead to changes in that material. Although these changes may not feel immediately welcome or gratifying—indeed, they may even feel regressive for a time—they do represent evolution, the "more" that every person is capable of experiencing.

Much of the therapist's task within E-H therapy is to facilitate this "more." In time, and as clients become aware of their wounds, they also tend to feel less daunted by those wounds, less imprisoned; they begin to realize, in other words, that they are *more* than their wounds, and through this process, that they are more than their "disorder." For example, Client X felt sure that he was despicable, plague-like, and demonic. His parents had convinced him so over a period of 18 years, and not through the usual route of abuse and punishment but exactly the opposite, through indulgence. Client X was led to believe he was a king, a seer, and a god. He was given "everything," and praised for virtually every routine move. The result: As soon as Client X hit adulthood, the trials and pressures of college, dating, and vocation, his bubble burst. No longer able to live under his former illusions, he now had to face his incompetencies, inabilities to compete, and his far from developed will. The convergence of these factors sent Client X into a tailspin. His view of himself completely reversed— such that he now (in his 30s) repudiated himself, whereas he had earlier glorified himself; and where he once saw a titan for whom every whim was fulfilled, he now saw an outcast for whom every desire was unreachable.

The work with Client X is highly illustrative of the trust dimension in the activation of presence. Although his self-hatred was formidable, it was not irrevocable. We spent many sessions on his anguish, self-pity, and searing guilt. There were many times when he could go only so far with these feelings, and had to warp back into the semblance of self and self-image that he had constructed as a defense. But there were times, increasingly productive times, when he could glimpse a counterpart. For example, in the midst of his self-devaluing, he might suddenly become frustrated and realize moments of self-affirmation, that is, times when he actually liked himself and liked being alive, regardless of the strokes he would receive from doting associates. At first this realization was fleeting, but eventually, as he stayed with it, it became the major counterpoint to his despairing self-reproach. Back and forth he would swing, between burning self-debasement and gleaming self-validation— including compassion, appreciation, and even exultation at being alive. This latter quality was also connected to his growing sense of outrage at not only his outdated sense of self but also his upbringing and well-intentioned but clueless parents. He began to realize that his lowliness, far from being an inherent defect, was a product of environment, circumstance, and, in part, choice.

To summarize, despite Client X's repeated resistance and readiness to give up, the therapist's empathic invitations to "give his hurt a few moments" or to "see what unfolds" were crucial to his reengagement with his larger self. And through this reengagement he began to discover that he was so much vaster than his stuck sense of unworthiness; he began to see that he was sensitive, alive, and resiliently mortal—and that these were enough.

The Interpersonal Activation of Presence

The activation of presence can also occur through the interpersonal route, or that which E-H therapists term the *encounter* (Phillips, 1980–1981; see also Krug, 2009), which is illustrated by E-H therapists in myriad and diverse forms. For example, the calling of attention to disturbances or undercurrents in the immediate relationship exemplifies the E-H concern with encounter, as does the recognition of transference and countertransference projections, as does the encouragement to explore the status of the therapeutic bond at given junctures. As a whole, E-H encounter is characterized by the following three criteria: (1) the real or present relationship between therapist and client (which can include past projections, but chiefly as they are experienced now rather than in the remoteness of reminiscences; e.g., the difference between reporting about and "living" transferential material); (2) the future and what is potential in the relationship (vs. strictly the past and what has already been scripted); and (3) the enactment or experiencing, to the degree possible, of relational material.

Attention to the encounter or *intersubjective,* as an emerging cadre of psychoanalysts have termed it (Stolorow, Brandchaft, & Atwood, 1987), is a vital part of E-H facilitation. The reason for this is that interpersonal contact has a uniquely intensive quality that both accentuates and mobilizes clients' presence. The encounter accentuates presence by awakening it to what is real, immediate, and directly personal, and it mobilizes presence by demanding of it a response, engagement, and address. There is something profoundly naked about the turn to an immediate interaction. It takes the parties out of their inward routine (assuming that is there) and focuses the spotlight on a new and utterly alternative reality— themselves. In short, there is something undeniably "living" about face-to-face interactions; they peel away the layers of pretense and expose the inflamed truth of embattled humanity (Krug, 2009). There are no easy exits from such interactions, and there are fewer "patch-up jobs" as a result.

Take the case of Elva. A thorny and self-aggrandizing widow, Elva spared few with her humor-laced vitriol. Yet Elva's battle was the profound sense of helplessness that underlay her bravado. Since the death of her husband, and despite her bouts with loneliness, Elva had been making a comeback through therapy. She was just beginning to reclaim her self-worth, and her jokes were becoming less caustic, when the bubble burst and she was mugged. The period following this attack, a callous purse snatching, was a trying one for Elva. She was retraumatized, and even her attempts at false bravado fell short.

Yet Elva's battle was clear—she was face-to-face with her worst fears of helplessness, and her wounds were exposed raw. It was at this critical juncture that Elva's therapist and author of this case, Yalom (1989), took a risk. Instead of encouraging her to report *about* her terrors, which might have alleviated some of her internal pressure but not genuinely confronted her wound, he invited her to experience her terrors directly with him. But instead of making it a one-sided exercise, he encouraged her disclosure with some disclosures of his own: "When you say you thought [the purse snatching] would never happen to you," Yalom confided to Elva, "I know just what you mean," he elaborated. "It's so hard for me, too, to accept that all these afflictions—aging, loss, death—are going to happen to me, too" (p. 150).

He went on: "You must feel that if Albert [her deceased husband] were alive, this would never have happened to you. . . . So the robbery brings home the fact that he's really gone" (p. 150). "Elva was really crying now," Yalom (1989) continued, "and her stubby frame heaved with sobs for several minutes. She had never done that before with me. I sat there and wondered, 'Now what do I do?'" But Yalom sensed "instinctually," just what to do. He took one look at her purse—"that same ripped-off, much abused purse" (p. 150), and challenged—"Bad luck is one thing, but aren't you asking for it carrying around something that large" (p. 150)?

This sardonic quip, which was also an offering to dialogue, set off a whole new direction for Elva and Yalom. Not only did she proceed to open up her purse to him, they shared intimately the discussion of its contents. Finally, "when the great bag had . . . yielded all," Yalom (1989) elaborated, "Elva and I stared in wonderment at the contents. . . . We were sorry the bag was empty and that the emptying was over" (p. 150). But what struck Yalom most of all was how "transforming" that engagement had been, for Elva, in his view, had "moved from a position of forsakenness to one of trust" (p. 150). That was "the best hour of therapy I ever gave" (p. 150), Yalom concluded.

Through sharing that bag, Elva accessed more vulnerability, more anxieties about trust, and more possibilities for risking, healing, and bridging than she would likely ever have, had she simply reflected on its contents.

Mutual confirmation, or what Buber calls an "I–thou" relationship, "a relationship of openness, presence, directness, and immediacy," is essential to the therapist's responsibility according to Friedman (2001, p. 344). Although there is a place, of course, for modulating this confirmation, and no professional relationship can be mutual in the sense of a friendship, such a notion is nevertheless a bellwether, a palpable and reliable indicator, of intensive therapeutic transformation. Why is this so? Because the further that one can be present to and work out differences with another, the more one can generally engage in the same relational dynamics toward oneself.

In her discussion of Sylvia, Molly Sterling (2001) articulates both sides of the responsibility question, and she does so poignantly and incisively. "My client leaned forward," Sterling begins her case presentation, "eyes intently on me, voice passionately intense, and said to me, 'I just want to be in your kitchen while you cook.'" "Inwardly," Sterling goes on,

> I froze. Not one therapist sinew, not one trained muscle of years of practice, flexed into action. Nowhere in me was there a standard response, and I parody our standard psychotherapeutic repertoire a bit here: "Tell me how that would be" or "You would like to be closer to me" or "Our meetings aren't enough for you" or just a genuinely open and quiet waiting for my client to continue." Instead I reacted viscerally," elaborated Sterling. "In my frozen moment, I saw the dishes left as I hurried out early that morning. I felt my pleasure in my own rhythm of my puttering about. I wondered how my family would take to this new person slipped into their lives. These images supplanted my unawareness that I could not sustain my client's intense pressure. I felt, in short, inadequate to her proposition. (p. 349)

Sterling (2001) took Sylvia's request as a "concrete proposition to which [Sterling] was called to give a concrete answer. . . . And so, the gist of [Sterling's] reply carried all of these [above] feelings and many more to which [she] was then blind: 'Oh, you might not like me so much if you were around me more.'" And "in one blind stroke," Sterling conceded, "I had cleaved open a chasm of distance, betrayal, shame, fury, and misconstrual" (p. 349).

Sylvia was a "successful . . . kind, intelligent, and savvy" therapy client, according to Sterling (2001, p. 349). She took "care of herself and her life everywhere but in her most private heart, where she [hid] shame, guilt, and grief," and where she "neither is loved nor loves (she believes)"(p. 349). To Sterling, her "blind remark" to Sylvia rejected Sylvia's "plea for abiding acceptance," and "violently broke open her heart" (p. 349). Sylvia "wanted something" from Sterling, according to Sterling, and she (Sterling) failed to provide it. Caught up in her own discomfiting anxieties about being wanted, needed, and accompanied, Sterling reacted—as would many therapists in similar situations—with modified, low-grade panic.

But, and this is where the existential, I–thou notions of encounter become so relevant, Sterling (2001) did not *desist* at the point of her anxiety. She did not "fold up" and revert to some stilted or rehearsed professionalism; nor did she abandon Sylvia, either physically or emotionally. To the contrary, she stayed profoundly with her evolving distress, immersed in it, took time to study it, explored it with Sylvia, and gradually, charily, fashioned a response to it.

The response that Sterling fashioned recognized both her own and Sylvia's shortcomings but also their humanity. Sterling *was* overwhelmed by Sylvia's neediness in her request, and she had a right to experience this sensibility; at the same time, Sylvia had a right to expect something more from Sterling, something that acknowledged her plea. Sterling took inspiration from the existential–phenomenological philosopher Levinas:

> The ability to respond is the primary meaning of responsibility. Levinas took this further to show that responsibility also carries the experience of being beholden to the other person. . . . Responsibility, for Levinas, meant that simply by the fact of the face of the other person, one is "taken hostage"—before thought, choice, or action. . . . It is this level of our human condition, brought into presence by our naked encounter, that Sylvia and I . . . had to reckon with. (2001, p. 351)

Although Sterling "failed" to meet the "obligation" of human encounter, in her very failure, she realized, were the seeds of her success. For as Sterling put it about her discouraging remark to Sylvia, "Sylvia *was* [nevertheless] in my kitchen with me—conflicts, mess, hurry, and all. At that moment, [Sylvia] had what she would get in my kitchen in actuality, if not what she wanted in feeling. I was as naked as she was, if only she (and I) could see it" (2001, p. 352).

But Sterling did see it. In time, she acknowledged how overwhelmed she was by Sylvia's fantasy. She opened up some about her own weaknesses, fears, and misgivings, and this, as Sterling put it, "altered" (2001, p. 352) their relationship. From that point on, Sylvia was freed to respond as a person to Sterling, because Sterling, in turn, had responded as a person with Sylvia. But by acknowledging her limits with Sylvia, both as person and professional, Sterling helped free Sylvia to respond to something else—her nurture of herself—and the challenge thereby to actualize that relationship.

To summarize, E-H encounter is a complex and dynamic process whereby the entire therapeutic context is taken into consideration; among the salient factors within this context are the client's desire and capacity for change, the therapeutic alliance, and practical considerations. The guiding therapeutic question is, to what extent does encounter further the cause of immersion in, engagement with, and integration of clients' intensive struggles; or, on the other hand, to what extent does encounter do the opposite and defeat or stifle facilitative processes?

The Struggle with Resistance (or "Protection")

When the invitation to explore, immerse, and interrelate, is abruptly or repeatedly declined by clients, then the perplexing problem of resistance, or "self-protection," as more E-H therapists are terming it, must be considered. Resistance is the *blockage* to that which is palpably (immediately, affectively, kinesthetically) significant within the client, and between client and therapist. Several caveats must be borne in mind when considering client resistance. First, therapists can be mistaken about resistance. What Therapist *A*, for example, labels an internal resistance may in fact be a refusal on the part of Client *B* to accept Therapist *A*'s agenda for him or her. Resistance may also be a safety issue for a given client, or an issue of cultural or psychological misunderstanding. From an E-H perspective, then, it is of utmost importance that therapists suspend their attributions of resistance and discern their relevant contexts.

Second, it is crucial to respect resistance from an E-H point of view. Resistance is a lifeline to many clients, and as miserable as their patterns may be, this lifeline represents the ground or scaffolding of an assured or familiar path. Although this path may seem crude or even suicidal to clients who experience it, it is starkly preferable to the alternatives (May, 1983, p. 28). Accordingly, it is important for E-H therapists to tread mindfully when it comes to resistance, acknowledging *both* its life-giving *and* life-taking qualities. It is also important to be cognizant of challenging clients' resistance prematurely, lest such challenges exacerbate rather than alleviate defensive needs.

From an E-H point of view, resistance work is mirroring work. By *mirroring work*, I mean the feeding back and elucidation of clients' monumental experiential battle. As suggested earlier, this battle consists of two basic factions: the side of the client that struggles to emerge (e.g., to liberate from, transcend, or enlarge his or her impoverished world), and the side that vies to suppress that emergence and revert. Whereas the activation of presence (e.g., the calling of attention to what is alive) mirrors clients' struggles to emerge, resistance work, as previously noted, elucidates clients' barriers to that emergence, and the ways and means they immobilize.

In summary, resistance work must be artfully engaged. The more that therapists invest in changing clients, the less they enable clients to struggle with change. By contrast, the more that therapists enable clients to clarify how they are willing to live, the more they fuel the impetus (and often frustration!) required for lasting change (Schneider, 1998a, 2008).

There are two basic forms of resistance work: vivification and confrontation. *Vivification of resistance* is the intensification of clients' awareness of how they block or limit themselves. Specifically, vivification serves three basic functions: (1) It alerts clients to their defensive worlds, (2) it apprises them of the consequences of those worlds, and (3) it reflects back the counterforces (or "counter-will," as Otto Rank, 1936, put it) aimed at overcoming those worlds. There are two basic approaches linked to vivifying resistance—noting and tagging. *Noting* apprises clients of initial experiences of resistance. Here is an illustration: "You suddenly get quiet when the subject of your brother arises" or "You laugh when speaking of your pain" or "We were just speaking about your anxieties working with me and you suddenly switched topics" or "I sense that you're holding down your anger right now."

In a distinctly dramatic illustration of noting resistance, Bugental (1976) reported a highly stilted, initial interview with a client, in which decorum rather than genuine feeling permeated. Laurence (Bugental's client) took extensive pains to show how competent he was, how many accolades he had won, and how important his life was. But after some period of this self-puffery, Bugental "took a calculated risk" (p. 16). Instead of placating his new client or emulating the standard intake role of detached observer, Bugental turned to Laurence, faced him directly and averred: "You're scared shitless"—and at that, Laurence shed his mask of bravado and began a genuine interchange with Bugental.

Sometimes noting resistance takes the form of nonverbal feedback. For example, just sitting with clients in their uncertainty at a given moment can feed back to them the realization that a change or mobilization of some sort is necessary in their lives. Or through the therapist's mirroring of clients' crossed arms or furrowed brow, clients may begin to become clearer about how closed they have been, or how tensely they hold themselves.

Tagging alerts clients to the repetition of their resistance. Examples of tagging include "So here we are again; at that same bitter place" or "Every time you note a victory, you go on and beat yourself up" or "You repeatedly insist on the culpability of others" or "What is it like to feel helpless again?" Like noting, tagging implies a subtle challenge, a subtle invitation to reassess one's stance. Implicitly, it enjoins clients to take responsibility for their self-constructions and to revisit their capacities to transform.

Revisitation is a key therapeutic dimension. Every time clients become aware of how they stop (or deter) themselves from fuller personal and interpersonal access, they learn more about their willingness to approach such situations in the future. Frequently, many revisitations are required before "stuck" experiences can be accessed; clients must revisit many frustrations and wounds before they are ready substantively to reapproach those conditions. Yet, as entrenched as their miseries may be, each time clients face them, they face remarkable opportunities for change; and each incremental change can become monumental—a momentum shift of life-changing proportions.

Another form of vivifying resistance, *tracing out,* entails encouraging clients to explore the fantasized consequences of their resistance. For example, I have encouraged obese clients who fear weight loss to review and grapple with the expectations of that weight loss, and not just intellectually but experientially, through dramatizing an anticipated scene; identifying the feelings, body sensations, and images associated with the scene; and encountering the fears, fantasies, and anticipated consequences of following the scene to its ultimate conclusion. Although clients often find such tracing out disconcerting, they also often find it illuminating, as it animates their overinflated fears, unexpected resources, and resolve, in addition to their harrowing frailties. The tracing out of *capitulation* to a behavior or experience is also highly illuminating. Such tracing out, for example, might take the form of foregoing weight loss and the anticipated fears, fantasies, and implications of maintaining the status quo. The question "Where does this (reluctance to lose weight) leave you?" or "How are you willing to respond (to such intransigence)?" can help elaborate these exercises.

When clients' stuckness becomes intractable, but with a potential for substantive change, a confrontation may be called for. *Confrontation* with resistance is a direct and amplified form of vivification. However, instead of *alerting* clients to their self-destructive refuges, confrontation *alarms* them, and in lieu of *nurturing* transformation, confrontation *presses* for and *demands* (or *requires,* to use Bugental's [1987] term) such transformation (Schneider, 2008). There are several caveats, however, about confrontation that bear consideration. First, confrontation may risk an argument or power struggle between client and therapist, versus a deepening or facilitative grappling. Second, confrontation risks the surrender of clients' decision-making power to therapists, with the resultant withdrawal of that decision-making power from clients' own lives. Third, confrontation risks alienating clients—not merely from an individual therapist but from therapy as a whole.

As unfortunate as these potentially calamitous outcomes may be, they are not by any means foreordained. Engaged optimally, confrontation requires not only careful and artful encouragements to clients to change but also, and equally important, a full appreciation for the consequences of such encouragements. Prior to decisions to confront, therefore, therapists must carefully weigh the stakes—such as their intervention's timeliness, their degree of alliance with clients, and their own personal and professional preparedness.

Bugental (1976) provides a keen illustration of confrontation with his case of Frank, who was an obstinate and reproachful young man. He repeatedly scorned life, yet refused to entertain its possibilities for betterment as well. At one peculiarly frustrating juncture,

Frank chastises Bugental: "Whenever you guys want to make a point but can't do it directly, you tell the sucker he's got some unconscious motivation. That way. . . . "

> [Bugental responds:] "Oh shee-it, Frank. You're doing it right now. I answer one question for you and get sandbagged from another direction. You just want to fight about everything that comes along."
>
> [Frank:] "It's always something I'm doing. Well, if you had to eat as much crap every-day as I do, you'd . . . "
>
> [Bugental:] "Frank, you'd rather bellyache about life than do something about it." [Frank's "pouting tone" changes.]
>
> [Bugental continues:] "Frank, I don't want all this to get dismissed as just my tired-ness or your sad, repetitive life. I am tired, and maybe that makes me bitch at you more. I'll take responsibility for that. But it is also true that somehow you have become so invested in telling your story of how badly life treats you that you do it routinely and with a griping manner that turns people off or makes them angry. You don't like to look at that, but it's so, and I think some part of you knows it." (p. 109)

This vignette illustrates several important points. First, by intensifying his description of Frank's behavior, Bugental stuns or gently shocks Frank into a potentially new view of himself—that of responsible agent rather than passive victim. By accenting Frank's "invest-ment" in complaining, he tacitly asks Frank to reassess that investment, and his entire stance, in fact, of treating himself as a victim. Second, the vignette illustrates how a therapeutic interaction can reflect a more general reality in a client's day-to-day world. As Bugental's comment makes plain, Frank's "griping" must turn off a lot of people, and, as in the case with Bugental, this reaction can only complicate, if not exacerbate, Frank's intransigent bitterness. Third, and by way of summary, Bugental's remarks challenge Frank to reassess his whole stance, the issues leading up to that stance, and the necessity of maintaining that stance. In effect, Bugental beseeches, "What is the payoff of staying bitter, and is it worth the price"?

On the other hand, there are notable times when such imploring (or even gentle inquiring) with clients is futile, if not outright hazardous. At such times, clients may feel sapped, "spent," or defiantly entrenched, and instead of confronting or challenging those states (which may have the unintended effect of threatening and thereby hardening intrac-table defenses), the best strategy from the E-H view may simply be to enable or allow those devitalizing realities (e.g., see Schneider, 1999). Frequently, for example, I have found that clients' investments in their resistance directly parallel my own investment in their over-coming that resistance. Furthermore, when I have pulled back some from my own intransi-gence, clients too have seemingly loosened up and pulled back. This dynamic makes sense; for what is being asked of clients, in effect, is to leap headlong into the doom that they have designed a lifetime to avoid. However, to the extent that such clients feel that they have room, can take their own pace, and can shift in their own time-tested fashion, they are often more pliable, flexible, and inclined toward change.

To summarize, resistance work is mirror work and must be skillfully facilitated. Vivifi-cation (noting and tagging) of resistance alerts, whereas confrontation alarms clients about their self-constructed plights. Presumptuousness, however, must be minimized in this work. Whereas some clients are amenable to the accentuation and vivification of their life pat-terns, others are more reticent, and such reticence should not be undervalued. It, too, can be informative and eventually facilitate a fuller and deeper stance.

The Coalescence of Meaning, Intentionality, and Awe

As clients are able to face and overcome the blocks to their aliveness, as they begin to *choose* rather than succumb to the paths that beckon them, they develop a sense of life meaning. This meaning is wrought out of struggle, deep presence to the rivaling sides of oneself, and embodied choice about the aspect of oneself that one intends to live out. The overcoming of resistance, in other words, is preparatory to the unfolding of meaning, and the unfolding of meaning is preparatory to revitalization.

Such revitalization, or what Rollo May (1969) terms "intentionality," is the full-bodied orientation to a given goal or direction. It is different from intellectual or behavioral change, because its impetus derives from one's entire being, one's entire sense of import, and one's entire sense of priority (see also the "I am" experience in May, 1983).

The coalescence of meaning and intentionality takes many forms. Sometimes clients find it on the job site, in the home, with friends, or with community. At times it takes the form of a sport or a class or a trip, and sometimes it is without form (e.g., the freedom to be). The pivotal issue here is attitude. To what extent does a client's life meaning align with his or her inmost aspirations, sensibilities, and values, and how much is the client willing to risk (take responsibility for) the consequences of those alignments?

The task of the therapist at this stage is to assist clients in their quest to *actualize their life meanings*. This assistance may take the form of a Socratic dialogue about possible ways to change one's lifestyle or relate to a partner, or begin a new project. It may be manifest as an invitation to visualize or role-play new scenarios, inner resources, or concerted actions. It may develop as a reflection on one's dream life and the symbols, patterns, and affects associated with the dream's message. It may take the shape of a challenge to try out newfound capacities in real-life circumstances—a desired encounter, a wished for avocation, a contemplated journey. Following each of these explorations, meaning is further cultivated by encouraging clients to sort through their experiential discoveries. For example, by attuning to the feelings, sensations, and general life impact of risking a new relationship, clients are in an enhanced position to evaluate the significance of that relationship.

While the coalescence of meaning and intentionality addresses a client's life priorities, it may sometimes lead beyond discernable priorities. This "beyond" I have come to call *awe*, which is the humility and wonder, thrill and anxiety, of simply life itself (Schneider, 2004, 2008, 2009). It is the capacity to experience the *adventure* of life, regardless of a particular mode or path. E-H therapy, in other words, forms a staging ground for not only attainment of particular goals but also the inner freedom to experience more fully and deeply the context within which goals operate, and this colors all of one's life experience. One result of E-H therapy, then, is that clients can experience the fuller ranges of life—both its vulnerable lows and its transcendent peaks. They become more "whole," but whole in the sense of being able to experience the great paradoxes of life—vulnerability and unsettlement, as well as resiliency and pluck—and they become less susceptible to polarizing identifications.

At the same time, one does not necessarily have to come through a formal therapeutic process to arrive at these awe-based realizations—Viktor Frankl (1963), for example, discovered them in a concentration camp. However, what one does need is the capacity for the cultivation of presence. Ultimately, E-H therapy is about "access and expressibility" (Bugental, 1987, p. 27)—the capacity to access and express the maximal range of ourselves, including ranges of spiritual depth.

A Note about the Social and Spiritual Dimensions of E-H Transformation

E-H therapy takes very seriously the question: On whose behalf does a therapist function—the culture, the organization within which he or she works, the demands of the health care industry, or the client him- or herself? Although none of these can be neglected from an E-H point of view, it is emphatically the client, and the profound subjective and intersubjective realizations of depth-experiential inquiry, that reflect E-H therapy's primary commitment. This person-centered priority, moreover, is not just for the revitalization of individuals; it is for the revitalization of their (our) community, culture, and indeed, world (e.g., Bugental & Bracke, 1992; Friedman, 2001; May, 1981). To put it another way, E-H therapy promotes depth inquiry, and depth inquiry promotes a sense of what deeply matters. Although such a sense does not always lead to social consciousness, in my experience—and that of many E-H practitioners—this is predominantly what results.

One point, therefore, must be underscored: One cannot simply heal individuals to the neglect of the social context within which they are thrust. To be a responsible practitioner, one must develop a vision of responsible social change alongside and in coordination with one's vision of individual transformation—and increasingly, E-H practitioners are becoming conscious of this interdependence (Hoffman, Stewart, Warren, & Meek, 2009; Mendelowitz, 2008; O'Hara, 2001; Schneider, 2004, 2009). Another area where such interdependence is key is that of spirituality. Although it is not often well publicized, spirituality has a long and venerated lineage within E-H therapy. This lineage dates back to the romantic philosophers of 18th- and 19th-century Europe, such as Johann von Goethe and Søren Kierkegaard, and wends its way into the 20th century through such luminaries as William James, Paul Tillich, Rollo May, and Ernest Becker (Elkins, 2001; Moss, 1999; Schneider, 1998b). The essence of this lineage is an appreciation of life's paradoxes: among them, our separateness from yet relatedness to others; our limitedness yet remarkable capacity to transcend.

In E-H therapy life's paradoxes, such as isolation and fusion, humility and boldness are central. Over and over again clients revisit these paradoxes, and persistently they emerge from them anew. The result is that over time, clients learn to be more present with themselves, more able to respond to rather than react against their paradoxical natures—and more able to be present to, or stand in awe of, the paradoxes of life (Hoffman, 2008, Mendelowitz, 2008; Schneider, 2008, 2009). This capacity to stand in awe, to experience the humility and wonder—or *adventure*—of life is perhaps the apex of E-H therapy; it is perhaps the apex of spiritual renewal.

CURATIVE FACTORS OR MECHANISMS OF CHANGE

As previously indicated, the core of E-H change processes is presence. Without presence, there may well be intellectual or behavioral or physiological change but not necessarily the sense of agency or personal involvement that core change requires. To put it another way, E-H therapy stresses presence to *what really matters*, both within the self and between the self and the therapist. This presence has two basic functions: (1) It reconnects people to their pain (e.g., blocks, fears, and anxieties), and (2) it attunes people to the opportunities to transform or transcend that pain.

Presence, then, is both the ground (condition, atmosphere) and the goal for E-H facilitation. As ground, presence holds and illuminates that which is palpably (immediately, affectively, and kinesthetically) significant within the client and between the client and therapist. Presence in this sense provides the holding environment whereby deeper and more intensified presence can take root. As goal, presence mobilizes clients. It accompanies them during their deepest struggles, their search to redress those struggles, and their day-to-day integration of those struggles (Bugental, 1987; May, 1981).

In addition to facilitating experiential forms of change, such as those previously mentioned, presence also guides and provides a container, where appropriate, for more behavioral or mechanistic levels of change. The question that presence illuminates is "What is really going on with this client, and how can I optimize my assistance to her?"; or to put it another way, "What is this client's desire and capacity for change?" (Schneider, 1995).

Insight in E-H therapy is more like "inner vision," as Bugental (1978) frames the term. Inner vision facilitates an *experience* of past, present, or future issues rather than an explanation or formulation *about* them. The end goal of inner vision is not so much to "figure issues out" as to stay with them, attend to their affective and kinesthetic features, and sort out how or whether one is willing to *respond* to them. To the degree that one can follow this process through, one can not only become more intentional (i.e., concerted, purposeful) in one's life, but also, and paradoxically, more flexible, tolerant, and capable of change.

Interpretations are provided in E-H therapy more to facilitate a deepening of experience than to strengthen analytical skills. Although a strengthening of analytical skills can certainly be of benefit over the course of an E-H regimen, the thrust of the work is toward empowering *clients* to find their logical or adaptive paths. In this sense, interpretations tend to take the form of mirroring responses in E-H therapy, reflecting and amplifying clients' rival impulses.

E-H change processes comprise both an intra- and interpersonal dimension. The intrapersonal aspect is facilitated through concerted efforts to survey the self, whereas the interpersonal dimension is facilitated through the naturally evolving "I–thou" dynamic of relationship. Although E-H practitioners tend to emphasize different aspects of intra- and interpersonal exploration, there is essential unanimity when it comes to the core of these emphases—immediacy and presence.

To summarize, E-H therapy has two essential aims: (1) to cultivate presence (i.e., attention, choice, and freedom), and (2) to cultivate responsibility (i.e., ability to respond) to that presence. These aims are fulfilled by therapists, through their capacity to attune to, tolerate struggle with, and vivify emergent patterns, and by clients, through their commitment to and capacity for change. Although E-H therapy parallels, and indeed grounds, many other intensive therapies (see the section "Research Support"), its emphasis on presence, struggle, and whole-bodied responsiveness renders it unique.

TREATMENT APPLICABILITY AND ETHICAL CONSIDERATIONS

As suggested earlier, E-H therapy applies to a diverse population of clients. Despite its high-brow image, E-H practice has been applied to substance abusers, ethnic and racial minorities, gay and lesbian clientele, psychiatric inpatients, and business personnel (Schneider, 2008; Schneider & Krug, 2010). Furthermore, E-H principles of presence, I–thou relationship, and courage have now been adopted by a plethora of practice orientations (see, e.g., Bunting & Hayes, 2008; Fosha, 2008; Portnoy, 2008; Stolorow, 2008; Wolfe, 2008). That said, however, the expansion and diversification of E-H therapy is a relatively recent phenomenon; most E-H practice still tends to take place in white middle- to upper-class neighborhoods with white middle- to upper-class clientele. Yet there is no necessary link between such clientele and successful E-H therapy; as E-H practitioners are discovering, the benefits of presence, I–thou encounter, and responsibility are cross-cultural, as well as cross-disciplinary (Rice, 2008; Vontress & Epp, 2001).

While E-H therapists realize that they cannot be "all things to all people," and that certain problems (e.g., circumscribed phobias and brain pathology) are best handled by specialists, a definite ecumenicism impacts contemporary E-H practice. This ecumenicism emphasizes cross-disciplinary openness, adaptations for diverse populations, and sliding-fee scales.

In the end, however, no formulaic guideline determines the course of E-H practice. Each client and therapist must have their say.

RESEARCH SUPPORT

Inasmuch as E-H therapy places a premium on common factors (e.g., the therapeutic alliance, empathy, and expressed emotion), it is now being recognized—at least partially—as an evidence-based approach (e.g., Elkins, 2007; Wampold, 2008). Not to be discounted, moreover, is E-H therapy's enduring tradition of eloquent case studies (e.g., Binswanger, 1958; Boss, 1963; Bugental, 1976; May, 1983; Schneider & May, 1995; Spinelli, 1997; Yalom, 1980). That said, however, the systematic, corroborative evidence for E-H therapy is relatively limited (Walsh & McElwain, 2002; Yalom, 1980). There are two major reasons for this situation. First, the E-H theoretical outlook has tended to attract philosophically and artistically oriented clinicians who are more at home with clinical practice or case study narratives than with laboratory procedures or controlled investigations (Wertz, 2001). Second, when E-H therapists or theorists have attempted to conduct research, they have found themselves facing an array of theoretical, practical, and political barriers. Among these barriers are the difficulties of translating long-term, exploratory therapeutic processes and outcomes into controlled experimental designs and requirements (Schneider, 1998b; Seligman, 1996), the problems of quantifying complex life issues (Miller, 1996a), and the hardships of obtaining research funds for "alternative" therapeutic practices (Miller, 1996b). Furthermore, the obstacles are even more daunting for those in the E-H therapy community who have called for qualitative (e.g., phenomenological) assessment of their practices. Although many consider such assessments more appropriate than their conventional counterparts to evaluate E-H subject matter, there are substantial barriers associated with their implementation (Wertz, 2001). Among them are not only perplexing theoretical and practical challenges but also, and no less confounding, disparagement from a quantifying, medicalizing research community (Wertz, 2001).

These difficulties, however, appear to be lessening. In the past decade, mainstream conceptions of therapeutic process and outcome research have undergone notable reevaluations, and models once considered invulnerable are now being revised. The randomized controlled trial, for example, once considered the "gold standard" of therapeutic evaluation research, has been criticized as well (see Bohart, O'Hara, & Leitner, 1998; Goldfried & Wolfe, 1996). Conversely, qualitative research, once considered practically and scientifically untenable, has attained professional legitimacy (Elliott, 2002; Wertz, 2001).

In light of these changes, E-H therapy has been accumulating a considerable base of empirical support. Although still comparatively small, this base is both rigorous and promising (Elkins, 2007; Walsh & McElwain, 2002); it also dovetails consistently with the latest findings about so-called "common factors" research, which shows convincingly the value of E-H practice principles for effective psychotherapy (Elkins, 2007; Wampold, 2008). In the domain of systematic quantitative inquiry, for example, there is growing support for key E-H principles of therapeutic rapport, attunement to clients' needs, facilitation of emotional expression, and personal accessibility (or genuineness). This support is reflected in both the "common factors" and "contextual factors" research that consistently upholds relationship as opposed to technical factors as the core facilitative condition (Elkins, 2007; Wampold, 2001, 2008). It is echoed in the research on therapeutic alliance (Hovarth, 1995), empathy (Bohart & Greenberg, 1997), genuineness and positive regard (Orlinsky, Grawe, & Parks, 1994), and clients' capacity for self-healing (Bohart & Tallman, 1999), and it is mirrored in the existing research on expressed emotion (e.g., Gendlin, 1996; Greenberg, Rice, & Elliott, 1993). Greenberg and colleagues, for example, demonstrated that E-H compatible facilitations such as evocative unfolding (or vivifying a problematic scene), empty-chair technique (role play with an imagined other), and experiential processing (which includes evoking awareness of experience, attendance to unclear or emergent experience, ownership of emotional reactions, interpersonal contact, development of a meaning perspective, and translation of emerging awareness into daily life) all correlated with positive outcome (see also Greenberg, 2007).

Finally, in a little known but provocative study of E-H therapy with patients diagnosed with schizophrenia and treated in the alternative, minimally medicating psychiatric facility Soteria House, Mosher (2001) reported that at 2-year follow-up, the experimental (E-H treated) population had significantly better outcomes regarding rehospitalization, psychopathology, independent living, and social and occupational functioning than their conventionally treated (medicated) counterparts over the same investigative period. The findings of this study were recently confirmed in *Schizophrenia Bulletin,* accompanied by an "urgent" recommendation to evaluate Mosher's approach further (Calton, Ferriter, Huband, & Spandler, 2008, p. 181).

On the qualitative side of the equation, Bohart and Tallman (1999), Rennie (1994), and Watson and Rennie (1994) have demonstrated the value of such E-H stalwarts as presence and expanding the capacity for choice in effective facilitation. Specifically, they showed that successful therapy, as understood by clients, necessitates "a process of self-reflection," consideration of "alternative courses of action, and making choices" (Walsh & McElwain, 2002, p. 261). In a related qualitative study, Hanna, Giordana, Dupuy, and Puhakka (1995) investigated what they termed "second order" or deep and sweeping change processes in therapy. Compatible with existential emphases on liberation, they found that "transcendence," or moving beyond limitations, was the essential structure of change. Furthermore, they found that transcendence comprises "penetrating, pervasive, global and enduringly stable" insight, accompanied by "a new perspective on the self, world, or problem" (p. 148).

Finally, in a study of clients' perceptions of their E-H–oriented therapists, Schneider (1985) reported that although techniques were important to the success of long-term (i.e., 2-year-plus) therapeutic outcomes, the "personal involvement" of the therapist— which comprised his or her genuineness, support, acceptance, and deep understanding—was by far the most critical factor identified. Such involvement, moreover, inspired clients to become more self-involved and to experience themselves as more capable, responsible, and self-accepting. (For a comprehensive review of these and other E-H therapeutic investigations, see Elkins, 2007; Elliott, 2002; Schneider & Krug, 2010; Walsh & McElwain, 2002; Watson & Bohart, 2001.)

To summarize, empirical investigation of E-H therapy is in a nascent but flowering stage. Many conceptual dimensions of E-H practice have been confirmed by both quantitative and qualitative investigation, and many remain to be more fully illuminated. Yet if the trends in therapy research continue, E-H practice may become a model, evidence-based modality that stresses three critical variables: (1) the therapeutic relationship, (2) the therapist's presence or personality, and (3) the active self-healing of clients. By implication, on the other hand, statistically driven manuals, programs, and techniques may become increasingly adjunctive, if not peripheral, in their facilitative role (Bohart & Tallman, 1999; Messer & Wampold, 2002; Westen & Morrison, 2001).

CASE ILLUSTRATION

Mary was a self-referred, 240-pound, single, European American sales clerk. She had a minimal 3-month history of "mental health" counseling (as a young adolescent), and no history of psychiatric medication. From the moment Mary stepped into my office, I could sense a deep connection with her, yet, at the same time, a curious reluctance on her part to engage.

Seduced and teased as a child, Mary had minimal trust in men, little trust in herself in the presence of men, and minute trust in the culture that tacitly assented to these conditions. Yet here she was, at 30 years old, declaring her commitment to reenvision and reassemble her life. Here she was—partly with my encouragement—dashing off reams of journal pages about the pain, injustice, and outrages of her life, but at the same time, about the dreams, desires, and possibilities that could be her life. She would read from, and we would share reflections about her entries, and she would scrap tirelessly with them. Back and forth, she would swing—between searing self-abasement and rising self-attunement, between depleting worry and replenishing confidence. Her struggle displayed all the earmarks of the depth excursion, the depth entanglement, that precedes restoration. She, like so many therapy clients, had to straddle contending life paths, to sift out the implications of those life paths, and to consolidate a plan, direction, and vision based on those implications. Following 3 years of such wrangling and deep experiential immersions, she gradually and doggedly reemerged. She found that capitulating to her father, the culture, and the taboo of asserting herself was no longer tolerable and that changes had to occur.

Her first step, which I encouraged, was to allow herself to be angry and indignant enough to halt her automatic bingeing and to peer into the void it replaced. Instead of instantly seeking food as a refuge, therefore, and based on my recommendation, she instituted a pause in her experience; she allowed the fears and hurts to percolate. Yet in this percolation were much more than fears and hurts. She realized, for example, that she did not have to be so readily panicked over being seen by others, that she would not inexorably be attacked by the person she feared, and that, greatest of all, she had a value and truth that she could not squander. Regardless of her obesity, Mary realized, *she* had worth; a tender, loving essence inside her, yearning to be felt, heard, and held.

Her second step, which we coordinated with a local weight loss clinic, was the long and arduous process of losing her excess girth and of confronting the barriers to this toilsome process. It is not that she felt an *obligation* to lose pounds or even that this ordeal was mandatory for her physical health. All these "supposed to's" were increasingly peripheral to her. By contrast, that which was mandatory for her was an internal rightness about losing her weight. She did not want to go into a program until she felt clearly that health, attractiveness, and integrity were necessary for *her*—not for some imagined other.

Following this clarification, Mary embarked on an 8-month trial with a powder diet as a replacement for meals. This course had its own thorny challenges, but she met them well. On the one hand, the powder was "easy" because it was readily available, habit forming, and required little forethought. On the other hand, precisely because it was *not* food, the powder presented Mary with opportunities to reassess her associations to food. Among these associations were the comfort value of food, the special linkages to sweets, and the pleasure of cooking. But chief among Mary's discoveries was that behind all these compelling features of food was the daunting capacity of food to protect. From the standpoint of protection, Mary realized, food was not simply a distraction or a pleasurable obsession; it was a refuge from perceived annihilation. By eating the powder, and particularly, by attending to the feelings, sensations, and images conjured up by her abstinence from food, Mary began to confront death, the "death" (or brutality) she associated with her nakedness, beauty, and rawness, removed from her culinary refuge. As a result, she began to cope better with that death anxiety. She became less anxious and acquired new patterns of self-support—such as speaking up for herself, or associating with caring company. She also found freedom in her newfound visibility, particularly the freedom to play. She indulged in play like a kid on her first visit to a beach. She ran, worked out, hiked, and simply reveled in her newfound (130 pound) mobility. She also reveled in her newfound attractiveness to men.

Despite these Herculean developments, however, and like so many who embark on the dieting path (see, e.g., Wadden & Stunkard, 1986), Mary emphatically relapsed. After 8 energizing months, and upon transitioning to real food, Mary discovered yet another layer to her ordeal: She had yet to confront her rage. Oh, Mary could get angry. She could rail at the indignities of life, the injustices of culture, the cruelty of her narrow-minded peers, and so on. Yet what she could not do earlier, in the ease and comfort of her powdered diet, was to rail at the chief source for her oppression—her incest-mongering father.

The reexposure to food then brought back a torrent of memories, hurts, and defenses for Mary. She conveyed a dream—early on in this transition—that coupled a hovering, heavily breathing face, with a tiny, prenatal body. I asked her to focus on the feeling tone of this dream and to explore its affective and kinesthetic associations. Although reluctant at first, she soon was able to "live out" the sequences of the dream and to "speak" from its urgent depths. The voice that stood out consequently was the prenatal voice, which was her voice, of course, struggling for its survival. But suddenly a shift occurred: The ostensibly fragile, prenatal cry, became a blood-curdling scream, and the scream became an attacking fist. But this sequence only lasted a few seconds. In moments, she would revert back again to a cry. Mary spent many subsequent months unpacking the above sequence, delving ever closer to her core battle. Repeatedly, we would call attention to her swings between abject timidity, helplessness, and vulnerability, and flagrant rebellion, vengefulness, and fury; then her fear and guilt would set in, and the whole cycle would be repeated.

The instantiation of this pattern was evident in Mary's daily life. Consistently she would oscillate between holing herself up in her house with bags of candy, to bulldozing her coworkers, to bloating and flagellating herself again with food. After 6 months of her transition back to food, Mary regained 60% of her postdietary weight loss (about 65 pounds).

There were, of course, livelier times for Mary, but at this juncture, they were mercilessly under siege. The encrusted layers of pain, dormant just 6 months ago (in association with her powder diet), now broke open into raw, exposed gashes; and although Mary empathized with these gashes, their intensity sometimes overwhelmed her. Binge eating, as noted previously, was one avenue of defense against this intensity, but so were vain efforts to gain control, such as bulimic purging and even mild cutting.

At one point I mirrored these patterns back to Mary. I echoed back to her what I experienced as her slow "suicide," her pull to "give up," and her readiness to defer her power. In turn, Mary bristled at my characterizations, denied that she was in crisis, and simmered in defiance. Yet, at the same time, Mary and I both knew that I had touched a chord at some level, that death was at her doorstep, and that time was slipping fast. It is during just such periods that clients stand before a crossroad in E-H therapy—the crossroad of life or death, possibility or foreclosure, and it is precisely the handling of that crossroad (by both therapist and client) that has an indelible impact on recovery. In light of these contexts, I concertedly invited Mary to stay present to herself, to reverberate to her agonizing dilemma, and to open to the possibilities, the "more" that her dilemma foretold. A part of this "more" encompassed Mary's relationship with me. To the degree that Mary and I could tussle with one another—could face one another's ire and awkwardness and discomfort—to that extent we could also begin to appreciate one another and the "truth" we separately offered to one another. Mary's truth, as I grew to appreciate it, was the stark terror of confronting and overcoming her father's wrath. It was the dread of change, and of becoming the "new" person who has to embody that change. The truth that I held for Mary, on the other hand, which she grew to appreciate, was the anguish, self-deprecation, and disability she countenanced by remaining in her father's thrall, and, conversely, the freedom, mobility, and life that awaited her on the other side of that thrall.

This I–thou meeting afforded Mary a chance to reappraise her relationship to herself, her father, and me. It helped her see—in vivid and experiential immediacy—that she was more than her paralyzing fragility, more than a rape victim, and even more than a victim of women-hating men but a person who could struggle and be vulnerable with another person, yet emerge with renewed vigor.

Gradually then, and with mounting force, the side of Mary that aspired to feel, deepen, and live began to predominate, whereas the regressive side, the side that pulled to hide, waned. (Although this was not a permanent state of affairs, it definitely set the tone for the future.)

These changes afforded Mary and me a chance to revisit the question of her transformation. The first step in our reassessment was to institute a stopgap measure; in order for Mary to reemerge, the "blood-letting" had to be stanched. Accordingly, Mary limited her bingeing, stopped her cutting, and ceased her purging. With my encouragement, furthermore, she enrolled in an intensive, yearlong rehabilitation program. This program—which comprised nutritional counseling, group therapy, and behavioral modification training—was aimed at curtailing her bingeing, bolstering her life-management skills, and strengthening her capacity to communicate.

Once Mary began stabilizing—which was about 8 months after her transition to food—and could learn to exercise some control over her external patterns, the long and continuing inner work could be engaged more fully. Her behavioral skills building, in other words, paved the way for the next and more pivotal phase of internal skills building, which illustrates the integrative dimension of E-H therapy.

In the final phase of our work, Mary focused on living while dieting rather than dieting to live. Over the course of her many ordeals, Mary had learned to grab into the life that awaits her *now* rather than postponing it for some unreachable ideal. In accord with this philosophy, and in the midst of her ongoing weight management, she began dating again, went on trips that she had deferred, and resumed her "working through" with her father. For example, to facilitate Mary's rising self-confidence in relation to her father, we worked with a variety of exploratory outlets—from role plays to drawings to rituals with effigies.

Yet, whereas these initial encounters with her father were imaginary, Mary soon began to shift her tack and contemplate an actual confrontation. She spent many weeks exploring the necessity of such a confrontation, but by closely attending to her experience—immediately, affectively, and kinesthetically—she emphatically arrived at a decision: She would write him a letter, spelling out her entire experience of him—decimating, as well as ambivalent and loving—and offer personally to discuss that letter at a location of her choosing.

This decision on Mary's part was a turning point of therapy. Regardless of how her father responded, in my view, Mary had turned the tide with this decision, from floundering panic to concerted choice, and from impotence to agency. As it turned out, Mary fulfilled her plan and met with her father. Although he was reportedly "shaken" by the ordeal, it did bring a renewed life to their relationship, and most important, it helped to restore Mary's life, the "life" that she could give to herself.

By the end of our work together—about 3½ years of therapy—Mary acquired a revivified sense of self. Although she continued to contend with weight issues (e.g., she was now about 30% overweight) and harbored residual anxieties, these no longer stifled her or prevented her from *concertedly* living. She enjoyed most of her food, ate healthfully, and began a promising romantic relationship. She also experienced a great deal more freedom in her life, and that sensibility paid off in her deepened friendships, expanded physical activities, and enhanced service to the community.

Finally, although Mary was "liberated," she did not completely eradicate her symptoms. What she did eradicate, on the other hand, was a corrosive view of life, which was a partial view that stressed helplessness over possibility and anxiety over courage. Like many E-H therapy clients, Mary formed a new relationship with her symptoms; she learned that she could expand beyond them and through that expansion discover new relationships to food, to her father, and even to existence itself.

Mary was not unlike another weight loss survivor, Karen, who, after about 3 years of her own therapy, declared:

> I wish I could tell you that being a size twelve is all wonderful but I'm finding out that being awake and alive is a package deal. I don't get to go through the line and pick only goodies. On one side is wonder, awe, excitement and laughter—and on the other side is tears, disappointment, aching sadness. Wholeness [or, I would say, the fuller experience of awe] is coming to me by being willing to explore ALL the feelings.
>
> So . . . 275 pounds later, my life is a mixture of pain and bliss. It hurts a lot these days but it's real. It's my life being lived by me and not vicariously through a soap opera. . . . I don't know where it's all heading, but one thing I know for sure, I'm definitely going. (in Roth, 1991, pp. 183–184)

Mary was a deeply troubled but extraordinarily dedicated E-H therapy client. She grappled with some of the most trying personal and social barriers with which humans must contend—incest, obesity, depersonalization—yet she comparatively and realistically triumphed. Beginning with her furious journal writing; our introductory struggles; and her fitful alignment with fears, desires, and outrages, Mary gradually reconstructed her life. Through my presence and our presence to each other, Mary was able to experience the safety to do more than merely report about her life but to "work out" that life amid torments of the past, promptings of the present, and callings of the future. Through invitations to stay present to herself—particularly the feelings, sensations, and images evoked within herself—she began to illuminate not only what she profoundly desired in her life (e.g., freedom, mobility, and intimacy) but also, and equally important, what separated her from those profound desires (e.g., terror of annihilation [her father, men], suppressed rage, and entrenched habits).

In the meantime, adjunctive therapies were employed at key stages throughout the E-H therapy process. These therapies, such as nutritional counseling and behavioral skills training, provided a key confidence-building component to the E-H work. At the same time that they helped Mary to stabilize, they also helped to empower her, and this empowerment translated into her willingness to take risks in depth therapy.

In short, E-H therapy provided a forum whereby presence and its activation through inner struggle, resistance work, and coalescence of meaning and awe, along with an adjunctive program of rehabilitation, could converge to reassemble a life. To the extent that such opportunities for meaningful convergence are being hampered by cost-control measures today, there are dwindling opportunities to reassemble lives, and this, lamentably, may be the direst legacy of market-driven mental health care.

CURRENT AND FUTURE TRENDS

The outlook for E-H therapy is both guarded and promising. It is guarded to the extent that all depth therapies are guarded and under threat today—by an encroaching medicalized ethos. Moreover, as students, instructors, and professional organizations acquiesce to and, in some cases, encourage the foregoing ethos, there is a decreasing incentive to teach, let alone apply E-H alternatives. On the other hand, the outlook for the future is not so one-sided as it may seem. As previously suggested, there are trends, such as the embrace of experientially informed practice, that run directly counter to the aforementioned scenario. These trends suggest that a backlash is building, and that E-H therapy is on its cutting edge. The recent inclusion of E-H therapy in the American Psychological Association monograph series *Theories of Psychotherapy* (Schneider & Krug, 2010) as well as in its companion video series *Psychotherapy Over Time* (Schneider, 2009) is further indication of E-H therapy's budding and intensifying renaissance. Finally, and not to be neglected, is the compatibility between E-H principles and the landmark research on common or contextual factors as key to effective psychotherapy. As Wampold (2008) puts it, "It could be . . . that an understanding of existential therapy is needed by all therapists, as it adds a perspective that . . . might form the basis of all effective treatments" (p. 6).

On the other hand, I do not want to sound glib about the difficulties E-H and related practice modalities face in the coming years. Medicalization and expedience are here to stay, and there are sound bases for their existence (e.g., Schneider, 2008). But what I do wish to emphasize is that with discernment, focus, and passion, a major transformation can be staged in psychology. This change will not be exclusivist—it will not reject conventional modalities—but it will widen, deepen, and integrate these modalities, and it will weave them into a liberating whole.

SUGGESTIONS FOR FURTHER STUDY

Recommended Reading

Bugental, J. F. T. (1976). *The search for existential identity: Patient–therapist dialogues in humanistic psychotherapy.* San Francisco: Jossey-Bass.—This book is a classic of the E-H case literature. In addition to lively and instructive case synopses, Bugental provides a rare glimpse of himself as he grapples personally with each of his encounters.

Schneider, K. J. (Ed.). (2008). *Existential–integrative psychotherapy: Guideposts to the core of practice.* New York: Routledge.—This edited volume extends E-H therapy to a new, more diverse generation of practitioners. In addition to elaborating an integrative framework for existential–humanistic practice, it also features 20 ethnically and diagnostically diverse case studies, including those by cognitive-behaviorists and psychoanalysts, as well as existential humanists. See also the predecessor of this book edited by Schneider and May, called *The psychology of existence: An integrative, clinical perspective* (1995).

Schneider, K. J., & Krug, O. T. (2010). *Existential–humanistic therapy.* Washington, DC: American Psychological Association.—This book covers the very latest in existential–humanistic theory, practice, and research. It is also highlighted by illuminating case vignettes. Finally, the book is distinguished by an emerging female voice within the movement—Orah Krug.

DVDs

Bugental, J. F. T. (1995). *Existential–humanistic psychotherapy in action.* San Francisco: Psychotherapy. Net. Available at *www.psychotherapy.net.*

May, R. (2007). *Rollo May on existential psychotherapy.* San Francisco: Psychotherapy.Net. Available at *www.psychotherapy.net.*

Schneider, K. J. (2006, 2009). *Existential–humanistic therapy* (Systems of Psychotherapy Video Series). Washington, DC: American Psychological Association. Available at *www.apa.org/videos.*

REFERENCES

Alsup, R. (2008). Existentialism of personalism: A Native American perspective. In K. J. Schneider (Ed.), *Existential–integrative psychotherapy: Guideposts to the core of practice* (pp. 121–128). New York: Routledge.

Ballinger, B., Matano, R., & Amantea, M. (2008). A perspective on alcoholism: The case of Charles. In K. J. Schneider (Ed.), *Existential–integrative psychotherapy: Guideposts to the core of practice* (pp. 177–185). New York: Routledge.

Becker, E. (1973). *Denial of death.* New York: Free Press.

Binswanger, L. (1958). The case of Ellen West. In R. May, E. Angel, & H. Ellenberger (Eds.), *Existence* (pp. 237–364). New York: Basic Books.

Bohart, A. C., & Greenberg, L. S. (Eds.). (1997). *Empathy reconsidered.* Washington, DC: American Psychological Association.

Bohart, A. C., O'Hara, M., & Leitner, L. M. (1998). Empirically violated treatments: Disenfranchisement of humanistic and other psychotherapies. *Psychotherapy Research, 8,* 141–157.

Bohart, A. C., & Tallman, K. (1999). *How clients make therapy work: The process of active self-healing.* Washington, DC: American Psychological Association.

Boss, M. (1963). *Psychoanalysis and daseinsanalysis* (L. B. Lefebre, Trans.). New York: Basic Books.

Bradford, G. K. (2007). The play of unconditional presence in existential-integrative psychotherapy. *Journal of Transpersonal Psychology, 39,* 23–47.

Brown, L. (2008). Feminist therapy as meaning making practice: Where there is no power, where is the meaning? In K. J. Schneider (Ed.), *Existential–integrative psychotherapy: Guideposts to the core of practice* (pp. 130–140). New York: Routledge.

Bugental, E. (2008). Swimming together in a sea of loss: A group process for elders. In K. J. Schneider (Ed.), *Existential –integrative psychotherapy: Guideposts to the core of practice* (pp. 333–342). New York: Routledge.

Bugental, J. F. T. (1976). *The search for existential identity: Patient–therapist dialogues in humanistic psychotherapy.* San Francisco: Jossey-Bass.

Bugental, J. F. T. (1978). *Psychotherapy and process: The fundamentals of an existential–humanistic approach.* New York: McGraw-Hill.

Bugental, J. F. T. (1987). *The art of the psychotherapist.* New York: Norton.

Bugental, J. F. T. (2008). Preliminary sketches for a short-term existential therapy. In K. J. Schneider (Ed.), *Existential–integrative psychotherapy: Guideposts to the core of practice* (pp. 165–168). New York: Routledge.

Bugental, J. F. T., & Bracke, P. (1992). The future of existential–humanistic psychotherapy. *Psychotherapy, 29,* 28–33.

Bugental, J. F. T., & Sterling, M. (1995). Existential psychotherapy. In A. S. Gurman & S. B. Messer (Eds.), *Essential psychotherapies* (pp. 226–260). New York: Guilford Press.

Bunting, K., & Hayes, S. C. (2008). Language and meaning: Acceptance and commitment therapy and the E-I model. In K. J. Schneider (Ed.), *Existential–integrative psychotherapy: Guideposts to the core of practice* (pp. 217–234). New York: Routledge.

Calton, T., Ferriter, M., Huband, N., & Spandler, H. (2008). A systematic review of the soteria program for the treatment of people diagnosed with schizophrenia. *Schizophrenia Bulletin, 34,* 181–192.

Churchill, S., & Wertz, F. J. (2001). An introduction to phenomenological research in psychology: Historical, conceptual, and methodological foundations. In K. J. Schneider, J. F. T. Bugental, & J. F. Pierson (Eds.), *The handbook of humanistic psychology: Leading edges in theory, practice, and research* (pp. 247–262). Thousand Oaks, CA: Sage.

Comas-Diaz, L. (2008). Latino psychospiritualiy. In K. J. Schneider (Ed.), *Existential–integrative psychotherapy: Guideposts to the core of practice* (pp. 100–109). New York: Routledge.

Cooper, M. (2003). *Existential therapies.* London: Sage.

Decker, L. (2007). Combat trauma: Treatment from a mystical/spiritual perspective. *Journal of Humanistic Psychology, 47,* 30–53.

Dorman, D. (2008). Dante's cure: Schizoprenia and the two-person journey. In K. J. Schneider (Ed.), *Existential–integrative psychotherapy: Guideposts to the core of practice* (pp. 236–245). New York: Routledge.

Elkins, D. N. (2007). Empirically supported treatments: Deconstruction of a myth. *Journal of Humanistic Psychology, 47,* 474–500.

Elliott, R. (2002). The effectiveness of humanistic therapies: A meta-analysis. In D. J. Cain & J. Seeman (Eds.), *Humanistic psychotherapies: Handbook of research and practice* (pp. 57–81). Washington, DC: American Psychological Association.

Fischer, C. T. (1994). *Individualizing psychological assessment.* Hillsdale, NJ: Erlbaum. (Original work published 1985)

Fosha, D. (2008). Transformance, recognition of self by self, and effective action. In K. J. Schneider (Ed.), *Existential–integrative psychotherapy: Guideposts to the core of practice* (pp. 290–320). New York: Routledge.

Frankl, V. (1963). *Man's search for meaning.* New York: Pocket Books.

Friedman, M. (1995). The case of Dawn. In K. J. Schneider & R. May (Eds.), *The psychology of existence: An integrative, clinical perspective* (pp. 308–315). New York: McGraw-Hill.

Friedman, M. (2001). Expanding the boundaries of theory. In K. J. Schneider, J. F. T. Bugental, & J. F. Pierson (Eds.), *The handbook of humanistic psychology: Leading edges in theory, practice, and research* (pp. 343–348). Thousand Oaks, CA: Sage.

Galvin, J. (2008). Brief encounters with Chinese clients: The case of Peter. In K. J. Schneider (Ed.), *Existential–integrative psychotherapy: Guideposts to the core of practice* (pp. 168–175). New York: Routledge.

Gendlin, E. T. (1996). *Focusing-oriented psychotherapy.* New York: Guilford Press.

Giorgi, A. (1970). *Psychology as a human science: A phenomenologically based approach.* New York: Harper & Row.

Goldfried, M. R., & Wolfe, B. E. (1996). Psychotherapy practice and research: Repairing a strained alliance. *American Psychologist, 51,* 1007–1016.

Greenberg, L. S. (2007). Emotion coming of age. *Clinical Psychology: Science and Practice, 14*(4), 414–421.

Greenberg, L. S., Rice, L. N., & Elliott, R. (1993). *Facilitating emotional change:The moment-by-moment process.* New York: Guilford Press.

Grondin, J. (1995). *Sources of hermeneutics.* Albany: State University of New York Press.

Hanna, F. J., Giordana, F., Dupuy, P., & Puhakka, K (1995). Agency and transcendence: The experience of therapeutic change. *Humanistic Psychologist, 23,* 139–160.

Heidegger, M. (1962). *Being and time* (J. Macquarrie & E. Robinson, Trans.). New York: Basic Books.

Hoffman, L. (2008). An EI approach to working with religious and spiritual clients. In K. J. Schneider (Ed.), *Existential–integrative psychotherapy: Guideposts to the core of practice* (pp. 187–201). New York: Routledge.

Hoffman, L., Stewart, S., Warren, W., & Meek, L. (2009). Toward a sustainable myth of self: An existential response to the postmodern condition. *Journal of Humanistic Psychology, 49,* 135–173.

Hovarth, A. O. (1995). The therapeutic relationship: From transference to alliance. *In Session, 1,* 7–17.

Husserl, E. (1962). *Ideas: General introduction to pure pheneomenology* (W. R. Boyce Gibson, Trans.). New York: Collier. (Original work published 1913)

James, W. (1936). *The varieties of religious experience.* New York: Modern Library. (Original work published 1902)

Jung, C. G. (1966). *Two essays on analytical psychology* (R. F. C. Hull, Trans.). Princeton, NJ: Princeton University Press.

Kierkegaard, S. (1944). *The concept of dread* (W. Lowrie, Trans.). Princeton, NJ: Princeton University Press. (Original work published 1844)

Krug, O. T. (2009). James Bugental and Irvin Yalom: Two masters of existential therapy cultivate presence in the therapeutic encounter. *Journal of Humanistic Psychology, 49,* 329–354.

Laing, R. D. (Speaker). (1985). *Theoretical and practical aspects of existential therapy* (Cassette Recording No. L330–W1A). The Evolution of Psychotherapy Conference, sponsored by the Erickson Institute, Phoenix, AZ.

Mahrer, A. R. (1996). *The complete guide to experiential psychotherapy.* New York: Wiley.

May, R. (1958). The origins and significance of the existential movement in psychology. In R. May, E. Angel, & H. Ellenberger (Eds.), *Existence* (pp. 3–36). New York: Basic Books.

May, R. (1972). *Power and innocence.* New York: Norton.

May, R. (1981). *Freedom and destiny.* New York: Norton.

May, R. (1983). *The discovery of being.* New York: Norton.

May, R. (2007). (Speaker). *Rollo May on existential psychotherapy* [DVD]. San Francisco: Psychotherapy. net.

Mendelowitz, E. (2008). *Ethics and Lao Tzu: Intimations of character.* Colorado Springs: University of the Rockies Press.

Merleau-Ponty, M. (1962). *The phenomenology of perception* (C. Smith, Trans.). London: Routledge & Kegan Paul.

Messer, S. B., & Wampold, B. E. (2002). Let's face facts, common factors are more potent than specific therapy ingredients. *Clinical Psychology: Science and Practice, 9*(1), 21–25.

Miller, I. J. (1996a). Managed care is harmful to outpatient mental health services: A call for accountability. *Professional Psychology: Research and Practice, 27,* 349–363.

Miller, I. J. (1996b). Time-limited brief therapy has gone too far: The result is invisible rationing. *Professional Psychology: Research and Practice, 27,* 567–576.

Monheit, J. (2008). A lesbian and gay perspective: The case of Marcia. In K. J. Schneider (Ed.), *Existential–integrative psychotherapy: Guideposts to the core of practice* (pp. 140–146). New York: Routledge.

Montuori, M., & Purser, R. (2001). Humanistic psychology and the workplace. In K. J. Schneider, J. F. T. Bugental, & J. F. Pierson (Eds.), *The handbook of humanistic psychology: Leading edges in theory, practice, and research* (pp. 635–644). Thousand Oaks, CA: Sage.

Mosher, L. (2001). Treating madness without hospitals: Soteria and its successors. In K. J. Schneider, J. F. T. Bugental, & J. F. Pierson (Eds.), *The handbook of humanistic psychology: Leading edges in theory, practice, and research* (pp. 389–402). Thousand Oaks, CA: Sage.

Moss, D. (Ed.). (1999). *Humanistic and transpersonal psychology: A historical and biographical sourcebook.* Wesport, CT: Greenwood Press.

Murray, H. A. (1938). *Explorations in personality*. New York: Oxford University Press.

Nietzsche, F. (1982). Twilight of the idols. In W. Kaufmann (Ed.), *The portable Nietzsche* (pp. 465–563). New York: Penguin. (Original work published 1889)

O'Hara, M. (2001). Emancipatory therapeutic practice for a new era: A work of retrieval. In K. J. Schneider, J. F. T. Bugental, & J. F. Pierson (Eds.), *The handbook of humanistic psychology: Leading edges in theory, practice, and research* (pp. 473–489). Thousand Oaks, CA: Sage.

Orlinsky, D. E., Grawe, K., & Parks, B. K. (1994). Process and outcome in psychotherapy—*noch einmal*. In A. E. Bergin & S. L. Garfield (Eds.), *Handbook of psychotherapy and behavior change* (pp. 270–378). New York: Wiley.

Phillips, J. (1980–1981). Transference and encounter: The therapeutic relationship in psychoanalytic and existential therapy. *Review of Existential Psychology and Psychiatry, 17*(2–3), 135–152.

Portnoy, D. (2008). Relatedness: Where humanistic and psychoanalytic approaches converge. In K. J. Schneider (Ed.), *Existential–integrative psychotherapy: Guideposts to the core of practice* (pp. 268–281). New York: Routledge.

Rank, O. (1936). *Will therapy* (J. Taft, Trans.). New York: Knopf.

Rennie, D. L. (1994). Storytelling in psychotherapy: The client's subjective experience. *Psychotherapy, 31*, 234–243.

Rice, D. (2008). An African American perspective: The case of Darrin. In K. J. Schneider (Ed.), *Existential–integrative psychotherapy: Guideposts to the core of practice* (pp. 110–121). New York: Routledge.

Roth, G. (1991). *When food is love*. New York: Plume.

Rowan, J. (2001). Existential analysis and humanistic psychotherapy. In K. J. Schneider, J. F. T. Bugental, & J. F. Pierson (Eds.), *The handbook of humanistic psychology: Leading edges in theory, practice, and research* (pp. 447–464). Thousand Oaks, CA: Sage.

Schneider, K. J. (1985). Clients' perceptions of the positive and negative characteristics of their counselors. *Dissertation Abstracts International, 45*(10), 3345b.

Schneider, K. J. (1995). Guidelines for an existential–integrative (E-I) approach. In K. J. Schneider & R. May (Eds.), *The psychology of existence: An integrative, clinical perspective* (pp. 135–184). New York: McGraw-Hill.

Schneider, K. J. (1998a). Existential processes. In L. S. Greenberg, J. C. Watson, & G. Lietaer (Eds.), *Handbook of experiential psychotherapy* (pp. 103–120). New York: Guilford Press.

Schneider, K. J. (1998b). Toward a science of the heart: Romanticism and the revival of psychology. *American Psychologist, 53*, 277–289.

Schneider, K. J. (1999). *The paradoxical self: Toward an understanding of our contradictory nature* (2nd ed.). Amherst, NY: Humanity Books.

Schneider, K. J. (2004). *Rediscovery of awe: Splendor, mystery, and the fluid center of life*. St. Paul, MN: Paragon House.

Schneider, K. J. (2008). *Existential–integrative psychotherapy: Guideposts to the core of practice*. New York: Routledge.

Schneider, K. J. (2009). *Awakening to awe: Personal stories of profound transformation*. Lanham, MD: Aronson.

Schneider, K. J., & Krug, O. T. (2010). *Existential-humanistic therapy*. Washington, DC: American Psychological Association Press.

Schneider, K. J., & May, R. (Eds.). (1995). *The psychology of existence: An integrative, clinical perspective*. New York: McGraw-Hill.

Seligman, M. E. P. (1996). Science as an ally of practice. *American Psychologist, 51*, 1072–1079.

Serlin, I. A. (1996). Kinesthetic imagining. *Journal of Humanistic Psychology, 36*(2), 25–34.

Spinelli, E. (1997). *Tales of unknowing: Therapeutic encounters from an existential perspective*. London: Duckworth.

Spinelli, E. (2001). A reply to John Rowan. In K. J. Schneider, J. F. T. Bugental, & J. F. Pierson (Eds.), *The handbook of humanistic psychology: Leading edges in theory, practice, and research* (pp. 465–471). Thousand Oaks, CA: Sage.

Sterling, M. (2001). Expanding the boundaries of practice. In K. J. Schneider, J. F. T. Bugental, & J. F. Pierson (Eds.), *The handbook of humanistic psychology: Leading edges in theory, practice, and research* (pp. 349–353). Thousand Oaks, CA: Sage.

Stolorow, R. D. (2008). Autobiographical and theoretical reflections on the "ontological unconscious." In K. J. Schneider (Ed.), *Existential–integrative psychotherapy: Guideposts to the core of practice* (pp. 281–290). New York: Routledge.

Stolorow, R. D., Brandschaft, B., & Atwood, G. E. (1987). *Psychoanalytic treatment: An intersubjective approach.* Hillsdale, NJ: Analytic Press.

Taylor, E. T. (1999). An intellectual renaissance in humanistic psychology? *Journal of Humanistic Psychology, 39*(2), 7–25.

Tillich, P. (1952). *The courage to be.* New Haven, CT: Yale University Press.

Thompson, M. G. (1995). Psychotic clients, Laing's treatment philosophy, and the fidelity to experience in existential psychoanalysis. In K. J. Schneider & R. May (Eds.), *The psychology of existence: An integrative, clinical perspective* (pp. 233–247). New York: McGraw-Hill.

Vontress, C. E., & Epp, L. R. (2001). Existential cross-cultural counseling: When hearts and cultures share. In K. J. Schneider, J. F. T. Bugental, & J. F. Pierson (Eds.), *The handbook of humanistic psychology: Leading edges in theory, practice, and research* (pp. 371–387). Thousand Oaks, CA: Sage.

Wadden, T. A., & Stunkard, A. J. (1986). Controlled trial of very low calorie diet, behavior therapy, and theier combination in the treatment of obesity. *Journal of Consulting and Clinical Psychology, 54*(4), 482–488.

Walsh, R. A., & McElwain, B. (2002). Existential psychotherapies. In D. J. Cain & J. Seeman (Eds.), *Humanistic psychotherapies: Handbook of research and practice* (pp. 253–278). Washington, DC: American Psychological Association.

Wampold, B. E. (2001). *The great psychotherapy debate: Models, methods, findings.* Mahwah, NJ: Erlbaum.

Wampold, B. (2008, February 6). Existential–integrative therapy comes of age [Review of *Existential–integrative psychotherapy: Guideposts to the core of practice*]. *PsycCRITIQUES, 53,* Release 6, Article 1.

Watson, J. C., & Bohart, A. C. (2001). Humanistic–experiential therapies in the era of managed care. In K. J. Schneider, J. F. T. Bugental, & J. E. Pierson (Eds.), *The handbook of humanistic psychology: Leading edges in theory, practice, and research* (pp. 503–517). Thousand Oaks, CA: Sage.

Watson, J. C., & Rennie, D. L. (1994). Qualitative analysis of clients' subjective experience of significant moments during the exploration of problematic experiences. *Journal of Counseling Psychology, 41,* 500–509.

Welwood, J. (2001). The unfolding of experience: Psychotherapy and beyond. In K. J. Schneider, J. F. T. Bugental, & J. F. Pierson (Eds.), *The handbook of humanistic psychology: Leading edges in theory, practice, and research* (pp. 333–341). Thousand Oaks, CA: Sage.

Wertz, F. J. (2001). Humanistic psychology and the qualitative research tradition. In K. J. Schneider, J. F. T. Bugental, & J. F. Pierson (Eds.), *The handbook of humanistic psychology: Leading edges in theory, practice, and research* (pp. 231–245). Thousand Oaks, CA: Sage.

Westen, D., & Morrison, K. (2001). A multidimensional meta-analysis of treatments for depression, panic, and generalized anxiety disorder: An empirical examination of the status of empirically supported theories. *Journal of Consulting and Clinical Psychology, 69,* 875–899.

Wolfe, B. (2008). Existential issues in anxiety disorders and their treatment. In K. J. Schneider (Ed.), *Existential–integrative psychotherapy: Guideposts to the core of practice* (pp. 204–216). New York: Routledge.

Yalom, I. (1980). *Existential psychotherapy.* New York: Basic Books.

Yalom, I. (1989). *Love's executioner.* New York: Basic Books.

PART V

SYSTEMS-ORIENTED APPROACHES

CHAPTER 9

Family Therapies

Nadine J. Kaslow
Jeshmin Bhaju
Marianne P. Celano

HISTORICAL BACKGROUND

The roots of family therapy are found in the social work, marriage and family life education, and marriage counseling movements of the late 1800s and early 1900s. In addition, family therapy has had origins in psychiatry. Many early theorists were psychoanalytically trained clinicians who began including family members in treating individuals. In response to their concerns that the patient's symptoms were maintained by dysfunctional family interactional patterns and that individual therapy was insufficient to change these patterns, they turned to general systems and communication theories to enhance their understanding of complex human interactions. Many present-day family therapy models are systemic and underscore the interrelatedness and reciprocal influences of the individual, family, and larger social system.

Early, first-wave research undergirding family theories and therapy, and stemming from clinician's observations, was conducted with adults with schizophrenia and their families. The seminal paper linking family communication patterns to the development of individual psychopathology was "Toward a Theory of Schizophrenia" (Bateson, Jackson, Haley, & Weakland, 1956). Bateson and colleagues asserted that the essential family determinant in the development of schizophrenia was double-bind communication, in which two or more contradictory messages from the same person require a response guaranteed to meet with disapproval. The double-bind concept is now considered more pertinent to the maintenance than to the etiology of schizophrenia, which is understood to be a biologically based disorder that may be exacerbated by environmental stresses. In addition to Bateson and colleagues and Virginia Satir at the Mental Research Institute in Palo Alto, California, other family therapy founders studied persons with schizophrenia and their families: (1) Theodore Lidz and coworkers Fleck, Cornelison, and R. Lidz; (2) Murray Bowen; (3) Lyman Wynne; (4) Ivan Boszormenyi-Nagy; and (5) Carl Whitaker and his colleagues Tom Malone and John Warkentin. Other early leaders were John Bell, one of the first to conduct

297

sessions with all family members, and Christian Midelfort, who authored the first book solely devoted to family therapy.

Family theories and interventions were applied to families in which the target was the child. Nathan Ackerman, a child psychiatrist and psychoanalyst, asserted that the family is the proper unit of diagnosis and treatment. His article "Family Diagnosis: An Approach to the Preschool Child" (Ackerman & Sobel, 1950) is considered the founding document of the family therapy movement. Consistent with this position and simultaneous with the foregoing developments in understanding family processes in schizophrenia, clinicians who felt frustrated or thwarted in their therapy with children turned their focus to the family as a locus of pathology and a unit for change. This paradigm shift emphasized greater attention to family processes, the interactional context in which individual behavior occurs, and reciprocal influences in families. Some early family research was conducted during this time in child guidance clinics. Salvador Minuchin and colleagues at the Philadelphia Child Guidance Center studied family therapy with delinquents, low-socioeconomic-status families, and psychosomatic families (Minuchin, Montalvo, Guerney, Rosman, & Schumer, 1967).

The second wave (1962–1977) began with the publication of *Family Process*, the first family therapy journal. Training centers were established throughout the country. Emphasis was placed on certification and licensure, with the American Association of Marriage and Family Therapy (AAMFT) recognized as the official accrediting agency for graduate training programs. This decade witnessed the development of competing schools of thought and training models, and an increasing clamor for outcome studies and interactional and process research. The end of this wave was marked by the establishment of the American Family Therapy Academy (AFTA).

The most recent chapter in the history of family therapy encompasses a number of changes. First, there has been an epistemological shift toward second-order cybernetics, which highlights the impact of the observer on his or her observations; thus, it is essential to consider each family member's and the therapist's construction of reality, and how these constructions are influenced by the social context and larger systems within society. According to this postmodern framework, reality is subjective, and there are no universal truths to be discovered by objective observers.

Second, integrative models have been developed that borrow from various family theories and other schools of therapy or are created as integrative approaches (Pinsof, 1995; Sprenkle, Davis, & Lebow, 2009). Third, and relatedly, there has been an increased emphasis on a biopsychosocial perspective (McDaniel, Campbell, Hepworth, & Lorenz, 2005). This focus is evidenced by trends such as attention to gene × environment interactions as related to family-based preventive interventions, consideration of constructs ranging from biology to spirituality in family work, conceptualization of illness within a biopsychosocial context, the well-established field of medical family therapy, and the marriage between pediatric and family psychology.

Fourth, the field has become more sensitive to the diversity of families, with particular emphasis on family organization, ethnicity/race, gender, sexual orientation, social class, and spirituality (Boyd-Franklin, 2003; Celano & Kaslow, 2000; McGoldrick, Giordano, & Garcia-Preto, 2005; McGoldrick & Hardy, 2008; Walsh, 2008). Culturally competent family therapists are cognizant that their interactions with families are informed by not only their professional knowledge, but also their own cultural values, attitudes, customs, beliefs, and practice. They recognize that clinical encounters reflect an engagement between the therapist's and the family's cultural constructions about family life and healthy–abnormal behavior.

Fifth, there have been interorganizational and interdisciplinary efforts to develop a classification schema on relational diagnosis (Beach, Wamboldt, Kaslow, Heyman, & Reiss, 2006). The fourth, text revised edition of the *Diagnostic and Statistical Manual of Mental Disorders* (DSM-IV-TR) includes a Global Assessment Scale of Relational Functioning. Future diagnostic classification schemas may include relational syndromes that are maladaptive in their own right, relational processes that are harmful only in the presence of an individual mental disorder, or relational processes that are relevant to the diagnosis or treatment of a disorder.

Sixth, increased emphasis on empirical study of family therapy principles and methods has been made possible by the development of reliable and valid assessment measures and interactional coding schemas, and the ability to track families and their therapists over the course of treatment. Family psychology has played a pivotal role in refining family research. The growth in complexity of outcome research has been accompanied by efforts to identify change mechanisms that underlie positive clinical outcomes. There has been progress toward establishing evidence-based treatments and ascertaining the effectiveness of family therapy. Importance has been placed on identifying evidence-based principles that guide the application of intervention (e.g., understanding the stages of therapeutic change). There is increased emphasis on qualitative research for understanding family processes and therapy outcomes.

Seventh, there has been a burgeoning of interest in family-oriented prevention efforts. Some of these efforts aim to prevent divorce through premarital programs; others attempt to promote resilience and optimal psychosocial development in children and adolescents at risk for maltreatment or who live with parents with psychiatric illness.

Eighth, ethical guidelines for doing family therapy have been set forth by the AAMFT (Gladding, 2006). Ethical guidelines have been offered to guide research (Hohmann-Marriott, 2001).

Ninth, there has been increased attention to family therapy training and supervision across multiple disciplines and theoretical perspectives. In recent years, training in family therapy generally, and within family psychology more specifically has become more competency-oriented (Celano, Smith, & Kaslow, 2010; Kaslow, Celano, & Stanton, 2005)

Tenth, the field of family psychology has emerged as a specialty during this time, and many family psychologists find their professional home in the Society of Family Psychology, a division of the American Psychological Association. Board certification in couple and family psychology is now available through the American Board of Professional Psychology.

Finally, recent years have witnessed the internationalization of the field, with the development of the International Family Therapy Association and the International Academy of Family Psychologists, and the publication of materials on international family therapy (Kaslow, 2009). Family therapy in the United States has been influenced increasingly by the clinical and theoretical developments throughout the world.

THE CONCEPT OF THE FAMILY

Family theory views the family as the primary unit of focus and interactions between individuals as key. Attempts have been made to integrate individual personality development, family development, and the sociocultural context.

The *nuclear family* traditionally was defined as a group of people connected by blood or legal bonds that shared a residence. This definition has evolved to include groups of people perceived to be a family, united by marriage, blood, or residence sharing. Stepfamilies, cohabiting heterosexual couples and families, same-sex couples and families, foster families, adoptive families, and commuter relationships represent variations of the modern family. Despite changes in the structure of families, the family's primary function continues to be mutual exchange among family members to meet the physical and emotional needs of each individual.

General systems theory (von Bertalanffy, 1950) provides the underpinnings for major family therapy models. A *system* is a group of elements that interact with one another. Families are ongoing and living systems that comprise networks of interrelated parts and are organized around these consistent relationships (*organization*). Families are part of the larger ecological context. Family units continually change and advance toward greater levels of organization and functioning (*anamorphosis*), simultaneously self-regulating to maintain equilibrium (*homeostasis*). When families experience disruption, members strive to regain homeostasis by activity mechanisms to reduce stress and restore stability. The balance between change and stability enables the family to function adaptively throughout the life cycle.

Family systems exchange information via *feedback loops,* circular patterns of responses in which there is a return flow of information within the system. Such information exchanges indicate that the family is experiencing disequilibrium and requires corrective actions to restore relationships to the a priori balanced state. *Positive feedback* increases deviation from the steady state, enabling the family to evolve to a new state and a greater level of change. *Negative feedback* counteracts or attenuates deviations in the system to restore homeostasis.

Family interactions reflect *circular causality* in which single events are viewed as both cause and effect and reciprocally related, with no beginning or end to the sequence of events. Families may be viewed in terms of *structure* and *function.* Structure refers to the family organization, the ways in which the subsystems are arranged, the power hierarchy or chain of command, and the ways in which the unit maintains itself cross-sectionally. The key structural property of the family is its *wholeness* (i.e., the whole is greater than the sum of its parts). The family comprises interdependent and coexisting subsystems that carry out distinctive functions and processes to maintain themselves and sustain the system as a whole. Each individual is his or her own subsystem. Each member belongs to several subsystems simultaneously, providing the basis for differential relationships with other members. Subsystems can be formed by generation, gender, interest, and/or function. The family unit also is a subsystem, as it interacts with the extended family, larger community, and outside world.

Subsystems are delineated by *boundaries,* invisible lines that separate them from their surroundings. Boundaries protect the subsystem's integrity while allowing interaction between subsystems. Boundaries can be more or less permeable and adapt to the changing needs of the family. Impairments in adaptive functioning arise if boundaries are too *rigid,* overly restrictive and not allowing adequate communication between subsystems, or too *diffuse,* overly blurred and allowing too much communication with other subsystems. Excessively rigid boundaries lead to disengagement, in which members are isolated from one another and function autonomously. Diffuse boundaries are associated with enmeshment, in which family members are overinvolved in one another's lives. Family systems have boundaries that regulate transactions with the outside world. An *open system* has flexible and permeable boundaries, permitting interaction with the outside community without compromising the integrity of the family. When families operate as open systems, they are receptive to new experiences and eliminate maladaptive interactional patterns. Conversely, a *closed system* has rigid boundaries, minimizing contact with the outside world. When families are closed, their boundaries are relatively impermeable, they are not able to benefit from what is important in the environment, and they mistrust the outside world. Families exist on the open–closed system continuum.

To maintain their structure, family systems have *rules*, operating principles that enable them to perform the tasks of daily living. Some rules are negotiated openly and are overt, whereas others are unspoken and covert. Healthy families have rules that are consistent, clearly stated, and fairly enforced over time yet can be adapted to the changing developmental needs of the family.

Each member plays a number of *roles*, exhibiting a predictable set of behaviors associated with his or her social position. One's family of origin, gender, and generation within the nuclear family influence role behavior. Roles may include partner, parent, child, sibling, victim, hero, caregiver, martyr, and scapegoat. Optimally, roles are negotiated to accommodate the needs of the unit and the developmental stages of the members, as well as to eliminate dysfunctional roles. Changes in gender roles as a result of societal changes have impacted family functioning as men and women negotiate new interactive patterns and at-home responsibilities.

Family rituals demark family transitions, such as beginnings, endings, separations, and unions, and provide a context within which to notice and honor these changes. They involve symbolic communication and signify the family's identity. Family rituals, along with routines, reflect the family life cycle, developmental regulation, and behavior change. Rituals can be prescribed to intervene in family patterns and promote change by challenging the status quo and opening up new options for family members (Imber-Black, Roberts, & Whiting, 2004).

Family Development

Family development refers to the growth of individual members; changes in the structure, tasks, and interactional process of the family unit over time; and reciprocally related sub-cycles involving the partnership–parental couple, sib-ship, and extended family. Passage through family life cycle stages includes continuous and discontinuous change. Each stage qualitatively is different; developmental tasks are negotiated in new ways. Successful passage depends on the effectiveness of developmentally appropriate negotiations of tasks and stressors. A number of characteristics influence family members' transitions through these family life cycle stages. A member's symptom may reflect the family's difficulty moving from one stage to the next. Interactions at any stage are influenced by interactions at earlier stages; thus, dysfunctional resolution at one stage increases the likelihood of further impairments.

Most families transition through expectable marker events or phases, often preceded by an event. Relationships shift during these various stages, and individuals transverse through various developmental tasks. Commonly reported family life cycle stages include (1) leaving home: single young adults; (2) the joining of families through marriage: the new couple; (3) families with young children; (4) families with adolescents; (5) launching children and moving on; and (6) families in later life (Carter & McGoldrick, 1998). These stages do not fit every family, and there are different development sequences in other families (e.g., single-parent led, divorcing, remarried, gay and lesbian) and in different sociocultural contexts (e.g., immigration).

Normal Family Functioning

Family theorists differ in their views of the applicability of the construct of normality to individual family members, units, or a combination of the two. Normal families (Walsh, 2003) may evidence (1) asymptomatic functioning, (2) optimal functioning (successful according to the values of a given conceptual paradigm), (3) average functioning (fits a typical or prevalent pattern and falls in the normal range), and/or (4) transactional family processes (adaptation over the family life cycle to a particular socioecological context).

Some theorists depict healthy families as comprising individuals who are healthy in physical, spiritual, contextual, nutritional, interactional, sensual, emotional, and intellectual domains. Just as various components of each person's functioning contribute to his or her overall sense of self, each member's sense of self contributes to the overall health of the family. Using a systemic perspective, researchers offer schemas (Beavers & Hampson, 2000) of healthy family functioning. The pattern of characteristics indicative of healthy functioning changes across the family life cycle and depends on the sociocultural context.

Optimally functioning families are cohesive and emotionally bonded, with a strong commitment of members to the unit and a clear yet flexible structure. Generational and individual boundaries are understood, allowing closeness and belonging to coexist, with respect for the privacy of the individual and the subsystems. Healthy families encourage age-appropriate autonomy, express well-modulated emotions, are supportive of and empathically attuned to one another, maintain a sense of humor even in the face of adversity, and are open to feedback. Family members enjoy spending time together, including leisure times. They share beliefs, enabling them to address existential concerns. These transcendent values are transmitted across generations. These families have a worldview that is optimistic, and they are cognizant of their place in the world.

Healthy families adapt their power structure, role relationships, and rules in response to demands and new information. Relatively equal power is the norm for the marital/partnership dyad. A clear power hierarchy exists between the parents and children, and control and authority dynamics are clear to all members. The power dynamics change throughout the family life cycle. Standards for controlling behavior are reasonable, and there is opportunity to modify these standards using negotiation and problem solving. Family functions are filled such that members are not overburdened with too many roles, and there is flexibility in roles played. These families manage stress and crises effectively and recognize when they need community assistance.

They have positive communication and communicate clearly and effectively about their feelings and practical matters. There is congruence between the content and process of the communications (*contextual clarity*), such that few double-binding messages occur. Members communicate appreciation, respect, and affection toward one another.

Attention has been paid to posttraumatic growth at the family systems level and family resilience in response to stress. According to this strengths-based perspective, families are resilient and can grow and evolve in the aftermath of trauma. *Family resilience* refers to successful coping in response to adversity, which enables the members to flourish with warmth, support, and cohesion. Resilient families are characterized by a positive outlook, family member accord, flexibility, adaptive family communication, effective handling of finances, and time spent together, including shared recreation, routines and rituals, and strong support networks.

Pathological or Dysfunctional Family Functioning

Psychiatric nomenclature is less relevant in understanding family pathology than are interaction patterns. The gap between the psychiatric and family systems views is evidenced by the lack of a family classification system in DSM-IV-TR, despite efforts of the Coalition on Family Diagnosis to implement a system (Kaslow, 1996). Instead, the Global Assessment of Relational Functional Scale (GARF; Group for the Advancement of Psychiatry Committee on the Family, 1996) developed by coalition members was included in the DSM-IV-TR appendix.

Recent efforts have been made to influence the DSM-V with regard to describing relationship problems (Beach et al., 2006). Four approaches for including relational issues have been proposed: (1) disordered and general relational processes; (2) nondisordered and general relational processes; (3) disordered and specific relational processes that are components of some disorders and that affect treatment and research for particular disorders; and (4) nondisordered and specific relational processes that affect treatment and research for particular disorders. We hope the proposed frameworks will guide future research and diagnostic efforts.

Family theorists' conceptualizations of dysfunction emphasize the development of family classification schemas or the linking of family interaction patterns to individual pathology. Researchers have described the functioning of family units from healthy/adaptive to severely dysfunctional/extreme along the dimensions of cohesion, change, and communication (Beavers & Hampson, 2000; Olson, 2000). Severely dysfunctional families are inflexible and not adaptable; they fail to change in response to environmental or situational demands or developmental changes. They tend to be undifferentiated and to have poor boundaries, and they fail to provide an environment conducive to the healthy development of each individual and the establishment of trusting relationships. Severely dysfunctional families have a poorly defined power structure, impaired communication, difficulties with problem solving and negotiation, and a pervasively negative affective quality, with minimal expressions of caring and warmth. They lack an appropriate level of cohesion, and are instead disengaged or enmeshed. Heterogeneity in the expression of the family pathology is dependent on the family's characterization on dimensions such as cohesion, adaptability, and communication style.

Although, historically, attention was paid to the etiological role of aberrant family patterns in the development of individual psychopathology, as more has become known regarding the genetic and biological bases of mental illnesses, it is clear that family patterns do not play an etiological role. Thus, there has been an increased focus on the interactive contributions of genes and environment. In addition, attention has been paid to family patterns associated with various disorders throughout the lifespan, without an implication that these patterns are causal, and with an appreciation of a mutual influence between an individual's symptoms and the family's interaction style. Although the initial research focused on families with a loved one with schizophrenia, investigators have established the relationship between family and parent–child interaction patterns and individual disorders (Hooley & Gotlib, 2000) in youth and adults (mood, anxiety, eating, attention deficit, conduct, schizophrenia, substance, personality).

Family patterns influence the course and symptom manifestation of a disorder. One quality that has received much attention is *expressed emotion*; individuals with various forms of psychopathology are vulnerable to relapse if they reside in a family characterized by high

levels of expressed emotion (i.e., critical, hostile, and emotionally overinvolved verbal attitudes expressed toward the child or adult individual with the psychiatric diagnosis; Hooley,
2007). Because the expressed emotion concept implies that part of the problem lies in the
negative attitudes and behaviors of family members, it has become controversial among
family members who feel blamed for their relative's disorder. Increasingly, these constructs
have been linked to the course rather than the etiology of disorders.

Investigators struggle to answer the question; Why are only some family members
symptomatic" Symptoms depend on characteristics of the individual, interactive effects,
and extrafamilial influences. Thus, an individual with considerable personal strengths and
external resources can reside in a dysfunctional family yet function adaptively over time,
whereas another family member who may have fewer strengths and/or resources may be
more vulnerable to developing psychopathology. Each family member's personal characteristics influence how other family members interact with him or her. These interaction patterns in turn affect the individual's level of functioning. Furthermore, individual biological
vulnerabilities also interact with these multiple levels of environmental stressors to create a
complex explanation of the etiology of the manifestation of symptoms in human behavior
and couple/family interactional patterns.

THE PROCESS OF CLINICAL ASSESSMENT

Ideally, assessment is integrated into the therapeutic process. It is cost-effective and yields
an overview of family dynamics, and is useful in problem identification, treatment selection,
evaluation of ongoing therapy, and determination of treatment efficacy. Clinical assessments ascertain appropriate treatment participants, family patterns to be addressed, and
interventions likely to be most effective. Over the course of therapy, assessment is ongoing
and guides the revision of systemic conceptualizations, leads to treatment modifications,
and examines progress.

The therapist's theoretical orientation guides the clinical assessment. Schools of
thought differentially emphasize assessing intrapsychic variables, behavioral functioning,
and systemic patterns. Clinical interviews focus on family history, family structure, family maladaptive behavioral patterns, current interactive patterns, ways in which individual
symptoms impact family functioning and vice versa, and members' view of their world.
Many family therapists agree that while a formal assessment is valuable, it is the process of
interacting with the family over time that yields the richest data.

Multisystem, Multimethod Approach

Family therapists vary on the extent to which they use formal approaches to assessment.
Formal assessments incorporate a multisystem, multimethod approach; evaluate the individual, various dyads, and the family system; and use clinical interview techniques and multiple standard assessment methods. Tools can be divided into self-report measures, observational data, and interactional coding schemas.

Self-Report Measures

Self-report measures are easy and inexpensive to administer and score, useful in assessing
family relations and processes, and can measure change and intervention effectiveness.

However, they do not adequately assess several key variables (e.g., family power), and they measure individual differences rather than a system and its interrelationships. The most frequently used and psychometrically sound self-report measures include the Family Assessment Device (Epstein, Baldwin, & Bishop, 1983), the Family Assessment Measure (Skinner, Steinhauer, & Sitarenios, 2000), the Family Environment Scale (Moos & Moos, 1994), the Family Adaptability and Cohesion Evaluation Scales (Olson, in press), and the Beavers Self-Report Family Inventory (Beavers, Hampson, & Hulgus, 1985).

Observational/Clinician-Rated Methods

Research over the last 25 years has evolved from self-report methodology focused on individuals to a multimethod approach that accommodates a systems perspective and integrates data gleaned from observation. Direct observation provides information regarding the complexities of the interactional processes of which family members may or may not be conscious. They offer an outsider's perspective on the family's functioning. Observational measurements are obtained by rating specified nonverbal and verbal interactions of given subsystems in response to a structured task completed in a standard setting. The resulting data are reduced via a coding schema to glean meaning from the complex set of behaviors exchanged among family members. Most coding schemas assess dimensions that discriminate between normal and dysfunctional families. Coding schemas assess family interactions from a microanalytic or macroanalytic perspective. Recently, family observational measures were assessed with regard to their evidence base. Five measures were deemed "well established" (Alderfer et al., 2007). These include the Beavers Interactional Scales (Beavers & Hampson, 1990), the McMasters Clinical Rating Scale (Miller et al., 1994), the Family Mealtime Interaction Coding System (Dickstein, Hayden, Schiller, Seifer, & San Antonio, 1994), the Circumplex Clinical Rating Scale (Olson & Gorall, 2003), and the Iowa Family Interaction Rating Scale (Melby et al., 1998).

FAMILY THERAPY MODELS

There is not one brand of family therapy; we would do a disservice to depict the practice of family therapy as homogenous. This section focuses on some of the most widely practiced and influential schools of family therapy. There is inconsistency regarding how to categorize the various approaches; our presentation reflects one possible division. These schools are presented in a sequence organized by the extent to which they emphasize the past versus the present, and intrapsychic versus interpersonal dimensions. The psychodynamically informed and intergenerational approaches emphasize primarily the past. However, the psychoanalytic perspective also primarily focuses on intrapsychic issues, whereas the intergenerational models address intrapsychic and interpersonal dimensions equally. Bowen therapy would ordinarily be included, but because it is couple-focused, it is discussed by Gurman in Chapter 10 (this volume). The experiential–humanistic brands of family therapy occupy the middle of both spectrums, placing relatively equal emphasis on past and present, and on intrapsychic and interpersonal dimensions. Strategic, systemic, structural, cognitive-behavioral, psychoeducational, multisystemic, and postmodern/social constructivist approaches focus on the present and on interpersonal factors. Integrative models vary on the extent to which they focus on the past versus the present, and on intrapsychic versus interpersonal variables. To facilitate comparison of the various schools, our presentation considers the basic structure of the therapy, goals, techniques and process of therapy, role of the therapist, curative factors, treatment applicability, and evidence base.

Psychodynamically Informed Family Therapy

As many family therapy pioneers were trained in the psychoanalytic tradition, psychodynamic concepts have been integral to the development of several family therapy models. However, given many family therapists' rebellion against the historically individual focus associated with the psychoanalytic tradition, continuities between psychoanalytic and family theories have been minimized. Psychodynamically informed family therapy is one of the only models that acknowledges its ties to psychoanalytic thinking, valuing the role of the unconscious and past history in determining behavior and motivations, the necessity of insight for behavior change, and the importance of transference and countertransference dynamics.

Ackerman, the "grandfather" of family therapy, is the most noted early, psychoanalytically oriented family therapist. Other early key figures include James Framo, Boszormenyi-Nagy, A. C. R. Skynner, Norman Paul, and John Bell. Recently, some writers have integrated psychoanalytic theory with family systems models, referring to their work as *object relations family therapy* (Scharff, 1989). Attention to patterns of attachment in family relationships lends an understanding of the interpersonal dynamics inherent in behavior. When family members respond inappropriately to attachment behavior, such as prematurely forecasting loss, there is a need to attend to these patterns. Therefore, psychodynamically oriented family therapists instill a sense of safety within the system to enable the family to explore new ways of relating. In bridging psychodynamic tenets and systems theory, these therapists attend to the complex interplay among each individual's personality and background, family interactional processes, and the sociocultural context.

Family-of-origin experiences provide the foundation for sense of self, internalized images of significant others (*introjects*), and expectations for close relationships. Symptomatic behavior represents unresolved conflicts that stem from one's family of origin and are reenacted with one's family of creation. Reenactment occurs via individuals' use of projection of introjected "bad objects" (negative internalized image of one's parent[s]) onto significant others in adult life. Interpersonal interactions unconsciously are interpreted to be consistent with one's inner object world of positive and negative introjects. Each person unconsciously seeks a mate who will be a willing recipient of lost and split-off introjects, resulting in a collusive partnership.

A family member's symptom becomes part of a recurring, predictable, interactional pattern that ensures equilibrium for the individual but impairs the family's ability to adapt to change due to rigid, stereotypical, or rapidly shifting family roles. Such role distortions and the breakdown of role complementarity are associated with intrapsychic and interpersonal conflicts, often occurring simultaneously and exacerbating each other. Unresolved conflicts often result in the unconscious placement of a family member in a role in which he or she is consistently exposed to criticism and blamed for the family tension (*scapegoating*). Scapegoating further validates negative introjects, thus exacerbating individual symptoms and family dysfunction.

Central to object relations theory is the idea that attachment as an infant determines personality development; therefore, the cultivation of secure attachment is central to an individual's sense of self. The assertion and resolution of needs over time within close family relationships lead to an individual's personality development or vulnerability to psychopathology. Understanding of attachment style and provision of a safe attachment or holding environment lend the essential information and the circumstances necessary to decipher dysfunctional patterns and address core dynamics responsible for these patterns.

Basic Structure of Therapy

Object relations family therapy is conducted weekly and is long term to address unresolved intrapsychic conflicts reenacted in one's current life and causing interpersonal and intrapsychic difficulties. Session membership may vary based on the presenting problem and goals of each phase of the work. Membership may include family of origin, family of creation, intimate partner dyad, and/or the individual. Concurrent treatments may be conducted. Sessions are relatively unstructured. Although the therapist provides the external structure, the family's interactions and comments provide the internal structure.

Goal Setting

The goals are relatively similar across families with a variety of problems and are implicit rather than overtly discussed and negotiated. Goals are not differentiated into intermediate- and long term. These therapies help family members achieve increased insight; strengthen ego functioning; acknowledge and rework defensive projective identifications; attain more mature self and object representations; develop more satisfying relationships supporting their needs for attachment, individuation, and psychological growth; and reduce interlocking pathologies among family members. The desired outcome is for members to have more access to their true selves, become more intimate with the true selves of significant others, and view others realistically rather than as projected parts of themselves. This enables the family to achieve a developmental level consistent with the needs of its members and the tasks to be addressed.

Techniques and Process of Therapy

In the initial phase, the therapist provides a frame, a *holding environment*, consisting of a specified time, space, and structure for the therapy. The therapist observes family interactions during an open-ended interview to ascertain members' level of object relations, predominant defense mechanisms, and the relation between current interactional patterns and family-of-origin dynamics. A comprehensive history is conducted with all members present, with attention to family-of-origin dynamics, early experiences, presenting problems, and treatment history. Object relations family therapists view the examination of family history as essential to the conceptualization of current family functioning.

Establishing a *therapeutic alliance* is key. Once established, the therapist interprets conflicts, defenses, and patterns of interaction. Interpretations address dynamics of individual members and/or various family subsystems. Interpretations link an individual or family's history with current feelings, thoughts, behaviors, and interactions, permitting more adaptive family interactional patterns and intrapsychic changes. In making empathic interpretations, the therapist relies on theoretical knowledge and affective responses to each person and the unit.

The primary techniques are *interpretations of resistance, defenses, negative transference*, and *interaction patterns* indicative of unresolved family-of-origin and intrapsychic conflicts. To facilitate change, therapists address external and internal resistances, and transference and countertransference dynamics. Therapists use their own reactions to family members' behavior and interaction patterns (*objective countertransference*) to understand empathically the shared yet unspoken experiences of each member regarding family interactional patterns (*unconscious family system of object relations*). Therapists employ their objective countertransference reactions to interpret interpersonal patterns in which one member is induced to behave in a circumscribed and maladaptive fashion (*projective identification*).

The therapist attends to termination each session and toward the end of the therapy. Time boundaries for ending sessions and the therapy course are respected, communicating the therapist's commitment as a consultant to the change process. The ending of each session raises issues of loss and separation that need to be worked through in preparation for termination. The therapist addresses how the family's history and present system of object relationships interfere with healthy, autonomous functioning. Discussions and interpretations regarding conflicts and feelings of separation and mourning precipitated by the finite nature of sessions help the family prepare for termination of the therapy. During the termination phase, salient conflicts are reviewed, and unresolved family transferences are reworked. There is an opportunity for mourning the loss of the therapist, who has become a significant attachment figure.

The Stance of the Therapist

Of utmost importance is the provision of a "good enough" holding environment, where the therapist enables family members to feel safe and secure, so that they can express openly their feelings and beliefs, and feel more intimate with one another, while maintaining a sense of self. The therapist functions as a "good enough" parent, reparenting the family by providing consistent nurturance, a secure attachment, and structure (e.g., limit setting) to enhance the development of individual members and the family unit.

Curative Factors

Therapy focuses on individuals' early family experiences, feelings about one another, and relationships. Primary mechanisms of change are interpretations of interpersonal patterns, including transference and countertransference dynamics, offered in the context of a positive working alliance and a safe holding environment. Interpretations help family members gain both historic–genetic and interactional insights into their psychological realities. Although the therapy does not directly teach more adaptive interpersonal skills, the development of these skills is an outgrowth of increased insight. Effective management of affects elicited during the termination process is considered crucial to a successful outcome, as it provides the individual an opportunity to rework unresolved separation issues related to family of origin.

There are specific techniques associated with object relations family therapy. Techniques, however, are considered secondary to the therapist–family relationship in defining this approach. Rather, the defining characteristic is the therapist's joining with the family and creating a safe holding environment in which family members rediscover each other and the lost parts of the self projected onto one another. Although most therapies emphasize the therapeutic relationship, psychodynamically oriented family therapists focus on the relationship as a curative factor and use transference interpretations as a cornerstone of the treatment. Given the importance of addressing countertransference dynamics, the therapist's psychological health and his or her family-of-origin dynamics influence the treatment process. The therapist needs to address unresolved intrapsychic and interpersonal conflicts in supervision and personal treatment.

Treatment Applicability

Clinicians typically use object relations family therapy with high-functioning families in which none of the members is severely disturbed. These families tend to be psychologically minded, educated, and interested in gaining insight, and they possess the resources necessary to engage in long-term treatment. Some also have advocated its use in families with a schizophrenic, borderline, or narcissistic family member (Scharff, 1989). This approach also has been practiced with families with young children, school-age children, and adolescents; families of divorce and remarriage; and families coping with trauma, loss, or death.

Evidence Base

The only family-based intervention that falls within the rubric of psychodynamically informed family therapy is attachment-based family therapy (ABFT), a semistructured, manualized treatment tailored specifically to the needs of depressed adolescents and their families (Diamond, Reis, Diamond, Siqueland, & Isaacs, 2002). This model seeks to repair ruptures in the attachment relationship and build trust between adolescents and parents. It uses five treatment tasks: relational reframing, alliance building with both parent and adolescent, reattachment (i.e., rebuilding an emotional family attachment bond), and promotion of competency. ABFT is a promising treatment for depressed adolescents. Compared to a minimal contact control group, ABFT was more successful in decreasing depression, anxiety, hopelessness, and suicidal ideation, and was linked to greater improvements in mother–adolescent attachments, with a medium effect size of 0.72 (Diamond et al., 2002). Data also support ABFT for anxious adolescents (Siqueland, Rynn, & Diamond, 2005). It is associated with reduced anxiety and depression, and appears to be as effective as cognitive-behavioral therapy for this population.

Intergenerational–Contextual Family Therapy

Intergenerational–contextual family therapy, associated with Boszormenyi-Nagy, Grunebaum, and Ulrich (1991), is an outgrowth of psychodynamically informed family therapy. It emphasizes both intrapsychic and interpersonal dynamics, focuses on both the past and the present, and stresses concepts of legacy, loyalty, indebtedness to one's family of origin, and the profound influence of one's biological roots. *Loyalties* are structured expectations to which family members are committed. One's fundamental loyalty is to the maintenance of the family, not to self-differentiation. Family members maintain a ledger of *merits* (investments into relationships) and *debts* (obligations) for each relationship. This ledger changes according to family members' *investments* (e.g., supporting others) and *withdrawals* (e.g., exploiting others). When perceived injustices occur, repayment of psychological debts is expected. Every family maintains a *family ledger,* a multigenerational accounting system of who owes what to whom. Obligations rooted in past generations covertly influence the behavior of family members in the present (*invisible loyalties*). Dysfunction results when individuals or families feel they have chronically imbalanced or unresolved ledgers. This diminishes the level of trust, which may result in destructive entitlement or overindebtedness, or in scapegoating of an identified patient. To understand the etiology, function, and maintenance of individual symptoms, one must consider the history of the problem, the family ledger, and unsettled individual accounts.

Basic Structure of Therapy

Intergenerational–contextual therapy is intensive, long-term therapy for individuals and families, and may include multigenerational family sessions. A cotherapy team can conduct this work most effectively, providing a balanced model to the family unit, complementing one another. The therapist maintains control of the sessions, encouraging members to express themselves openly and validating each individual's worth.

Goal Setting

The goals are universal and not dependent on family characteristics. The therapy aims to identify and address invisible or hidden loyalties within the family; recognize unsettled individual and family accounts; rebalance in actuality one's obligations (*rejunction process*) to repair ruptured or strained relationships, and develop adaptive ways of relating, more trusting relationships, and an equitable balance of give and take among family members; and develop a preventive plan for current and future generations. Although symptom alleviation and amelioration of distress are important intermediate goals, developing self–object delineation and responsible engagement within relationships (*self-validation*) are the overriding aims.

Techniques and Process of Therapy

Assessment involves creating a trusting atmosphere, so that family members feel safe to express their sense of entitlement and indebtedness. One method used to develop a trusting therapeutic environment, *multidirected partiality*, refers to the therapist's acknowledgment of each individual's perspective on an issue. Having one's views acknowledged leads to an increased capacity to communicate and listen to others. A comprehensive history is taken, focusing on facts, psychology, interactional patterns, and relational ethics. Emphasis is placed on the construct of the *genogram* (McGoldrick, Gerson, & Petry, 2008), a graphic depiction of a historical family system that can be useful in understanding family patterns. A three-or-more-generation genogram enables the therapist(s) to help the family ascertain the fairness and violations of fairness between family members and generations. In contrast to other family therapists with practices rooted in psychoanalytic theory, intergenerational–contextual family therapists conceptualize assessment as integral to developing a trusting relationship with the family and to the ongoing therapeutic process.

During the working-through phase, the therapist acknowledges the family's defenses and resistances. Family interactions during sessions are discussed in light of each individual's object relations. Techniques include the therapists' siding with each member to maintain multidirectional partiality, crediting each member for efforts to help the family, encouraging mutual accountability to replace mutual blame, and using the *rejunction process* of giving due credit. Issues of loss, separation, and abandonment are discussed during the termination phase. Successful termination occurs when individuals face invisible loyalties in the family and rebalance unsettled accounts.

Throughout the treatment the cotherapists facilitate the work via empathic involvement in the family, acknowledgment of each member's contribution, and investment in the trustworthiness of familial relationships. Although the cotherapists are catalysts for the change process, the actual work done by the family may include meetings at home, family rituals, and other activities between sessions. Coaching may be used to help individual members change themselves in the context of their family of origin, and define themselves proactively in their relationships without emotionally disengaging or giving in. Coaching involves teaching members to observe and research their own role in their family patterns, enabling them to be genuine in their family interactions. Homework (e.g., writing letters, visiting one's family of origin) may be assigned to help members develop more positive and trusting relationships. The most common resistances occur when the family remains fixated in symbiotic or distanced relationships and the regressive forces of therapy are experienced as intolerable. In such instances, therapy is rejected.

Less serious resistance is evident when members find the in-depth reworking of family relationships too painful and prefer only the alleviation of the presenting problem. Although this goal is acceptable, the therapists communicate that lasting change requires successful rebalancing of individual and family ledgers. As is the case with all insight-oriented therapies, other common resistances include the mobilization of defense mechanisms, failure to develop new insights, and an unwillingness to be accountable. Family members are encouraged to face the relational ethical issues from which their resistances derive, define their positions regarding these issues, and move toward multilateral consideration of one another's interests.

The Stance of the Therapist

The therapy typically is conducted by cotherapists who align with the healthy aspects of the family. The cotherapy team communicates empathy, compassion, flexibility, complementarity, creativity, and a concern for members' capacities for individuation and relatedness. The therapists are catalysts for the work, take an active role in the process, and communicate that members can help heal one another. They encourage the family to rebalance accounts and suggest alternative interaction patterns. However, the therapeutic task belongs to the family, and members are held accountable for their actions.

Curative Factors

The primary curative mechanism is the development of a trusting alliance between the family and the therapists, a process that may be enhanced by pertinent self-disclosures on the part of the therapists. Reframing the presenting problem as reflecting unbalanced family ledgers or loyalty conflicts is an additional mechanisms for change. Reframing paves the way to the redressing of the imbalances in the nuclear and extended family.

Individuals are helped to face their distortions about family members by learning more about their histories. This knowledge enables them to have more compassion for family members, and to exonerate their parents and rebalance their relational account of debts and merits. This work frequently includes the involvement of the parental and grandparental generation to rebalance one's accounts. In these multigenerational sessions, feelings are openly expressed to develop a more meaningful dialogue and more positive interactions, which relieves the grandchildren of the burden of unsettled accounts passed through the generations.

Insight into family-of-origin dynamics is crucial to the change and healing process. Insight is achieved through dialogic relating induced by the therapist. Insight is not sufficient for change; rather, lasting change entails efforts at rejunction, or giving due credit. Enhanced relational capacities, a vital outcome of the work, are not conceptualized as skills that can be taught. Rather, it is assumed that individuals benefit from the rewarding interactions that are an outgrowth of the rejunction process, which in turn enables them to relate in a healthier fashion.

The most important transference distortions are between family members. Transference reactions may occur between family members and therapists, in which the therapists are seen as the parents. The therapists manage this transferential process by helping members understand and modify their relationships, and by underscoring the importance of family roles. This occurs in a context of nurturance in which the therapist reparents to support the rejunction process.

The therapist's personal maturity and the degree to which he or she has worked through a sense of entitlement and is conscious of family loyalties influences his or her capacity for multidirectional partiality, which affects the effectiveness of the rejunction process and thus the therapy. Countertransference reactions are resources for deepening one's engagement in the multilateral process and, if well understood, can enhance the rejunction process.

Treatment Applicability

Intergenerational–contextual family therapy is applicable to many clinical problems. However, it may be most efficacious in conjunction with other established treatments for individual symptoms (e.g., medications, substance abuse treatment).

Evidence Base

There are no empirical studies of the efficacy of this family therapy approach.

Experiential and Humanistic Family Therapies: Symbolic–Experiential Family Therapy

Experiential and humanistic family therapies conceptualize dysfunctional behavior as a failure to fulfill one's potential for personal growth. These therapies emphasize family members' present experiences and affects, and their associated meanings. A number of theorists have been identified with the experiential–humanistic school, most notably Whitaker and Keith (Keith, Connell, & Connell, 2001; Whitaker & Keith, 1981), and Satir (1988). Although these individuals have worked with families differently, they share common philosophical tenets. First, all believe that change results not from emotional catharsis or insight, but from the immediacy of the relationship and process cocreated by the family and an involved therapist. Second, they strive to behave as real, authentic individuals in their interactions with clients, a stance that promotes spontaneity as well as idiosyncratic interventions. Finally, all emphasize choice, free will, human capacity for self-determination, and self-fulfillment. Whitaker's approach is detailed here; Satir's contributions to couple therapy are addressed by Gurman in Chapter 10 (this volume).

Symbolic–experiential family therapy (SEFT) was developed by Whitaker and associates at Emory University in Atlanta and later at the University of Wisconsin–Madison. Whitaker's approach is atheoretical; theory is viewed as a hindrance to clinical practice. His views, however, on the healthy family and the dysfunctional family have been articulated, particularly as they influence the therapy process (Roberto, 1991).

Basic Structure of Therapy

SEFT is time-unlimited and of intermediate duration. It is conducted at a variable frequency, usually weekly or biweekly, with monthly sessions in the latter phases. Sessions optimally include the symptomatic family member, nuclear family residing with the symptomatic person, extended families, and the index person's social support network. Therapy usually is conducted by a cotherapy team or a therapist and a consultant.

Goal Setting

The ultimate goals of SEFT apply to all dysfunctional family units. The operationalization of these goals is developed by the family and the cotherapy team based on the family's relational patterns. Ultimate goals are to (1) increase members' perceptions of belongingness and cohesion, (2) help the family facilitate each member's individuation and completion of developmental tasks, and (3) foster the creativity ("craziness") and spontaneity of the family and its members. Mediating goals include disorganizing rigid recycling of interaction to allow for more adaptive responses; activating and allowing constructive anxieties by positively refraining symptoms as efforts toward competence; expanding the presenting problem to include each members' role in the dysfunction; encouraging and supporting new decisions; creating transgenerational boundaries, and creating a therapeutic suprasystem in which the family and cotherapy team develop a shared meaning system and inter-member alliances.

Techniques and Process of Therapy

During the beginning phase, therapists engage the family in a nonthreatening manner, using metaphors, reframing, and humor. The *battle for structure* and the *battle for initiative* must be fought before the family trusts the cotherapists enough to allow them to help the family reorganize (Whitaker & Keith, 1981). The battle for structure is the conflict over rules about treatment structure, session membership, scheduling, and fees. This battle is completed when a minimum of a two-generational structure to the therapy is established, with the therapist(s) in charge and having maximal freedom to move in and out of the family system. If successfully won, this battle induces regression in the family, engenders an intense transference relationship, and communicates that therapy is "serious business." In the battle for initiative, which occurs after the therapeutic structure is established, the cotherapy team encourages the family to take initiative for their own growth, and responsibility for life decisions. This battle is resolved when the cotherapy team establishes an existential adult-to-adult relationship with each member, with involvement in the therapeutic exchange by all participants.

In the middle phase, the family addresses its life difficulties with the help of the cotherapists, who have become personally involved with family members. Throughout this phase, techniques are imlemented to facilitate change and create alternative interaction patterns that reduce scapegoating and blame of the caretaking parent. These techniques include redefining symptoms as efforts toward growth; explicating covert conflict; separating interpersonal and internal stress, and modeling fantasized alternatives to stress; the therapists' use of self, including unconscious material, absurdity, and "acting-in" (affective confrontation of family members by the therapist); involving grandparents and other extended family members in treatment; and reversing roles (Roberto, 1991). More recently, attention has been paid to the use of play with families during this phase, in a modality referred to as *family play therapy* (Gil, 1994). The middle phase may yield positive results, with the family working effectively in the therapy or solving problems effectively on their own, or lead to an impotence impasse, in which the family does not change or take responsibility for its own problems. This impasse is successfully negotiated when decisions about treatment are mutually agreed on between the family and the cotherapy team.

In the end phase, the cotherapy team disentangles itself from the family and takes a more peripheral role, intervening only when necessary. The family observes its own functioning and takes responsibility for solving problems. Thus, the cotherapy team and the family work as equal partners. This relational shift is facilitated by several techniques, including therapists' spontaneous self-disclosure, expression of grief regarding termination, and requests for feedback about the therapy. The family and cotherapy team part with the recognition of mutual interdependence and loss. Termination is indicated when members appear self-confident and the family demonstrates that it possesses the resources to resolve problems and tolerate life stress.

The Stance of the Therapist

SEFT is typically conducted by a cotherapy team, enabling each therapist to perform unique functions and to interchange these functions when indicated. The cotherapy team models adaptive interpersonal relationships and provides experiential alternatives for family interactions. SEFT therapists are actively engaged in the family's interactional process, yet do not direct the therapy. They listen, observe, attend to their own affective reactions, and intervene to change the family's functioning without focusing on etiology. These therapists openly express warmth and caring for the family and use their personalities (true self) in sharing their internal processes with the family without losing their differentiated sense of self. They are like "coaches" or surrogate grandparents, roles that require structure and discipline, as well as caring and availability. Emphasis on participant observation underscores the family's responsibility for change, even though the therapists are responsible for the interventions. Resistances are considered inevitable in the change process and are not interpreted. Rather, they are managed with a combination of challenge, support, and humor.

Curative Factors

The basic assumption of SEFT is that families change as a result of experiences, not through education or interpretation. Chief mechanisms for change are the experience of new relational stances with family members, the expression of strong emotions, and the challenging of current interactional patterns, all of which lead to interactional insights. Interactional insights are considered more prominent and effective than are historical insights. The therapists' own roles within their families of origin and creation affect their interactions with the family and the cotherapist. Therefore, family therapy for the therapist is strongly encouraged.

Treatment Applicability

SEFT has been used with families in which the index person presents with a range of problems, including severe psychopathology. However, it is difficult to use this approach with families with a member with a severe personality disorder. For families coping with a trauma, this treatment may be emotionally overwhelming and thus contraindicated.

Evidence Base

Empirical studies of this approach have not yet appeared. The conduct of such research largely runs counter to the experiential and humanistic nature of the approach.

Strategic Family Therapy

A number of family therapists can be classified as strategic family therapists: (1) the communications school of the Mental Research Institute (MRI) group and, later, the Brief Therapy Center in Palo Alto, California, which initially included Gregory Bateson, Don Jackson, John Weakland, Jay Haley, and Virginia Satir and later added Paul Watzlawick, Richard Fisch, and Arthur Bodin; and (2) Haley (1976) and Madanes's (1991) *problem-solving therapy*. Strategic therapy approaches are influenced heavily by Bateson's focus on communication processes and the strategic therapy of Milton Erickson. These approaches view problems as maintained by maladaptive family interaction sequences, including faulty and incongruent hierarchies and malfunctioning triangles. The behavioral sequences observed in the family's attempts at problem resolution are assumed to perpetuate the problem. These sequences are viewed as complex and circular rather than linear; therefore, change within the family system is a necessary prerequisite for individual change.

Strategic approaches are ahistorical, emphasizing present interactions and communications rather than the past. They attend to metacommunications among family members, focusing on the covert, nonverbal messages that amplify or change the meaning of overt, verbal messages. The presenting problem is an analogical message, a metaphor for underlying dysfunction. For example, siblings' arguments over trivial matters may reflect their power and/or attachment struggles. Haley and Madanes's model is described as illustrative of strategic approaches.

Basic Structure of Therapy

Strategic therapies are brief interventions that may include the whole family or only one or two members. Sessions occur weekly or biweekly and are conducted by a single therapist. The approach is structured, as the therapist directs the questioning, gives directives, and intervenes actively.

Goal Setting

The primary goal is solving the family's presenting problem. Initial goals are formulated as increases in positive behaviors rather than reduction of problematic behaviors. This formulation helps the family feel motivated, as success seems possible. Long-term goals include altering the interaction sequences maintaining the problem and helping members resolve a crisis and progress to the next stage of the family and individual life cycle.

Successful strategic therapy achieves *second-order change*, fundamental changes in the family system's structure and functioning, rather than *first-order change*, superficial modifications that do not affect the structure of the system itself. In a family with an oppositional adolescent son, first-order change occurs when the parents become more lenient and the son becomes more willing to comply with parental requests. In contrast, second-order change is evident when the son demonstrates more responsible behavior in the context of age-appropriate separation from the parents, and the parents no longer need to triangulate their son in their relationship. In such cases, the strengthening of executive power hierarchy is concurrent with an increased level of intimacy within the marital/partnership subsystem, and the adolescent forms more age-appropriate peer relationships without engaging in self- or other-destructive behavior.

Techniques and Process of Therapy

The therapy occurs in stages until the presenting problem is resolved and other treatment goals are achieved. The first stage encompasses the initial interview, in which the problem and the context within which it is embedded are ascertained. This interview includes five stages: (1) *social stage*—therapist makes direct contact with each member, makes initial hypotheses, and matches the family's mood; (2) *problem stage*—therapist asks questions regarding the problem; (3) *interaction stage*—therapist asks members to talk with one another about the problem and observes communication patterns; (4) *goal-setting stage*— therapist specifies the desired changes in behavioral terms; and (5) *task-setting stage*—therapist gives the family a directive designed to alter dysfunctional interaction sequences.

Once the problem and goals are defined, the therapist formulates a therapeutic approach consisting of an overall plan for a series of tactical interventions (*directives*). Directives are used to change the underlying interaction sequences maintaining the problem; to intensify the therapeutic relationship; and to gather information about family members, particularly their resistance to change. Straight directives, designed to elicit the family's cooperation with the therapist's request, are useful in crisis situations or with family members committed to change. They attempt to alter out-of-session interaction patterns.

Other techniques to alter dysfunctional behavioral sequences include *paradoxical directives* (a directive that will be resisted, therefore producing change in the desired direction); *reframing* (providing a new meaning for the symptom, such as relabeling the problem behaviors in a positive light); *ordeals* (recommending that a member engage in a behavior he or she dislikes but one that would improve a family relationship); *pretending* (directing a member to "pretend" to exhibit his or her symptom, casting the symptom as voluntary and thus altering members' reactions); *unbalancing* through creating alternative coalitions; and prescribing *homework*. There are many forms of paradoxical interventions: (1) therapeutic use of *double-bind communication*; (2) *positioning*, in which the therapist accepts and exaggerates family members' position, underscoring its absurdity and therefore forcing them to consider a different view; (3) *restraining*, in which the therapist discourages change by enumerating its dangers; and (4) *symptom prescription*, in which the therapist provides a compelling rationale for the family member to practice his or her symptom.

The time-limited nature and problem-solving focus of this therapy make termination a natural process. Families are ready to terminate when significant and durable improvements in the presenting problem have occurred, and family members handle their problems without the therapist's help. During the termination phase, the family is given credit for progress, yet cautioned against developing false optimism that problems will not return.

For families hesitant about terminating, termination may be framed as a break from therapy in which gains are consolidated.

The Stance of the Therapist

Strategic therapists are active and present in a powerful, authoritative, and charismatic fashion, using their powers of persuasion to convince a family to follow a precise directive, whether straightforward or paradoxical. These therapists have been considered by some to be manipulative in implementing their interventions, as is the case when they recommend that a couple chronically in conflict fight at planned times during the day for a specified period. The therapist intervenes when he or she chooses rather than when the family requests participation. Strategic therapists avoid being aligned with one family faction; however, they voluntarily take sides to overcome an impasse.

Curative Factors

Techniques are of paramount importance in effecting change. Curative factors include correcting the hierarchy by encouraging the parental subsystem to utilize its power effectively and appropriately, helping family members negotiate agreements, and reuniting family members in an effort to heal old wounds. Insight is not valued, and interpretations are rare. Family members are not educated directly in interpersonal skills, yet the directives often require the development of a more adaptive interpersonal style. Change in the index person's problem behavior is inextricably interwoven with systemic changes.

Treatment Applicability

Haley's problem-solving therapy and the MRI group's strategic therapy approaches have been applied successfully to families in which members suffer from schizophrenia, anorexia, substance abuse, violence, or anxiety disorders. Madanes adapted strategic family therapy for incestuous families and developed an intervention for reparation.

Evidence Base

Although few controlled studies have addressed efficacy, there is empirical support for the use of brief strategic approaches with high-risk Latino youth (Kazdin, 2002). Szapocznik and colleagues' brief strategic family therapy (BSFT), based on structural and strategic principles (see "Integrative Models") reduces behavior problems and improves family interactions in Latino families (Szapocznik & Willliams, 2000). Interventions integrating strategic and structural approaches effectively reduce adolescent drug abuse.

Systemic Family Therapy

Systemic family therapy was pioneered in Italy by the Milan group, originally consisting of Mara Selvini-Palazzoli and colleagues Luigi Boscolo, Gianfranco Cecchin, and Guiana Prata (Boscolo, Cecchin, Hoffman, & Penn, 1987; Selvini-Palazzoli, Boscolo, Cecchin, & Prata, 1978). In 1980, the group divided, with Selvini-Palazzoli and Prata focusing on research and clinical endeavors, and Selvini-Palazzoli proposing a systemic model of psychotic processes in families. Boscolo and Cecchin emphasized training in systemic therapy, asserting that optimal interventions should remain flexible and tailored to the family. This therapy has been popularized in the United States by Lynn Hoffman at the Ackerman Institute and in Amherst, Massachusetts, and by Peggy Papp, Olga Silverstein, and their colleagues at the Ackerman Institute in New York. Recently, many systemic therapists have integrated a postmodern perspective (see "Postmodern Family Therapy"). These systemic family therapists refer to themselves as post-Milan and incorporate new techniques and perspectives along with the original concepts set forth by the Milan group.

The systemic model is the purest application of Bateson's *circular epistemology*. The Milan model focuses on process rather than structure. Consistent with the beliefs posited by the MRI group, the systemic approach views the family and therapist as an ecosystem in which each member affects the health of all other members over time. Thus, symptomatic behavior is perpetuated by *rule-governed transactional patterns*. The symptom keeps the family system in a homeostatic state. Systemic therapists view the family as a nonlinear and complex cybernetic system, with interlocking feedback mechanisms and repetitive patterns of behavior sequences. Systemic therapists are unified in their efforts to comprehend the meaning of *second-order cybernetics* (the cybernetics of cybernetics) and to use this understanding as a basis for practice.

Basic Structure of Therapy

This therapy is conducted with all family members present. Sessions frequently are spaced at monthly intervals, allowing time for the intervention to take effect and elicit change throughout the system. Typical courses of therapy are between three and 20 sessions, with 10 sessions being modal. The number of sessions is agreed on in advance and adhered to rigidly. A single therapist or cotherapy pair conducts the sessions, with other members of the therapy team providing live supervision through a one-way mirror. Observers behind the mirror enhance the objectivity of the therapist(s) working directly with the family. The therapists are responsible for structuring the process of the sessions.

Goal Setting

The therapist's goals are to create a context within which the family's belief system can be explored and change can occur. To do this, the therapist maintains a systemic view of the family and offers a new conceptualization of the family's problems. However, family members determine the specific goals, and how the family changes is their responsibility. If the therapist does not agree with the family's goals, he or she respects the family's wishes, unless the family's choices may be harmful to one or more members.

Techniques and Process of Therapy

Systemic therapists assert that problematic behaviors emerge when the family's *epistemology* (rules and conceptual framework for understanding reality) is no longer adaptive. Thus, they attempt to create an environment in which new information inviting spontaneous change is introduced to facilitate an alternative epistemology. Sessions follow a standard format, including (1) *the presession*, during which therapists gather information; (2) *the session*, during which therapists give information, elicit discussion, and observe transactional patterns; (3) *discussion of the session* in a separate room by the therapists and observers, culminating in a systemic hypothesis and associated intervention; (4) *rejoining the family* by the therapists to offer a comment and a prescription (typically a paradoxical directive) for an outside the session task; and (5) *the postsession* therapy team discussion of the family's reaction to the intervention and a written formulation summarizing the session.

Systemic therapists use many techniques described in the strategic therapy section. They begin with a *systemic hypotheses*, which creates a framework from which to ask questions and devise interventions. An effective diagnostic technique associated with the Milan school is *circular questioning*, in which one member is asked to comment on the interactional behaviors of two other members. Circular questioning addresses members' differential perceptions of events and relationships, enabling participants to view differences nonjudgmentally and conceptualize problems systemically. In *positive connotation*, the therapist labels a problem behavior as positive because it maintains family homeostasis and cohesion. Positive connotation fosters members' acceptance of interventions and curiosity about why symptomatic behavior is essential for cohesion. *Rituals*, designed to address the conflict between unspoken and spoken family rules, are prescriptions directing family members to change their behavior, leading to modification of associated cognitive maps. *Counterparadoxical interventions* occur when the therapist places the family in a therapeutic double bind to counteract their pattern of paradoxical communications. The use of counterparadoxical interventions, in which the therapist overtly directs the family not to change, is based on the assumption that symptomatic behavior maintains the homeostasis. Rather than give prescriptions that elicit resistance, therapists offer prescriptions that provide information about family connectedness. Taken together, these interventions uncover family games, introduce a new cognitive map, and engender the family to discover solutions via transformation in family rules and relationships.

Because behavioral goals are not specified, it is often unclear when the therapy should be terminated. Termination occurs when therapist and family agree that the problem is alleviated or the family no longer perceives the behavior to be a problem. The therapist may recommend that the family return for a review session at a later time.

The Stance of the Therapist

Systemic therapists take a neutral, objective, and nonreactive stance, and do not become a part of any family alliance or coalition. This neutrality allows maximum leverage for achieving change, as the therapist is free to attend to the system in its entirety, without being pulled into the family's repetitive patterns of interaction. The therapist develops a relationship with each member, openly shares hypotheses about family processes, and minimizes the use of paradoxical techniques. Consistent with the cybernetics of cybernetics, the referring source and the therapy team are considered integral parts of the coevolving ecosystem, affecting each other in circular feedback loops.

Curative Factors

Mechanisms of change include interviewing the family in a manner that permits individuals to develop new connections between events and their meanings, and creating a new meaning system that leads to the development of alternative behaviors and interaction patterns. The value of insight is minimized, and interpretations are not utilized. The therapist's personality is important insofar as it enables him or her to relate attentively, while simultaneously entertaining systemic hypotheses. Although the therapist's personality may influence the work, it is not considered central to the change process. Therapy is most efficacious when there is a good fit between the therapist and the family, with the family permitting the therapist to question its belief system, and the therapist providing feedback in a challenging yet respectful manner.

Treatment Applicability

The Milan group's systemic approach has been used with families with a variety of severe emotional problems, most notably psychosomatic and psychotic symptoms. The Milan approach is appropriate for any family whose solution to its problems has become interwoven with the family's meaning system, such that alternative solutions for problem solving are limited.

Evidence Base

Evaluations of treatment efficacy are sparse. One outcome study comparing problem-solving versus systemic family therapy found that while both yielded significant symptom reduction, families completing the systemic treatment evidenced a broader systemic perspective regarding their family's functioning (Bennum, 1986). Another study reported that families receiving Milan family therapy exhibited more change among family members and required less time for treatment than families that received standard child outpatient treatment (Simpson, 1991). A more recent study (Bressi, Manenti, Frongia, Porcellana, & Invernizzi, 2008) found that systemic family therapy following the Milan School model yielded an improved clinical course and better pharmacological compliance in the first year of follow-up than routine psychiatric treatment for patients with schizophrenia. Efforts to conduct controlled comparative outcome studies have been hampered by poor specification of the intervention, but Pote, Stratton, Cottrell, Shapiro, and Boston (2003) have developed a manual and adherence protocol for systemic family therapy, perhaps paving the way for more methodologically rigorous evaluation of this approach in the future.

Structural Family Therapy

Minuchin and colleagues (e.g., Edgar Auerswald, Branlio Montalvo, Harry Aponte, Jay Haley, Lynn, Hoffman, and Bernice Rosman) founded the structural model (Minuchin, 1974), which serves as the basis for much of the family therapy conceptualized and practiced today. The model was an outgrowth of the authors' work at the Philadelphia Child Guidance Clinic, where they worked with conduct disordered youth and their low-socioeconomic-status families that were predominantly African American. The model continues to be utilized and expanded for the African American population as it incorporates an ecostructural perspective in which the family's transactions with outside agencies and systems are the focus of concern.

Structural family therapy, a theoretically based approach for intervening with children/adolescents and their families, incorporates structuralist conceptualizations. Adaptive and maladaptive functioning are described in terms of the organized patterns of interactions among individuals, their families, and the environment. This model uses concepts about structure, communication patterns, and expression of affect to explain the family's organization, coping patterns, and adaptation to developmental transitions. *Boundaries* demarcate *subsystems* and are the rules that define who participates and how in various tasks and activities. Families are *hierarchically organized*, with caregivers positioned in the executive subsystem above their children. *Alignment* refers to the joining or opposition of one member to another in carrying out an operation. Under the rubric of alignment are the concepts of *coalition* (a covert alliance between two family members against a third) and *alliance* (two individuals share a common interest not held by a third person). *Power* has been defined as the relative influence of each family member on the outcome of an activity. The structural dimensions of boundaries and alignments depend on power for action and outcome.

Dysfunctional families fail to adapt to stressors in a developmentally appropriate manner. Families show maladjustment when they rigidly cling to familiar interaction patterns that are no longer adaptive. The nature of the family dysfunction may be categorized according to the structural dimensions of boundary, alignment, and power that are most salient. The terms *enmeshment* and *disengagement* refer to maladaptive expressions of family boundaries and reflect extreme points on a continuum. Another impairment in family boundaries occurs when one family member inappropriately intrudes into the domain of other members, as in the case of the parental or parentified child. Common dysfunctional family alignments include stable coalitions, detouring coalitions, and triangulation. *Stable coalitions* are those in which two family members are consistently in agreement against a third person. When the two allies agree that the third person is the source of their problem, a *detouring coalition* is formed to reduce the stress in the dyad, giving the impression of harmony. *Triangulation* occurs when an opposing family member (frequently one of the parents) demands that a third person (typically a child) side with him or her against the opposing party. This process emotionally paralyzes the triangulated individual, resulting in symptomatic behavior.

Dysfunctional family patterns relevant to the power dimension may reflect the inability of members to utilize their authority to implement their assigned roles, such as when the parental subsystem fails to exert the force required to guide the children. Families deficient on all three structural domains are underorganized, with limited coping strategies and structure that is employed rigidly yet inconsistently. In contrast, healthy families have well-defined, elaborated, flexible, and cohesive family structures that accommodate the changing roles of individual members, the various family subsystems, and the sociocultural environment.

Basic Structure of Therapy

The structure is flexible in terms of number of therapists; which family members participate; and location, length, and frequency of interviews. Typically, however, structural family therapy is a brief intervention (5–7 months on average) whose primary participants are family members who interact daily. A single therapist usually conducts this therapy, because the presence of a cotherapy dyad makes it difficult to exert maximal control over the family's transactional patterns. Rather than a focus predominantly on the content of family communication, the primary focus is on verbal and nonverbal interactional processes, as they reflect the family structure.

Goal Setting

The primary goal negotiated between the therapist and the family is resolution of the presenting problem. The family may desire resolution of the problem, with a focus on the index person and a lack of attention to underlying structural patterns. However, the therapist asserts that this goal can only be attained by restructuring the family unit, so that more adaptive interaction patterns prevail. A second important aim of the work is to change the family's construction of reality; the therapist helps members to develop an alternative explanatory model for the problem, enabling them to develop more adaptive family transactions.

Techniques and Process of Therapy

This approach entails three cyclical and overlapping stages: *joining, assessing,* and *restructuring.* The therapist joins the family rapidly and in a position of leadership. To facilitate the joining process, the therapist utilizes three procedures: *maintenance* (supporting the existing structure of the family); *tracking* (following the content of the family's communication with minimal intervention), and *mimesis* (adopting the style and affective experience of the family). The therapist initially accepts the family's view of the presenting problem and designs interventions to ameliorate the problem by changing the family structure. As symptom reduction proceeds, the family gains more confidence in the therapist's expertise may be more inclined to address underlying structural issues.

The assessing stage focuses on six domains of family functioning: (1) structure, boundary quality, and resonance (sensitivity to the actions of members and tolerance for deviation); (2) flexibility and capacity for change; (3) interaction patterns of the spousal/intimate partnership, parental, and sibling subsystems; (4) role of index person and how his or her symptom maintains family homeostasis; (5) ecological context within which the problem develops and is maintained; and (6) developmental stage of the family and its members. This assessment enables the therapist to conceptualize how structural problems and current symptoms are interrelated.

The third phase, restructuring, redresses the structural difficulties noted during the assessment. With enmeshed families, the goal is to increase age-appropriate separation–individuation; with disengaged families, the restructuring process entails enhancing family attachments. A number of techniques serve the restructuring process. The therapist facilitates structural change through the use of *enactments,* in which the therapist promotes the family's acting out of dysfunctional and habitual transactional patterns during the session. Additional techniques include escalating stress, boundary marking, unbalancing the family alignments, assigning homework tasks, and providing support, education, and guidance.

According to Minuchin, symptoms are indicative of dysfunctional family patterns for managing stress. He recommends escalating stress within the family to help the system develop more effective interaction patterns. Strategies for escalating stress include prolonging an enactment, introducing new variables (e.g., new family members), blocking typical patterns of relating, challenging the communication rules and structure of the family, or suggesting alternative transactions in session that may facilitate change outside the session. Spatial interventions, including rearranging the seating and removing members from the room temporarily to observe the interactions from behind a one-way mirror, are also used to alter the perspectives of family members and improve interpersonal boundaries. Tasks are assigned to the family, both inside and outside the session. Tasks are diagnostic probes that yield valuable information about the family's openness to change and serve to alter maladaptive communication patterns and structure. Tasks may be assigned in a direct fashion and/or paradoxically.

The Stance of the Therapist

Minuchin considers the role of the therapist as that of a distant and friendly relative who takes an active and authoritative stance by asking probing questions and giving homework assignments. Consistent with his persona, the therapist is often colorful and dramatic. He or she demands that members accommodate to him or her to facilitate therapeutic progress, and communicates his or her expertise in helping the family mobilize adaptive resources to facilitate change.

Curative Factors

Emphasis is on interactions occurring in the present, and the therapeutic task is one of behavior change as opposed to development of insight. The structural approach is more symptom-oriented than are the psychoanalytic schools, yet less symptom-focused than are strategic therapies. Techniques are considered important in achieving change. This approach incorporates a developmental perspective in understanding the association between life-stage transitions and dysfunction, conceptualizes transactional patterns in terms of both cybernetic properties and organizational structure of the family, and takes into account the therapist's impact on the family in the data-gathering process. Resistance to change is either circumvented through the use of enactments or challenged by escalating the stress within the family. However, resistances to change are not typically interpreted by the therapist. Genuine change in the index person occurs only when the family structure is transformed.

   The effective use of structural family therapy techniques requires both clarity of purpose and a complex balancing of a commitment to change, with sensitivity to corrective feedback from the family. Other aspects of the therapist's psychological health and personality are not specifically highlighted. This is not surprising given that transference and countertransference dynamics are not considered integral to the curative process.

Treatment Applicability

The structural approach has been applied successfully to a range of families with a wide variety of problems and symptoms (e.g., externalizing behavior disorders; psychosomatic illnesses such as eating disorders; and substance abuse). Additionally, this approach has been used with multiproblem, disorganized families experiencing family violence, and with families in the process of divorce or rebuilding a remarried, blended, or stepfamily. Developed primarily for low-income African American families, structural family therapy is also implemented with other ethnic/minority populations, such as Latino families.

Evidence Base

Minuchin's uncontrolled case studies provided preliminary evidence of the promise of structural therapy, and controlled empirical research conducted over the past three decades has demonstrated its efficacy for specific populations and problems. Stanton and Todd (1982) found that young adult heroin addicts receiving structural family therapy combined with methadone showed greater improvement than addicts receiving individual therapy combined with methadone. Currently, structural approaches are included in several evidence-based, integrative family therapy interventions for adolescents with alcohol, drug, and disruptive behavior problems (see "Integrative Models").

Cognitive and Behavioral Family Therapies

Behavioral family therapies are predicated on social learning theory and behavior exchange principles derived from classical and operant conditioning approaches, whereas cognitively oriented approaches view family distress and conflict as influenced by an interaction of cognitive, behavioral, and affective factors. The philosophy and procedures for cognitive and behavioral family therapies (CBFTs) are based on the logical positivist research tradition for the scientific study of human behavior; that is, the conduct of CBFTs is similar to a scientific experiment and includes (1) a testable, well-articulated conceptual framework; (2) hypotheses derived from, and consistent with, the conceptual model; (3) interventions that can be replicated and tested; and (4) objective measurement of outcome. CBFTs began with Robert Liberman's *conjoint behavioral family and couple therapy* (Liberman, Mueser, & Glynn, 1988), James Alexander's *functional family therapy* (see "Integrative Models"), Luciano L'Abate's *structured enrichment for families* (L'Abate & Weinstein, 1987), Nathan Epstein's (2002) *McMaster problem-solving model*, Gerald Patterson's *behavioral parent training* (Patterson & Forgatch, 1987), and Sheila Eyberg's *parent–child interaction therapy* (Brinkmeyer & Eyberg, 2003).

Despite differences in the techniques associated with the various forms of CBFT, all approaches are built on research findings. Current advances incorporate theoretical constructs and research findings from the areas of social and cognitive psychology, sociology, and pathophysiology. Therefore, unlike other models that are tied in part to charismatic leaders and their clinical and theoretical contributions, the progress of CBFTs has depended primarily on collaborations between researchers and clinicians.

The behavioral approach to the assessment and treatment of family problems reflects an expansion from the traditional individual approach to behavioral treatment based on principles from operant and classical conditioning. According to this approach, maladaptive behavior is generated and maintained by environmental contingencies, including one's learning history. Interpersonal interactions reflect reciprocal patterns of behavior in which one person's behavior reinforces the other's behavior, and circular and potentially escalating patterns of interaction emerge. With its emphasis on environmental, situational, and social determinants of behavior, the behavioral perspective is well suited to addressing problematic behavior in a family context. Behavioral family therapists attend to environmental events that precede and follow problem behaviors to determine how the behaviors have been learned and reinforced. They underscore the family as a system, emphasizing the interdependent behavioral patterns between family members. Historically, behavioral approaches have not considered the role of relationship problems in the development and maintenance of the child's difficulties or the impact of the child's behavioral problems on the intimate partnership. More recently, however, behaviorally oriented family therapists have focused on not only the reciprocal influences of the child's behavior problems and the parent's relationship but also the influence of the community on family and individual behavior.

Cognitive approaches to family therapy, outgrowths of individual cognitive therapy and rational-emotive therapy, assume that one's cognitive processing influences family members' behaviors, transactions, and emotional and behavioral reactions. Each family member experiences external events, including other family members' behaviors, the combined effects of several members' behaviors toward him or her, and his or her observations of interactions among family members. As family members cognitively appraise these events, they develop cognitions regarding self, the relationship between self and family members, and interrelationships among family subsystems. In healthy families, perceptions are positive, realistic, and open to change via direct verbal communication. In dysfunctional families, perceptions tend to be distorted.

Basic Structure of Therapy

CBFTs are brief, time-limited, and typically conducted by a single therapist. Membership varies from attendance by caregivers only (e.g., parent training) to the whole family, depending on the reason for referral. Extended family members are not likely to be included. The therapy is relatively structured, with the structure provided by the therapist.

Goal Setting

A hallmark of CBFTs is developing specific and measurable treatment goals. Goal setting follows a functional analysis that assesses maladaptive affective and instrumental behaviors and the environmental contingencies supporting these behaviors, and the ways in which family members' reciprocal interactions affect their relational satisfaction. Based on the functional analysis, the therapist and family together delineate specific treatment goals. The intervention is discussed, and the therapist obtains a commitment from the parties to participate in a specified treatment plan. This commitment may be formalized in a treatment contract.

Although treatment goals are tailored to the specific problems of the family, general goals of CBFT include changing maladaptive behaviors by modifying environmental contingencies, facilitating flexible behavior control, increasing positive interactions between family members, altering environmental conditions that interfere with positive interactions, teaching more adaptive behaviors, and facilitating the maintenance and generalization of newly acquired behavioral changes. In addition, CBFTs aim to change the cognitive processing and behavior of each family member such that relationship and family satisfaction is improved.

Techniques and Process of Therapy

CBFTs include a diverse array of approaches and techniques (Falloon, 1991). The first descriptions were case studies of parents' implementation of behavioral interventions for their child's problem. Change strategies addressed a particular target behavior elicited by one member (typically a child); the role of other family members was to eliminate the contingencies maintaining the problematic behavior and to initiate different contingencies to support more desirable behaviors that were incompatible with the deviant behavior. This behavior modification approach was further developed by Patterson, who recognized that the nature of family interaction patterns made the implementation of operant strategies much more difficult in the home than in the laboratory (Patterson & Yoerger, 1993). Attention was focused on effectively implementing behavioral assessment and intervention strategies in the home environment. The CBFTs practiced today are built on the groundbreaking work of Patterson and coworkers. A major example is parent training.

In *parent training*, the therapist provides information and imparts skills to parents to better equip them to address their child's problematic behaviors. Therapists coach parents in new skills and ways of interacting with their child, and supervise caregivers' implementation of these skills at home. Caregivers are recognized as offering unique and intimate insights into the day-to-day routines, behaviors, and emotions of their child. Caregivers and therapist work together and share their expertise to help the caregivers better help the child. This short-term intervention approach is accessible, understandable, maintainable, generalizable, ecologically valid, and time- and cost-efficient. As a result, adults are likely to seek out this treatment, adhere to the protocol, and continue to apply skills learned over time. Parent training has been advocated for parent–child relationship disorders and for parents of children who manifest externalizing behavior disorders, such as attention-deficit, disruptive behavior, developmental, and habit disorders. We describe one parent training approach, parent–child interaction therapy (PCIT).

PCIT is an evidence-based, manualized behavioral family treatment for disruptive behavior in preschoolers. Developed and refined by Eyberg (Brinkmeyer & Eyberg, 2003; Eyberg & Robinson, 1982), PCIT draws on attachment and social learning theories to help parents achieve *authoritative parenting*, a parenting style characterized by high levels of control and warmth. As it is assumed that a secure, nurturing relationship is a necessary foundation for effective limit setting and consistent discipline, PCIT progresses in two theory-based phases. In the first phase, *child-directed interaction* (CDI), the parent learns to follow the child's lead in play by applying specific communication skills (giving labeled praise, or reflecting the child's comments) often used by play therapists. In the second phase, *parent-directed interaction* (PDI), the parent learns specific behavior management techniques based on social learning theory, such as how to give a direct command, reinforce compliance, and remove attention in response to noncompliance. Most PCIT sessions are devoted to coaching the parent to demonstrate the communication skills (CDI) or behavioral management techniques (PDI) *in vivo* with the child.

PCIT begins with a targeted assessment of the parent–child interaction. An empirically supported behavioral observation system, the Dyadic Parent–Child Interaction Coding System (DPICS), rates key parent and child behaviors in three consecutive situations with progressively greater demand for parent control: child-led play, parent-led play, and a cleanup task. Ratings from the DPICS and the parent-rated Eyberg Child Behavior Inventory guide each session, the progress through the phases, and assess clinical outcome. Although the full DPICS (five 5-minute tasks) is conducted at the beginning and end of treatment, a 5-minute observation period is conducted at the beginning of all CDI sessions to ascertain the parent's progress.

PCIT differs from other behavioral family interventions in its format and utilization of specific toys and recording/coaching equipment. Coaching takes place in a playroom containing toys appropriate for CDI, a time-out chair for PDI, and a one-way mirror and "bug-in-the-ear" system for helping the parent to use the desired skills. Coaching consists of frequent, brief statements designed to give parents immediate feedback, suggestions, or gentle corrections. At the end of each session, the therapist reviews with the parents the summary sheet from the 5-minute observation period, showing them their progress and identifying skills needing additional work. The parent must demonstrate specific phase-dependent skills to move from CDI to PDI, and to finish PDI. As treatment progress depends on parent mastery of CDI or PDI criteria, PCIT is open-ended, with an average length of 12–16 sessions. Throughout treatment, the therapist acts as a positive and supportive coach to the parent, with minimal interaction with the child. The focus is on specific behavioral skills implemented *in vivo* by the parents toward the target child. If both parents participate, they are coached separately, often with one parent behind the one-way mirror with the therapist.

The Stance of the Therapist

Those who practice CBFTs function as scientists, collaborators, educators, role models, and teachers in the Socratic tradition. Therapists are active, directive, and present-focused, and provide didactic information to teach the family about processes associated with the maladaptive behavior. They direct the treatment process, taking responsibility for setting the agenda, reviewing homework, and enforcing the treatment contract. The therapist can serve as a consultant as family members test their perceptions, and generate and rationally assess alternative hypotheses regarding individual and relational functioning. Because the approach is geared to the building of adaptive skills (communication, assertiveness, problem solving, conflict resolution, and negotiation), the therapist serves as a teacher who supervises the family's rehearsal of new behaviors. Although a collaborative working alliance is essential for behavior change, transference is not addressed specifically or considered important.

Curative Factors

The mechanisms of change in CBFTs are related to the specific techniques used to attain treatment goals. For most families, learning new interpersonal skills (e.g., communication and conflict resolution) is curative. Reality testing is viewed as essential for behavior change. The focus is on the present, and insight is not viewed as central for accomplishing behavioral change. The relationship between the therapist and family members does not play a direct role in bringing about change. However, a therapist who has difficulty structuring the sessions or helping family members to challenge their distorted cognitions is unlikely to be successful in effecting behavior change or improving relationship satisfaction.

Treatment Applicability

CBFTs have been applied to a broad range of problems (e.g., affective disorders, internalizing and externalizing child behavior problems, and substance abuse). CBFTs have been implemented in multiple countries, and though developed primarily for young children with disruptive behavior disorders, they have been tailored and adapted to new populations, including physically abusive parents, foster parents, and children with internalizing and autism spectrum disorders.

Evidence Base

Behavioral parent training has been shown to be effective for managing disruptive behavior disorders, antisocial behavior, elimination disorders, and anxiety disorders. A meta-analysis provided support for the short-term effectiveness of behavioral parenting training in modifying children's behavior and enhancing parental adjustment (Serketich & Dumas, 1996). CBFTs decrease the rate of relapse in adults with psychiatric disorders such as schizophrenia (Doane, Goldstein, & Miklowitz, 1986) and bipolar disorder (Miklowitz et al., 2004) and have proven effective for remarried families, families with older adults, addicted individuals, suicidal and depressed persons, and adults with sexual dysfunctions.

PCIT is a probably efficacious treatment for disruptive behavior disorders among 3- to 6-year-olds (Eyberg, Nelson, & Boggs, 2008). PCIT outcome studies reveal significant improvements in parents' behavior toward their children. Although PCIT is a dyadic intervention, its positive effects have been found to generalize to untreated siblings. While PCIT has also been demonstrated to be superior to group parent training, relatively few studies compare PCIT to an alternative treatment or placebo condition. While most findings have been based on samples that were primarily European American, PCIT has been adapted for Mexican American, African American, and Puerto Rican families.

Psychoeducational Family Therapy

Psychoeducational family therapy was first used with individuals with schizophrenia and their families by William McFarlane (1991) and Carol Anderson, David Reiss and Gerald Hogarty (1986), and due to its efficacy in reducing relapse has been adapted for individuals with other serious psychiatric and medical illnesses. Family psychoeducational models, designed to remediate individual and family difficulties and enhance functioning, train family members to be helpers to their loved ones; teach family members communication, problem-solving, and conflict resolution skills; and prevent the emergence of problems in order to enhance the quality of family life.

Psychoeducational approaches are based on a multitude of theoretical perspectives but some are atheoretical. Psychoeducational programs have been developed for such diverse areas of focus as parent training, and marriage and family enhancement and enrichment. Medical family therapy emphasizes the importance of educating the family, so that its members can be informed consumers, collaborators in the treatment process, and better able to cope effectively with the demands of their loved one's illness. The following comments focus on psychoeducational interventions for families with a loved one with a schizophrenia spectrum disorder.

Basic Structure of Therapy

This structured treatment can be conducted with an individual family or in a multiple-family group format. Session frequency depends on the stage of the work and status of the patient's illness. The treatment may take a few years, with longer intervals between sessions during the latter phases.

Goal Setting

The intermediate goals are stabilizing the patient, involving all members in the psychoeducation process, educating the family about illnesses and medications, establishing a treatment team that includes family members and emphasizes continuity of care, encouraging the use and development of the social support network, helping the family cope with the burdens associated with a prolonged disorder in a family member, and teaching adaptive family stress management. The long-term goals are preventing relapse and integrating the patient into the community. Goals are explicit and openly negotiated with all participants throughout the therapy.

Techniques and Process of Therapy

Single-family and multiple-family psychoeducation approaches consist of a number of phases. The first phase begins at the time of the family member's first psychotic episode or relapse, typically an acute episode necessitating hospitalization or day treatment. The therapists (typically two clinicians) rapidly form an alliance with all relevant family members. Family meetings occur frequently, often without the patient, to allay the family's anxiety and decrease distressing interactions. Separate therapist–patient meetings foster a supportive working relationship and help the patient understand the approach. The assessment entails evaluating the present crisis; eliciting reactions to the patient's disorder and the treatment system; and examining the family's structure, coping resources, and social support network. This phase culminates with the development of a contract.

The second phase consists of an educational workshop(s) for family members and friends, and sometimes concurrent sessions for patients in a group format. Educational workshops are didactic, with a lecture (with accompanying handouts) and a discussion format. The intervention presumes that the patient's disability is caused by biological factors, and that interpersonal and environmental stresses are risk factors for relapse. The therapists educate the family to reduce expectations for rapid progress; use a relaxed manner of relating to the patient; reduce external stimulation in the patient's environment; set limits on the patient's disruptive, bizarre, or violent behavior; ignore symptoms that cannot be changed; use clear and simple communications; comply with the recommended treatment plan; maintain routine daily activities; help the patient avoid substance use; and ascertain warning signs suggestive of relapse. As time progresses, sessions are held less frequently, typically biweekly, and continue for at least 12 months. The clinicians meet with a single family, including the patient, or with multiple families.

In the last phase, rehabilitation, the clinicians and family collaborate to increase the patient's adaptive functioning. Decisions to reduce the frequency of the sessions and terminate are based on the patient's improvement, family preference, and, in the case of multiple family psychoeducation, group members' need for continued social support. Social support is crucial in helping families and patients maintain treatment gains.

Clinicians adhere to the following steps: (1) socialize with family and patient; (2) review the outcome of the task assigned in the previous meeting; (3) review the week's events, particularly those that may be characterized as stressors; (4) reframe the family's reported stressors in the context of the realities of the patient's illness and integrate this with the guidelines presented during the educational component of the intervention; (5) educate the family in adaptive problem-solving and communication skills; and (6) underscore the importance of medication compliance.

The Stance of the Therapist

The therapists create a collaborative relationship with the patient, family, and other team members. They provide direct advice, guidance, and information. They communicate their expertise in managing psychiatric disorders, while recognizing the patient's and family's knowledge about the patient's unique psychiatric presentation and their resources to solve family problems creatively. The clinicians' role differs depending on the phase of the work. During joining, they actively establish rapport with the family. In the educational phase, they present themselves as teachers and experts in managing psychiatric disorders and may facilitate the development of a social support network among families in the multiple-family groups. During rehabilitation, they help the family use problem-solving and communication techniques to monitor the patient for relapse and increase independent functioning.

Curative Factors

Because researchers have linked specific types of family interaction characterized by high expressed emotion to the course of schizophrenia and bipolar disorder, intervention helps family members communicate without blame, make clear requests for behavior change, and achieve consensus on conflict management and problem solving. The focus is on helping the family provide a supportive environment for the patient and cope with the stress of having a family member with a psychiatric disorder. Change is brought about by increased knowledge, skills, and use of social support. Given the persistent nature of the psychiatric disorders for which this approach was developed, continuity of care is key, and termination is not stressed. Many families, particularly those in family groups, participate indefinitely.

Treatment Applicability

Psychoeducational approaches have been used most with persons with schizophrenia spectrum disorder and their families. More recently, they have also been used with families in which an adult or child has a mood disorder.

Evidence Base

The evidence in support of psychoeducational approaches has been growing. Reviews of randomized controlled trials show that family psychoeducation is the treatment of choice for schizophrenia (McFarlane, Dixon, Lukens, & Lucksted, 2003). These interventions have proven effective for other mental illnesses, such as bipolar disorder (Miklowitz et al., 2004; Miklowitz, George, Richard, Simoneau, & Suddath, 2003). Another psychoeducational intervention, multifamily psychoeducational groups, have been examined with youth with bipolar disorder or major depressive disorder/dysthymic disorder, and the findings are quite promising (Fristad, Verducci, Walters, & Young, 2009).

Postmodern Family Therapy

Postmodern thought in the human sciences represents a paradigm shift that disputes the notion that reality is fixed and knowledge is an obtainable entity. "Postmodern" refers to a family of concepts that challenge the certainty of objective truths, the relevance of universal narratives, and language as an agent of the truth. Social construction posits that truth, knowledge, and reality are the product of language, experience, culture, and context. Language is considered the vehicle through which people know and attribute meaning to their lives and solutions to their problems. Problems do not reside within individuals, families, or the larger system; instead, they are social and linguistic constructions amenable to change through dialogue. This philosophy poses challenges for the traditions of the helping professions. Unlike therapies that target dysfunctional family patterns, postmodern approaches hold that problems are context-bound constructions cocreated by family members' interpretations and linguistic accounts of their social, cultural, and historic experiences. This therapy helps family members change their story of the problem by focusing on positive elements and unseen resources. As objective knowledge and universal truth are viewed skeptically, therapist authority and application of expert knowledge is eschewed in favor of the therapist's nonjudgmental, nonpathological view of problems and an egalitarian relationship between therapist and clients.

Postmodern and social construction ideology-informed approaches can be applied to individuals, couples, families, and groups. The goal of therapy is to create a relational and dialogical context for outcomes and solutions to emerge. *Transformation*—the evolving of new outcomes and solutions—is unique to the participants in therapy and therefore cannot be determined ahead of time. Several examples of postmodern therapies include solution-focused brief therapy developed by Steve de Shazer (1988) and colleagues solution-oriented therapy developed by Bill O'Hanlon and Michelle Weiner-Davis (1989), and narrative therapy developed by Michael White (White & Epston, 1990).

Basic Structure of Therapy

Postmodern therapies tend to be brief and have been praised for their simplicity and criticized for their lack of focus on long-term outcomes. They are typically conducted by a single therapist, but some postmodern therapists use a *reflecting team* (Anderson, 1995). The reflecting team technique involves the facilitation of conversation through a two-way mirror, in which there is open dialogue between the therapist and family, and a consultant team watching the therapy through a one-way mirror, and later dialoguing about the session while the family watches through the one-way mirror. Most postmodernists encourage as many family members as can to attend sessions, and the therapist may ask others in the community or system who may be a part of the problem to attend a given session. The structure of sessions is guided by questions initiated by the therapist; however, the focus is on dialogue generated by family members. There is no assumption that the views of either the therapist or any family member have greater value than any other person's views.

Goal Setting

While the primary goal negotiated between the therapist and the family varies according to the type of postmodern therapy practiced, the overarching aim is for family members and therapist to challenge the meaning surrounding the problem. Using direct (solution-focused therapy) or indirect (collaborative therapy, narrative therapy) means, the therapist focuses on the presenting concerns through dialogue. There is no direct effort to address family structure, roles, transference, or dysfunction.

Techniques and Process of Therapy

Several assumptions distinguish postmodern therapies from other models. First, the therapist is not considered the "expert" on the problem; families are empowered to find alternative accounts of their situation. Second, issues surrounding cultural diversity are more likely to be taken into consideration, as the family determines the nature of the collaborative dialogue by generating their own solutions. In fact, one postmodern approach, narrative therapy, has a clear social and political agenda: to help clients liberate themselves from the problem stories created by the dominant culture, and to construct new stories that give more possibilities to their lives. Third, the therapists do not consider their actions as techniques but as a philosophical stance or way of thinking about, experiencing, being in relationship with, and talking and responding to clients. Thus, the primary therapy activity is creating a space and facilitating a process for dialogical conversations and collaborative client–therapist relationships. Family members engage in dialogue about their problems and are empowered to change by becoming aware of and accommodating to each others' needs and belief systems. Most postmodern therapists are not invested in a particular out-come; rather, they favor mutual inquiry or co-construction of narratives in the service of new meaning and action. A notable exception is solution-focused brief therapy (SFBT), in which therapists steer families toward a specified behavioral goal and discussion of solutions.

SFBT is influenced by the brief therapy model of the MRI, Erikson's strategic therapy, and social constructivism. de Shazer, a leading figure, claimed that solutions do not need to have any relation to the problem. He argued that the client is the expert on his or her life and should have a large role in directing therapy. Accordingly, SFBT aims to help families construct a new use of their existing abilities and resources to solve a specific problem.

SFBT therapists negotiate well-formed and achievable goals with the family, shifting the conversation from "problem talk" to "solution talk." This approach assumes that family members can discover the solution to their problem through creating a new context within which the solution can be enacted. Like other postmodern approaches, SFBT avoids the use of complex, previously constructed interventions in favor of dialogue to help clients uncover solutions to problems based on their existing resources. Nevertheless, SFBT thera-pists use three types of questions to guide the family's search for solutions: the miracle question, the exception-finding question, and the scaling question. The *miracle question* asks members to imagine that a miracle occurs in the middle of the night and upon waking, their problem is solved. The therapist asks them to describe how they would know that the problem is resolved and what would be different. The *exception-finding question* asks about situations in which the problem does not occur, so that family members can identify solu-tions based on their own successful experiences controlling these problems. The *scaling question* asks members to rate their problem on a 1- to 10-point scale, and uses this rating to encourage its resolution through monitoring and forecasting progress. The therapist may ask family members what it would take to move the rating 1 point up or down, or what accounts for changes in the rating as therapy progresses. SFBT sessions usually conclude with a "consulting break," in which the therapist constructs a message for the family that includes compliments and a homework task.

The Stance of the Therapist

The stance is that of a nonhierarchical collaborator and a creative agent working with the family to cocreate alternative meanings that lead to solutions for change. The first step involves joining the "meaning systems" of the family, inviting members to explore these systems, challenging members to expand these systems, and validating and stabilizing the new system that support resolution of the problem. The therapist sets the stage, stating the expectation for change, eliciting collaborative participation, and reflecting new perspec-tives that support solutions. The therapist assumes a stance of "not knowing," which entails being curious, impartial, and conveying a lack of full understanding. "Not knowing" invites the therapist's active and responsive listening, and inquiry into the situation with an attitude of respectful confidence in the client. This position is in contrast to the role of a detached outside observer commenting on family process. The collaboration between therapist and family reflects the notion that there are many ways to perceive a situation. This cooperative stance empowers family members to engage in the search for more adaptive solutions. In addition, therapists examine the cultural influences on their own perceptions and actions, and they openly disclose their beliefs and biases about problems and therapy.

Curative Factors

The primary curative factor is deconstructing (challenging) the problem story and its supporting assumptions, so that individuals can reenvision their past and future, create "preferred" stories, and discover solutions. Most postmodern therapists promote small changes that they believe will lead to larger changes in the system. These therapies focus on engaging in dialogue to create more adaptive solutions and identities.

Treatment Applicability

Postmodern approaches have grown in popularity over the past three decades, particularly among practitioners. SFBT's clear and concrete guidelines for treatment make it a favorite among clinicians and managed care organizations, as evidenced by the websites of the Solution-Focused Brief Therapy Association (*www.sfbta.org*) and the European Brief Therapy Association (*www.ebta.nu*). Postmodern approaches have been applied to a variety of presenting problems (e.g., child maltreatment, domestic violence, eating disorders, alcohol and substance abuse, war trauma, psychosis) and populations (children, patients in outpatient and inpatient psychiatric settings, court-mandated patients).

Evidence Base

There has been little research demonstrating the efficacy of these therapies, in part because conventional quantitative research methods privilege therapists' conceptualizations of successful outcomes. In contrast, a collaborative therapist–client relationship places equal (if not more) importance on clients' perceptions and evaluations of therapy and what therapists can learn from them. Thus, most evidence of the effectiveness of postmodern therapy is found in anecdotal reports and case studies. A review of 15 outcome studies provided preliminary support for the efficacy of individual or group SFBT (Gingerich & Eisengart, 2000); empirical evidence of its efficacy as a family intervention is lacking.

Integrative Models

While distinct schools characterized the family therapy field in its early years, current practice is dominated by integrative approaches that meld two or more schools into a unifying conceptual framework that guides treatment. The term *integration* has been contrasted with *eclecticism,* which describes a pragmatic, case-based approach in which the strategies or interventions from different approaches are applied, without attempts at conceptual unification (Lebow, 2003). Integrative models are either broadly targeted, describing theories and practice that apply to all client problems and populations, or specific to a given problem or population.

Although integrative models vary in theoretical constructs and strategies for intervention, they share a number of features: (1) theory of change or an algorithm for when to use specific techniques; (2) attention to multiple levels of human experience; (3) consideration of common factors across schools; (4) understanding of the presenting problem in systemic terms and of the family system as a vehicle for change; (5) incorporation of psychoeducation and skills development; (6) descriptions of the intervention and change process that transcend theoretical orientation; (7) tailoring of interventions to specific populations;

(8) utilization of data to organize, build, and evaluate the model; (9) practical approach of achieving change through the simplest strategy available; and (10) a focus on client strengths (Lebow, 2003). Integration also applies to session formats; who is seen in a given session is generally dictated by pragmatic considerations and phase-specific goals. Despite compelling arguments for integrative approaches, no single integrative model has emerged as the standard of practice..

Integrative Problem-Centered Therapy

Integrative problem-centered therapy (IPCT; Pinsof, 1995) is a metamodel that organizes family, individual, and biological therapies to address a presenting problem. IPCT is comprehensive, in that it can be applied to any problem for which patients seek therapy. It evolved from William Pinsof's personal and professional experiences, Gestalt therapy, and object relations models. IPCT is grounded in systems theory and the concepts of interactive constructivism and differential causality.

IPCT is organized by the patient's presenting problem. The *patient system* consists of everyone involved in maintaining and resolving the problem; different problems are associated with different patient systems. Problems are conceptualized in terms of cycles or sequences. Therapy replaces the problem sequence with an alternative adaptive sequence that competes with the problem behavior and is consensually determined by patients and the therapist. The problem behavior might be parental conflict about child discipline, and the alternative behavior might be parents' enforcement of mutually negotiated consequences for a child's acting out.

IPCT involves three stages: identification of the problem cycle, implementation of the alternative adaptive sequence, and termination. Assessment is the formulation of the *problem maintenance structure* (PMS), the set of constraints within the patient system that prevent it from solving its problem. IPCT conceptualizes these constraints along six levels: *social organization, biological, meaning, families of origin, object relations*, and narcissistic vulnerabilities from the *selves* of key patients. This formulation is based on the patient system's responses to therapy.

Intervention draws on six orientations (*behavioral, biobehavioral, experiential, transgenerational, psychodynamic, self psychological*) and three assessment/intervention contexts (*family/community, couple, individual*). The six orientations correspond to the levels of PMS constraints. The problem-centered principle guides decisions about which orientations and intervention contexts to employ with a given family. According to this principle, therapy progresses in a "failure-driven" (trial and error) sequence from the interpersonal to the individual, from the here and now to the past, from transactions between individuals to processes within individuals. Failure of any one intervention is a useful learning experience in revealing new aspects of the PMS not previously apparent. The principle of application in IPCT sequences the orientations and contexts from the simplest, most direct, and least expensive to the most complex, indirect, and expensive.

During termination, the therapist helps patients develop a narrative about the change processes in therapy that will empower them to solve similar problems on their own in the future. Depending on the problem, the duration of therapy varies from several weeks to years. As a problem-centered approach, IPCT is episodic, with the door always open for future work.

Multisystemic Therapy

Multisystemic therapy (MST; Henggeler, Schoenwald, Rowland, & Cunningham, 2002) was developed in the context of the system of care reforms in children's mental health service and consumer and family advocacy efforts. Scott Henggeler's MST is predicated on both general systems theory and Bronfenbrenner's (1979) theory of social ecology, buttressed by research on the correlates and causes of adolescent mental health problems. MST redresses three weaknesses of early approaches by assuming that the child is embedded within multiple, interrelated systems (e.g., peer, school); by considering developmental perspectives; and by utilizing empirically based nonsystemic strategies to help families change. It provides a comprehensive framework that can integrate specific, individualized interventions into a unified, methodical treatment plan.

Given the focus on individualized treatment, MST assessment and interventions are guided by nine treatment principles rather than a manualized plan. According to the first treatment principle, assessment is a dynamic and continuous process in which the therapist, in collaboration with the family, sets "overarching goals," and attempts to identify characteristics of the youth's ecology ("fit factors") that are maintaining the problem behavior. Short-term, intermediary goals are developed to target prioritized fit factors, and specific interventions are selected to achieve these goals. The remaining eight principles stipulate that MST interventions (1) emphasize the positive and leverage systemic strengths for change; (2) promote responsible behavior and decrease irresponsible behavior among family members; (3) are present-focused, targeting specific and well-defined problems; (4) target sequences of behavior within or between multiple systems that maintain the identified problems: (5) are tailored to the developmental needs of the adolescent and the family; (6) require daily effort by family members; (7) are evaluated continuously for effectiveness, with the therapist assuming accountability for overcoming barriers to success; and (8) promote generalization and long-term maintenance of treatment gains. Interventions are consistent with the nine core principles, evidence-based whenever possible, and target behavior change in the youth's natural environment. MST treatment plans incorporate behavioral and cognitive-behavioral strategies, psychopharmacology, and techniques from structural and strategic models. Thus, MST can combine individual, couple, family, and sibling therapy, as well as group work and systems consultation.

MST differs from other models in its intensity, venue of service delivery, and quality assurance system. The treatment is typically delivered by a master's-level therapist with a caseload of four to six families, supported by a team of full-time therapists, a supervisor, and appropriate organizational support. Therapeutic contacts occur several times per week, and the therapist is available to the family 24 hours/7 days a week to react to crises that threaten goal attainment. Treatment is time-limited (3–5 months) to promote cost-effectiveness and family self-sufficiency. MST uses a home-based model to reduce barriers to access and to increase family engagement. Extensive quality assurance procedures have been developed to enhance fidelity and support effective implementation in community sites. MST has been transported to community settings throughout the world; sites are licensed through MST Services, Inc. (*www.mstservices.com*), which has the exclusive license for transport of MST technology and intellectual property (Henggeler, Sheidow, & Lee, 2009).

MST has been shown to be more effective than usual community services in improving family functioning, reducing rearrests, and decreasing drug use (Henggeler, Clingempeel,

Brondino, & Pickrel, 2002). Independent evaluations in community settings provide similar support for treatment effectiveness, though follow-up periods to date are limited to 2 years (Timmons-Mitchell, Bender, Kishna, & Mitchell, 2006). There is evidence for MST's efficacy with juvenile sex offenders, youth with serious mental health problems, maltreating families, and youth with complex health problems.

Multidimensional Family Therapy

Multidimensional family therapy (MDFT; Liddle, 2009) is an empirically supported, manualized, family intervention for adolescent substance abuse and related mental health problems. Related to structural–strategic family therapy, Howard Liddle's MDFT integrates a contextual framework with developmental psychopathology to guide assessment, interventions, and outcome evaluation. It intervenes in four domains: (1) adolescent, (2) parent(s), (3) family interaction, and (4) extrafamilial social systems. Motivation to enter treatment or change is assumed to be malleable; the therapist accepts responsibility for promoting participation, motivation, and behavior change.

Treatment is phasic, interventions are individualized, case formulations are revised on the basis of feedback, and therapists advocate for both the adolescent and the parent (*balanced alliance*). MDFT values both individual and family meetings as part of assessment. Typically, therapists meet first with the entire family to understand how members contribute to the adolescent's circumstances. Separate individual meetings with the adolescent and the parent(s) clarify their unique perspectives. Adolescents give their life story and draw an ecomap. In the parents' session, the therapist assesses their emotional investment in the adolescent, their own family experiences, parenting strengths and weaknesses, and mental health and substance use. Assessment also includes gathering of information about multiple extrafamilial influences (e.g., youth's educational/vocational placement). The goal of the initial assessment is to identify risk and protective factors for substance abuse and related problems in the four domains.

The therapist implements interventions to decrease risk and enhance protective processes, first within the most accessible and malleable domains. MDFT is unique in that substantive time is spent working with the teen alone. These individual sessions have alliance-building value; reveal history and feeling states not always forthcoming in family sessions; and can be leveraged to create content, motivation, and readiness to address problems in joint sessions. Sessions with the parents may include strategies to enhance parents' emotional connection to the child, to validate parents' past efforts, to acknowledge current difficult circumstances, and to generate hope. In family sessions, therapists may use structural therapy techniques to coach constructive family interactions. As MDFT is a therapy of subsystems, decision rules specify which family members should be present for a given session, according to the goals of that session or intervention and the stage of treatment. Urine screening procedures to detect illicit drug use are integrated into the treatment.

MDFT has been investigated in efficacy/effectiveness randomized controlled trials (RCTs; Liddle, Rowe, Dakof, Henderson, & Greenbaum, 2009), process studies (Diamond & Liddle, 1996), and implementation studies examining the intervention's transportability to community settings (Liddle et al., 2006). MDFT achieves greater reduction in adolescent substance use and related problems compared to other active treatments for adolescent drug abuse, including peer group treatment and individual cognitive-behavioral therapy. The efficacy of MDFT has been supported by independent reviews (Waldron & Turner,

2008), and its average weekly costs are less than for community-based outpatient treatment (Liddle, 2009).

Functional Family Therapy

Functional family therapy (FFT; Sexton & Alexander, 1999) is an evidence-based, manual-driven, therapy designed to treat a wide range of problems affecting adolescents and families. FFT is best characterized as a systemic clinical model that evolved from a dynamic process of model integration incorporating clinical experience, integrated theory and scholarship, and empirical evidence. In FFT, the presenting problem is seen as embedded within a core family relational pattern, that, over time, becomes stable and serves to maintain the problem behavior. These family relational patterns are in turn maintained and supported by the ways in which relationships "function" within the system. The term *relational function* refers both to the internal experiences of the individuals in the relational pattern and to the outcome of the patterned sequences, such as relational connection or control.

What makes FFT unique is its conceptualization of relational functions as ideographic (i.e., different behaviors can produce the same functional outcomes) and adaptive for an individual family. Rather than targeting relational functions for change, FFT therapists identify behavioral targets "matched" to functions. For example, a parent who achieves relational control of an adolescent through violence is assisted to do so instead via authoritative parenting and nurturance. This focus on the *expression* of functional outcomes, rather than the outcomes themselves, allows therapists to individualize behavioral change strategies to fit the family's relational functions. For example, improved parent–child communication strategies might take the form of collaborative negotiation for a family with a high degree of relatedness and increased exchange of information via texts and e-mails for a family with a low degree of relatedness.

FFT, a short-term treatment (12–16 sessions over 3–6 months) implemented by one therapist, is based on four integrated principles: (1) Change is predicated on alliance-based motivation; (2) behavior change cannot proceed without meaning change; (3) goals are obtainable and appropriate for the family's culture, abilities, and context; and (4) intervention strategies match and respect the unique characteristics of the family. FFT conceptualizes a successful therapeutic alliance as one in which the therapist and family develop a positive bond and a shared sense of hope, responsibility, and expectation for change. The therapist has the same level of working alliance with the parents and youth (balanced). Practitioners achieve meaning change through reframing, which reduces family members' negative attributions and emotionality about the presenting problem, instead creating an alternative definition of the problem in terms of its meaning or relational focus. *Reframing* is an interactive process in which FAMILY members' responses and ideas are incorporated into the therapist's developing explanation for the problem behavior. Ultimately the constructed, family-focused problem definition becomes an organizing theme that explains problematic interactions and guides behavior change efforts.

Goals in FFT are behavioral changes obtainable for a specific family given its resources, cultural values, and unique circumstances. FFT practitioners do not try to change families to fit a theoretical construct of "healthy functioning," or to reconstruct the personalities of the individuals. FFT negotiates the dialectic between model theory/goals and individual differences across families by "matching to" the relational functions and the family's abilities, social context, and cultural values. Resistance is viewed as family members' perception that the offered activity or attribution does not fit their belief system or perceived circumstances.

During assessment, the therapist determines the interactional sequences in which problems are embedded and the functions served by the behavioral sequences. In addition, the therapist evaluates individual characteristics of family members that may constrain or facilitate change. FFT includes three phases of intervention: *engagement and motivation, behavior change,* and *generalization.* Goals of the engagement and motivation phase are development of a balanced alliance, reduction of negativity and blame, and formulation of the presenting problems in relational terms. In the behavior change phase, the therapist identifies risk factors that contribute to the problem behavior and targets these for change in a way that matches the relational functions of the family. Desired outcomes typically include improved parent–adolescent communication, developmentally appropriate problem solving or conflict management, and negotiation of rewards and punishments for youth behavior. Interventions include contingency contracting and management, modeling, systematic desensitization, time-out procedures, communication skills training, assertiveness training, and problem-solving training. Goals of the generalization phase are to maintain treatment gains by using relapse prevention techniques, supporting the family's use of newly acquired skills in addressing other problems, and linking the family with necessary community resources and support.

FFT has been applied to adolescents with conduct disorder, substance abuse, and delinquency, with high engagement rates (Barnoski, 2004). A cost-effective intervention, FFT has been identified as an evidence-based program in independent reviews, resulting in is broad national and international dissemination. To guide these dissemination efforts, FFT developers designed a manualized approach to clinical supervision and a computer-based quality improvement system to promote transportability and treatment fidelity (Sexton, 2009).

Brief Strategic Family Therapy

Brief strategic family therapy (BSFT), which incorporates structural and strategic approaches, is a systemic treatment for youth behavior problems developed by Jose Szapocznik and colleagues (Szapocznik, Hervis, & Schwartz, 2003) from an integrated program of theory development, clinical practice, and research primarily with Latino youth and their families. BSFT sessions include the entire family and occur once per week for 8–16 weeks. Regular, frequent phone contact with the family is encouraged to reengage, coach, support, and acknowledge treatment gains. Sessions take place in the clinic or in the family's home. BSFT is focused on the "here and now." The therapist facilitates interactions to understand strengths and weaknesses in relationships, and to create opportunities to bring about new relational patterns. BSFT therapists attempt to balance their connection with individual family members, particularly those in overt conflict with one another, because families at greatest risk for dropping out of treatment are those in which the therapeutic alliance is unbalanced between the mother and the adolescent.

Family interaction is assessed along five interactional dimensions: *organization or structure, resonance, developmental stage, identified patienthood,* and *conflict resolution.* Diagnosis is based on family interaction patterns observed in sessions. Assessment data are integrated into a clinical formulation that explains the presenting symptom in terms of family interaction patterns. The goal of treatment is to change these maladaptive patterns to a more adaptive set of interactions. Interventions include the structural techniques of enactments, reframing, and working with boundaries and alliances.

BSFT has been applied to families of low to moderate income, with target youth between 6 and 18 years of age. Presenting problems among adolescents generally include conduct disorders, delinquent behavior, association with antisocial peers, and alcohol and drug use. Given its initial focus on Cuban refugee families in a particular sociopolitical context, BSFT has always attended to cultural issues as a part of treatment. BSFT has demonstrated efficacy with Latino youth with externalizing behavior problems and/or drug abuse (Szapocznik et al., 2004; Szapocznik & Williams, 2000). BSFT with specialized engagement strategies has proven superior in preventing premature termination compared to BSFT with engagement-as-usual strategies or community control conditions for culturally diverse Hispanic samples.

Common Factors

Common factors (Sprenkle et al., 2009) offers a paradigm for understanding therapeutic change, with the view that therapy efficacy is due to mechanisms that cut across all models of psychotherapy. Categorization of common factors can be broad, including nonspecific change mechanisms (e.g., therapeutic alliance) and dimensions inherent in the therapy process itself (e.g., client factors, therapist factors), or narrow, focusing on common aspects of interventions found in different models, often under different names. Adherents assert that different models conceptualize the same systemic processes underlying dysfunction and recommend similar interventions to help a family move from dysfunction to health. Common factors for family therapy include (1) conceptualizing problems in relational terms; (2) disrupting dysfunctional relational patterns; (3) expanding the direct treatment system to include family members of the index patient; and (4) expanding the therapeutic alliance to include each individual, various subsystems, the whole family, and the indirect treatment system.

The application of the common factors paradigm to family therapy has sparked debate that is complicated by the heterogeneity of positions. Those with a radical position believe that common factors are the essence of psychotherapy, in which one treatment is as good as any other, and place a primary emphasis on the therapeutic relationship over the specific treatment model. Those with a moderate position support treatment models demonstrated to be efficacious or based on sound psychological principles but understand treatment efficacy in terms of the model's ability to activate the relevant common factors and give the therapist a conceptual map to organize treatment. The promise of the paradigm is its potential to serve as a metamodel to guide change in family therapy regardless of which model is being utilized.

Research on specific common factors in family therapy is in its infancy. Data indicate that therapeutic alliance, the most studied factor in family therapy, contributes to successful outcomes in all effective models. For example, balanced alliances appear to be more important to treatment outcome than the strength of the alliance (Robbins, et al., 2008). Although there is no direct evidence for other specific common factors, there is indirect evidence for factors such as systemic conceptualization of presenting problems, disruption of dysfunctional relational patterns, and expansion of the treatment system (Celano et al., 2010).

CONCLUSION

The evolution of family therapy has been the product of several historical trends involving a focus on family and interpersonal process, structure, and interaction. Sociocultural, philosophical, economic, and scientific influences have contributed to the development of more divergent practices, which has resulted in greater diversity among models. This growth has broadened the concept of family intervention, which has enhanced the utility, flexibility, and adaptability of family-based treatment. Many models originated from the unified theories of charismatic leaders, yet have been integrated with other theories, adapted to account for sociocultural differences, evaluated using family-oriented assessment devices, held accountable for producing meaningful outcomes, applied to prevention, and focused on contemporary societal problems. Although family therapy models have grown more divergent in some cases, there has been a greater move toward integrative approaches in practice and research. Family therapists have articulated philosophies and standards of practice, supervision, and training.

The central unifying concept remains general systems theory. A family therapist not only takes into account systemic forces in accounting for problem behavior but also engages these forces to create change. Differences in models not only involve therapist conceptualization of problem behavior but also focus on distinct methods of interacting that will lead to therapeutic change. As these models are applied to contemporary problems and settings and evaluated for their efficacy, they will continue to evolve. The integration of various perspectives offered through these distinct approaches will continue to advance the work of family therapists.

SUGGESTIONS FOR FURTHER STUDY

DVDs

Lebow, J. (2007). *Integrative family therapy* (Relationships Video Series). Washington, DC: American Psychological Association.—Multimodal approach to addressing multilayered family difficulties.

McDaniel, S. (2009). *Family therapy over time* (Psychotherapy in Six Sessions Video Series). Washington, DC: American Psychological Association.—Addresses current and multigenerational factors with a common parent–adolescent problem.

REFERENCES

Ackerman, N., & Sobel, R. (1950). Family diagnosis: An approach to the preschool child. *American Journal of Orthopsychiatry, 20,* 744–753.

Alderfer, M. A., Fiese, B. H., Gold, J. I., Cutuli, J. J., Holmbeck, G. N., Goldbeck, L., et al. (2007). Evidence-based assessment in pediatric psychology: Family measures. *Journal of Pediatric Psychology, 33,* 1046–1061.

Anderson, C. M., Reiss, D. J., & Hogarty, G. E. (1986). *Schizophrenia and the family: A practitioner's guide to psychoeducation and management.* New York: Guilford Press.

Anderson, H. (1995). Collaborative language systems: Toward a postmodern therapy. In R. H. Mikesell, D. D. Lusterman, & S. H. McDaniel (Eds.), *Integrating family therapy: Handbook of family psychology and systems theory* (pp. 27–44). Washington, DC: American Psychological Association.

Barnoski, R. (2004). *Outcome evaluation of Washington State's research-based programs for juvenile offenders.* Olympia: Washington State Institute for Public Policy.

Bateson, G., Jackson, D. D., Haley, J., & Weakland, J. (1956). Toward a theory of schizophrenia. *Behavioral Science, 1,* 251–264.

Beach, S. R. H., Wamboldt, M. Z., Kaslow, N. J., Heyman, R. E., & Reiss, D. (2006). Describing relationship problems in DSM-V: Toward better guidance for research and clinical practice. *Journal of Family Psychology, 20,* 359–368.

Beavers, R., & Hampson, R. B. (2000). Empirical approaches to family assessment. *Journal of Family Therapy, 22,* 128–143.

Beavers, W. R., & Hampson, R. B. (1990). *Successful families: Assessment and intervention.* New York: Norton.

Beavers, W. R., Hampson, R. B., & Hulgus, Y. F. (1985). Commentary: The Beavers systems approach to family assessment. *Family Process, 24,* 398–405.

Bennum, I. (1986). Evaluating family therapy: A comparison of the Milan and problem-solving approaches. *Journal of Family Therapy, 8,* 235–242.

Boscolo, L., Cecchin, G., Hoffman, L., & Penn, P. (1987). *Milan systemic family therapy: Conversations in theory and practice.* New York: Basic Books.

Boszormenyi-Nagy, I., Grunebaum, J., & Ulrich, D. (1991). Contextual therapy. In A. S. Gurman & D. P. Kniskern (Eds.), *Handbook of family therapy* (Vol. 2, pp. 200–238). New York: Brunner/Mazel.

Boyd-Franklin, N. (2003). *Black families in therapy: Understanding the African American experience* (2nd ed.). New York: Guilford Press.

Bressi, C., Manenti, S., Frongia, P., Porcellana, M., & Invernizzi, G. (2008). Systemic family therapy in schizophrenia: A randomized clinical trial of effectiveness. *Psychotherapy and Psychosomatics, 77,* 43–49.

Brinkmeyer, M. Y., & Eyberg, S. M. (2003). Parent–child interaction therapy for oppositional children: Evidence-based psychotherapies for children and adolescents. In A. E. Kazdin & J. R. Weisz (Eds.), *Evidence-based psychotherapies for children and adolescents* (pp. 204–223). New York: Guilford Press.

Bronfenbrenner, U. (1979). Contexts of child rearing: Problems and prospects. *American Psychologist, 34,* 844–850.

Carter, B., & McGoldrick, M. (Eds.). (1998). *The expanding family life cycle: Individual, family, and social perspectives* (3rd ed.). New York: Prentice-Hall.

Celano, M. P., & Kaslow, N. J. (2000). Culturally competent family interventions: Review and case illustrations. *American Journal of Family Therapy, 28,* 217–228.

Celano, M. P., Smith, C. O., & Kaslow, N. J. (2010). A competency-based approach to couple and family therapy supervision. *Psychotherapy: Theory, Research, Practice, and Training, 47,* 35–44.

de Shazer, S. (1988). *Clues: Investigating solutions in brief therapy.* New York: Norton.

Diamond, G., & Liddle, H. A. (1996). Resolving a therapeutic impasse between parents and adolescents in multidimensional family therapy. *Journal of Consulting and Clinical Psychology, 64,* 481–488.

Diamond, G. S., Reis, B. F., Diamond, G. M., Siqueland, L., & Isaacs, L. (2002). Attachment-based family therapy for depressed adolescents: A treatment development study. *Journal of the American Academy of Child and Adolescent Psychiatry, 41,* 1190–1196.

Dickstein, S., Hayden, L. C., Schiller, M., Seifer, R., & San Antonio, W. (1994). *The Family Mealtime Interaction Coding System.* Providence, RI: Brown University School of Medicine: Bradley Hospital.

Doane, J. A., Goldstein, M. J., & Miklowitz, D. J. (1986). The impact of individual and family treatment on the affective climate of families of schizophrenics. *British Journal of Psychiatry, 148,* 279–287.

Epstein, M. B., Baldwin, C. M., & Bishop, D. S. (1983). The McMaster Family Assessment Device. *Journal of Marital and Family Therapy, 9,* 171–180.

Epstein, N. B. (2002). Couple and family therapy. In M. A. Reinecke & M. R. Davison (Eds.), *Comparative treatments of depression* (pp. 358–396). New York: Springer.

Eyberg, S. M., Nelson, M. M., & Boggs, S. R. (2008). Evidence-based psychosocial treatments for children and adolescents with disruptive behavior. *Journal of Clinical Child and Adolescent Psychology, 37,* 215–237.

Eyberg, S. M., & Robinson, E. A. (1982). Parent–child interaction training: Effects on family functioning. *Journal of Clinical Child and Adolescent Psychology, 11,* 130–137.

Falloon, I. R. H. (1991). Behavioral family therapy. In A. S. Gurman & D. P. Kniskern (Eds.), *Handbook of family therapy* (Vol. 2, pp. 65–95). New York: Brunner/Mazel.

Fristad, M. A., Verducci, J. S., Walters, K. L., & Young, M. E. (2009). Impact of multifamily psychoedu-cational psychotherapy in treatment children aged 8 to 12 years with mood disorders. *Archives of General Psychiatry, 66*, 1013–1021.

Gil, E. (1994). *Play in family therapy.* New York: Guilford Press.

Gingerich, W. J., & Eisengart, S. (2000). Solution-focused brief therapy: A review of the outcome research. *Family Process, 39*, 477–498.

Gladding, S. T. (2006). *Family therapy: History, theory, and practice.* Englewood, NJ: Prentice-Hall.

Group for the Advancement of Psychiatry Committee on the Family. (1996). Global Assessment of Relational Functioning Scale (GARF): I. Background and rationale. *Family Process, 35*, 155–172.

Haley, J. (1976). *Problem solving therapy.* San Francisco: Jossey-Bass.

Henggeler, S. W., Clingempeel, W., Brondino, M., & Pickrel, S. (2002). Four-year follow-up of multi-systemic therapy with substance-abusing and substance-dependent juvenile offenders. *Journal of the American Academy of Child and Adolescent Psychiatry, 41*, 868–874.

Henggeler, S. W., Schoenwald, S., Rowland, M., & Cunningham, P. (2002). *Multisystemic treatment of children and adolescents with serious emotional disturbance.* New York: Guilford Press.

Henggeler, S. W., Sheidow, A. J., & Lee, T. (2009). Multisystemic therapy (MST). In J. Bray & M. Stanton (Eds.), *The Wiley-Blackwell handbook of family psychology.* West Sussex, UK: Wiley.

Hohmann-Marriott, B. E. (2001). Marriage and family therapy research: Ethical issues and guide-lines. *American Journal of Family Therapy, 29*, 1–11.

Hooley, J. M. (2007). Expressed emotion and relapse of psychopathology. *Annual Review of Clinical Psychology, 3*, 329–352.

Hooley, J. M., & Gotlib, I. H. (2000). A diathesis–stress conceptualization of expressed emotion and clinical outcome. *Applied and Preventive Psychology, 9*, 135–151.

Imber-Black, E., Roberts, J., & Whiting, R. (Eds.). (2004). *Rituals in families and family therapy* (rev. ed.). New York: Norton.

Kaslow, F. W. (1996). *Handbook of relational diagnosis and dysfunctional family patterns.* New York: Wiley.

Kaslow, F. W. (2009). International family psychology. In J. H. Bray & M. Stanton (Eds.), *The Wiley–Blackwell handbook of family psychology* (pp. 684–701). West Sussex, UK: Wiley.

Kaslow, N. J., Celano, M. P., & Stanton, M. (2005). Training in family psychology: A competencies-based approach. *Family Process, 44*, 337–353.

Kazdin, A. E. (2002). Psychosocial treatments for conduct disorder in children and adolescents. In P. E. Nathan & J. M. Gorman (Eds.), *A guide to treatments that work* (pp. 57–85). London: Oxford University Press.

Keith, D. V., Connell, G. M., & Connell, L. C. (2001). *Defiance in the family: Finding hope in therapy.* Philadelphia: Brunner-Routledge.

L'Abate, L., & Weinstein, S. E. (1987). *Structured enrichment programs for couples and families.* New York: Brunner/Mazel.

Lebow, J. L. (2003). Integrative approaches to couple and family therapy. In T. L. Sexton, G. R. Weeks, & M. S. Robbins (Eds.), *Handbook of family therapy: The science and practice of working with families and couples* (pp. 201–225). New York: Routledge.

Liberman, R. P., Mueser, K., & Glynn, S. (1988). Modular behavioral strategies. In I. R. H. Falloon (Ed.), *Handbook of behavioral family therapy* (pp. 27–50). New York: Guilford Press.

Liddle, H. A. (2009). Multidimensional family therapy: A science-based treatment system for adoles-cent drug abuse. In J. Bray & M. Stanton (Eds.), *The Wiley–Blackwell handbook of family psychology* (pp. 341–354). West Sussex, UK: Wiley.

Liddle, H. A., Rowe, C. L., Dakof, G. A., Henderson, C. E., & Greenbaum, P. E. (2009). Multidimen-sional family therapy for young adolescent substance abuse: Twelve-month outcomes of a ran-domized controlled trial. *Journal of Consulting and Clinical Psychology, 77*, 12–25.

Liddle, H. A., Rowe, C. L., Gonzalez, A., Henderson, C. E., Dakof, G. A., & Greenbaum, P. E. (2006). Changing provider practices, program environment, and improving outcomes by transporting multidimensional family therapy to an adolescent drug treatment setting. *American Journal on Addictions, 15*(Suppl.), 102–112.

Madanes, C. (1991). Strategic family therapy. In A. S. Gurman & D. P. Kniskern (Eds.), *Handbook of family therapy* (Vol 2, pp. 396–416). New York: Brunner/Mazel.

McDaniel, S. H., Campbell, T. L., Hepworth, J., & Lorenz, A. (2005). *Family oriented primary care* (2nd ed.). New York: Springer.

McFarlane, W. R. (1991). Family psychoeducational treatment. In A.S. Gurman & D.P. Kniskern (Eds.), *Handbook of family therapy* (pp. 363–395). New York: Brunner/Mazel.

McFarlane, W. R., Dixon, L., Lukens, E., & Lucksted, A. (2003). Family psychoeducation and schizophrenia: A review of the literature. *Journal of Marital and Family Therapy, 29*, 223–245.

McGoldrick, M., Gerson, R., & Petry, S. (2008). *Genograms: Assessment and intervention* (3rd ed.). New York: Norton.

McGoldrick, M., Giordano, J., & Garcia-Preto, N. (Eds.). (2005). *Ethnicity and family therapy* (3rd ed.). New York: Guilford Press.

McGoldrick, M., & Hardy, K. V. (Eds.). (2008). *Reenvisioning family therapy: Race, culture, and gender in clinical practice* (2nd ed.). New York: Guilford Press.

Melby, J., Conger, R. D., Book, R., Rueter, M., Lucy, L., Repinski, D., et al. (1998). *The Iowa Family Interaction Rating Scales.* Ames, IA: Institute for Social and Behavioral Research.

Miklowitz, D. J., Axelson, D. A., Birmaher, B., George, E. L., Taylor, D. O., Schneck, C. D., et al. (2004). Family-focused treatment for adolescents with bipolar disorder: Results of a 2–year randomized trial. *Journal of Affective Disorders, 82*(Suppl. 1), S113–S128.

Miklowitz, D. J., George, E. L., Richard, J. A., Simoneau, T., & Suddath, R. L. (2003). A randomzied study of family-focused psychoeducation and pharmacotherapy in the outpatient management of bipolar disorder. *Archives of General Psychiatry, 60*, 904–912.

Miller, W., Kabacoff, R. I., Epstein, N. B., Bishop, D. S., Keitner, G. I., Baldwin, L. M., et al. (1994). The development of a clinical rating scale for the McMaster model of family functioning. *Family Process, 33*, 53–69.

Minuchin, S. (1974). *Families and family therapy.* Cambridge, MA: Harvard University Press.

Minuchin, S., Montalvo, B., Guerney, B., Rosman, B., & Schumer, F. (1967). *Families of the slums.* New York: Basic Books.

Moos, R. H., & Moos, B. S. (1994). *The Family Environment Scale Manual* (3rd ed.). Palo Alto, CA: Consulting Psychologists Press.

O'Hanlon, W. H., & Weiner-Davis, M. (1989). *In search of solutions: A new direction in psychotherapy.* New York: Norton.

Olson, D. H. (2000). Circumplex model of marital and family systems. *Journal of Family Therapy, 22*, 144–167.

Olson, D. H. (in press). FACES IV and the circumplex model: Validation study. *Journal of Marital and Family Therapy.*

Olson, D. H., & Gorall, D. M. (2003). Circumplex model of marital and family systems. In F. Walsh (Ed.), *Normal family processes* (3rd ed., pp. 514–547). New York: Guilford Press.

Patterson, G. R., & Forgatch, M. S. (1987). *Parents and adolescents living together: The basics (Vol. 1).* Eugene, OR: Castalia.

Patterson, G. R., & Yoerger, K. (1993). Developmental models for delinquent behavior. In S. Hodgins (Ed.), *Mental disorder and crime* (pp. 140–172). Thousand Oaks, CA: Sage.

Pinsof, W. M. (1995). *Integrative problem-centered therapy: A synthesis of family, individual, and biological therapies.* New York: Basic Books.

Pote, H., Stratton, P., Cottrell, D., Shapiro, D., & Boston, P. (2003). Systemic family therapy can be manualized: Research process and findings. *Journal of Family Therapy, 25*, 236–262.

Robbins, M. S., Szapocznik, J., Dillon, F. R., Turner, C. W., Mitrani, V. B., & Feaster, D. J. (2008). The efficacy of structural ecosystems therapy with drug-abusing/dependent African American and Hispanic American adolescents. *Journal of Family Psychology, 22*, 51–61.

Roberto, L. G. (1991). Symbolic–experiential family therapy. In A. S. Gurman & D. P. Kniskern (Eds.), *Handbook of family therapy* (Vol. 2, pp. 444–476). New York: Brunner/Mazel.

Satir, V. (1988). *The new peoplemaking.* Palo Alto, CA: Science and Behavior Books.

Scharff, J. S. (Ed.). (1989). *Foundations of object relations family therapy.* Northvale, NJ: Aronson.

Selvini-Palazzoli, M., Boscolo, L., Cecchin, G., & Prata, G. (1978). *Paradox and counterparadox.* Northvale, NJ: Aronson.

Serketich, W. J., & Dumas, J. E. (1996). The effectiveness of behavioral parent training to modify antisocial behavior in children: A meta-analysis. *Behavior Therapy, 27*, 171–186.

Sexton, T. L. (2009). Functional family therapy: Traditional theory to evidence-based practice. In J. H. Bray & M. S. Stanton (Eds.), *The Wiley–Blackwell handbook of family psychology* (pp. 327–340). West Sussex, UK: Wiley.

Sexton, T. L., & Alexander, J. F. (1999). *Functional family therapy: Principles of clinical intervention, assessment, and implementation.* Henderson, NV: RCH Enterprises.

Simpson, L. (1991). The comparative efficacy of Milan family therapy for disturbed children and their families. *Journal of Family Therapy, 13,* 267–284.

Siqueland, L., Rynn, M., & Diamond, G. S. (2005). Cognitive behavioral and attachment based family therapy for anxious adolescents: Phase I and II studies. *Journal of Anxiety Disorders, 19,* 361–381.

Skinner, H., Steinhauer, P., & Sitarenios, G. (2000). Family Assessment Measure (FAM) and process model of family functioning. *Journal of Family Therapy, 22,* 190–210.

Sprenkle, D. H., Davis, S. D., & Lebow, J. L. (2009). *Common factors in couple and family therapy: The overlooked foundation for effective practice.* New York: Guilford Press.

Stanton, M. D., & Todd, T. C. (1982). *The family therapy of drug abuse and addiction.* New York: Guilford Press.

Szapocznik, J., Feaster, D. J., Mitrani, V. B., Prado, G., Smith, L., & Robinson-Batista, C. (2004). Structural ecosystemic therapy for HIV-seropositive African American women: Effects on psychological distress, family hassles, and family support. *Journal of Consulting and Clinical Psychology, 72,* 288–303.

Szapocznik, J., Hervis, O. E., & Schwartz, S. (2003). *Brief strategic family therapy manual.* Rockville, MD: National Institutes of Health.

Szapocznik, J., & Williams, R. A. (2000). Brief strategic family therapy: Twenty-five years of interplay among theory, research and practice in adolescent behavior problems and drug abuse. *Clinical Child and Family Psychology Review, 3,* 117–134.

Timmons-Mitchell, J., Bender, M. B., Kishna, M. A., & Mitchell, C. C. (2006). An independent effectiveness trial of multisystemic therapy with juvenile justice youth. *Journal of Clinical Child and Adolescent Psychology, 35,* 227–236.

von Bertalanffy, L. (1950). The theory of open systems in physics and biology. *Science, 111,* 23–29.

Waldron, H. B., & Turner, C. W. (2008). Evidence-based psychological treatments for adolescent substance abuse. *Journal of Clinical Child and Adolescent Psychology, 37,* 238–261.

Walsh, F. (Ed.). (2003). *Normal family processes: Growing diversity and complexity* (3rd ed.). New York: Guilford Press.

Walsh, F. (Ed.). (2008). *Spiritual resources in family therapy* (2nd ed.). New York: Guilford Press.

Whitaker, C. A., & Keith, D. V. (1981). Symbolic–experiential family therapy. In A. S. Gurman & D. P. Kniskern (Eds.), *Handbook of family therapy* (Vol. I, pp. 187–225). New York: Brunner/Mazel.

White, M., & Epston, D. (1990). *Narrative means to therapeutic ends.* Adelaide, South Australia: Dulwich Centre.

CHAPTER 10

Couple Therapies

Alan S. Gurman

HISTORICAL BACKGROUND

Significant cultural changes in the last half-century have had enormous impact on marriage and the expectations and experiences of those who marry or enter other long-term committed relationships. Reforms in divorce law (e.g., no-fault divorces), more liberal attitudes about sexual expression, the increased availability of contraception, and the growth of the economic and political power of women have all increased the expectations and requirements of committed relationships to go well beyond maintaining economic viability and assuring procreation. Most couple relationships nowadays are also expected to be the primary source of adult intimacy, support and companionship, and a facilitative context for personal growth. At the same time, the "limits of human pair-bonding" (Pinsof, 2002, p. 135) are increasingly clear, and the changing cultural expectations of couple relationships have led the "shift from death to divorce" (p. 139) as the primary terminator of marriage.

With changing expectations of not only committed relationships but also their permanence, the public health importance of the "health" of such relationships has understandably increased. Through divorce or chronic conflict, the breakdown of couple relationships exacts enormous costs. Recurrent couple conflict and divorce are associated with a wide variety of problems in both adults and children (Gurman, 2008b). Divorce and couple problems are among the most stressful conditions people face. Partners in troubled relationships are more likely to suffer from anxiety; depression and suicidality; substance abuse; and both acute and chronic medical problems and disabilities, such as impaired immunological functioning and high blood pressure; and health risk behaviors, such as susceptibility to sexually transmitted diseases and accident-proneness. Moreover, the children of distressed couple relationships are more likely to suffer from anxiety, depression, conduct problems, and impaired physical health.

Although physical and psychological health are affected by relational satisfaction, there are more common reasons why couples seek, or are referred for, conjoint therapy (Gurman, 2008b). These concerns usually involve matters such as emotional disengagement and waning commitment, power struggles, problem-solving and communication difficulties, jealousy and extramarital involvements, value and role conflicts, sexual dissatisfaction, and abuse and violence.

What Is Couple Therapy?

The term *couple therapy* has recently increasingly replaced the historically more familiar term *marital therapy*, because of its emphasis on the relational bond between two people, whether or not it recognized legally. In the therapy world, the terms are usually used more or less interchangeably. Whether therapeutic methods operate similarly with "marriages" and with "couple" relationships in which there is commitment but no legal bond, is unknown, but is assumed here.

Psychotherapy aimed at improving some aspects of a couple's relationship can be, and often is, provided as an aspect of individual and family therapy treatment formats. For practical purposes, however, it seems reasonable to consider couple therapy as involving the presence of both relationship partners, and not to include clinical methods in which the focus or emphasis is on child or adolescent problems, or parent–child interaction.

This chapter focuses on *couple therapy* in the sense in which that term is usually used (i.e., in reference to *conjoint therapy*, a term coined by Don Jackson (1959), a Sullivanian-trained psychiatric pioneer of family therapy, and popularized by the charismatic Virginia Satir (1964). Some approaches use more "combined" conjoint and individual session formats. Although all who regularly treat couples inevitably practice some sort of "divorce therapy," this practice does not constitute a distinct therapeutic form or "school" of treatment, and therefore is not addressed here. Likewise, sex therapy, a domain of obvious relevance to couple therapists, has generally not intersected with the world of couple and family therapy, and its principles and practices are also not considered. Finally, preventive intervention programs, such as those developed to promote healthy couple functioning for couples at risk for divorce, have expanded rapidly recently but are not the mainstay of more remedially oriented clinicians.

Relationship to Family Therapy

Nathan Ackerman, the unofficial founder of family therapy, once identified "the therapy of marital disorders as the core approach to family change" (1970, p. 124). Despite this early assertion, and the fact that family and couple therapy traditionally "draw from the same body of concepts and techniques" (Fraenkel, 1997, p. 380), the field of family therapy has historically failed to embrace the practice of couple therapy as central to its identity and, in fact, has usually placed it in quite a marginalized conceptual and professional position (Gurman & Fraenkel, 2002). This marginalized position is universally reflected in most textbooks of family therapy, which devote only a small fraction of their pages to couple therapy, despite the fact that surveys repeatedly show that couple problems exceed whole-family problems in the practices of family therapists (Doherty & Simmons, 1996; Rait, 1988). Influential contemporary couple therapy approaches have derived at least as much from clinical extensions of social learning theory/behavior therapy, psychodynamic theory, and humanistic/experiential theory, as from family systems theory and general systems theory (Gurman, 1978), the conceptual soils in which dominant family therapy approaches were planted and have grown.

The Evolution of Couple Therapy

Gurman and Fraenkel (2002) have provided a comprehensive historical account of the evolving theory and practice of couple therapy, describing four conceptually distinctive but chronologically overlapping phases in that history. The first phase, "Atheoretical Marriage Counseling Formation," lasted from approximately 1930 to 1963. This period began with the opening of "marriage counseling" centers in several American cities and Great Britain, and culminated in the first legal recognition of the marriage counseling profession in California (1963). The only national professional organization in the field in this period was the American Association of *Marriage* Counselors, which changed its name first to the American Association of Marriage *and Family* Counselors, and finally, in 1978, to the American Association for Marriage and Family *Therapy*. These name changes reflected significant political accommodation to, and attempts to merge with, the emerging and clearly more powerful field of family therapy.

Marriage counseling was a service-oriented profession, populated mostly by obstetricians, gynecologists, clergy, social workers, and family life educators. Their clinical work, which did not regularly include conjoint therapy until well into the 1970s, focused on helping couples adjust to culturally dominant marital roles, and giving advice and information about practical aspects of married life, including sexuality and parenting. Marriage counselors did not work with couples in severe conflict, or with significant individual psychopathology, but changed their "counseling" moniker to "therapy" only to be more widely accepted among the traditional mental health professions. Couple therapy in this first phase, appropriately characterized by Manus (1966) as a "technique in search of a theory" (p. 449), did not produce any influential clinical theorists.

Couple therapy's next phase (1931–1966), "Psychoanalytic Experimentation," began with challenges by psychiatrists such as Mittelman (1948) and Oberndorf (1934) to the conservative and dominant psychoanalytic tradition against the inclusion of analysands' relatives in treatment. Noticing the apparent "interlocking neuroses" of married partners in psychoanalysis, and the inconsistencies in their stories in analyses with the same analyst, such innovators began experimenting with different combinations and sequences of working with both partners, including some work with the conjoint approach (Greene, 1965). Even as the conjoint approach to couple therapy within psychoanalytic circles became more commonplace late in this period (Sager, 1966), the treatment focus remained largely on the partners as individuals, not on their jointly constructed dyadic system, and on the patient–therapist transference (e.g., Sager, 1967). Psychoanalytic couple therapists had not yet recognized "the healing power within couples' own relationships" (Gurman & Fraenkel, 2002, p. 208).

Just at the time when a more interactional awareness was beginning to emerge within this approach, the conceptual cutting edge of psychoanalytic couple therapy was significantly dulled by the rapidly accelerating family therapy movement, most of which disavowed most psychoanalytic/psychodynamic principles in favor of a more mechanistic "black box" understanding of human behavior. Psychodynamically oriented couple therapy, with rare exceptions (e.g., Framo, 1965), went underground but has resurfaced in important ways during couple therapy's current phase of development due especially to growing interest in object relations and attachment theory.

In couple therapy's third phase (1963–1985), "Family Therapy Incorporation," a few prominent voices within the family therapy field who had a major impact on couple therapy from the "family systems" perspective. Don Jackson, of the Mental Research Institute

(MRI) in California, and Jay Haley, also of the MRI and later the famous Philadelphia Child Guidance Clinic, who both exemplified the "system purists" (Beels & Ferber, 1969), and Murray Bowen, at the Menninger Clinic and later the National Institute of Mental Health and Georgetown University, showed little interest and at times even disdain for the psychology of the individual's unconscious motivation and anything that smacked of the theories of mainstream psychoanalysis and psychiatry. Jackson (1959, 1965), a founder of the MRI Interactional Approach, and Haley (1963), a pioneer in the Strategic approach, emphasized the interpersonal functions of symptoms and the power and control dimensions of couple relationships, and Bowen (1978) created the first multigenerational family and couple therapy approach. Although none of these influential perspectives ever resulted in a discernible "school" of couple therapy, many of their central concepts have trickled down to and permeated the thinking and practices of most psychotherapists who regularly treat couples.

The one major family therapy figure in this period who was not at all a "system purist," not insignificantly, was a woman and a social worker, Virginia Satir. Her 1964 classic *Conjoint Family Therapy* exuded a humanistic and experiential sensitivity, and an emphasis that was hard to find in most family therapy quarters during this period. Satir emphasized patients' self-esteem and both individual and relationship growth, and of all the important family therapy pioneers has probably had the most enduring effects on couple therapy.

Couple therapy's current phase, "Refinement, Extension, Diversification, and Integration" (1986–present) has been marked by continual and significant modification of therapy theory, research, and practice. The "Refinement" component of this phase has been evidenced primarily in the development of three treatment models: Behavioral Marital Therapy (BMT), Emotionally Focused Couple Therapy (EFT), and Insight-Oriented Marital Therapy (IOMT). BMT has evolved from a "behavior exchange phase," emphasizing couples' contracted trading of desired behavior (e.g., Stuart, 1969), to a "skills training phase," emphasizing teaching couples communication and problem-solving skills (e.g., Jacobson & Margolin, 1979), to the current "acceptance phase," balancing the earlier focus on behavior change with a new interest in enhancing partners' abilities to accept inevitable and unresolvable perpetual difficulties (Christensen, Babcock, & Jacobson, 1995). EFT (Johnson, 2004; Greenberg & Johnson, 1986) has reacquainted the couple field with Satir's humanistic–experiential psychotherapy tradition and has singlehandedly exposed clinicians to the relevance of attachment theory for couples (Bowlby, 1988). IOMT (Snyder, 1999; Snyder & Mitchell, 2008) is an empirically supported approach that draws upon psychodynamic object relations theory, interpersonal role theory, and social learning theory, with a developmental emphasis.

Couple therapy's recent "Extension" has seen a dramatic shift from marriage counseling's exclusive attention to minimally troubled, "normal" couples, to partners suffering with significant psychiatric disorders, such as depression, bipolar illness, anxiety disorders, alcoholism, and violence, with BMT (e.g., O'Farrell & Fals-Stewart, 2006), EFT (e.g., Whiffen, 2003), and IOMT (e.g., Snyder, Schneider, & Castellani, 2006) clearly leading the way in this direction. Couple therapy's recent "Diversification" refers to its increasing attention to multiculturalism (i.e., recognizing the role of ethnicity, race, social class, religion, and sexual orientation) in couple relationships and couple therapy (e.g., Rastogi & Thomas, 2009). "Diversification" also includes incorporation of feminist social values and awareness, especially regarding salient couple issues such as gender, power, and intimacy. Finally, couple therapy's "Integration" refers to the revision of clinical theory and practice in the movement toward theoretical and technical integration (Gurman, 2008c), with the most common integrative approaches emphasizing combinations of behavioral and psychodynamic concepts and methods. The integrative thrust in couple therapy includes awareness (e.g., Fishbane, 2007) of the biological bases of behavior relevant to couple relationships.

Common Characteristics of Contemporary Couple Therapy

Contemporary couple therapies have been significantly influenced by psychodynamic (especially object relations) theory, humanistic theory, and cognitive and social learning theory; more recent perspectives provided by feminism, multiculturalism, and postmodernism; as well as basic principles of family systems theory (Gurman, 2010b). Despite this array of influences on the theory and practice of couple therapy, a number of central characteristics are held in common by almost all currently influential approaches (Gurman, 2001): (1) clinical parsimony and efficiency, with an emphasis on what maintains current difficulties; (2) the adoption of a developmental perspective on the source of clinical problems, along with attention to current problems; (3) a balanced awareness of patients' strengths and weaknesses; and (4) a deemphasis on the centrality of treatment and the therapist in patients' lives compared to the couple's real-life interaction. These attitudes overlap some of the core treatment attitudes of brief individual therapists (Budman & Gurman, 1988) and contribute to most couple therapies being quite brief.

Functional versus Dysfunctional Relationships

It is hardly surprising that therapists of varying theoretical orientations define couples' core problems quite differently, ranging from couples' self-defined problems to relationship skill deficits to maladaptive ways of thinking and restrictive narratives about relationships, to problems of self-esteem, to unsuccessful handling of normal life cycle transitions, to unconscious displacement onto the partner of conflicts with one's family of origin, to the inhibited expression of normal adult needs, to the fear of abandonment and isolation. Such varying views lead to a diversity of clinical interventions focusing on behavior patterns, belief systems, and historical and wider contextual factors, the most influential of which are the focus of this chapter.

Despite these varied views of what constitutes the core of couple difficulties, in recent years couple therapists of different orientations have sought a clinically meaningful description of functional versus dysfunctional intimate relationships that rests on a solid research base (Lebow, 1999). Perhaps uniquely in the world of psychotherapy, basic science research on couple health and dysfunction, especially through the work of John Gottman (e.g., 1979, 1999), has provided such a base. For example, his studies of hundreds of couples show that ailing relationships, compared to healthy ones, can be reliably described as suffering from problems in three areas. In the interactive realm, these include showing more negativity than positivity, especially during conflict; more contempt, criticism, stonewalling, and defensiveness; more emotional disengagement; more gridlock centered on perpetual issues involving core personality characteristics and vulnerabilities; and poor conflict management. In the perceptual realm, these include more negative attribution about one's partner's personality and more negativity in partners' narratives about the history of their relationship. In the physiological realm, difficulties involve more chronic diffuse arousal and difficulties in soothing both oneself and one's partner. Findings such as these have been incorporated into the treatment models of a wide array of couple therapies, including eclectic, cognitive-behavioral and behavioral, humanistic, experiential, psychodynamic, transgenerational, and feminist (Gurman, 2010a). Nevertheless, therapists of different orientations make sense of these findings in their own ways, and complement them with ideas about relational health in ways that are specific to their own perspectives. These school-specific perspectives on couple function and dysfunction are addressed in the following section on the practice of varied couple therapies.

THE PRACTICE OF COUPLE THERAPY

Psychotherapists of every theoretical orientation work with couples. While their methods may overlap more than proponents of particular approaches might wish or assert (Gurman, 2010a), there are nonetheless a number of discernibly different models of couple therapy that vary in their conceptualization of the nature of problematic relationships, and of useful ways to reduce couple conflict and enhance relational resilience and connectedness. Here, I describe the conceptual and technical attributes of the couple therapy approaches that have had the greatest influence on training and clinical practice, ranging from early but enduring contributions, such as Bowenian, psychodynamic, structural, strategic, and Satirian, to more recent approaches, such as behavioral, emotionally focused, integrative, and postmodern. These models are presented more or less in the order in which they first appeared, with temporal sequencing at times compromised for the sake of presenting philosophically similar approaches together.

Transgenerational Approaches

Roberto-Forman (2008) provides a comprehensive analysis of the four influential transgenerational approaches to family therapy (i.e., those that emphasize the understanding of couple problems within the long-term, developmental context of the larger family systems from which the couple partners come). Of these, which include Symbolic-Experiential Therapy (Whitaker & Keith, 1981) and Contextual Therapy (Boszormenyi-Nagy & Ulrich, 1981), Bowen Family System Therapy and Object Relations Couple Therapy have developed the clearest models of couple functioning and couple therapy, and have had the greatest impact on clinical practice and training.

Bowen Family Systems Therapy

The father of transgenerational approaches, Murray Bowen, created a conceptual approach referred to as Bowen Family Systems Therapy (BFST) and a body of clinical theory that pervades clinical practice, even among therapists who do not consider themselves "Bowenians." His transgenerational thinking, most prominently set forth in *Family Therapy in Clinical Practice* (Bowen, 1978), originated in the 1950s in research at the National Institute of Mental Health, while he worked to understand the role of family-of-origin interactions in the development of schizophrenia. Bowen (1976a) emphasized that "practically, the two spouses are usually the only ones who are important enough to the rest of the family and who have the motivation and dedication for this kind of [therapeutic] effort" (p. 392). Thus, working with the marital couple was Bowen's preferred therapy format, even when the presenting problem was not marital conflict, but, the symptom of one partner, or even of a child.

Bowen's central construct is *differentiation of self* and its opposite, *fusion*. Differentiation involves the ability both to distinguish emotional states from intellectual processes within oneself and one's own experience from that of significant others. Differentiation from others depends on self-differentiation. Differentiation is a precondition for relational health, and allows internal direction, autonomy, and thus the possibility of intimacy. Poor differentiation manifests in defensiveness, externalization, and discrediting of one's partner. Such fusion is reflected in a couple or family's *emotional stuck-togetherness* or *undifferentiated family-ego mass*.

In common with object relations theorists, Bowen believed that people choose partners at the same level of differentiation, partners who repeat early familial experience and experience-of-self, who show complementary overt behavior styles (e.g., the classic "obsessive–compulsive" husband and "histrionic" wife), and who expect their mates to make up for their own developmental failures. Such fusion can take four forms: emotional distance (*emotional cutoff*), marital conflict, one spouse's symptoms, or the scapegoating of a child (*family projection process*). Conflict ensues when the anxiety level of one or both partners rises due to factors external to the relationship or within the relationship. In such circumstances, partners almost inevitably recruit a third factor (e.g., an affair, a political cause, a symptom) to stabilize the unsteady dyad (*triangulation*). For Bowen, however, couple conflict points not only to problems in the dyad but also more prominently to problems in the larger family systems of the partners, that is, their families of origin (*multigenerational transmission process*). Dysfunctional relationships bespeak undifferentiation not only within the partners but also from their families of origin.

THE PRACTICE OF THERAPY

Structure of Therapy. BFST is carried out with both partners by a solo therapist. Although often presented as a very long-term treatment, BFST also may be conducted on a short-term basis, and with varying intervals between sessions.

Goal Setting. The focus in BFST is on modifying the recurrent cycling of symptoms and problems between the partners and key extended family members, accomplished by increasing each partner's differentiation both within-self and from one's family of origin, resulting in greater acceptance of individual differences. Anxiety reduction usually is sought before experimenting with direct interactions with partners' families of origin.

Techniques and Process of Therapy. Bowen's (1978) central principle for therapeutic change is that "conflict between two people will resolve automatically if both remain in emotional contact with a third person who can relate actively to both without taking sides with either" (p. 177). The techniques of BFST derive directly from the approach's theory of dysfunction and flow directly from the required stance of the therapist.

The Bowen couple therapist assumes a role of "coach" and actively controls the flow of the session. The overriding process aim is to keep sessions calm. To this end, partners are usually encouraged to communicate through the therapist rather than to each other. Little interest is shown in the couple's in-session interaction, and relationship skills are not taught directly. The therapist is generally quite cerebral and intellectual, regulating his or her own emotional reactivity, without judging the partners. More important than any specific therapeutic techniques is the therapist's capacity to stay in a position of *detriangula-*

tion (emotional neutrality) vis-à-vis the couple, often expressed as taking "I-positions" and avoiding side taking.

Two interventions associated with BFST are prominent and common. *Family genograms*, three-generational (or more) maps of families, help partners objectively identify multigenerational family patterns and, in so doing, understand their current difficulties in a new context, thus facilitating the aim of increased differentiation. Genograms visually depict core family patterns, and, in their most complex and sophisticated versions, include wide-ranging information such as family members' names, dates of birth and death, religion, geographical location, socioeconomic status, marriages and divorces, major life events (both positive and negative), cultural and ethnic identities, personality characteristics, and frequency of contact. Visits to partners' families of origin are often encouraged and coached after partners have achieved at least a moderate level of differentiation and decreased emotional reactivity. These visits can include the goal of reconnecting with family members with whom one has had an emotional cutoff, promoting one's own differentiation by not being pulled into historically problematic patterns of relating with family members, or merely observing existing family patterns as an aid to increasing one's objectivity.

Therapist's Role and Mechanisms of Change. The BFST clinician's capacity for maintaining objectivity and his or her knowledge of (Bowenian) family systems principles provide the central forces for therapeutic change. Unlike most other therapeutic approaches, BFST calls on the therapist to teach actively, directly, and didactically about the functioning of emotional systems. BFST asserts that partners cannot achieve higher levels of differentiation than their therapist has achieved. Therapy sessions always include a good deal of attention to defining and clarifying the relationship between the partners, and emphasize isolating "the more prominent stimulus–response mechanisms and teaching the spouses to be observers" (Bowen, 1976b, p. 262). The therapist asks each partner about his or her reactivity, feelings, and thoughts about the other's behavior and expressions. The process goal is for partners to examine the process between them, not to enact it. Thus, the therapist helps each partner become more aware of his or her contribution to problematic couple chain reactions. The process emphasis on changing self and managing emotional reactivity is both facilitated and modeled by the therapist's consistent style of relating to each partner, and may be complemented by the use of relaxation training or mindfulness training to improve affective self-regulation.

Applicability. While conjoint treatment is preferred by BFST, partners may be seen alone if therapy sessions are unmanageably volatile (e.g., Titelman, 2010). Some aspects of BFST may be experienced as quite aversive by members of cultural/ethnic groups (e.g., Middle Eastern, Asian, Southeast Asian) for whom examining multigenerational transmission processes may be experienced as blaming the family (especially elders) for current relationship difficulties (Roberto-Forman, 2008).

Object Relations Couple Therapy

Of the many variants of psychoanalytic thought, object relations theory has had the most pervasive influence on the theory and practice of couple therapy. Challenging classical Freudian theory, object relations theory (e.g., Winnicott, 1960) asserts that the main drive in human experience is to be connected with a "mothering" (nurturant, responsive) person, not struggling with sexual and aggressive impulses.

Despite early forays into couple work by researchers like Mittelman (1948), not until the mid-1960s did analytically oriented couple therapists work conjointly on a regular basis. Even as conjoint therapy became more common, it remained oriented toward the two individuals. As Clifford Sager (1967), the most influential psychoanalytic couple therapist of the 1960s and 1970s, wrote, "I am not primarily involved in treating marital disharmony, which is a symptom, but rather in treating the two individuals in the marriage" (p. 185). Therapy emphasized the interpretation of defenses and the use of free association, dream analysis, and catharsis, and the transference was still the major focus of the therapist's attention.

Because of its inherently marginalized position in the broader family therapy field, psychoanalytically oriented couple therapy receded from visibility during family therapy's "golden age" (roughly 1975–1985; Nichols & Schwartz, 1998, p. 9), although some important contributions came forth in this period (e.g., Framo, 1981). Psychodynamic couple therapy reemerged in the 1980s, partly because of growing interest in integrative models of treatment (see below), partly because of the long-dormant "self in the system" (Nichols, 1987) being reawakened in the family therapy field, and partly because of the creative efforts of a number of clinical theorists working independently to refine their approaches to couple problems (e.g., Willi, 1982). Jill and David Scharff (Scharff & Scharff, 1991, 2008) of the International Institute of Object Relations Therapy in Washington, D.C. have made particularly valuable contributions to Object Relations Couple Therapy (ORCT) over the last 2 decades.

Object relations theory, as applied to clinical work with couples, rested upon the conceptual groundwork of Henry Dicks's classic, *Marital Tensions* (1967). The central lesson from Dicks that led object relations therapists away from traditional psychoanalytic ideas was expressed cogently by Skynner (1980), a British family therapist: "The unconscious conflicts are already fully developed in the mutual projective system between the couple, and could be better dealt with directly rather than by the indirect methods of 'transference'" (pp. 276–277). The aim of therapy, then, was that of "getting the projections (in the marriage) back somehow into the individual selves" (Skynner, 1976, p. 205).

In object relations theory, the core source of couple dysfunction is partners' failure to see both themselves and each other as whole persons. Conflict-laden aspects of oneself, presumably punished or aversively conditioned earlier in life, are repudiated and *split off* from conscious experience; that is, these unwanted, anxiety-laden aspects of self are *projected* onto the mate, and attacked in the mate, who in turn "accepts" the projection (i.e., behaves in accordance with it). For example, a husband who was socialized to be "a real man" finds it unacceptable in himself to be "dependent" by asking for his wife's emotional support even when he is very distressed. His wife, in turn, socialized not to be comfortable with her own competence, frequently asks her husband for advice on matters about which she is quite knowledgeable. He criticizes her for her "neediness," and she sulks in the face of his criticism, for which he also criticizes her as being "too sensitive." She angrily responds that the problem is not that she is "too sensitive," but that her husband is "too self-reliant" and, thus, distant from her. This two-way process of *projective identification* is further complicated by *collusion*, an implicit, unspoken "agreement" not to talk about the unconscious agreement. Projective identification and collusion involve a shared avoidance, a joint defense mechanism that protects each partner from unexpressed and often not consciously experienced fears and impulses (e.g., of merger, attack, or abandonment). Highly or chronically conflicted couples tend to see each other, consciously or unconsciously, in terms of past relationships instead of as "real contemporary people" (Raush, Barry, Hertel & Swain, 1974).

Such rigidity leads to polarized psychological roles, reducing a couple's capacity to respond effectively to new developmental circumstances and to accommodate to other necessary changes and requests for change.

THE PRACTICE OF THERAPY

Structure of Therapy. ORCT is preferably conducted as a long-term experience, with sessions held once or twice a week over a 2-year period or longer (Scharff & Scharff, 2008). ORCT can be used as the basis of a short-term approach, but with more limited aims, such as crisis management. In either situation, in ORCT, very little structuring of the sessions is provided by the therapist, who prefers to follow the lead of the couple, much as a psychoanalytic therapist would do in working with individuals.

Goal Setting. The ORCT therapist does not attempt to impose an agenda on therapy, or to emphasize highly specific therapy goals, which are believed to be too restrictive. Symptom reduction, while desirable, is not a priority, because symptoms are seen as useful in allowing a therapeutic focus on the defenses that produce them. The ORCT clinician's overriding goals are (1) to help the partners reduce the maladaptive controlling power of their collusive arrangement, primarily by improving their *holding capacity* (i.e., their joint ability to receive projections without counterprojection) by listening to the partner's feelings empathically without experiencing intolerable anxiety; and (2) to improve their capacity for *containment* (i.e., the ability to experience, acknowledge, and regulate their own affective experience, allowing painful feelings and thoughts into consciousness, without the need to project them onto the mate). If the partners remain unable to identify with each other's feelings, they are more likely to show reciprocal and often rapidly escalating problematic behavior.

Techniques and Process of Therapy. As noted, therapy sessions in ORCT are not actively controlled by the therapist. Rather, he or she listens nondirectively, maintaining simultaneously an awareness of both partners' transferences toward him or her, and of the mutually transferential projective system within the dyad. The therapist provides a clear and consistent environment to explore one's self and that of one's partner (*setting the frame*). He or she identifies and points out repetitive couple interaction patterns, paying particular attention to those that seem to be fueled by defensiveness. As the patient–therapist alliances deepen, the therapist is more likely to interpret partners' resistance to change, including self-exploration. The ORCT therapist prizes therapeutic neutrality with regard to both partners' choices and values, and avoids siding with either partner. In this process, the therapist's use of self is a central technique. Described as the ability not to need to impose meaning or to "know," it is achieved by not doing too much in sessions (e.g., taking too much responsibility), and by remaining open to one's own internal experience. This *negative capability* facilitates the therapist's capacity to take in the partners' transference reactions, and to experience his or her own *countertransference* as a way of understanding both the partners as a couple, and each partner in the relationship.

A central technical therapist activity in ORCT involves the *interpretation* of patient defenses in general, especially defenses against intimacy. These might be expressed in the emerging session themes, silences, nonverbal behavior, and patients' expressed fantasies and dreams (about which the interpersonal meaning is emphasized). Termination is deemed appropriate when partners have developed adequate holding capacities and can relate more intimately. The couple decides when termination should occur. Separating from the therapist is considered a significant part of the therapeutic process, and is treated as such.

Therapist's Role and Mechanisms of Change. In ORCT, the therapeutic alliance is fortified primarily by the therapist's ability to tolerate the partners' anxiety in an adequate *holding environment*. Although mostly nondirective, the therapist is not a caricatured psychoanalytic "blank screen." Whereas the ORCT therapist generally follows rather than leads, he or she is confrontative at times, as the mood of the session and the couple's needs (and avoidances) require. Therapeutic change is mediated through the patient–therapist relationship, and projectively distorted perceptions of both the therapist and one's partner are examined, interpreted as to both their current avoidance function and their historical origins, and reworked many times over the course of treatment. Clearly, the ORCT therapist must be skilled at maintaining appropriate affective boundaries, capable of holding a neutral stance, and composed in the face of the couple's anxiety in response to the therapist's low level of structuring.

Applicability. Psychological mindedness is a fundamental characteristic of couples who are appropriate for ORCT, especially long-term ORCT. As Scharff and Bagnini (2002) state it, "Object relations couple therapy is indicated for couples that are interested in understanding and growth. It is not for couples whose thinking style is concrete" (p. 77). Contraindications in ORCT are common to other types of couple therapy (e.g., those engaged in ongoing affairs or with severe psychiatric disorder or uncontrollable volatility in sessions). Couples who are most appropriate for ORCT are seeking personal and relational growth more than symptom reduction alone. In addition to its relevance to ordinary couple tensions, ORCT has been reported to be helpful in dealing with grief and mourning, lack of sexual intimacy, and a variety of individual symptoms that predate but are now affecting, the relationship.

Structural and Strategic Approaches

While not originally developed to treat couple problems, these "system purist" approaches (Beels & Ferber, 1969) have played major roles in the training of tens of thousands of couple and family therapists, and elements of these approaches are regularly incorporated into the clinical practices of many psychotherapists who have other primary theoretical allegiances.

Structural–Strategic Couple Therapy

Structural Therapy, developed by Salvador Minuchin (1974; Minuchin & Fishman, 1981), and Strategic Therapy, developed by Jay Haley (1974) and Cloe Madanes (1981), involve couple therapy methods that evolved out of what have been among the most influential approaches to family therapy. Although structural therapy offers a very important perspective on couple difficulties, very little has been published on this approach to treating couples (cf. Aponte & DiCesare, 2000; Simon, 2008), whereas such writings about strategic therapy (e.g., Haley, 1963, 1974; Madanes, 1990) are plentiful. While often presented as separate "schools" of therapy, the two approaches share overlapping and complementary constructs about couple functioning and couple therapy. Strategic therapy is often seen as putting somewhat greater emphasis on clinical technique than on a theory of intimate relationships, and structural therapy is often seen the other way around.

Both therapies are present-oriented, emphasizing how committed relationships, and the broader families and social contexts within which they operate, are organized. They epitomize the maxim, "The system is its own best explanation" (i.e., the patterned regularities of the system as it now operates explain its behavior better than can be done by invoking any set of constructs that lie outside the system, such as inferential attributions of therapists). Still, these approaches have a very strong interest in the developmental or *family life cycle* context in which problems arise, not for the purpose of excavating the past, but for understanding the meaning and place of problems in the current developmental functioning of the couple and family as a system that evolves over time. Structural–Strategic therapists believe that symptoms often signal a developmental impasse in couple life, and that symptoms are both systems-*maintained* and systems-*maintaining*. A central tenet of Structural–Strategic Couple Therapy (SSCT) is that symptoms maintain couple systems by serving a protective, *homeostatic* function for the relationship, by deflecting conflict away from its real sources. For example, a wife who feels disempowered in her marriage becomes quite depressed, leading the couple's life to become increasingly organized around "her problem," while her lack of a voice in the marriage is not addressed or even identified.

In SSCT, formulations about the etiology of problems are secondary to consideration of how problems are maintained. SSCT clinicians are concerned with the *structure* of a couple's relationship, including its repeating interactions over time with others (e.g., the partners' families of origin). Although the emphasis in SSCT has become more muted, for many years, the central relational dynamic of couple relationships was thought to be power and control. As Haley (1963) said, "The major conflicts in marriage center in the problem of who is to tell whom what to do and under what circumstances" (p. 227). For Haley, problems arise when the hierarchical structure is unclear, when there is a lack of flexibility, or when the relationship is marked by *rigid symmetry* or *complementarity*. Symptoms represent ways in which couples are organized by a *dysfunctional incongruity*, with the symptom-bearer maintaining relational power through his symptoms. Haley's (1963) classic article "Marriage Therapy" presented his "first law of human relations" to explain the resistance to change so common in relationships: "When one individual indicates a change in relation to another, the other will respond in such a way as to diminish that change" (p. 234). Couples with a symptomatic partner and couples with recurrent conflict have problems establishing and maintaining appropriate couple boundaries. Too much overinvolvement or *enmeshment* (e.g., anxiously attempting to direct too many aspects of the partner's life) limits individual growth and freedom of expression, while too much being out of emotional contact or *disengagement* (e.g., showing little awareness of or interest in noncouple aspects of the partner's life) may lead to an inability to empathize or involvement in affairs. Such couples also often have maladaptive boundaries with others outside their relationship (e.g., when excessive attention by one parent focused on a child *detours* the couple away from their tensions, or when one partner's overinvolvement with the family of origin creates a problematic *cross-generational coalition*).

In SSCT, the focus is more on how a couple is "stuck" than on how it is "sick," so that few couple structures are seen as inherently unhealthy. The emphasis is on whether the current structure allows the relationship to be flexible enough for its members to meet their individual needs, as well as the needs of the relationship at its particular developmental juncture.

THE PRACTICE OF THERAPY

Structure of Therapy. Therapy sessions are usually weekly or biweekly. Conjoint sessions dominate SSCT practice, but portions of sessions may be used to work with the individual partners to obtain necessary information or to resolidify a therapeutic alliance. On average, SSCT lasts about 8–10 sessions, but there are no formal time limits. Therapists usually work alone, because cotherapy may raise issues about maintaining therapeutic focus and a consistent therapist stance (e.g., whether to use direct or indirect interventions; see below).

Goal Setting. The strategic influence in SSCT emphasizes resolution of the couple's presenting problem, while the structural influence emphasizes reworking of underlying structural problems. Although there are some common universal goals in SSCT, such as increased couple intimacy, a better balance of power, and improved dealings with "third parties" to the relationship, each course of SSCT includes the creation of an explicit, couple-specific treatment contract that specifies the roles of both the therapist and each partner in attempting to achieve these goals.

Techniques and Process of Therapy. The emphasis in SSCT is not on seeking the "truth" but on doing "what works." Interpretation is offered by the therapist not to develop "insight" but to relabel the meaning, and thus the function, of behavior to induce observable change. The therapist is held more responsible for inducing change than in most other approaches to couple therapy. The overriding principle by which this happens is through the therapist's planful (hence, "strategic") interventions to interrupt, redirect, and change problem-maintaining sequences in the couple's interaction, especially through the use of tasks and directives. In-session tasks are more associated with the structural influence in SSCT, and out-of-session tasks with strategic influences. Likewise, whereas direct interventions (e.g., asking the partners to talk to each other about a specific topic; nonverbally interrupting a husband's frequent interruptions of his wife) tend to be more structural, indirect interventions (e.g., via the use of "paradoxical" interventions; see below) tend to be more strategic.

The integrative structural–strategic approaches of M. Duncan Stanton (1980) and Thomas Todd (1986) encourage sequential integration, with structurally oriented interventions being attempted first, followed by a more strategic approach when structural intervention is not helpful. Strategic work is done from the outset if there are good reasons to expect that a structural emphasis would not be effective (e.g., numerous previous treatment failures, or a history of previous noncompliance). In practice, most structural–strategic couple work is an admixture of both of these therapeutic styles.

A hallmark of SSCT is the use of *directives,* which Keim and Lappin (2002) define as "a communication by the therapist suggesting that a client experience, think, and/or behave differently" (p. 102). Many directives have been associated with structural and, especially, strategic therapy (see, Keim, 1999, for a listing of the most common directives). Although structural–strategic therapists are very respectful of "client-inspired" directives (e.g., wife suggests a novel way for herself and her husband to handle a recurrent problem), SSCT is more readily identified with *therapist-inspired directives,* which can be direct (more "structural") or indirect (more "strategic"), and can be focused more on in-session couple behavior (more "structural") or out-of-session behavior (more "strategic"). *Direct directives* often emphasize the structurally derived interventions of joining and restructuring. *Joining* is often misunderstood as being equivalent to empathy. While joining includes empathic relatedness, it also implies the therapist's capacity to form working alliances without being induced into the couple's dysfunctional patterns, roles, and interactions (Simon, 2008). Joining is actually *joining with the transaction*, implying the therapist's connection to the couple as a dyad, as well as to individuals, and is as much an attitude as a technique. As therapy progresses, joining merges into *tracking* (i.e., the use of patient language, idiom, and worldview to prepare for a more change-focused intervention).

Restructuring involves a number of suboperations, especially enactment and unbalancing. In *enactment*, the therapist deals directly with dysfunctional patterns rather than talking about them. He or she encourages the couple to deal with their problems in their usual ways in the session in order for the therapist to see the problem around which he or she wishes to shift the couple's interaction. Enactments allow the therapist opportunities to substitute functional for dysfunctional behavior. Enactment may include the therapist's *boundary marking*, by challenging the couple's psychological proximity (e.g., overtly identifying the couple's usual patterns of overinvolvement and underinvolvement as maladaptive and encouraging new alternatives). *Unbalancing* interventions challenge rigid couple hierarchical relationships by supporting one partner (e.g., by entering into a temporary *coalition* with one partner to empower that person or create new interactive possibilities). *Intensification* of the couple's interaction may also be used to restructure problem-maintaining behavior (e.g., by emphasizing differences between enmeshed partners who avoid conflict; by drawing out and developing implicit couple conflicts; and by *relabeling* the purpose, function, or intention of a recurrent behavior in order to shift a partner's attributions about that behavior). Homework tasks, a common direct intervention, are usually meant to challenge existing problematic structures and to increase adaptive behavior.

Indirect directives are more defiance-based than direct directives, in that they assume individual and/or couple resistance to change and fall under the rubric of what are often called *paradoxical interventions*. They direct the partners to continue their dysfunctional thinking or overt behavior rather than to discontinue it, the stance a psychotherapist is generally assumed to favor. When such techniques focus on cognition, they are called reframing, and when they focus on observable behavior, they are considered directives. *Reframing* means labeling a behavior in such a way as to give it a new and usually more acceptable meaning, such as when a therapist uses *positive connotation* or *positive interpretation* (e.g., asking a couple to consider the theretofore unseen beneficial effects of a problem), or *ascribing noble intention* (e.g., attributing an acceptable motivation to an unwanted partner behavior).

Paradoxical interventions that focus on out-of-session behavior may involve prescribing the symptom, restraint, ordeals, and pretending. *Prescribing the symptom*, including *symptom scheduling*, calls for the therapist to present a rationale for a partner to intentionally "do" her clinical symptom or undesired behavior, especially if it is experienced as "involuntary," thus bringing it under more voluntary control. The therapist may also *restrain change* by warning the partners to *go slow*, noting the unacknowledged "dangers" of rapid improvement that would be worse than their present difficulties. *Therapeutic ordeals* call on the therapist to urge a partner to carry out behavior he or she strongly dislikes, but which is purported to have ultimate benefit for the couple. Finally, *pretending* calls on the therapist to (often playfully) instruct a partner to "pretend" to have dysfunctional behavior, be it symptomatic behavior or nonsymptomatic behavior that is aversive to his or her partner, and, if challenged by the mate about the authenticity of his or her behavior, to deny that any pretending is occurring.

Therapist's Role and Mechanisms of Change. In SSCT, change occurs by restructuring both short and long couple sequences that constitute the problems and, in the case of a symptomatic partner, reinforce the problem. The SSCT therapist must be able to "read" the level of active influence needed by a given couple in order to change, and be comfortable giving both direct and indirect directives. This needed range of therapist styles parallels the need for the structural–strategic therapist to be flexible by moving between a challenging stance and a supportive stance, at times with great and serious intensity, and at other times with an ironic sense of humor (Simon, 2008).

Applicability. Because of SSCT's present and future focus, couples who prefer to talk about the past may have limited success in this approach. Partners with incompatible goals may have difficulty insofar as SSCT calls for many therapist directives, and devising directives that are responsive to the needs of partners with very different therapeutic aims can be difficult. Because of SSCT's emphasis on a conjoint experience and collaborative effort, this approach may have limited value for separated couples who do not interact a good deal outside therapy.

Brief Strategic Couple Therapy: The MRI Approach

Another influential approach to treating couple problems that emerged within the family therapy movement is the Brief Problem-Focused Therapy of the MRI in Palo Alto, California, originally developed by John Weakland, Richard Fisch, Paul Watzlawick, and Arthur Bodin (1974), also called the "Palo Alto approach" (Shoham, Rohrbaugh, & Cleary, 2008). This approach, presented in the classic, *Change: Principles of Problem Formation and Problem Resolution* (Watzlawick, Weakland, & Fisch, 1974) and in *The Tactics of Change* (Fisch, Weakland & Segal, 1982), is also referred to as "Brief Strategic Therapy," thus possibly leading to misidentification as synonymous with the strategic therapy of Haley and Madanes just described (and because Haley was an early member of the Brief Therapy Center of the MRI). But the approaches differ in two reliable ways: one practical, the other conceptual. While Haley-type strategic approaches set no time limit on treatment, the MRI approach often sets a definite and almost standard time limit of 10 sessions, and is the only influential method of couple therapy to do so (Gurman, 2001).

More significant is the difference in how these approaches understand clinical problems. Haley-type strategic therapists and structural–strategic therapists view problems and symptoms as serving protective functions in relationships. MRI-style therapists reject the symptom-as-function view, and have little interest in notions such as implicit couple and family processes, or underlying relationship structures. In the MRI approach there is no effort to define what constitutes a "normal" couple relationship. The form or topography of couple relationships is largely irrelevant (with obvious exceptions, e.g., violence), so that if there is no complaint about the relationship, there is no relationship problem. The MRI approach is constructivist, seeing problems not as being "discovered" but as socially "constructed" (i.e., perceived and created through attribution and meaning giving).

The MRI model views problems as the result of misguided efforts to solve *difficulties*, usually everyday life situations that are typically either solvable by using common sense, or that must be accepted as inherently unsolvable. *Problems,* on the other hand, are patterns of ongoing, deadlocked, impasse-laden mishandling of difficulties, called *ironic processes,* that is, when particular attempts to solve a problem actually make it worse (i.e., when the "solution *is* the problem"). Such processes create *vicious cycles*, positive feedback loops between a problematic behavior and the actions taken to change that behavior. The misguided actions of vicious cycles are called *attempted solutions*, and therapy aims to replace such cycles with *virtuous cycles*, resolving the problem by doing "less of the same (attempted solution)" rather than repeating the unsuccessful "more of the same" approach.

There are three types of problems. Type-I problem-solving errors, known as *terrible simplifications*, occur when action is necessary but is not taken (i.e., a difficulty is dealt with as though it does not exist). Type II problem-solving errors constitute the *utopian syndrome*, when action is taken but is not really necessary, as in trying to change a nonexistent difficulty or what is unchangeable. The third maladaptive problem-solving pattern is called *paradox*, when action is called for but is taken at the wrong level of change. This happens when couple partners attempt *first-order change*; that is, when behavior changes but follows the original relationship rules (e,g., husband now does more household tasks, but wife still has the responsibility of seeing to it that household tasks are being done) when actually *second-order change* (basic change in relational structure or underlying assumptions) is required (e.g., husband now does more household tasks because he has a new attitude about men's and women's relationship roles), or vice versa. A common example of the latter in couple therapy is the *be spontaneous! paradox*, in which misguided attempts to control naturally occurring behavior *is* the problem.

THE PRACTICE OF THERAPY

Structure of Therapy. MRI couple therapy is often time-limited, with a maximum of 10 sessions. If treatment ends without all 10 sessions being used, they are kept "in the bank" for the future. Treatment ends when goals are reached and change seems stable. In institutional settings, where MRI couple therapy is typically practiced, behind-the-mirror peer consultants often participate in therapy, phoning in suggestions as needed. MRI therapists often begin with weekly meetings but soon move to longer intervals. Since the MRI approach was not created specifically for couple (or family, or individual) therapy per se, MRI therapists often meet with individuals with relationship problems. This notion of *customership* refers to who is most motivated for change. In order to maximize *maneuverability*, the therapist may see the partners separately instead of, or in addition to, conjointly. This stance notwithstanding, recent research on the MRI approach in fact seems to support the common clinical view that couple therapy is more effective when both partners participate (Shoham et al., 2008).

Goal Setting. The MRI approach emphasizes solving presenting problems as quickly as possible. It does not seek insight, the enhancement of relationship skills, or personal growth. The overriding goal is the interdiction of vicious cycles that maintain the problem. Problems are defined in precise behavioral terms, as are relevant *problem–solution loops*. Aiming for second-order change, the therapist's intent is to correct "corrective" behavior. The origins of the problem are not of interest except insofar as they may clarify unfortunate attempted solutions. The MRI therapist pays a good deal of attention to the client's use of language and views of the problem (e.g., whether it is seen as internal vs. external, or as voluntary vs. involuntary). Awareness of such nuances helps to plan the selection and use of change-oriented interventions.

Techniques and Process of Therapy. Before actively intervening to disrupt a problem–solution loop, the MRI couple therapist assesses previously attempted solutions that have failed. The goal is to induce the partners, or even one of them, to do "less of the same" behavior that is intended by them to solve the problem but actually reinforces it.

MRI techniques and tactics include both *general* and *specific* interventions. General interventions are relevant to work with most couple problems and reflect the basic MRI stance of encouraging *therapeutic restraint.* By urging couples to *go slow,* the therapist anticipates and absorbs clients' natural tendencies to resist change, and reduces their uneasy sense of urgency to resolve their problems. Likewise, the therapist may *caution about the dangers of improvement,* pointing out heretofore unforeseen negative consequences to positive changes. Or the therapist may offer suggestions about *how to make the problem worse.*

Interventions with distressed couples emphasize the distinction between complementary and symmetrical relationship patterns. *Complementary interactions,* and prevailing relationship styles, involve maximizing differences. In these relationships, negative behavior evokes different counterresponses from one's partner. In *symmetrical interactions,* there is a minimization of differences, and negative behavior by one partner evokes the same kind of behavior in his or her mate (e.g., both partners withdraw from a fight; yelling by one leads to yelling by the other). Symmetrical relationships are not only often competitive relationships but are also more likely to keep conflict covert. As a result, they are less common among clinical couples.

Interventions, while decided on a case-by-case basis, include some relatively predictable motifs, such as the well-known *pursuer–distancer* or *demand–withdraw* pattern, which may take the form of demand–refuse, discuss–avoid, criticize–defend, accuse–deny. In a demand–refuse situation, the MRI therapist may encourage the demander to do less demanding, thus changing his or her "solution" to the problem (e.g., of the partner's uncommunicativeness), perhaps by having him or her "merely" observe the partner in problem-evoking situations, without commentary or insistence on change. In cases heavy with criticism–defense behavior, the defending partner may be encouraged to do something different when criticized, (e.g., acknowledge the criticizer's point of view rather than explaining away his or her own behavior). Accusation–denial pairings (e.g., about dishonesty) may be helped by *jamming.* The therapist asks the accusee to do the suspicion/accusation-evoking behavior randomly (e.g., talking to strangers in public or on the telephone), while asking the accuser to see if he or she can figure out what the accused partner is up to (e.g., is this "real" or feigned suspicious behavior?). Both keep written notes on these exchanges, to be shared at the next therapy session. These interdictions decrease the information value of the interchanges and introduce novel elements into an all-too-familiar maladaptive interaction.

While MRI interventions are sometimes seen as manipulative, in fact, to be effective, they require a highly refined sensitivity to client needs and individual differences. Effective restraining or paradoxical interventions call for finely tuned appreciation of the *patient position,* how each partner sees him- or herself and the relationship, and how each partner uniquely uses language to express his or her self-view and view of the world. The reframing of the meaning of client behavior and potential consequences of behavior change is done, not to induce insight, but to induce cooperation with the therapist's directives for out-of-session behavior. Thus, any reframing the partners find plausible is acceptable, without regard to its inherent "truth." Consistent with the overriding attitude of therapeutic restraint, positive changes in the course of therapy are met with cautious optimism.

Therapist's Role and Mechanisms of Change. The therapist's role in MRI couple therapy is to induce change from the "outside," but to do so by tuning in to the partners' "insides." The therapeutic relationship, in its usual sense, is not heavily weighted as a vehicle for change. While respectfulness and empathy are essential in MRI therapy, the therapist–client relationship is not at all seen as healing, and as Fisch et al. (1982) have said,

> In doing therapy briefly . . . termination is not viewed as such a special event. The brevity of treatment and the problem-solving approach leave little room for "developing a relationship" between patient and therapist; thus, there is little sense of a wrenching from treatment or a cutting the patient adrift to fend for himself. (pp. 175–176)

Healing or change comes about by the therapist's interruption/interdiction of ironic couple processes. The therapist must avoid ironic therapeutic processes by not engaging in the same failed "solution" errors of either partner, thereby maintaining therapeutic maneuverability. Accomplishing this often leads to the therapist's *taking a one-down position* (e.g., by soft-selling an idea or suggestion) to promote cooperation with directives and receptivity to reframing.

Applicability. MRI couple therapy is especially indicated when a couple has a very specific and clear complaint, or when the partners are likely to engage reluctantly with more direct interventions, or resist them altogether. MRI couple therapy is contraindicated when couples seek personal growth and self-awareness. A potential constraint in practicing MRI therapy is that the therapist must be willing to limit therapeutic attention to what the partners complain about, and resist temptations to broaden the scope of clinical attention.

Experiential–Humanistic Approaches

The three most influential experiential–humanistic approaches to couple therapy are the Satir (1964, 1972) Model, also called "Family Reconstruction," one of the earliest couple treatment methods; Emotionally Focused Couple Therapy (Greenberg & Johnson, 1986; Johnson, 2004), one of the most influential methods; and the Gottman Method Couple Therapy (Gottman, 2004; Gottman & Gottman, 2008), the most empirically derived method.

The Satir Model

Satir was the most visible and influential popularizer of couple and family therapy among both professional and lay audiences from the mid-1960s until about the mid-1970s. Her legacy in the field remains strong, although currently there is probably no discernible "school" of Satir therapy. The author of such classic books as *Conjoint Family Therapy* (1972), Satir held a unique place among the pioneers of family therapy, in that she was the only nationally and internationally influential female clinician in the field. Although the titles of most of her published works referred to family rather than couple therapy, most of her systems-oriented therapeutic contributions were about dyads, especially the marital dyad. Satir was a cofounder (1959) of the MRI in Palo Alto, California, and established its first family therapy training program. She left the MRI, in 1966, to become the first director of the famous personal growth center known as the Esalen Institute. Her increasing involvement in the "human potential movement" of humanistic–experiential therapists such as

Carl Rogers and Fritz Perls pulled her outside the mainstream of systems therapy. More-over, her contributions were undoubtedly undervalued by the "systems purists" of her era, with their emphasis on family structures, boundaries, power and, for some, therapeutic indirectness.

Satir became the MRI's first director of training. She gave primary emphasis to the func-tioning and experiencing of the individual, as much as to the individual-in-relational con-text. She viewed the roles people assume in close relationships (e.g., "placator," "rescuer"), and the dysfunctional communication styles they exhibit as fundamentally expressions of low self-esteem and poor self-concept (Satir, 1964). From Satir's experiential perspective, the main goal of couple therapy was to foster greater self-esteem and self-actualization by increasing the congruence and clarity of self-expression about relational needs, self-perceptions, and perceptions of one's partner; increasing self-awareness; removing protec-tive "masks" that shield authentic self-revelation; and accepting and valuing differences. Toward these ends, a wide variety of techniques was used, ranging from verbal methods, such as an emphasis on talking *to* rather than *about* one's mate, and direct expression of feelings to nonverbal methods, such as "family sculpting" and dance movement. Among the most influential values Satir represented were the centrality of authentic communication and self-disclosure, the salience of relational closeness and security over and above mere problem resolution, and belief in the restorative potential of committed couple relation-ships. In these respects, her contributions lay the cornerstone for later influential models of couple therapy grounded in attachment theory and focused on the expression of emotional vulnerability. Satir never lost sight of what Nichols (1987) called "the self in the system."

Emotionally Focused Couple Therapy

Emotionally Focused Couple Therapy (EFT), a synthesis of experiential and systemic tradi-tions in psychotherapy, was created by Canadian psychologists Susan Johnson and Leslie Greenberg. The name of this approach was chosen as a statement of the belief in the cen-trality of emotion in intimate relationships and as a counterposition to the overwhelming absence of attention to emotion in the "black box" couple and family therapy field of the early 1980s.

EFT adheres to humanistic–experiential therapy principles: (1) The therapeutic alli-ance can itself be healing; (2) the inherent validity of the patient's experience is central to change, and is fostered by the therapist's authenticity and transparency; (3) given the opportunity to do so, people have the ability to make healthy choices; (4) both the inner and outer realities of people's lives need to be attended to; and (5) therapy can provide opportunities for direct, in-session, corrective emotional experiences. EFT is also linked to systems theory principles, such as the circularity of behavior and the idea of behavior being communicative. It differs from most other systemically oriented methods in its cen-tral attention to the role of emotion to break maladaptive, repetitive cycles of couple inter-action. Recently, Greenberg and Goldman (2008) have proposed a modification of EFT that emphasizes affect regulation skills more than in the original model.

What especially sets EFT apart from other approaches is the prominence of *attachment theory* (Bowlby, 1988) in its understanding of couple tension and creation of a therapeutic emphasis. EFT emphasizes emotional "bonds" over "bargains" to be negotiated (Johnson, 1986) as the basis for committed relationships. Following Bowlby, EFT holds that all human beings have an innate need for consistent, safe contact with responsive and caring others. Such bonds create a mutual sense of safety, which in turn help partners regulate emotions effectively, deal with differences, and communicate clearly. Research consistently has shown that relationship security predicts high levels of closeness, trust, and satisfaction (Cassidy & Shaver, 1999).

Couple disharmony is usually signaled by expressions of anger, which is seen as a *secondary emotion* experienced and shown in reaction to some other, more vulnerable, *primary emotion* (e.g., sadness or fear). When expressions of anger do not elicit emotional responsiveness in the partner, a downward-spiraling process is set in motion, from coercion to clinging to depression and despair. EFT views such eventual disengagement as a cumulative stressor.

THE PRACTICE OF THERAPY

Structure of Therapy. Nothing inherently limits EFT's duration, but most EFT lasts about 8–15 sessions. Therapy usually begins with one or two joint sessions, followed by individual sessions with each partner to intensify the therapeutic alliance and gather potentially relevant data on partners' relationship histories.

Goal Setting. EFT has two basic aims: exploring partners' views of self and other, as organized by their immediate (in-session) affective experience, and helping partners access previously unacknowledged (often to oneself, as well as to one's mate) feelings, so that they may be expressed directly in the moment of the therapy session. These aims are fostered in the context of addressing the particular difficulties and goals of each couple.

Techniques and Process of Therapy. The overall corrective emotional experience sought in EFT is achieved through a mixture of some Gestalt and general "systemic" interventions, with client-centered reflection of partners' immediate experience central to promoting a degree of sustained empathic focus and level of affective immediacy that is higher than in most couple therapies. The focus is on the present, and interpretation of unconscious motivation is used sparingly, if at all. Such corrective experiences increase mutual empathy, decrease defensiveness, and lead to an increased capacity for problem solving. Interpersonal skills are not taught directly. EFT therapists restructure interpersonal patterns to incorporate each partner's need for secure attachment.

The EFT model has been clearly described, especially in Johnson's (2004) *The Practice of Emotionally Focused Marital Therapy* and *Becoming an Emotionally Focused Couple Therapist: The Workbook* (Johnson, Bradley, Furrow, & Lee, 2005). Stage One, "Cycle Deescalation," emphasizing assessment and the deescalation of painful relational cycles, includes four steps: (1) creating a working alliance and delineating core conflict issues and themes; (2) mapping the recurring problematic interactions patterns in which the central problems appear; (3) accessing relevant and previously unacknowledged or insufficiently acknowledged feelings behind each partner's behavioral contribution to the problematic cycles; and (4) reframing the meaning of problems in light of the underlying emotions and each partner's attachment needs and fears. Stage Two, "Changing Interactional Patterns," includes three steps: (1) encouraging each partner to "own" previously disowned attachment needs; (2) encouraging acceptance of each partner's emotional experience; and (3) supporting the direct expression of other specific needs in the relationship. Stage Three, "Consideration and Integration," includes two steps: (1) developing new solutions to old problems, and (2) reviewing the successes achieved in therapy and helping the partners generalize their experiences.

EFT therapists have identified a number of core interventions to aid exploring and reformulating emotional experience, and restructuring couple interactions: (1) reflecting emotional experience, which focuses the session and builds alliances; (2) reframing in the context of the central cycles and attachment needs, which connects "undesirable" partner responses to new, affect-based meanings and softens the view of one's partner; and (3) restructuring and shaping interactions via enactment and the therapist's choreographing or guiding specific new pieces of couple interaction, which increases accessibility and responsiveness.

Therapist's Role and Mechanisms of Change. EFT does not emphasize increased insight, problem-solving skill, or emotional catharsis. The central change mechanism invoked by EFT therapists is each partner's enhanced attunement to aspects of his or her own relationally relevant emotional experience. It is such self-attunement that softens anger, increases affective responsiveness, and heightens couple bonding. In these opportunities for self-attunement, the acceptance and validation of each partner by the EFT therapist is essential. The EFT therapist is active and authentic, and always on the alert for breaks in the therapeutic alliance, which must serve as the secure base on which new partner–partner interactions rest.

Applicability. The main contraindications to EFT involve clinical presentations in which heightened vulnerability would be inappropriate, such as domestic violence and ongoing affairs, since it requires a relatively high level of partner–partner trust. EFT has been used successfully in patients with varied clinical problems such as depression and posttraumatic stress disorder (e.g., childhood sexual abuse), for which enhancing the couple bond may have particular healing value, because both inherently involve violations or losses of attachment bonds.

Gottman Method Couple Therapy

Gottman Method Couple Therapy (GMCT; Gottman, 2004; Gottman & Gottman, 2008) rests on a foundation of descriptive research on more than 700 couples on what differentiates the "masters" and the "disasters" of relationships. Gottman's data (e.g., 1979, 1999) constitute the Sound Relationship House theory, also called the Sound Marital House theory, which emphasizes how couples sustain their friendship, manage conflict, and create a shared sense of meaning. GMCT interventions are tied directly to the data on couple interaction, mutual perception, and physiological arousal, summarized earlier in this chapter.

THE PRACTICE OF THERAPY

Structure of Therapy. GMCT averages 15–20 sessions for distressed couples, and 25–50 sessions when recent extramarital affairs are involved. Sessions usually last 80 minutes and are typically conducted by solo therapists. Couples are often followed at wider intervals for up to 2 years posttermination on an as-needed basis. Concurrent individual therapy is common.

Goal Setting and the Techniques and Process of Therapy. Because the many techniques of GMCT are so inextricably tied to the data-based building blocks of the seven hierarchical "levels" of sound relationship house theory, goal-setting and interventions are discussed here together. In a full course of GMCT, all seven levels of couple relating are addressed, more or less in the sequence described here.

The first three levels provide the foundation for later work and are generally geared toward reconnecting (typically disengaged) partners to each other's inner experiences about a wide variety of matters (by building *love maps*; e.g., by showing appreciation and curiosity), rebalancing partners' microbehaviors to build more general positivity (by building the *fondness and admiration* system; e.g., by showing caring and respect in everyday interactions), and responsiveness (by improving the balance of partners' *turning toward* each other's *bids* for connection, whether verbal or nonverbal).

Taken together, these three domains of change help to reestablish trust and friendship, thus fostering greater *positive sentiment override*, partners' reduction of negative attributional bias ("give the benefit of the doubt") in the face of neutral or even undesirable mate behavior, and work against partners' prejudging each other's intentions, motivations, and meanings.

The fifth level of GMCT focuses on conflict management and usually constitutes the lion's share of the therapy. Three important microfoci are to help couples compromise more, to use gentler *startup* when raising problems, and to *accept being influenced* (e.g., acknowledging the validity of each other's views).

The core of Level 5 intervention emphasizes taming the relationship-eroding "*Four Horsemen of the Apocalypse*": *contempt, criticism, stonewalling,* and *defensiveness.* This can be accomplished by encouraging "I" versus blaming statements; by partners' assumption of personal responsibility for recurrent problems; by reducing sarcasm and insults; and by promoting sustained engagement, even in hot-topic conversations. Level 5 work also focuses on teaching partners effective way to reduce the diffuse physiological arousal that characterizes conflicted couples. *Physiological soothing* of both self and partner is facilitated by the use of techniques such as guided imagery, mindfulness coaching, and breathing training. Soothing one's partner is aided by an emphasis on the use of empathy and *repairing ruptures* in conversations (e.g., by returning wandering exchanges to their initial focus); by using non-sarcastic humor; or by appropriate apology for one's own contribution to the emotional escalation process.

The most salient component of Level 5 work is teaching partners to distinguish between problematic events (which are short-term, situational, and solvable) and *perpetual problems* (which Gottman empirically estimates to comprise 69% of couple difficulties). Perpetual problems derive from central lifestyle and value differences, and especially from core personality differences and recurrent emotional vulnerabilities (e.g., about closeness–distance). Such core problems never truly "resolve" but reappear in many forms over time. Fostering empathy and acceptance, and learning to value differences may help couples not only tolerate unresolveable differences but also grow from such differences.

The sixth and seventh levels of GMCT focus on *honoring each other's dreams*, often facilitated by discovering the "dreams" hidden within couples' conflicts, and on *creating shared meaning* by strengthening the couple's formal and informal use of rituals of emotional connection, and supporting each other's life roles. While GMCT is eclectic in its use of numerous methods to address Levels 1 through 5 of the sound relationship house, it is these last two elements in particular that locate the approach within the experiential–humanistic domain.

Therapist's Role and Mechanisms of Change. The GMCT therapist serves as a coach and facilitator of relational change, and there is little explicit attention to therapist–partner interactions. As a relationship coach, the therapist's responsibility is to teach partners the couple skills, attitudes, and styles of behavior that characterize stable, healthy intimate relationships.

Applicability. GMCT is contraindicated when there is an ongoing extramarital affair or recurrent couple violence.

Behavioral Approaches

All variations of behavioral couple therapy (BCT) express the core philosophy of clinical behaviorism: the central role of the environment in shaping and maintaining behavior; the importance of operationally defined constructs; and the scientific testing of hypotheses and clinical interventions. The first two phases of BCT correspond to Traditional Behavioral Couple Therapy (Christensen et al., 1995), and include the "behavior exchange phase," and the "skills training phase." The first phase was marked by Richard Stuart's (1969) understanding of couple problems based on social exchange theory (i.e., that the success of a marriage depends on the frequency and variety of positive behaviors that are reciprocated). Treatment emphasized partners' specification (*objectification*) of desired positive changes from their mates, with various reinforcements of desired behavior change, leading to *behavioral exchanges*.

This simple, direct approach soon evolved into the "skills training phase" of BCT, ushered in by Neil Jacobson and Gayla Margolin's (1979) groundbreaking treatment manual, *Marital Therapy: Strategies Based on Social Learning and Behavior Exchange Principles.* In this phase, research on the differences between happy and unhappy couples flowered. Couples in unsatisfying relationships were found to communicate and to problem-solve less effectively than satisfied couples, to use coercive rather than positive approaches to influence, and generally to engage in less positive, and more negative, behavior. Treatment emphasized assumed "skill deficits" and included training in communication and problem solving. Another area of "deficits" and "excesses" attracting attention was the cognitive domain, with an emphasis on partners' interpretations and evaluations of their own and each other's behavior (Baucom, Epstein, La Taillade, & Kirby, 2008) based on maladaptive information processing, leading to problematic appraisals of relationship events and interactions.

The third phase in BCT saw the development of "Integrative Behavioral Couple Therapy" (Christensen et al., 1995), set forth in *Integrative Couple Therapy* (Jacobson & Christensen, 1996), but includes other developments as well. Having found that the outcomes of traditional BCT were not as positive as they had at first appeared, and that many couples were primarily dealing with inherently unresolvable "perpetual problems" à la Gottman (1999), Jacobson and Christensen (1996) moved from a skills training emphasis to mutual acceptance of such irreducible differences through affective and cognitive shifts in partners' frames of reference for understanding and empathically tuning into important reasons why their mates behave as they do.

The most recent extension of IBCT and CBCT emphasizes the role of self-regulation in couple difficulties and is central to BCT's important contributions to the development of a couple therapy adaptation (Fruzzetti & Fantozzi, 2008) of Dialectical Behavior Therapy for highly dysregulated couples.

THE PRACTICE OF THERAPY

Structure of Therapy. While BCT is very goal-focused, it is not inherently time-limited, typically lasting about 8–20 sessions. Behavioral couple therapists differ from adherents to other approaches by including comprehensive individual assessment sessions with each partner at the beginning of therapy, and in providing a very thorough, systematic, and structured feedback session with the couple after the initial three or four meetings in order to form a treatment contract.

Goal Setting. Although BCT emphasizes individualized treatment goals via functional analysis, some common goals are considered, with their choice depending on the conceptual emphasis of the therapist (more or less skills-oriented, more or less cognitively oriented, more or less acceptance-oriented), and characteristics of the couple (severity of conflict, collaborative capacity, level of trust, etc.). Generally, behavioral exchange (BE) and communication and problem-solving training (CPST) occur early in therapy with more compatible, flexible, and regulated couples. Emotional acceptance strategies usually appear earlier with more combative, mistrustful, or disengaged couples, though elements of both styles appear in most BCT.

Functional analysis is key to BCT and is concerned not with the topography, or form, of behavior, but with its effects. The goals of functional analysis are to identify patterns of behavior of concern and the conditions (behavioral, cognitive, affective) that maintain these patterns, to select appropriate interventions, and to monitor the progress of treatment. The function of behavior is understood by identifying the factors that control the behavior. Assessment requires a description of the problem behavior, including its frequency, the conditions under which it is more and less likely, and its consequences. BE and skills training emphasize the content of behavior. In setting treatment goals, skills-oriented and BE-oriented therapists focus more on specific behavioral events, while acceptance-oriented therapists focus more on problematic relationship themes, called *functional classes* or *response classes*, in which behaviors that have different forms share the same function. For example, the husband works longer hours, reads the newspaper during marital conversations, increases his volunteer work, and spends many weekend hours in his garage workshop. The behaviors differ but serve the same function: reducing anxiety associated with closeness.

Common BCT goals are increasing overall positivity in the relationship; decreasing overall negativity; teaching problem-solving and communication skills; changing from negative (e.g., coercion, punishment) to positive (e.g., appreciation, acknowledgment) styles of influencing one's partner; modifying dysfunctional attitudes, assumptions, expectations and relationship standards, and attributions about one's partner; modifying emotional reactivity; and enhancing empathic attunement to foster mutual acceptance around unresolveable incompatibilities and differences, often involving dominant personality styles or long-term emotional vulnerabilities.

Techniques and Process of Therapy. BCT sessions initially unfold with the couple raising an issue for discussion, one partner's recounting of a recent conflict situation, and so forth. Some sessions, or parts of sessions, are very structured and closely directed by the therapist (e.g., when teaching interpersonal skills or new cognitive appraisal strategies) but most of the time, with most couples, are more conversational, with the therapist doing as much following as leading. BCT typically involves both behavior change interventions and acceptance-enhancing interventions.

BE asks the partners to specify behaviorally (*pinpoint*) what behaviors they would like to see increased in each other. Point-for-point ("tit for tat") exchanges are discouraged, as they imply mistrust and caution. Each person commits to the therapist to make changes based on the partner's list but is not required to make any particular change from that list. The use of BE procedures requires active therapist structuring, guidance, and feedback, as does the use of CPST. Communication skills taught include, for the speaker or sender: the use of "I" statements rather than blaming "you" statements; measured honesty in the expression of feelings rather than "letting it all hang out"; and checking to see that the message sent or intended matches the message received. For the listener or receiver, the skills taught include paraphrasing and reflecting the speaker's expressions to maintain adequate understanding rather than interrupting or reacting defensively, and validating and empathizing rather than discounting or trivializing the speaker's feelings.

Common targets for improved problem solving include discussing one (agreed upon) topic at a time and not allowing sidetracking; identifying problems in terms of behavior rather than personality traits or character; avoiding "mind reading"; requesting positive ("more of") behavior change rather than negative ("less of") behavior change; emphasizing present- and future-oriented solution possibilities rather than (usually hostilely) rehashing the past; brainstorming a variety of potential behaviorally specific solutions and evaluating the pro's and con's for each such possibility; implementing an agreed upon solution; and evaluating the effectiveness of the solution chosen.

The therapist very actively structures and guides, modeling or role-playing desired behavior, providing feedback to the partners on their behavior, and explaining the rationale for particular behavioral principles and alternatives. Many behaviorally oriented couple therapists also use cognitive restructuring techniques derived from cognitive therapy and others modified specifically for use with couples (Baucom et al., 2008) (e.g., challenging automatic thoughts, examining the probabilities of certain outcomes, reconsidering the implicit meaning of behavior, examining the evidential basis for certain conclusions).

While earlier BCT methods emphasized changes in rule-governed behavior, the newer *acceptance-oriented* approach emphasizes changes in contingency-shaped behavior. *Rule-governed behavior* occurs in response to explicit verbal rules, with consequences determined by the degree to which behavior matches the rule, not by consequences (contingencies) occurring in the natural environment (e.g., the wife watches more sports on television with her husband, because the therapist says the couple should spend more time together). BE and CPST both involve rule-governed changes.

In contrast, *contingency-shaped behavior* is strengthened or weakened as a result of natural consequences. Changes generated in this way (e.g., wife spends more TV sports time with husband because he is friendly and affectionate to her at those times) tend to feel more authentic (vs. "You're only doing this because the therapist said you should") and are likely to generalize outside the treatment context, since they are not merely under the *stimulus control* of the therapist. Indeed, many common couple problems cannot be meaningfully changed by rule-governed methods (e.g., spontaneity, trust or sexual interest). The most important tactical change in acceptance-oriented intervention, and its central technique, is *empathic joining around the problem*, which involves the therapist's reformulation (reattribution) of the problem, from seeing behavior as "bad" to seeing it as understandable in light of the partners' vulnerabilities or other heretofore unexpressed factors that influence the "bad" behavior, and allowing the motivation (controlling consequences) to be seen in a new light by the partner. Such a shift is achieved by helping the "offending" partner identify and express "the feeling behind the feeling," or the feelings behind the undesirable behavior. Such *softening* self-disclosures facilitate empathic responses, help to decrease the aversiveness of the behavior at issue, and allow new responses by the receiving partner.

Other acceptance-oriented techniques include *unified detachment*, in which the couple is encouraged to discuss problems in a more intellectual, descriptive manner, as though the problem is an external "it", and *tolerance building*, in which the pain caused by a partner's behavior is reduced, even though the behavior may not change a great deal. Tolerance may be enhanced by pointing out possible positive (and unrecognized) aspects of undesirable behavior (producing a cognitive shift), by practicing the undesirable behavior in the session (desensitization), by faking or pretending undesirable behavior at home (thus bringing it under voluntary control), and by increased self-care (filling more of one's own needs).

Finally, affective self-control, or self-regulation, strategies focus on altering one's response to the partner's undesired behavior, changing one's approach to trying to gain cooperation from one's partner regarding changes, and using stimulus control methods to limit and contain conflict (e.g., discussing "hot" topics only at predetermined times).

Therapist's Role and Mechanisms of Change. In BCT, the therapist assumes a great deal of responsibility for the outcome of treatment, based at first on a thorough functional analysis in the initial assessment, and later ensuring that the direction and topical focus of the unfolding therapy process remains thematically consistent. As in all couple therapies, a supportive, empathic attitude toward the couple is essential for developing trust and collaboration. More than in many other couple treatment approaches, the therapist in BCT may take on a decidedly instructional, didactic coaching role, especially when using BE, cognitive restructuring, and CPST methods. The therapist must be flexible enough to adopt different stances with the couple as both the overall focus of the therapy and the exigencies of the moment require.

Applicability. There are few specific contraindications to BCT, with the main exceptions being spousal battering, significant substance abuse, and ongoing extramarital affairs. Various components of BCT have been studied and found to be helpful for general couple distress and dissatisfaction, with acceptance-based methods possibly being more effective. BCT has also been found to be effective in treating conflicted couples with comorbid depression, agoraphobia, and alcoholism.

Integrative Approaches

Just as eclecticism is the most common theoretical orientation among individual psychotherapists, so it appears to be among couple therapists (Rait, 1988). Indeed, Lebow (1997) has noted that the integrative "revolution" in couple (and family) therapy, is "so much a part of our work that it largely goes unrecognized" (p. 1). Couple therapy integrations have brought together structural and strategic approaches (e.g., Keim & Lappin, 2002; Todd, 1986), and behavioral and systemic approaches (e.g., Birchler & Spinks, 1980; Weiss, 1980), but the most common conceptual combinations have been behavioral and psychodynamic (e.g., Gurman, 1981, 2008c; Luquet, 2007; Segraves, 1982; Snyder & Mitchell, 2008; Weeks, 1989). One of the most empirically supported approaches, Integrative Behavioral

Couple Therapy (Dimidjian, Martell, & Christensen, 2008), in fact is not "integrative" as that term is usually defined, emphasizing the combined use of interventions that focus on both change and acceptance within couples' relationships, but all from a consistently functional-analytic, social learning perspective.

Douglas Snyder's (1999; Snyder & Mitchell, 2008) "Affective Reconstruction Approach," also known as Insight-Oriented Marital Therapy (IOMT; Snyder & Wills, 1989), is one of the most sophisticated integrative couple models to date and emphasizes relational dispositions of individuals and their associated core individual intimate relational themes over time, including family of origin. IOMT promotes awareness of the contradictions and incongruencies within people about their relational needs and expectations, and attends to partners' behavior, feelings, and cognitions in both present and historical terms. IOMT draws upon psychodynamic (mostly object relations), experiential, and cognitive and behavioral techniques. Insight, affective immediacy, and modification of partners' problematic attributions about each other, as well as indirect skills enhancement, are all valued in IOMT. IOMT is a pluralistic, theoretically eclectic approach (Fraenkel & Pinsof, 2001) that uses different theoretical perspectives, even within the same clinical case, at different phases of therapy. The most common sequencing in IOMT is from more present-centered, pragmatic, and problem-focused emphases toward increasingly more historical/multigenerational understanding.

Integrative Couple Therapy: An Illustration

Alan Gurman's (1981, 1992, 2008c) Integrative Couple Therapy (ICT), which attends simultaneously to both interpersonal and intrapersonal factors, is used to illustrate the principles and practices of the integrative practice of couple therapy.

ICT emphasizes how repetitive cycles reciprocally include both intrapsychic processes (conscious and unconscious) and overt behavior (i.e., how deep structures and surface structures of intimate relationships influence each other). Object relations theory provides the base for mapping deep structures. Conflict is seen as arising when the implicit "rules" (unspoken agreements) of the relationship that are central to either partner's sense of self or core schema for close relationships are violated. ICT emphasizes *implicit behavior modification* (i.e., partners' unwitting reinforcement of undesired behavior in their mates), and punishment of behavior for which they consciously wish. Such reinforcing and punishing contingencies occur in circular relationship and can be triggered internally, between the partners, or by external events.

ICT aims for change in both interaction patterns and inner representational models of intimate relationships, and using both direct and indirect methods. In addition to its object relations base, ICT relies heavily on functional analysis for a more fine-grained, ongoing assessment of couple problems. As noted earlier, functional analysis is concerned not with the form of behavior but with the factors that maintain problematic patterns, be they interactional, cognitive, affective, or biological. It does not assume a priori that any particular class of events has more influence than any other over a couple's difficulties. Behavior is behavior (is behavior), and in ICT, behavior is pragmatically construed broadly to include unconscious experience. Treatment is usually organized around a small number of dominant themes, and ICT's emphasis on the function of behavior over its form allows the use of a wide variety of change methods.

THE PRACTICE OF THERAPY

Structure of Therapy. ICT emphasizes the healing power of the couple's own relationship above and beyond the patient–therapist relationship; thus, individual sessions are almost never held, except when the volatility of joint sessions cannot be limited. Sessions are usually biweekly, and most ICT lasts 8–20 visits. The therapist almost always begins sessions by asking, "What would you (two) like to focus on today?" The content and direction of the session is chosen by the couple, but the therapist is responsible for guiding the couple in ways that stay on a central thematic track.

Goal Setting. The goals of any particular course of therapy vary. Still, there are certain overriding goals across couples, such as more accurate self-perception and self-acceptance, more accurate perception of and acceptance of one's partner, and resolution of both presenting problems and emergent problems.

Techniques and Process of Therapy. ICT requires behavioral specification of projective processes, among others. These processes can be identified by some predictable patterns, for example, when partners fail to see aspects of each other's behavior (including positive changes) that are perceptible to a third person; when partners reinforce in each other the very behavior they complain about; when partners fail to see their own contributions to the couple problems; or when partners exaggerate differences and minimize similarities.

To counter collusive processes, ICT inculcates systemic awareness, teaching and evoking relationship skills as needed, and challenging dysfunctional implicit relationship rules by actively interrupting and modifying collusive processes in session, linking individual and interactional experience, and creating therapeutic tasks. Interruption and modification of collusive processes is accomplished, for example, by therapist *blocking interventions*, designed to interrupt couple enactments of habitual unconscious shared avoidance agreements (e.g., via "anticollusive questions," such as "How do you protect each other from even worse pain?"; "Even though you often complain about *X* in your mate, do you find that you sometimes do *X* yourself?"; "What stops you from accepting what your mate is giving you, since it seems to be what you're asking for?"; or "What do you do to get your mate to behave in ways that, ironically, bother *you* so much?"), and by goal-directed, strategic *instigative interventions* to effect a particular change, in contrast to more exploratory, process-oriented interventions. Tasks can occur both in session and out of session.

Therapist's Role and Mechanisms of Change. The therapist's role is to facilitate the partners' experiencing of themselves and each other as whole persons, in a safe yet challenging environment that works against the joint avoidances that reciprocally reinforce, and are reinforced by, problematic interaction patterns. The therapist closely tracks his or her alliances with each partner but focuses on the partner–partner alliance. Both affect-eliciting, interpretive, and direct behavior change methods are used. Indeed, the familiar behavior therapy idea of exposure to fearful stimuli is a principle that often guides the therapist's choices about where, when, and how to intervene. Thus, in effect, ICT often uses active methods to achieve psychodynamic goals.

Applicability. The principles and core techniques of ICT are applicable both to psychologically minded and more pragmatically oriented couples. While interpretive activity by the therapist certainly can deepen the treatment experience, it is the therapist's understanding and tracking of the interactions between conscious and unconscious experience, and between observed and inferred relationship events, that allow for direct, practical interventions to serve object relational aims. Because ICT does not a priori pay more attention to particular aspects of experience, the possibilities for helpful intervention at multiple levels of experience, using a broad array of methods, are enhanced.

Postmodern Approaches

Most approaches to psychotherapy are based on implicit worldviews inherent in *modernism*, a belief that there exists a knowable, observable, measurable, objective reality that exists independently of how it is perceived, and that discernible laws of how it operates that can be discovered through scientific investigation. *Postmodernism*, in contrast, questions the possibility of knowing absolute "truth" and discovery of universal laws or principles to explain human behavior. Unquestioned givens in knowledge systems are *deconstructed* (i.e., their assumptions are extracted and identified).

Within the postmodern clinical movement has emerged the perspective of *social constructionism*, with a central tenet that reality does not exist "out there," but rather is socially constructed (this is different from another postmodern perspective, *constructivism*, which emphasizes how people actively construct meaning and reality). Given the relativistic, contextualistic view that there is no one "truth," only multiple realities, it follows that, in the therapy context, participants, including therapists, cannot be "experts" on reality but are merely collaborative co-inquirers, co-investigators, or co-constructors (Dickerson & Crocket, 2010). The antireductionistic bias in social constructionism also leads to an emphasis on unique patient experience and meanings rather than research-based descriptions of problems, "types" of relationships, and the like. The most influential and visible postmodern couple therapy approaches have been Solution-Focused Couple Therapy and Narrative Couple Therapy.

Solution-Focused Couple Therapy

Of the existing postmodern approaches to couple therapy, Solution-Focused (or Solution-Oriented) Couple Therapy (SFCT) has the most direct connections with more traditional methods of couple and family therapy. Indeed, the work of SFCT's creator, Steve de Shazer (1985, 1988), trained at the MRI, and that of his colleagues (e.g., Weiner-Davis, 1992) at the Brief Family Therapy Center in Milwaukee, Wisconsin, reflects many central MRI beliefs and values. Like the MRI approach, SFCT has little interest in a couple's joint history or the histories of each partner; is nonpathologizing, in that it believes there is no absolute reality and, thus, ideas of "normality" are irrelevant; is more interested in how problems continue than in how they arose; deals only with the complaints patients bring to therapy, and thus does not investigate "underlying issues"; believes that problems are usually maintained by constraining definitions; and is pragmatic and time-sensitive. In contrast to the MRI model, SFCT emphasizes solutions more than problems, places more emphasis on cognitive than behavioral change, and emphasizes patients' resources as more central to good outcomes than therapists' personal attributes.

For the postmodern solution-focused couple therapist, the notion that reality is constructed rather than discovered leads to a profound shift of emphasis from that of the MRI (and most other therapies, as well). Since problems are believed only to "exist in language," the therapist unhesitantingly emphasizes *solution talk* rather than *problem talk* (which, of course, includes talk about the history of the problem).

THE PRACTICE OF THERAPY

Structure of Therapy. Solution-focused therapists, like MRI therapists, are open to work-ing with the most motivated persons (*customers*), not necessarily with *complainants* (those who complain but appear unmotivated to change), although a good deal of their couple-oriented work occurs conjointly. Unlike the MRI approach, SFCT sets no fixed therapy limit, although it tends to be extremely brief, often in the range of five to seven sessions, and the therapist and couple negotiate whether to meet again at the end of each session.

Goal Setting. The goals of SFCT are to resolve the presenting problem(s) by shifting how these problems are "languaged." Therapy aims for "solution sight" (Hoyt, 2002) rather than insight. Process goals emphasize eliciting patient competencies and resources, which solution-focused couple therapists believe people have within themselves and, thus, do not need coaching, therapist interpretations, or skill training.

Techniques and Process of Therapy. Although solution-focused therapy has developed a more recent interest in the therapeutic relationship as a core component of clinical change (Miller, Duncan, & Hubble, 1997), it is still largely identified with its *formula tasks*, therapist interventions that are used with everyone. In the *formula first session task* (called the *skeleton key question* because it fits all "locks"), presented at the end of the first session, the therapist asks the partners to observe, between sessions, what about their relationship they would like to continue, despite their current problems (thus, shifting attention to the positive). With the *miracle question*, the therapist asks, "If a miracle happened, and your problem dis-appeared, how would you know? What would be different? What else would be different?" (This defines the problem clearly, demonstrates how problem definition may get in the way of partners behaving in ways they would prefer, and implies hopefulness). With *exceptions questions*, the therapist asks the couple to identify times when the problem is usually not present, and what happens differently at those times, and/or what the couple does differ-ently when the problem arises but handles better than usual. Such questions imply that the partners already know but are insufficiently using, their own solutions, and that they have the capacity to make the problem not happen.

Scaling questions are designed to emphasize solution-finding and -building, and to moti-vate patients toward change (e.g., "On a scale from 1 to 10, 1 being no [hope, relationship commitment, treatment motivation, judgment of therapeutic progress, or any other issue of interest], and 10 being complete [hope, etc.], how would you rate yourself today?"). *Coping* (or *endurance*) *questions* focus on patient strengths and encourage hopefulness by asking, for example, "Despite these couple problems, how do you still hang in there? How do you keep things from getting even worse than they've been?" And *agency* (or *efficacy*) *questions* highlight patients' ability to make change happen (e.g., "How did you do that/make that happen/decide to do that?"). Different types of solution–talk questions are more appropri-ate to different stages of therapy, but as a group, they are intended to identify problems, the conditions under which they occur, and the probable consequences of their elimination; to broaden the partners' view of their overall relationship beyond the problem; to reinforce the partners' awareness of their own problem resolution capacities; and to support the couple's hopefulness about change.

Therapist's Role and Mechanisms of Change. SFCT disavows interest in notions such as "mechanisms of change," which assume an objectivist, modernist, "normal science" per-spective. Ideas about "curative factors," suggestive of "the medical model," are shunned.

The solution-focused approach emphasizes collaborative, conversational meaning making and insists that changes in perceptions lead to changes in behavior, and that all such changes occur primarily, if not exclusively, through language. Solution-focused therapists also believe that it is not necessary to know why or how something works in therapy for it to be effective. The therapist's central role is to facilitate conversations that take into account patients' motivations, goals, values, and so forth, in order to find ways to maximize patients' cooperation with change.

Applicability. Solution-focused couple therapists appear to see no inherent applicability limits for their approach beyond those common to almost all methods of couple treatment (e.g., violence and major psychiatric impairment).

Narrative Couple Therapy

The therapeutic approach in the postmodern domain that has attracted the most attention in the past two decades is Narrative Couple Therapy (NCT), based on the seminal work of Michael White (e.g., White & Epston, 1990), and most recently refined by Jill Freedman and Gene Combs (2008), and Victoria Dickerson (e.g., Dickerson & Crocket, 2010).

The narrative couple therapist, questioning established mental health diagnostic systems, asserts that problems exist in cultural discourses and are seen as the effects of constraining discourses. The personal and shared *narratives* or *stories* about ourselves and the world that we experience do not merely influence our lives (e.g., by determining our behavior and perceptions), they *are* our lives. The types of culturally constructed narratives that are particularly relevant to couple therapy involve gender and socially constructed power. Indeed, these dimensions of relational experience are seen by NCT as important in almost all couple therapy situations, regardless of the content of couples' presenting problems. NCT regularly assumes that gender is involved in most couple problems, whether the couple (or therapist) recognizes its role or not. Thus, NCT is a decidedly and intentionally political (and politicizing) therapy, designed to liberate relationship partners from the restrictive, limiting, and oppressive assumptions of the larger culture, especially those involving traditional notions of maleness and femaleness. This thematic emphasis often extends to matters of race, social class, and other domains of dominant cultural values and institutions. NCT is probably the most explicit "therapy of social justice" (Nichols & Schwartz, 1998, p. 418) for couples that exists.

THE PRACTICE OF THERAPY

Structure of Therapy. NCT does not adhere to principles of systems theory and, in fact, is often individually focused. Because NCT seeks to help people change their most salient self- and worldviews, conjoint therapy is not required, and partners are seen alone if conditions warrant. In the conjoint format, the basic structure is that one partner explores his or her stories (*telling*) while the other listens (*witnessing*), then comments on what has been said. These roles then are switched. All the while, the therapist is active in helping partners elucidate, elaborate, and modify their stories.

Goal Setting. Goals, as usually thought of in psychotherapy, are not in the lexicon of NCT. Rather than narrowing the therapeutic focus, narrative therapists attempt to broaden it. Thus, "goals" are referred to as *projects* or *directions in life*. This is no mere hairsplitting, for the aim in NCT is to transform partners' individual and relational identities, not primarily to "solve problems." NCT seeks to "separate the problem from the person" by constructing new individual and shared stories. It is a psychopolitical endeavor, aimed at freeing people from oppressive cultural assumptions, and empowering them to live out their *preferred stories*. NCT projects can last a few sessions or a few years.

Techniques and Process of Therapy. To convey to couples at the outset of therapy that the narrative therapist is not to be seen as an "expert," the therapist *situates* him- or herself as a person in the collaboration in the first session by inviting the couple to ask questions about him or her, so as to minimize power differentials. For the same reason, the therapist also requires his or her own transparency (e.g., often by sharing the reasoning behind his or her questions over the course of therapy).

NCT has come to be identified with a number of distinctive therapeutic techniques (called *practices*) that are quite out of the ordinary in the world of mainstream psychotherapy and couple therapy. The central therapeutic change strategy involves *externalizing conversations*, in which the aim is linguistically to separate the person from the problem, in part by tracing the sources of the values that unproductively support and reinforce the patient's *problem-saturated* or *problem-laden stories*. For example, while being helped to trace the origins of a relationally problematic view of women, a husband may be encouraged to think of the problematic view as an "it" that acts upon him but *is* not him. The therapist may attribute intentionality to the problem, again relating to the problem as a reified "it." The therapist poses *effects questions* (e.g., "What effect does this problem have on your relationship?"), designed to lead the partners to perceive negative experiences of themselves and each other, and their relationship as the effects, or results, of the problem, not as its cause. He or she may also *construct problems* by giving them names (e.g., "`Distance' keeps getting in your way"). The essential NCT maxim is that the person is not the problem, but the problem is the problem, so that the couple has a "relationship" with "it" and may work to join together to oppose "it" having so much control in their lives.

The *reauthoring* of new stories with previously *subjugated narratives* (more productive, alternative stories) includes a good deal of attention to *unique outcomes* (i.e., times when the partners do not yield to the problem or behave in ways that would not be predicted in light of their dominant problem-saturated story). Therapist questions about unique outcomes include *landscape of action questions* (about sequences of behavior involved in the unique outcome) and *landscape of consciousness questions* (about the meanings, beliefs, values, and intentions of a person that are implied by the unique outcome). *Thickening new plots* as an element of the reauthoring process involves connecting unique outcomes to the past and to an extended future story in which the partner (or relationship) is seen as more potent than the problem. As the couple's thickened stories are further established, the therapist urges the *documentation and circulation of new stories* that involve varied methods designed to reinforce therapeutic gains and generalize them outside the therapist's office (e.g., presenting the couple a certificate to acknowledge a particular change; creating videotapes for partners' own use, in which they talk about the progress they have made; writing letters to the partners designed to thicken recently discussed unique outcomes by asking them new questions; and encouraging the partners to share these documents with important people in their lives).

Therapist's Role and Mechanisms of Change. In NCT, therapists participate not as professional experts with special knowledge but as people with the ability to foster collaborative "projects," to a significant extent, by asking questions that thicken new, adaptive, alternative stories about oneself and one's relationship. In the NCT view, significant change occurs via the *performance of meaning* (i.e., the repeated enactment, especially in everyday life, of reworked new stories).

Applicability. NCT sees traditional individual or couple diagnosis as totally irrelevant to its work and rejects the common criteria by which most therapists evaluate their work. Narrative therapists identify for whom their approach is "applicable" not by their own criteria, but by learning from couples in the process of therapy whether the work is helpful.

RESEARCH SUPPORT

From the earliest (Gurman, 1973) to the most recent (Snyder, Castellani, & Whisman, 2006) examinations of the pertinent empirical literature, and those in between (e.g., Baucom, Shoham, Meuser, Daiuto, & Stickle, 1998; Christensen & Heavey, 1999; Lebow & Gurman, 1995), research has consistently demonstrated the efficacy of conjoint couple therapy, with positive outcomes in about two-thirds of couples. This overall improvement rate affirms that the average treated couple is better off at termination than about 70–80% of untreated couples, which parallels the results for individual therapy. Every controlled, randomized clinical trial of couple therapy to date has found treatment to be superior to no treatment. These efficacy studies have shown treatment effects that exceed those of individual therapy for couple problems, and almost always in brief therapies of 12–20 sessions. Couple therapy has also been shown to play a significant remedial role in the treatment of depression, alcohol abuse, and anxiety disorders, problems traditionally thought to be treated appropriately by individual therapy (Snyder & Whisman, 2006).

Among the many approaches to couple therapy, those with the largest cumulative research base to date are Behavioral (including cognitive-behavioral) Couple Therapy (Shadish & Baldwin, 2005) and Emotionally Focused Couple Therapy (Johnson, Hunsley, Greenberg, & Schindler, 1999). Insight-Oriented Marital Therapy has also shown very strong treatment effects that endure at long-term (4-year) follow-up. None of the most influential integrative models of couple therapy discussed earlier have been studied empirically, but all draw heavily upon treatment components and principles present in models of therapy (BMT, EFT, IOMT) that have received substantial research support. Structural–strategic (e.g., Leff et al., 2000) and MRI-style therapies (e.g., Goldman & Greenberg, 1992), though studied infrequently, have received a modicum of empirical support. There is no evidence to date of differential efficacy or effectiveness among couple therapy methods. Finally, BFST, ORCT, GMCT, SFCT, and NCT have not yet been formally tested in controlled studies.

Efforts have recently been made to improve the empirical basis for evaluating couple (and family) therapy beyond familiar reliance on randomized controlled trials. Sexton et al. (2010) have proposed a multitiered "levels of evidence" approach that promotes diverse research methods and varied methodological criteria needed to answer questions specific to different clinical contexts (e.g., practice-related decisions vs. institutional policymaking). They argue that it is important to close the traditional research–practice gap and to foster ecologically meaningful research. For example, it is important to study clinical populations that reflect the most common reasons for which couples seek therapy, often without a diagnosed "patient" (e.g., struggles with divorce decisions, conflicting parenting values, and general couple distress, problems that are almost always excluded from funded research studies).

CURRENT AND FUTURE TRENDS

Couple therapy has come a very long way since its early peripheral position in the world of mental health and even its long-term marginalized position of more recent times. The overall efficacy of couple therapy is well established; it has become the dominant clinical practice within the broad field of family therapy; it is practiced by clinicians in all mental health fields; and it has been widely applied both to the treatment of individual disorders that impact and are impacted by couple relationships and "garden variety" couple distress and dissatisfaction.

Given the field's inherent interest in the organization and functioning of interpersonal systems, couple therapy perhaps inevitably continues to expand its integrative emphasis. While there are still discernible conceptual and technical differences among the major schools of therapy (Gurman, 2008a), there is clearly a pervasive trend toward the assimilation of disparate methods, prescriptive matching of problems and interventions, and an increasing awareness of the role of therapeutic common factors (e.g., Spenkle, Davis, & Lebow, 2009), including therapist factors and the therapeutic alliance, that transcend differences among "schools."

In addition to this evolving integrationism among couple therapy approaches, the field has recently pursued and is likely to continue to actively pursue the integration of clinically relevant knowledge from a variety of other fields and perspectives. For example, at the macrosystemic level, feminism (Nichols, 2008) and multiculturalism (Rastogi & Thomas, 2009) have enriched the practice of couple therapy by expanding therapists' awareness of how societal beliefs about gender, power, and intimacy influence both relational expectations and therapeutic processes.

At a more midrange level, basic research on developmental attachment theory (Cassidy & Shaver, 1999; Whiffen, 2003); healthy versus unhealthy couple interactional patterns (Gottman, 1999), and the role of individual psychological disorders (Snyder, Schneider, & Castellani, 2006) in couple conflict have increasingly informed both theory development and clinical practice. And at a more microsystemic level, clinically relevant data from the burgeoning field of affective neuroscience and "interpersonal neurobiology" (Fishbane, 2007) have deepened our understanding of how the human brain is "wired" through close relationships, how relationships affect brain functioning, and how various clinical methods can evoke the neuroplastic potential of the adult brain, while simultaneously expanding couples' options and flexibility for emotionally safe and collaborative connections. Such research has already influenced the clinical practices of couple therapists of many theoretical orientations (Gurman, 2010b).

In summary, despite its humble beginnings, couple therapy continues to evolve into a robust and respected collection of clinical methods that are increasingly integrative and genuinely multisystemic.

SUGGESTIONS FOR FURTHER STUDY

Recommended Reading: Case Studies

Gurman, A. S. (Ed.). (1985). *Casebook of marital therapy.* New York: Guilford Press.—Fourteen authors present in-depth case illustrations across a wider range of marital and couple problems than in most related books.

Gurman, A. S. (Ed.). (2010). *Clinical casebook of couple therapy.* New York: Guilford Press.—Eighteen authors present detailed clinical case studies exemplifying all major approaches to couple therapy.

Recommended Reading: Historical Review/Comparative Analysis

Gurman, A. S. (2008). A framework for the comparative study of couple therapy: History, models and applications. In A.S. Gurman (Ed.), *Clinical handbook of couple therapy* (4th ed., pp. 1–26). New York: Guilford Press.

Gurman, A. S., & Fraenkel, P. (2002). The history of couple therapy: A millennial review. *Family Process, 41*, 199–260.—Comprehensive in-depth review of the theoretical and clinical history of the field. Includes an historical account of trends in research since the inception of couple therapy.

DVDs

Jacobson, N. (1997). *Behavioral couples therapy: Integrating change and acceptance.* Alexandria, VA: American Association for Marriage and Family Therapy. Available at *www.aamft.org/familytherapyresources.*

Johnson, S. M. (2009). *Re-engaging withdrawers* (emotionally focused couple therapy). Ottawa: International Centre for Excellence in Emotionally Focused Therapy. Available at *www.iceeft.com/dvda.htm.*

REFERENCES

Ackerman, N. W. (1970). Family psychotherapy today. *Family Process, 9*, 123–126.

Aponte, H. S., & Di Cesare, E. J. (2000). Structural therapy. In F. M. Dattilio & L. J. Bevilacqua (Eds.), *Comparative treatments for relationship dysfunction* (pp. 45–57). New York: Springer.

Baucom, D. H., Epstein, N., La Taillade, J. J., & Kirby, J. S. (2008). Cognitive-behavioral couple therapy. In A. S. Gurman (Ed.), *Clinical handbook of couple therapy* (4th ed., pp. 31–72). New York: Guilford Press.

Baucom, D. H., Shoham, V., Meuser, K. T., Daiuto, A. D., & Stickle, T. R. (1998). Empirically supported couple and family interventions for marital distress and adult mental health problems. *Journal of Consulting and Clinical Psychology, 66*, 53–88.

Beels, C. C., & Ferber, A. (1969). Family therapy: A view. *Family Process, 8*, 280–318.

Birchler, G., & Spinks, S. (1980). A behavioral-systems marital and family therapy: Intervention and clinical application. *American Journal of Family Therapy, 8*, 6–28.

Boszormenyi-Nagy, I., & Ulrich, D. N. (1981). Contextual family therapy. In A. S. Gurman & D. P. Kniskern (Eds.), *Handbook of family therapy* (pp. 159–225). New York: Brunner/Mazel.

Bowen, M. (1976a). Principles and techniques of multiple family therapy. In P. J. Guerin, Jr. (Ed.), *Family therapy: Theory and practice* (pp. 388–404). New York: Gardner.

Bowen, M. (1976b). Family therapy and family group therapy. In D. H. L. Olson (Ed.), *Treating relationships* (pp. 219–274). Lake Milla, IA: Graphic.

Bowen, M. (1978). *Family therapy in clinical practice.* New York: Aronson.

Bowlby, J. (1988). *A secure base.* New York: Basic Books.

Budman, S. H., & Gurman, A. S. (1988). *The theory and practice of brief therapy.* New York: Guilford Press.

Cassidy, J., & Shaver, P. (Eds.). (1999). *Handbook of attachment: Theory, research and clinical applications.* New York: Guilford Press.

Christensen, A., Babcock, J. C., & Jacobson, N. S. (1995). Integrative behavioral couple therapy. In N. S. Jacobson & A. S. Gurman (Eds.), *Clinical handbook of couple therapy* (2nd ed., pp. 31–64). New York: Guilford Press.

Christensen, A., & Heavey, C. L. (1999). Interventions for couples. *Annual Review of Psychology, 50*, 165–190.

de Shazer, S. (1985). *Keys to solution in brief therapy.* New York: Norton.

de Shazer, S. (1988). *Clues: Investigating solutions in brief therapy.* New York: Norton.

Dicks, H. V. (1967). *Marital tensions.* New York: Basic Books.

Dickerson, V. C., & Crocket, K. (2010). *El tigre, el tigre*: A story of narrative practice. In A. S. Gurman (Ed.), *Clinical casebook of couple therapy* (pp. 153–180). New York: Guilford Press.

Dimidjian, S., Martell, C. R., & Christensen, A. (2008). Integrative behavioral couple therapy. In A. S. Gurman (Ed.), *Clinical handbook of couple therapy* (4th ed., pp. 73–106). New York: Guilford Press.

Doherty, W. J., & Simmons, D. S. (1996). Clinical practice patterns of marriage and family therapists: A national survey of therapists and their clients. *Journal of Marital and Family Therapy, 22*, 9–25.

Fisch, R., Weakland, J. H., & Segal, L. (1982). *The tactics of change: Doing therapy briefly.* San Francisco: Jossey-Bass.

Fishbane, M. D. (2007). Wired to connect: Neuroscience, relationships and therapy. *Family Process, 46*, 395–412.

Fraenkel, P. (1997). Systems approaches to couple therapy. In W. K. Halford & H. J. Markman (Eds.), *Clinical handbook of marriage and couples interventions* (pp. 379–414). New York: Wiley.

Fraenkel, P., & Pinsof, W. M. (2001). Teaching family therapy-centered integration: Assimilation and beyond. *Journal of Psychotherapy Integration, 11*, 59–85.

Framo, J. L. (1965). Rationale and techniques of intensive family therapy. In I. Boszormenyi-Nagy & J. L. Framo (Eds.), *Intensive family therapy* (pp. 143–212). New York: Harper & Row.

Framo, J. L. (1981). The integration of marital therapy with sessions with family of origin. In A. S. Gurman & D. P. Kniskern (Eds.), *Handbook of family therapy* (pp. 133–158). New York: Brunner/ Mazel.

Freedman, J., & Combs, G. C. (2008). Narrative couple therapy. In A. S. Gurman (Ed.), *Clinical handbook of couple therapy* (4th ed., pp. 229–258). New York: Guilford Press.

Fruzzetti, A. E., & Fantozzi, B. (2008). Couple therapy and the treatment of borderline personality and related disorders. In A. S. Gurman (Ed.), *Clinical handbook of couple therapy* (4th ed., pp. 567–590). New York: Guilford Press.

Goldman, A., & Greenberg, L. (1992). Comparison of integrated systemic and emotionally focused approaches to couple therapy. *Journal of Consulting and Clinical Psychology, 60*, 962–969.

Gottman, J. M. (1979). *Marital interaction: Empirical investigations.* New York: Academic Press.

Gottman, J. M. (1999). *The marriage clinic: A scientifically based marital therapy.* New York: Norton.

Gottman, J. M., & Gottman, J. S. (2008). Gottman method couple therapy. In A. S. Gurman (Ed.), *Clinical handbook of couple therapy* (4th ed., pp. 138–166). New York: Guilford Press.

Gottman, J. S. (Ed.). (2004). *The marriage clinic casebook.* New York: Norton.

Greenberg, L. S., & Goldman, R. N. (2008). *Emotion-focused couples therapy.* Washington, DC: American Psychological Association.

Greenberg, L. S., & Johnson, S. M. (1986). Emotionally focused couples therapy. In N. S. Jacobson & A. S. Gurman (Eds.), *Clinical handbook of marital therapy* (pp. 253–278). New York: Guilford Press.

Greene, B. L. (Ed.). (1965). *The psychotherapies of marital disharmony.* New York: Free Press.

Gurman, A. S. (1973). The effects and effectiveness of marital therapy: A review of outcome research. *Family Process, 12*, 145–170.

Gurman, A. S. (1978). Contemporary marital therapies: A critique and comparative analysis of psychoanalytic, behavioral and systems theory approaches. In T. J. Paolino & B. McCrady (Eds.), *Marriage and marital therapy* (pp. 445–566). New York: Brunner/Mazel.

Gurman, A. S. (1981). Integrative marital therapy: Toward the development of an interpersonal approach. In S. H. Budman (Ed.), *Forms of brief therapy* (pp. 415–462). New York: Guilford Press.

Gurman, A. S. (1992). Integrative marital therapy: A time-sensitive model for working with couples. In S. H. Budman, S. Friedman, & M. Hoyt (Eds.), *The first session in brief therapy* (pp. 186–203). New York: Guilford Press.

Gurman, A. S. (2001). Brief therapy and family/couple therapy: An essential redundancy. *Clinical Psychology: Science and Practice, 8*, 51–65.

Gurman, A. S. (Ed.). (2008a). *Clinical handbook of couple therapy, 4th ed.* New York: Guilford Press.

Gurman, A. S. (2008b). A framework for the comparative study of couple therapy: History, models and applications. In *Clinical handbook of couple therapy* (4th ed., pp. 1–26). New York: Guilford Press.

Gurman, A. S. (2008c). Integrative couple therapy: A depth-behavioral approach. In *Clinical handbook of couple therapy* (4th ed., pp. 383–428). New York: Guilford Press.

Gurman, A. S. (Ed.). (2010a). *Clinical casebook of couple therapy.* New York: Guilford Press.

Gurman, A. S. (2010b). The evolving practice of couple therapy. In *Clinical casebook of couple therapy* (pp. 1–20). New York: Guilford Press.

Gurman, A. S., & Fraenkel, P. (2002). The history of couple therapy: A millennial review. *Family Process, 41,* 199–260.

Haley, J. (1963). Marriage therapy. *Archives of General Psychiatry, 8,* 213–234.

Haley, J. (1974). *Problem-solving therapy.* San Francisco: Jossey-Bass.

Hoyt, M. F. (2002). Solution-focused couple therapy. In A. S. Gurman & N. S. Jacobson (Eds.), *Clinical handbook of couple therapy* (3rd ed., pp. 335–369). New York: Guilford Press.

Jackson, D. D. (1959). Family interaction, family homeostasis and some implications for conjoint family psychotherapy. In J. Masserman (Ed.), *Individual and family dynamics* (pp. 122–141). New York: Grune & Stratton.

Jackson, D. D. (1965). Family rules: The marital quid pro quo. *Archives of General Psychiatry, 12,* 589–594.

Jacobson, N. S., & Christensen, A. (1996). *Integrative couple therapy: Promoting acceptance and change.* New York: Norton.

Jacobson, N. S., & Margolin, G. (1979). *Marital therapy: Strategies based on social learning and behavior exchange principles.* New York: Brunner/Mazel.

Johnson, S. M. (1986). Bonds or bargains: Relationship paradigms and their significance for marital therapy. *Journal of Marital and Family Therapy, 12,* 259–267.

Johnson, S. M. (2004). *The practice of emotionally focused marital therapy.* New York: Brunner/Routledge.

Johnson, S. M., Bradley, B., Furrow, J., & Lee, A. (2005). *Becoming an emotionally focused couple therapist: The workbook.* New York: Brunner/Routledge.

Johnson, S. M., Hunsely, J., Greenberg, L., & Schindler, D. (1999). Emotionally focused couples therapy: Status and challenges. *Clinical Psychology: Science and Practice, 6,* 67–79.

Keim, J. (1999). Brief strategic marital therapy. In J. Donovan (Ed.), *Short-term couple therapy* (pp. 265–290). New York: Guilford Press.

Keim, J., & Lappin, J. (2002). Structural–strategic marital therapy. In A. S. Gurman & N. S. Jacobson (Eds.), *Clinical handbook of couple therapy* (3rd ed., pp. 86–117). New York: Guilford Press.

Lebow, J. L. (1997). The integrative revolution in couple and family therapy. *Family Process, 36,* 1–17.

Lebow, J. L. (1999). Building a science of couple relationships: Comments on two articles by Gottman and Levenson. *Family Process, 46,* 27–57.

Lebow, J. L., & Gurman, A. S. (1995). Research assessing couple and family therapy. *Annual Review of Psychology, 46,* 27–57.

Leff, J., Vearnals, S., Brewin, C. R., Wolff, G., Alexander, B., Asen, K., Dayson, D., et al. (2000). The London Depression Intervention Trial: Random/old controlled trial of antidepressants v. couple therapy in the treatment and maintenance of people with depression living with a critical partner: Clinical outcome and costs. *British Journal of Psychiatry, 177,* 95–100.

Luquet, W. (2007). *Short-term couples therapy: The imago model in action.* New York: Routledge.

Madanes, C. (1990). *Sex, love, and violence: Strategies for transformation.* New York: Norton.

Manus, G. (1966). Marriage counseling: A technique in search of a theory. *Journal of Marriage and the Family, 28,* 449–453.

Miller, S. D., Duncan, B. L., & Hubble, M. A. (1997). *Escape from Babel: Toward a unifying language for psychotherapy practice.* New York: Norton.

Minuchin, S. (1974). *Families and family therapy.* Cambridge, MA: Harvard University Press.

Minuchin, S., & Fishman, C. (1981). *Family therapy techniques.* Cambridge, MA: Harvard University Press.

Mittelman, B. (1948). The concurrent analysis of married couples. *Psychiatric Quarterly, 17,* 182–197.

Nichols, M. P. (1987). *The self in the system.* New York: Brunner/Mazel.

Nichols, M. P., & Schwartz, R. (1998). *Family therapy: Concepts and methods.* Boston: Allyn & Bacon.

O'Farrell, T. J., & Fals-Stewart, W. (2006). *Behavioral couples therapy for alcoholism and drug abuse.* New York: Guilford Press.

Oberndorf, C. P. (1934). Folie à deux. *International Journal of Psychoanalysis, 15,* 14–24.

Pinsof, W. M. (2002). The death of til death do us part: The twentieth century's revelation of the limits of human pair-bonding. *Family Process, 41*, 135–157.

Rait, D. (1988). Survey results. *Family Therapy Networker, 12*(1), 52–56.

Rastogi, M., & Thomas, V. (Eds.). (2009). *Multicultural couple therapy.* Los Angeles: Sage.

Rausch, H. L., Barry, W. A., Hertel, R. K., & Swain, M. A. (1974). *Communication, conflict and marriage.* San Francisco: Jossey-Bass.

Roberto-Forman, L. (2008). Transgenerational marriage therapy. In A. S. Gurman (Ed.), *Clinical handbook of couple therapy* (4th ed., pp. 196–228). New York: Guilford Press.

Sager, C. J. (1966). The development of marriage therapy: An historical review. *American Journal of Orthopsychiatry, 36*, 458–467.

Sager, C. J. (1967). Transference in conjoint treatment of married couples. *Archives of General Psychiatry, 16*, 185–193.

Satir, V. (1964). *Conjoint family therapy.* Palo Alto, CA: Science and Behavior Books.

Satir, V. (1972). *Peoplemaking.* Palo Alto, CA: Science and Behavior Books.

Scharff, D. E., & Scharff, J. S. (1991). *Object relations couple therapy.* New York: Aronson.

Scharff, J. S., & Bagnini, C. (2002). Object relations couple therapy. In A. S. Gurman & N. S. Jacobson (Eds.), *Clinical handbook of couple therapy* (3rd ed., pp. 59–85). New York: Guilford Press.

Scharff, J. S., & Scharff, D. E. (2008). Object relations couple therapy. In A. S. Gurman (Ed.), *Clinical handbook of couple therapy* (4th ed., pp. 167–195). New York: Guilford Press.

Segraves, R. T. (1982). *Marital therapy: A combined psychodynamic behavioral approach.* New York: Plenum Press.

Sexton, T., Gordon, K. S., Gurman, A. S., Lebow, J. L., Johnson, S. M., & Holtzworth-Munroe, A. (2010). *Evidence-based treatments in couple and family psychology* (Report of the Task Force on Evidence-Based Treatments in Family Psychology, Division 43, American Psychological Association). Washington, DC: American Psychological Association.

Shadish, W. R., & Baldwin, S. A. (2005). Effects of behavioral marital therapy: A meta-analysis of randomly controlled trials. *Journal of Consulting and Clinical Psychology, 73*, 6–14.

Shoham, V., Rohrbaugh, M. J., & Cleary, A. A. (2008). Brief strategic couple therapy. In A. S. Gurman (Ed.), *Clinical handbook of couple therapy* (4th ed., pp. 299–322). New York: Guilford Press.

Simon, G. M. (2008). Structural couple therapy. In A. S. Gurman (Ed.), *Clinical handbook of couple therapy* (4th ed., pp. 323–352). New York: Guilford Press.

Skynner, A. C. R. (1976). *Systems of family and marital psychotherapy.* New York: Brunner/Mazel.

Skynner, A. C. R. (1980). Recent developments in marital therapy. *Journal of Family Therapy, 2*, 271–296.

Snyder, D. K. (1999). Affective reconstruction in the context of a pluralistic approach to couple therapy. *Clinical Psychology: Science and Practice, 6*, 348–365.

Snyder, D. K., Castellani, A. M., & Whisman, M. A. (2006). Current status and future directions in couple therapy. *Annual Review of Psychology, 57*, 317–344.

Snyder, D. K., & Mitchell, A. E. (2008). Affective reconstruction: A pluralistic, developmental approach. In A. S. Gurman (Ed.), *Clinical handbook of couple therapy* (4th ed., pp. 353–382). New York: Guilford Press.

Snyder, D. K., Schneider, W. J., & Castellani, A. M. (2006). Tailoring couple therapy to individual differences: A conceptual approach. In D. K. Snyder & M. Whisman (Eds.), *Treating difficult couples* (pp. 27–51). New York: Guilford Press.

Snyder, D. K., & Wills, R. M. (1989). Behavioral versus insight-oriented marital therapy: Effects on individual and interspousal functioning. *Journal of Consulting and Clinical Psychology, 57*, 39–46.

Snyder, D. K., & Whisman, M. A. (2006). *Treating difficult couples.* New York: Guilford Press.

Sprenkle, D. H., Davis, S. D., & Lebow, J. L. (2009). *Common factors in couple and family therapy.* New York: Guilford Press.

Stanton, M. D. (1980). An integrated structural/strategic approach to family therapy. *Journal of Marital and Family Therapy, 7*, 427–439.

Stuart, R. B. (1969). Operant–interpersonal treatment of marital discord. *Journal of Consulting and Clinical Psychology, 33*, 675–682.

Titelman, P. (2010). A clinical format for Bowen family systems therapy with highly reactive couples. In A. S. Gurman (Ed.), *Clinical casebook of couple therapy* (pp. 112–133). New York: Guilford Press.

Todd, T. C. (1986). Structural-strategic marital therapy. In N. S. Jacobson & A. S. Gurman (Eds.), *Clinical handbook of marital therapy* (pp. 71–99). New York: Guilford Press.

Watzlawick, P., Weakland, J. H., & Fisch, R. (1974). *Change: Principles of problem formation and problem resolution*. New York: Norton.

Weakland, J. H., Fisch, R., Watzlawick, P., & Bodin, A. (1974). Brief therapy: Focused problem resolution. *Family Process, 13*, 141–168.

Weeks, G. R. (Ed.). (1989). *Treating couples: The Intersystem Model of The Marriage Council of Philadelphia*. New York: Brunner/Mazel.

Weiner-Davis, M. (1992). *Divorce-busting: A revolutionary and rapid program for staying together*. New York: Simon & Schuster/Fireside.

Weiss, R. L. (1980). Strategic behavioral marital therapy: Toward a model for assessment and Intervention. In J. P. Vincent (Ed.), *Advances in family intervention, assessment and theory* (pp. 229–271). Greenwich, CT: JAI Press.

Whiffen, V. E. (2003). What attachment theory can offer marital and family therapists. In S. M. Johnson & V. E. Whiffen (Eds.), *Attachment processes in couple and family therapy* (pp. 389–398). New York: Guilford Press.

Whitaker, C. A., & Keith, D. V. (1981). Symbolic–experiential family therapy. In A. S. Gurman & D. P. Kniskern (Eds.), *Handbook of family therapy* (pp. 187–225). New York: Brunner/Mazel.

White, M., & Epston, D. (1990). *Narrative means to therapeutic ends*. New York: Norton.

Willi, J. (1982). *Couples in collusion*. Claremont, CA: Hunter House.

Winnicott, D. W. (1960). The theory of the parent–infant relationship. *International Journal of Psychoanalysis, 41*, 585–595.

PART VI

OTHER INFLUENTIAL MODELS
OF THERAPEUTIC PRACTICE

CHAPTER 11

Brief Psychotherapies

Michael F. Hoyt

> I think the development of psychiatric skill consists in very considerable
> measure of doing a lot with very little—making a rather precise move
> which has a high probability of achieving what you're attempting to
> achieve, with a minimum of time and words.
> —HARRY STACK SULLIVAN (1954, p. 224)

We first consider some general principles of brief therapy, then turn our attention to several approaches developed specifically to address issues of length of treatment: (1) brief psychodynamic therapy, (2) brief redecision therapy, and (3) brief Ericksonian, strategic, and solution-focused therapy. Before turning to specifics, let us first consider what different brief therapies have in common.

THE CONCEPT OF BRIEF THERAPY

When a therapist and patient endeavor to get from Point A (the problem that led to therapy) to Point B (the resolution that ends therapy) via a direct, parsimonious, and efficient route, we say that they are deliberately engaging in *brief therapy*. The approach is intended to be quick and helpful, nothing extraneous, no beating around the bush. Another closely related term is *time-limited therapy*, which explicitly emphasizes the temporal boundedness of the treatment. Synonymous with *brief therapy* is the term *planned short-term therapy*, meaning, literally, a "deliberately concise remedy/restoration/improvement." As Bloom (1992, p. 3) has written: "The word *planned* is important; these works describe short-term treatment that is intended to accomplish a set of therapeutic objectives within a sharply limited time frame." This is how de Shazer (1991a, pp. ix–x) describes it:

> 'Brief therapy' simply means therapy that takes as few sessions as possible, not even one
> more than is necessary. . . . 'Brief therapy' is a relative term, typically meaning: (a) fewer ses-
> sions than standard, and/or (b) a shorter period of time from intake to termination, and/
> or (c) a lower number of sessions and a lower frequency of sessions from start to finish."

Brevity and *shortness* are watchwords signaling efficiency, the contrast being the more intentionally protracted course of traditional long-term (usually psychodynamic) therapy. Actually, most therapy is de facto brief, by default or design, meaning a few sessions, weeks to months. As numerous studies (see Messer, 2001a) have reported, the average length of treatment is three to eight sessions. The modal or most common length of treatment is actually only one session. Even with this "briefest of brief" duration, many successful outcomes are reported (e.g., Bloom, 2001; Slive & Bobele, 2010; Talmon, 1990, 1993).

Various authors have offered different definitions of what constitutes brief therapy. Some have emphasized a number of sessions, such as "5–10," "12," or "up to 20"; others have emphasized certain types of problems they attempt to address; still others have focused more on the idea of the passage of time being a contextual pressure. Budman and Gurman (1988), for example, eschew a specific number of sessions in their definition, instead referring to deliberate or planned brief therapy as "time-sensitive" or "time-effective" treatment. Setting a specific number of sessions may at times be helpful, however, to provide structure or to deliberately stimulate a termination process (Mann, 1973). Attention to temporal parameters is important since Parkinson's Law ("Work expands or contracts to fit the allotted time") may operate in psychotherapy (Appelbaum, 1975). Generally, the focus should be on making the most of each session. Focused intentionality is the key. Get to it; make everything count; don't be wasteful.

Planned brief therapy is predicated on the belief and expectation that change can occur *in the moment,* particularly if theoretical ability, practical skill, and interest in efficacy are brought to bear. As Lazarus and Fay (1990, p. 40) have expressed it, "Effective treatment depends far less on the hours you put in, than on what you put into those hours." The work is not superficial or simply technique-oriented; it is precise and beneficial, often yielding enduring long-term benefits as well as more immediate gains. Most patients want efficient help. Even if longer-term therapies sometimes do produce results that may be preferable (see Seligman, 1995), evidence (e.g., Lambert, 2001) shows that many patients respond quickly, even in therapies not specifically designed or planned to be brief. Given the social and professional imperative to provide psychological services to the wide range of persons who might need and benefit from mental health care, why not try a short-term approach first?

BASIC BELIEFS THAT CAN PROMOTE OR IMPEDE EFFECTIVE BRIEF THERAPY

The fundamental assumption of all forms of deliberate brief therapy is an attitude and expectation—supported by various theories, methodologies, and findings—that significant and beneficial changes can be brought about relatively quickly. The brief therapist recognizes that there is no time but the present. Whatever the therapist's particular theoretical orientation, primary effort is directed to help the patient recognize options in the present that can result in enhanced coping, new learning, growth, and other beneficial changes. Yapko (1990) has noted three factors that determine whether a patient will benefit from brief therapy interventions: (1) the person's primary temporal orientation (toward past, present, or future); (2) the general value given to "change," whether he or she is more invested in maintaining tradition or seeking change; and (3) the patient's belief system about what constitutes a complete therapeutic experience.

This fundamental assumption—that with skillful facilitation, useful changes can be set into motion relatively quickly, and that patients can then maintain and often expand

TABLE 11.1. Comparative Dominant Values of the Long-Term and Short-Term Therapist

Long-term therapist	Short-term therapist
1. Seeks change in basic character.	Prefers pragmatism, parsimony, and the least radical intervention; does not believe in the notion of "cure."
2. Believes that significant change is unlikely in everyday life.	Maintains an adult developmental perspective from which significant psychological change is viewed as inevitable.
3. Sees presenting problems as reflecting more basic pathology.	Emphasizes patients' strengths and resources.
4. Wants to "be there" as patient makes significant changes.	Accepts that many changes will occur "after therapy."
5. Sees therapy as having a "timeless" quality.	Does not accept the timelessness of some models of therapy.
6. Unconsciously recognizes the fiscal convenience of long-term patients.	Fiscal issues often muted, either by the nature of the practice or the organizational structure.
7. Views therapy as almost always benign and useful.	Views therapy as sometimes useful and sometimes harmful.
8. Sees therapy as being the most important part of the patient's life.	Sees being in the world as more important than being in therapy.
9. Views therapist as responsible only for treating a given patient.	Views therapist as having responsibility for treatment of a population.

Note. From Budman and Gurman (1988, p. 11). Copyright 1988 by The Guilford Press. Reprinted by permission.

the benefits on their own—underlies the "universal elements" or "common ingredients" of brief treatment. Budman, Friedman, and Hoyt (1992; also see Gurman, 2001; Messer, 2001a) highlight the most frequently cited generic components of brief therapy:

1. Rapid and generally positive working alliance between therapist and patient.
2. Focality, the clear specification of achievable treatment results and goals.
3. Clear definition of patient and therapist responsibilities, with a relatively high level of therapist activity and patient participation.
4. Emphasis on the patient's strengths, competencies, and adaptive capacities.
5. Expectation of change, the belief that improvement is within the patient's (immediate) grasp.
6. Here-and-now (and next) orientation, the primary focus being on current functioning and patterns in thinking, feeling, and behaving—and their alternatives.
7. Time sensitivity, making the most of each session, as well as the idea of intermittent treatment replacing the notion of a once-and-for-all definitive "cure."

This set of defining characteristics is reflected in the comparison of the dominant values of long-term and short-term treatment presented in Table 1.11.

Many of these same value differences can also be detected in the "resistances" or contrary attitudes some therapists hold about brief or short-term therapy (e.g., Hoyt, 1985; also see Messer & Warren, 1995, pp. 43–49):

1. *The belief that "more is better,"* often held despite the lack of evidence justifying the greater expense of long-term or open-ended treatment.

2. *The myth of the "pure gold" of analysis* (to use Freud's [1919/1955] term for idealized insight and interpretation) and the faulty assumption that change and growth necessarily require "deep" examination, and that anything else is dismissible as "superficial" or "merely palliative."

3. *Belief in the inappropriateness of greater therapist activity,* including the need to be selectively focused, confrontative, directive, and risk taking.

4. *The confusion of patients' and therapists' interests,* the tendency of therapists to seek and treat perfectionistically putative "complexes" and underlying personality issues rather than attend directly to patients' complaints and stated treatment goals. Most patients seek therapy because of a specific problem and want the most succinct help available.

5. *Financial pressures,* the temptation to hold on to that which is profitable and dependable, as well as other incentives such as the pleasures of intimate conversation and the lure of vicariously living through an extended relationship.

6. *Countertransference and termination problems,* including the need to be needed and difficulties saying good-bye.

7. *Psychological reactance,* the interesting response of valuing something more if one cannot have it (Brehm, 1966). Being told that one has to treat a patient with brief therapy (e.g., because of insurance restrictions or simply because that is what the patient wants) may trigger resentment and the thought, "No one is going to tell me what to do. I'm a professional." The fact is, however, that restrictions such as patients' willingness and ability to pay, insurance limits, and clinic policies regarding possible length of treatment do get imposed. There is also the social responsibility to provide needed services to the many rather than many services to the privileged few.

The foregoing notwithstanding, there are certainly times when short-term therapy is not adequate and appropriate—including treatment of severe psychiatric disorders, instances when a longer process is required for the patient to make desired changes, or when ongoing support is required to maintain a tenuous psychosocial adjustment. "Brief" really means "time sensitive" or "time efficient," not always "rapid" or "quick," and for those patients who truly require ongoing (continuous or intermittent) treatment, the basic attitudes of making the most of each session, accessing strengths and resources, and taking as few sessions as possible are still valuable. Indeed, if the needs of more than a handful of patients are to be served, the skillful application of brief therapy methods whenever possible is necessary to make longer-term treatments available for those who truly need them.

WHY DO PATIENTS/CLIENTS COME TO THERAPY?

Most patients or clients come to therapy because they hope that working with a psychotherapist will soon relieve some state of unhappiness, distress, or dysfunction that has become so troublesome that professional consultation appears preferable to continuing the status quo. The person feels that something timely has to be done. As Budman and Gurman (1988) have articulated it, five interrelated themes or foci can often be addressed productively in brief therapy: loss, developmental dysynchronies (life cycle transitions or passages for which the patient is not well prepared), interpersonal conflicts, specific symptoms, and personality issues.

It is helpful to keep in mind the idea that the word *diagnosis* comes from Greek and Latin words (*via gnosis*) meaning "the way of knowing," and this is just what a good functional diagnosis should do: provide information that illuminates a path (Hoyt, 1989). Pathology-oriented nosology may contain some important information, but it is seldom enough. Important data may be summarized in DSM-IV-TR (American Psychiatric Association, 2000) and may be especially useful for communicating with insurance companies and clinical researchers, as well as for differentially diagnosing whether medication is likely to be of help, but reviewing the axes also reveals a potentially discouraging orientation toward "disease" and "sickness." Information about potential suicidality and alcohol and substance abuse can be vital, but we also need to focus on the patient's strengths and capacities, and his or her beliefs, resources, and motivations for treatment to proceed successfully.

A therapist wanting to do effective brief treatment needs to accomplish a number of tasks early on with a patient:

1. Make contact and establish rapport.
2. Define the purpose of the meeting.
3. Orient and instruct the patient on how to use therapy.
4. Create an opportunity for the patient to express thoughts, feelings, and behavior.
5. Assess the patient's problems, strengths, motivations, goals, and expectations.
6. Establish realistic (specific and obtainable) treatment goals.
7. Make initial treatment interventions, assess effects, and adjust accordingly.
8. Assign tasks or "homework" as appropriate.
9. Attend to business matters such as future appointments and fees.

It is important in the first session to engage the patient and to introduce some novelty. In virtually all successful brief therapies, something new happens in the first meeting. As the old saying goes, "If you don't change directions, you'll wind up where you're heading!" More of the same (behavior, outlook, defense, etc.) does not produce change. Effective therapy involves breaking such patterns, doing something different. The novelty may come by seeing oneself and one's situation differently, by practicing a new way of transacting with others, by experiencing unacknowledged feelings, or by utilizing strengths and abilities that were overlooked previously or are newly learned. Whatever the means, the brief therapist looks for ways to start or amplify the patient's movement in the desired direction as soon as possible.

Alliance involves forming a union or connection ("They won't care about what you know until they know that you care"). Attending carefully to the early identification of specific, achievable goals promotes effective brief work. Operational definitions contribute to treatment accountability, counter the temptation to diffuse/confuse/refuse focality, and help to assure that genuinely obtainable results are not replaced with vague or unrealistic "missions impossible" or "therapeutic perfectionism" (Malan, 1976). Questions such as the following help to focus treatment and involve the patient:

- "What problem are you here to solve?"
- "If you work hard and make some changes, how will you be functioning differently?"

- "What are the smallest changes you could make that would tell that you are heading in the right direction?"
- "At those times when the problem is not so bad or is absent, what are you doing?"
- "What will tell us we're done? How will we know when to stop meeting like this?"
- "How might therapy help, and how long do you expect it to take?"

Treatment revolves around what the patient wants to accomplish plus the answers to three interrelated transtechnical, heuristic questions (Hoyt, 1995a, 2000a):

1. "How is the patient 'stuck' [what is the problem or pathology?]?"
2. "What does the patient need to get 'unstuck' [sometimes detected by identifying what the patient is doing differently at times when he or she is not 'stuck']?"
3. "How can I, as therapist, facilitate or provide what is needed?"

The good brief (or any) therapist needs to be multitheoretical (and multiculturally competent), able to conceptualize and reckon from a variety of perspectives lest patients be forced into the Procrustean bed of a pet theory or technique, or be dismissed and blamed for being resistant, unmotivated, or ego-deficient. The therapist wishing to be parsimonious (brief and effective) may need to choose which conceptualization(s) allow for the best chance of a change-producing intervention. Should the approach be toward revealing the intrapsychic domain of warded-off feelings, modifying the patient's typical way of viewing and meeting the world, altering the social skills with which the patient interacts, or changing the rules of the labyrinthine games that ensnare patients into maintaining the status quo? Or what else? And how to do so? Education and skill instruction? Cognitive-behavioral techniques? Psychodynamic interpretations? Solution-focused questions? Systemic interviewing and strategic interventions? Hypnosis? Commonsense appeals or wise exhortations? The brief therapist asks: *What would be likely to work with this patient and this therapist in this context at this time?*

INTERLUDE: A BRIEF HISTORY OF BRIEF THERAPY

People have been having problems and getting help since time immemorial, although the history of psychotherapy as a practice and a profession is considered to have begun in earnest only about 100 years ago (Freedheim, 1992). Sigmund Freud, usually thought of as the founder of psychoanalysis, was also the father of brief therapy. Reading his early cases (Breuer & Freud, 1893–1895/1955), one finds him working actively with patients and treating them in days, weeks, and months rather than years. Psychoanalysis was also a research instrument, however, and treatment became longer and longer as the early pioneers became fascinated with the psychological phenomena that emerged (e.g., Oedipal fantasies and transference neuroses) if the therapist remained a relatively inactive and neutral "blank" screen while the patient freely associated. An early effort to experiment with more active methods in treatment was made by Ferenczi and Rank (1925), but some of their methods were questionable and the time for revisionism was not right, since psychoanalysis was still struggling to establish itself. At the end of his life, Freud (1937/1953) expressed his frustration about the limited therapeutic benefits of psychoanalysis and called for the development of new methods based on the psychoanalytic understanding of transference, resistance, and unconscious material.

World War II intervened, with many consequences for the practice of brief (and other) psychotherapy. Prior to the war, psychological treatment usually had been a long-term luxury of the privileged and had fallen under the purview of the psychoanalytic and psychiatric–medical establishment. There were so many soldiers needing services, however, that (1) psychologists and clinical social workers were finally recognized as bona fide psychotherapy providers rather than being relegated to their respective "auxiliary" roles as psychometric testers and home visitors; (2) group therapy was greatly expanded as a treatment of choice (and necessity) rather than being an isolated and rare specialty; (3) the Veterans Administration medical system emerged as a training ground for mental-health professionals; and (4) interest was spurred in treatment methods that would help soldiers quickly reduce symptoms and return to function either in the combat zones or back in civilian life. Psychoanalytic theory continued to predominate, but "reality factors" were becoming increasingly influential— harbingers of what today is called "accountability" (Johnson, 1995; Cummings, 2000).

In 1946, Alexander and French published *Psychoanalytic Therapy: Principles and Applications*. The book was extraordinary, revisiting and updating many of the ideas of Ferenczi and Rank (1925) regarding the use of greater therapist activity, and suggesting that the length and frequency of sessions might be varied, both from case to case and within the same patient's treatment, to avoid excessive dependency in the patient that prolonged therapy and to bring about what Alexander and French referred to as a "corrective emotional experience." Many successful brief therapies were reported. Still, the politics of psychoanalysis were not yet ripe for change, and it remained for two leading psychoanalytic figures of the time, Bibring (1954) and Gill (1954), to publish their seminal papers about modifying the parameters of treatment and to call it psychoanalytically-*oriented* therapy (and not psychoanalysis) before attempts at psychodynamic modifications were recognized as legitimate by the mainstream.

By the early 1960s, a number of workers were exploring what could be done using psychodynamic principles in more active and shorter treatment. In London, Balint, Ornstein, and Balint (1972) and Malan (1963, 1976) were developing "focal psychotherapy"; in Boston, Sifneos (1972) was beginning to experiment with "short-term anxiety-provoking psychotherapy"; and in New York, Wolberg (1965) was investigating various ways of shortening the length of treatment, including use of hypnotherapy to work through patients' resistances more quickly. At the same time, several other important figures were becoming disenchanted with psychoanalysis and began to originate other, more active methods for bringing about psychological change more rapidly. Perls, Hefferline, and Goodman (1951) began to develop the theory and techniques of Gestalt therapy; Wolpe (1958) and Wolpe and Lazarus (1966) were developing behavior therapy; Ellis (1962) began to develop rational-emotive therapy, the first systematic form of what is now called "cognitive therapy"; and Berne (1961, 1972) began to develop transactional analysis. In Palo Alto, California, the innovative psychiatrist and pioneering family therapist Don Jackson founded the Mental Research Institute (MRI), which in 1966 became the home of the Brief Therapy Center. Concurrently, the psychiatrist Milton Erickson (1980) was still working in relative obscurity in Phoenix, Arizona, but his uniquely creative uses of hypnosis and strategic interventions to capitalize on patients' existing capacities would soon be recognized (especially with the 1973 publication of Jay Haley's *Uncommon Therapy: The Psychiatric Techniques of Milton H. Erickson, M.D.*) and contribute greatly to both the emerging family therapy movement and to various schools of strategic and systemic therapy.

Writing about the expanding spectrum of brief therapies, Barten (1971) underscored the convergence of a number of historical developments, including a growing professional commitment to providing appropriate mental health services to all segments of the community; an increasing shift from psychoanalysis to more ego-oriented techniques; and a recognition of the value of limited therapeutic goals, diversification of the roles of mental health professionals, long overdue recognition of the special needs of the disadvantaged, and increased consumer demand for economically feasible services. The community mental health movement of the 1960s and the federal Health Maintenance Organization (HMO) Act of 1973 gave further mandate to brief treatment. In 1988, a conference entitled "Brief Therapy: Myths, Methods and Metaphors," sponsored by the Milton H. Erickson Foundation, was held in San Francisco, with several thousand mental health professionals attending (Zeig & Gilligan, 1990); several such conferences have been held since (see *www.erickson-foundation.org*).

The recent enormous acceleration in various forms of managed mental health care—which by 1992 covered approximately 100 million Americans, by year 2000 covered approximately 160 million American, and with further heath care reform may provide some services for almost everyone—has given further impetus to the development and expansion of various forms of brief therapy. However, while various managed-care organizations, insurance companies, HMOs, clinics, counseling services, and consumers all desire, and often require, brief treatment, it is important not to conflate the terms *brief therapy* and *managed care*. There are numerous ethical and practical problems with the way some managed care organizations go about their business, including undertreatment of some patients (see Hoyt, 1995a, 2000a). As Steve de Shazer, the co-originator of solution-focused therapy, remarked, "We are *not* a response to managed care. We've been doing brief therapy for 30 years. We developed this a long time before managed care was even somebody's bad idea" (quoted in Short, 1997, p. 18, emphasis in original).

THE STRUCTURE OF BRIEF THERAPY

Brief psychotherapy can be conceptualized as having a structure of five sequenced phases. In actual practice, of course, the phases blend into one another rather than being discretely organized. The structure tends to be *epigenetic* or *pyramidal*; that is, each phase builds on the prior phase, so that successful work in one is a precondition for the next (e.g., the patient electing treatment and the therapist applying selection criteria and accepting the patient precedes forming a working alliance, which precedes focusing and making a contract, which precedes change-amplifying intervention, which precedes continuing work and following through).

As noted elsewhere (Gustafson, 1986; Hoyt & Miller, 2000), there is often an interesting parallel between the process of each individual session and the structure of the overall course of treatment: Like the idea of ontogeny recapitulating phylogeny, each session and each therapy involves connecting, working, and closing.

The questions one asks, beginning with the first, do much to set the theme and temporal orientation of each session and the overall treatment (Goulding & Goulding, 1979; Hoyt, 1990, 2006). Asking "What's better?" moves the focus more toward strengths and competencies, whereas asking "What's wrong?" invites *problem talk* rather than *solution talk* (de Shazer, 1988; Furman & Ahola, 1992). Similarly, if one asks, for example, "How have things gone?", the direction is largely toward reviewing the *past*. If one instead asks, "What are you experiencing?" or "What are you willing to change today?", the direction is more *present* centered. Asking "What do you need to discuss to do well next week?" or "How will you be different when the problem is solved?" points to the *future*.

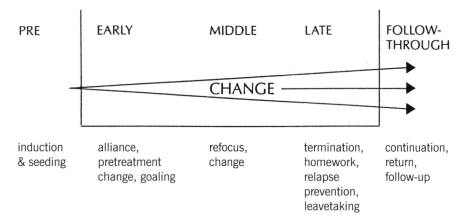

FIGURE 11.1. The temporal structure of brief therapy. From Hoyt (2000b, p. 218). Copyright 2000 by Michael F. Hoyt. Reprinted by permission.

As seen in Figure 11.1, each phase of treatment has its special issues:

1. *Pre: Election and selection.* Even before the first session occurs, change often begins with the recognition of a problem and the decision to seek therapy. Can the therapist capitalize on this? How? What may need to happen before change is possible? Is the patient ready, and what will circumstances permit? Is the patient a willing customer, an unwilling complainant, or simply a visitor (de Shazer, 1988)? Looked at from a somewhat different perspective, we can recognize the importance of the patient's stage of change: Is the patient in the precontemplation, contemplation, planning, action, or maintenance stage (Prochaska, DiClemente, & Norcross, 1992; Hoyt & Miller, 2000)? It is also good to remember that there are some patients—spontaneous improvers, nonresponders, and negative therapeutic reactors—for whom "no treatment" may be the prescription of choice (Frances & Clarkin, 1981).

2. *Early.* Key issues involve forming a working alliance; assessing patients' strengths, weaknesses, and motivations; finding a psychological focus, establishing achievable goals and forming a treatment plan and contract; introducing novelty and getting the patient actively involved in treatment; and attending to business matters. No mean feat!

3. *Middle phase.* This is the "working through" stage, which means staying on task, doing homework, and applying the lessons of therapy in real life, as well as possibly increasing insight into the original and present-day sources of problems. Maintenance and possible refinement of a central theme/focus/goal occur here.

4. *Late phase.* This includes termination and possible arousal of underlying separation–individuation issues in both patient and therapist, with possible return of symptoms and temptations to avoid ending; the need to subtract the therapist from the successful equation (Gustafson, 1986); maintaining gains, goal attainment assessment, possible homework or tasks, continuing change, and avoiding possible backsliding or "self-sabotage"; relapse prevention; inviting a follow-up or "check-in" appointment, with the possibility of later return to treatment; and leavetaking. Careful attention is paid to ending not too soon but not later than necessary.

5. *Follow-through.* This includes continuation of psychological work and change beyond the formal ending of therapist–patient contact. Internalization of favorable aspects of the treatment occurs here. In short-term therapy, much more than in longer treatments, change processes may be started or amplified without being completely worked through during the course of formal treatment. This is consistent with the distinction between treatment goals and life goals (Ticho, 1972). There is also, of course, the possibility of intermittent, episodic, serial, catalytic, or distributed therapy—the patient can return later for additional treatment as needed.

SOME SPECIFIC MODELS OF BRIEF THERAPY

There are various models or "schools" of brief therapy (see Bloom, 1992; Budman et al., 1992; Carlson & Sperry, 2000; Hoyt, 2009). Although each case is different and the skillful application of psychological principles is part of what makes therapy an interesting and artful endeavor, there are broad general guidelines in theory and practice that distinguish different forms of brief treatment. We highlight and illustrate a few of them here, but the reader should keep in mind two important caveats: (1) no summary or case presentation can do more than suggest a few broad brushstrokes of a particular approach; and (2) most therapy is eclectic and integrative, drawing ideas and methods from a range of sources rather than adhering to one particular theory.

Short-Term Psychodynamic Psychotherapies

Beginning with Freud, numerous theoreticians and clinicians have applied the psychoanalytic concepts of the unconscious, resistance, and transference to brief forms of treatment. Various short-term dynamic methods have been developed to bring the patient to a greater awareness of his or her maladaptive defenses, warded-off feelings, and counterproductive relationship patterns. The emphasis in all of the various short-term dynamic psychotherapies has been on increased therapist activity within a limited, central focus. There has been a general recognition that relative inactivity on the part of the therapist in the face of increasing resistance leads to prolonged and diffuse treatment. Brief dynamic therapists endeavor to promote change within a focalized area of conflict via an admixture of de-repression and affective release, corrective emotional experience and internalization of a benign therapist–patient relationship, relearning, and application of the patient's will.

Let us sketch a few of the main short-term psychodynamic approaches in terms of their central characteristics of focus, primary techniques, and length of treatment; we then consider a case vignette.

1. *Short-term anxiety-provoking psychotherapy* (Sifneos, 1987, 1992). This approach is primarily for carefully selected patients with Oedipal conflicts. Anxiety-provoking confrontations and transference interpretations are made by a teacher/therapist endeavoring to produce emotional relearning. Length of treatment varies but is typically about 6–15 sessions.

2. *Brief dynamic psychotherapy* (Malan, 1963, 1976). This method also focuses on issues of Oedipal conflict and loss, with research evidence indicating a positive correlation between therapy outcome and therapist emphasis on interpretive links between transference and

past (i.e., parents) relationship issues, and between outcome and the therapist emphasizing issues of termination and loss. Treatment is typically 30–40 sessions.

3. *Intensive short-term dynamic psychotherapy* (Davanloo, 1978, 1980, 1991; Malan, 1980; McCullough-Vaillant, 1997). The therapist functions as a "relentless healer," vigorously confronting and interpreting defenses, until there is an "unlocking of the unconscious" and a breakthrough into true feelings. The focus is broad, with strong emphasis on characterological defenses as they are manifested within the basic psychoanalytic "triangle of conflict" (impulse–feeling/anxiety/defense) and "triangle of persons" (transference/current significant persons/past significant persons), with special attention directed toward an experience in the transference. As McCullough (2000, p. 130) has written: "The core maladaptive conflict can be thought of as an affect phobia (i.e., fear of one's own emotional responses because of conflictual feelings associated with them). The treatment can be conceptualized as an exposure (to conflicted feelings) and response prevention (of defensive avoidance) to achieve desensitization of the feared but adaptive affects." Treatment length generally varies from five to 40 sessions, with progress expected to be evident early on.

4. *Stress response therapy and microanalysis* (Horowitz et al., 1984). The focus is on the patient's "states of mind," "self-schemas," "role-relationship models," and information-processing styles (couched in an explicitly cognitive language) to help the patient rework and emotionally master a recent stress event (e.g., the death of a loved one). Patients typically alternate between "intrusive–repetitive" and "denial–numbing" phases as they work through their stress response, usually over the course of 12 sessions.

5. *Time-limited dynamic psychotherapy* (Strupp & Binder, 1984; Levenson, 1995). A "cyclical maladaptive pattern" is identified and interpreted, involving acts of self, expectations of others, acts of others, and actions of the self toward the self. The therapist is empathic, appreciating the pull of countertransference as an opportunity to provide insight and a corrective emotional experience. Research on this method consistently indicates that "the quality of the therapeutic relationship, established early in the interaction, proved to be an important predictor of outcome. In particular, therapy tended to be successful if by the third session the patient felt accepted, understood, and liked by the therapist" (Binder & Strupp, 1991, p. 157). Treatment is usually 25 sessions.

6. *Time-limited psychotherapy* (Mann, 1973; Mann & Goldman, 1982). A firm 12-session treatment framework is established, with an emphasis on the patient's poor sense of self and his or her "present and chronically endured pain." The preset termination date focuses conscious and unconscious attention on the passage of time, creating a context in which the empathic therapist helps the patient look at and master underlying separation issues that become manifest in terms of themes of unresolved mourning, activity versus passivity, independence versus dependence, and adequate versus diminished self-esteem.

Messer and Warren (1995; also see Messer, 2001b) characterize the first three approaches listed earlier (Sifneos, Malan, Davanloo) as "the drive/structural model"; the next two approaches (Horowitz, and Strupp and Binder) as "the relational model" (in which they also include the work of Luborsky & Crits-Christoph, 1990, and of Weiss, Sampson, & the Mt. Zion Psychotherapy Research Group, 1986]); and the last approach (Mann) as "an integrative psychoanalytic model." As Messer and Warren (1995, p. 46) note, "The techniques employed by the drive/structuralist therapists, especially Davanloo and Sifneos, include direct confrontation of patients' defenses, which requires a rather bald show of therapist authority and assertiveness." Critics of these methods (e.g., Gustafson, 1986; Westen, 1986) perceive them as authoritarian. What is at stake here is more than "style." Drive/structural model therapists consider their view to be "The Truth"—"not hypothesis, metaphor, or construct, but an obvious and proven fact" (Messer & Warren, 1995, p. 113). Messer and Warren contrast this *correspondence* theory to "the *coherence* theory of truth, which posits that there is more than one true description of the world" (p. 113).

There have been many reports of how different forms of brief psychodynamic therapy have helped people come to grips with warded-off intrapsychic and interpersonal conflicts, thus achieving greater peace of mind, happiness in relationships, success at work, and the ability to say good-bye. Although the data are not without complication, the general thrust of the evidence is clear: Many patients benefit from brief, focused, psychodynamic therapy (Leichsenring, Rabung, & Leibing, 2004; Messer & Abbass, 2010).

Short-term dynamic psychotherapy, of course, is not for everyone. As research suggests, it requires a reasonably functional and psychologically minded patient with a grip on reality and an ability to tolerate painful emotional material. The patient also has to be available to attend sessions regularly. It is also not a panacea, since many biological, social, situational, and existential factors besides intrapsychic dynamics may require clinical attention. It is also important to remember that for psychodynamic psychotherapy to be effective, regardless of whether it is short-term or more extended, insight must serve as a vehicle and not as a final destination; that is, the real question is not how far back does a problem go but how far it will be carried forward.

The following case vignette illustrates some aspects of an integrated short-term psychodynamic approach.

THE CASE OF THE FORLORN LOVER

David was a 52-year-old man who sought therapy a few months after his lover died of AIDS. On the telephone, he tensely asked whether I was prejudiced against working with homosexuals. When I answered that I was not, he said he would see me at the appointment time I had offered.

He arrived a few minutes early, neatly dressed in tie and coat, coming from his job as manager of an office where he had worked for many years. He spoke slowly with great control—formal, severe, constricted—as he described his dilemma. He had never been close to anyone, he reported. He had grown up in an emotionally cold European household and had then spent many years as a monk in a religious order. Finally, he had left and eventually made his way to San Francisco. He was accepting of his sexual orientation and spent most of his off-work time among gays and lesbians because of greater compatibility and to avoid discrimination. He had adopted a lifestyle of occasional brief sexual encounters until he met Richard. It was difficult for him even to speak his late friend's name, the loss was so painful. Several times he started to choke up, would put his hand over his face, and recompose himself.

Near the end of our first session, I asked him why he had come to therapy, what did he want to accomplish? "The pain is so great I can't stand it, but damn him, he made me feel and now I don't want to go back to that cold life I had before. I'm lost." He cried a bit, then pulled himself together. He remarked that he found me kind and easy to talk with, and that he was relieved I had directly answered his question about possible antigay prejudice, because his insurance restricted whom he might be able to see. He asked if he could have an appointment to come back. When I agreed and asked when he would like to return, he indicated that his work schedule would require a 2-week interval between sessions. We set an appointment. (This time frame would also allow him to regulate better the intensity of whatever might transpire in our meetings, I thought, but I did not share this with him.)

Over the next three sessions, David gradually told me more about his relationship with Richard. The telling was slow and painful. Several times, when he felt a wave of emotion, he would either close his eyes and tremble until it passed, or set his jaw and actively suppress his feelings. He was grieving at a pace that seemed tolerable for him, while I mostly listened and occasionally asked leading questions. His level of tension and control was remarkable. He would make sure that the sessions stopped exactly on time. When I was a few minutes late to begin, he became especially cold and distant. When I commented that he seemed "somewhat tense," he paused until he was composed, then told me that he was "furious inside." I said I was sorry for the lateness and added:

THERAPIST: It is remarkable how you are able to keep your feelings in.

PATIENT: Yes, I can eliminate someone from my emotions. I am well trained not to feel.

THERAPIST: Yes, but to do that would render me useless to you. And that wouldn't be good for you.

He looked at me and palpably reconnected.

In the next two sessions, David hesitantly revealed more details about Richard, including various complaints about his drinking and bouts of irritability. David then became increasingly unforthcoming. I asked why.

PATIENT: If I talk more about him and let myself grieve, then the images and memories might fade and I will have nothing left. . . . (*Silence*)

THERAPIST: You're trying to hold on to him in your mind the way some people keep a room exactly like it was the day someone died. It's like a museum, as though time can be frozen. . . . But it can't.

PATIENT: Oh, God, yes, that's it. (*Cries and then recomposes himself.*)

THERAPIST: So, what are you going to do?

PATIENT: I want to go forward, but I don't know how. Oh, I do, there are other people, but I'm scared.

THERAPIST: Of what?

PATIENT: Of getting hurt again.

THERAPIST: Then go slow, when you're ready. But life is in front of you.

David continued his mourning process. He also began to experiment over the next several weeks by attending a dance club, having supper with someone, even asserting himself at his workplace and refusing to acquiesce to things he felt were unfair. He was well aware of his pattern of "stuffing" his feelings and still often did so when threatened or hurt, but with increased cognizance, he also sometimes expressed himself more. He even occasionally smiled and told stories that revealed a growing tenderness in his relations with others, including a new willingness to forgive and to remain involved with people rather than "eliminating" them if they were sometimes inconsiderate or annoying. He began to exercise and lost a few "extra" pounds that he had been carrying, all in preparation for the possibility of finding a new mate.

Follow-Up and Comment. This case might best be described as "eclectic–integrative" (Messer & Warren, 1995) and as falling within the "expressive–supportive" range of brief dynamic therapies (Pinsker, Rosenthal, & McCullough, 1991). Attention was paid to exploring the patient's warded-off feelings, his images of self and others, and ways his defenses and relationship patterns were repeated with the therapist. Although he was largely resistant to discussing possible connections between his family-of-origin experiences and his current functioning, he gained some insight, experienced support and a renewed connection with another (male) human being, and learned to tolerate some of the painful feelings he had tried to stifle. As one might expect, therapy termination was not easy for David. Relinquishing the therapist reminded him of losing Richard and also meant giving up a person he had learned to trust and with whom he felt at ease talking, but by the 12th therapy session he felt strong enough to go forward and so stopped treatment as planned. Consistent with Mann's (1973) model, themes of unresolved mourning, activity versus passivity, and independence versus dependence were prominent throughout the therapy, and especially during the explicit termination phase. Indeed, there was a countertransference "pull" to extend treatment, but I did not yield to that impulse, and we ended our meeting. David largely accomplished his goals for treatment—to get through the pain and to resume moving toward people rather than retreating into isolation. I encouraged him to return to therapy as needed, and he agreed to do so.

Redecision Therapy and Transactional Analysis

Eric Berne (1961, 1972) originated the transactional analysis (TA) school of therapy out of his desire to help patients see more quickly their own role in their personal difficulties. He had been trained as a psychoanalyst but found the psychoanalytic process too slow and ineffective. Although TA involves a complicated and comprehensive model of human development, intrapsychic organization, and interpersonal dynamics, there are three popular and readily accessible ideas from TA with which Berne is most identified: (1) the "I'm OK, You're OK" matrix of existential positions pertaining to how one regards self and others (actually developed by Robert Goulding in a discussion with Berne; see Hoyt, 1995b); (2) the Parent–Adult–Child conceptualization of personality "ego states" (the progenitor of various "Inner Child" theories); and (3) the "Games People Play" (Berne, 1964) idea of recognizing the ulterior motivations behind dysfunctional relationship patterns.

Combining some of the theory of TA with Gestalt techniques, plus many of their own innovations, Robert and Mary Goulding (1978, 1979) developed what they call *redecision therapy*. Until then, although TA was more empowering of clients, in that it emphasized choice and ego functions, it still lacked an "action" component and largely involved "talking about" problems. The Gouldings' unique "redecision" approach is built on the theory that, as children, people often adopt certain attitudes, making key life decisions (e.g., "Don't feel," "Don't think," "Don't be a child," "Don't grow up," "Don't be close," "Don't be important," "Don't enjoy," and "Don't be") in order to survive or adapt to perceived and often veridical parental pressures. In their model of therapy, the patient reenters and reexperiences the pathogenic childhood scene via imagery and Gestalt work, and with the encouragement and support of the therapist makes a redecision that frees him or her from the pernicious injunction that he or she had earlier accepted and internalized. Rather than working within a psychodynamic transference model, in which the therapist becomes a participant-observer "object," the patient is encouraged to do two-chair Gestalt work in which he or she "becomes" the pathogenic parent (extrojecting the introject, so to speak) and then engages in a powerful dialogue in which he or she experiences and reclaims a sense of power, self-determination, and well-being: "I'm OK and will take care of myself even if you don't think I'm OK." Implicit is the idea of state-dependent learning (and relearning), with the work conducted in the voice of the present tense in order to bring to life how the patient is carrying the conflict. A powerful combination of affect and insight is involved, with support and behavioral anchors to maintain the gains achieved.

The Gouldings (1979; Goulding & Goulding, 1986) describe a thinking structure to guide work in redecision therapy. Although many important details go beyond the scope of this discussion, it should be noted that each of the following main headings is an essential feature for making this approach brief and effective:

1. *Contact*, forming an alliance with the patient.
2. *Contract*, constructing the focus or goal of treatment in a way that can be specified and achieved.
3. *Con*, emphasizing patients' power and responsibility by confronting their efforts to disown autonomy through various ways they attempt to fool ("con") themselves and therapists into believing that others control their thoughts, feelings, and behavior, or with disingenuous claims of "trying" to make changes.
4. *Chief bad feelings, thoughts, behaviors, and psychosomatics,* identifying the painful or problematic counterproductive symptoms.
5. *Chronic games, belief systems, and fantasies,* clarifying the interpersonal and intrapsychic ways symptoms are maintained.
6. *Childhood early decisions,* bringing to vivid awareness a reexperience of childhood feelings via the imaginal reliving of an early pathogenic scene, including recognition of the chief parental messages (injunctions and counterinjunctions), childhood script formation, and stroking (reinforcement) patterns.
7. *Impasse resolution,* including redecisions, ego-state decontamination and reconstruction (involving the strengthening of distinctions between Parent–Adult–Child functions), reparenting, and other techniques.
8. *Maintaining the victory,* including anchoring the patient's new and healthier ways of responding, making changes in stroke (reinforcement) patterns, and forming plans for how to use the redecision in the future.

Consistent with the question Eric Berne would ask himself before each session, "What can I do to cure this patient today?" (reported in Goulding & Goulding, 1979), the Gouldings have developed Berne's concept of *contractual therapy* and ask patients, as they begin each treatment session, "What are you willing to change today?" In this one pithy sentence (from Hoyt, 1990, pp. 125–126), most of the key elements of brief therapy occur:

What [specificity, target, focus]
are [active verb, present tense]
you [self as agent, intrapsychic, personal functioning]
willing [choice, responsibility, initiative]
to change [alter or be different, not just "work on" or "explore"]
today [now, in the moment]
? [inquiry, open field, therapist receptive but not insistent]

The question focuses the therapist and the patient on making rapid changes. Although the therapist plays an important role in skillfully setting the context and guiding the client, there is a strong, ever-present emphasis on here-and-now patient autonomy and empowerment—it is the patient who sets the contract, the patient who does the work, and the patient who reaps the benefits. The following vignette illustrates this approach, which combines the theory of injunctions with Gestalt techniques "so that the patient does a great deal of experiential work *and* has a good understanding of his place in his life script, [and thus] is more likely to change both his behavior and his feelings" (R. Goulding, 1983, p. 634). As Mary Goulding (1990) has written, attention to contract plus redecision helps get the important work done fast.

THE CASE OF THE WOMAN WHO STOOD UP FOR HERSELF

Maria, who was 25 years old, came to therapy complaining of "insecurity" and "low self-esteem" in both her relationships with men and in her work performance. She needed to gather her confidence to move on in her adult life. She already had some understanding that many of her insecurities stemmed from her relationship with her verbally abusive, highly critical father. "I know he did this to me," she said, "but what can I do about it?" It appeared that she needed an experience that would separate her from her past, that would "empower" her to shift out of the "victim" position. She "knew" her father was still living in her head ("It's an old tape"), but so what?

By the end of our first meeting she had achieved several important steps:

1. Good contact with the therapist, establishing a sense of safety and a working alliance.
2. Increased awareness that her pattern of low self-esteem was a carryover from how her father had treated her.
3. A greater sense of her present role or personal autonomy; that is, she could see more clearly that she did the putdowns to herself, that the origin of her problem may have been in her childhood with her father, but that he was not "making" her feel bad now—she was.

As the session drew near an end, I remarked: "So what you want to do, so to speak, is to get his critical voice out of your head, right?" She agreed, and the contract was made specific: to stop putting herself down and, instead, to give herself due credit and not let others demean her.

Conditions were ripe for redecision work. At our second meeting, I reiterated the contract to make sure it was still what she wanted. Maria was then asked to give an example of a recent time when she felt lacking in confidence and self-esteem. She did, and was then asked how she felt in that situation and what she had said in her head about herself and the other person. She had felt scared, she had said to herself, "I can't do anything right," and she had said about the other person, "He is mad and doesn't like you." I then said: "You feel scared, you think you can't do anything right, and he is mad at you. How does that fit in with your childhood? What do you think of?"

Maria recalled a time when she was about 6 years old. She had spilled juice in the living room, and her father was chastising her for it. I asked her to stay with the scene, to imagine it vividly, to really get into it. "Let yourself be 6 years old again and go back there. See the room and the juice on the rug and all the details, and feel yourself being that scared 6-year-old girl." Maria paused and as she recalled and "got into" the scene, one could see her get smaller and shrink into herself.

Then, using the two-chair technique, I said to her, "Now sit in this other chair over here [Maria changed seats], and in this chair be your father, looking at the juice on the rug and being furious." With a little prompting, Maria got into the role. I then proceeded to conduct a brief "Parent interview" (McNeel, 1976), asking the "Father" his name and occupation, and questions to evoke "his" feelings and thoughts about the little girl who, in the scene, would be cowering in front of him. "He" was angry and did not like to have to clean up the mess, but as he talked more, it became clear that he was not all that ferocious and that he actually did love the girl, too.

I then had Maria switch back to the 6-year-old's seat and from there tell her father that she was scared and did not like it when he yelled at her. "I'm only a little kid and I make mistakes, but I'm not bad, and you shouldn't yell at me," she spontaneously added. "Yeah," I said. "Good. That's right. Stand up and tell him again. Let him know that he's not going to hurt you, and that you're OK even if you sometimes make mistakes." The little girl stood up for herself.

When she seemed done, I said, "Good job. Notice how strong you feel. Now, as you come back to yourself in the present you'll remember, whenever you need to, how it feels to stand up."

Follow-Up and Comment. The role playing had a powerful effect. Using the three questions—"How do you feel? What do you say about yourself? What do you say about the other person?"—as a kind of affect bridge back to an early scene often works rapidly to access a pathogenic (perhaps screen) memory, taking a different and quicker route than waiting for a transference neurosis to bloom fully. The two-chair work then allows a reworking or redecision, a new and healthier resolution of the impasse. For Mary, this was a turning point, a casting off of the "Don't be a child" and "Don't be important" injunctions she had earlier internalized. Therapy continued for another three visits, with the first two occurring weekly and the last occurring a month later, as the patient made plans and applied (worked through) her "breakthrough" in a variety of current life situations. With support, reminders, and practice, Mary learned to discount herself less and less. Her treatment goals of enhanced confidence and self-esteem were well met and demonstrated in a variety of contexts.

As the title of the Gouldings' 1978 book put it, *The Power Is in the Patient.* The client is seen as competent to resolve her own problem, without having to rely upon an outside expert to explain or reveal "The Truth." Explanation may lead to recognition, but experience leads to change. Can one really "go back"—via role playing, imagery, or transference enactment? Of course not—there is no time but the present. But "what is important," as Mary Goulding (1997, p. 87) has written, "is that the client recover from the past, real and imagined, and go on to a fulfilling life."

Ericksonian, Strategic, and Solution-Focused Approaches to Brief Therapy

We now consider a number of creative methods that, in varying ways, derive their inspiration from the life and work of the remarkably innovative psychiatrist-psychologist Milton H. Erickson, who seems to have emerged *sui generis* as a therapeutic genius (see Haley, 1973, 1994). They all have in common the idea that the client's complaints and symptoms should be taken seriously as the target of treatment, not just as a "symbol" or "screen" for something else (which the therapist would divine). Unlike most clinicians of his time, who felt that the therapist should *not* deliberately attempt to influence the patient, Erickson held that it was the therapist's responsibility to direct the client and to "make something happen" that would promote the client's treatment goals.

Milton H. Erickson: The Man and His Approach

Erickson (1901–1980) overcame great personal adversities (e.g., paralytic polio) to develop a hypnosis-based approach oriented toward growth and problem solving via utilization of whatever assets the patient might bring to therapy. Erickson's work has directly or indirectly had a tremendous influence on many schools of therapy, including hypnotherapy, family therapy, and various strategic interactional approaches (e.g., see Erickson, 1980, as well as Haley, 1973; Haley & Richeport-Haley, 1993; O'Hanlon & Hexum, 1990; Short, Erickson, & Klein, 2005).

It is especially difficult to summarize Ericksonian strategic therapy, because it is so individualistically based on the talents of particular patients and therapists—a situation that also makes systematic research quite problematic. Erickson focused on both the activation and transformation of patients' inner worlds of experience and personal meaning as well as their outer worlds of behavior and social community (Gilligan, 1997). Ericksonian approaches emphasize creative reorganization of relationships rather than a resistance-stimulating focus on diagnosing pathology.

What characterizes Ericksonian work? Lankton (1990, p. 364) explains:

> Therapy goals are built upon the intelligence and health of individuals. It [the approach] works to frame change in ways that reduce resistance, reduce dependency upon therapy, bypass the need for insight, and allow clients to take full credit for changes. Most problems are not viewed as internal pathologies but as the natural result of solving developmental demands in ways that do not fully work for the people involved. The Ericksonian strategic approach is distinctive in that it is associated with certain interventions upon which it relies heavily during extramural assignments and therapy sessions. These include skill building homework, paradoxical directives, ambiguous function assignments, indirect suggestions, hypnosis, reframing metaphors, and therapeutic binds. These are not so much interventions as characteristic parts of the therapist's interactions with clients. As such they are used to motivate clients to actively participate in changing the way they live with themselves and others.

For Lankton (1990), Erickson's work has seven defining characteristics:

1. *Non-pathology-based model.* Problems are seen as part of, and a result of, attempts at adaptation; symptoms are essentially natural (but limiting) responses of unique individuals.
2. *Indirection.* This concerns itself with helping an individual or members of a family discover talents and resources, options, and answers, seemingly without the aid of the therapist and without stimulating undue resistance or reactance.
3. *Utilization.* Whatever the patient brings to the office (understandings, behaviors, motivations) is used as part of the treatment.
4. *Action.* Clients are expected and encouraged to get quickly into actions related to desired goals—a basic ingredient of most successful brief therapies regardless of theoretical orientation (Budman et al., 1992).

5. *Strategic.* The therapist takes responsibility for influencing the patient and is active in setting or initiating the stages of therapy.
6. *Future orientation.* The focus is on action and experience in the present and future rather than the past.
7. *Enchantment.* Treatment engages the mind, appeals to the patient, and captures the ear of the listener.

Short et al. (2005) describe six core Ericksonian strategies:

1. *Distraction.* Shifting the client's attention away from self-defeating experiences to ones that promote health and success, particularly useful for countering the effects of self-fulfilling prophecies or highly conditioned responses to feared stimuli.
2. *Partitioning.* Breaking down of negative association by dividing a boundless problematic reality into smaller, more easily assimilated parts.
3. *Progression.* Building on a series of small gains, creating increased hope for continued accomplishments.
4. *Suggestion.* Collecting and guiding the patient's expenditure of energy, with or without hypnosis, to elicit a response that somehow exceeds the bounds of what the patient believed to be possible prior to therapy.
5. *Reorientation.* Providing the patient with a new perspective, a view of the situation that reduces the amount of subjective distress.
6. *Utilization.* Attending to the goodness of the patient's mind and body, using his or her energy, preferences, point of view, skills, and potentials.

An "Ericksonian" perspective can be appeciated in a wide variety of interventions:

1. The indirection of a police officer asking for a cup of coffee as a way of separating a domestically disputing couple (Everstine & Everstine, 1983); or the charming Japanese folktale (retold by de Shazer, 1991b) of a villager who, unable to warn his neighbors of an impending tidal wave, sets their hillside terraces on fire so that they will rush up the mountain to battle the flames and thus inadvertently be saved from drowning; or drawing into therapy a resistant husband by making statements about him that would require him to come to sessions "to set the doctor straight."
2. The use of imagery and hypnosis (e.g., Erickson & Rossi, 1979; Lankton & Lankton, 1983; Ritterman, 2005) and neurolinguistic programming (e.g., Andreas, 2006; Bandler & Grinder, 1982) to construct more useful realities.
3. Instructing and motivating with teaching stories and metaphoric communications (e.g., Battino, 2002; Rosen, 1982).
4. The use of provocation to challenge and motivate patients, including a last-ditch (and successful) effort to motivate a prideful patient out of a deep funk with humiliating taunts (Haley, 1973, pp. 270–273).
5. Prescribing ordeals and symptoms (e.g., Haley, 1984) to get patients to abandon undesirable behaviors.
6. Assigning tasks, the purpose and meaning of which are unclear to the client (e.g., having a couple climb a nearby peak or visit a botanical garden) in order to structure a decision-making experience or elicit an unconscious understanding (e.g., Furman & Ahola, 1992; Lankton & Lankton, 1986).
7. Using a psychiatric hospital patient's belief that he was Jesus Christ by having him

do work in the carpenter shop (!) and directing an isolated woman with a "green thumb" to grow and give African violet plants to thousands of people in order to reconnect them to the larger community (Haley, 1994; O'Hanlon & Hexum, 1990).

The basic principle underlying all these techniques and methods is *utilization*. The essential paradigmatic shift is from deficits to strengths, from problems to solutions, from past to future (Fisch, 1982, 1990), utilizing whatever the patient brings in the service of healthful change. "Whatever the patient brings is *not* grist for the mill. *It is fuel to propel forward into new space*. The patient's values can be utilized; the patient's situation can be utilized; the patient's resistances can be utilized; the patient's symptom can be utilized" (Zeig, 1992, p. 261, emphasis in original). Ericksonian epistemology is pragmatic and "emergent" (Lankton & Lankton, 1998), with therapist and client cocreating a useful worldview. For Erickson, the basic problem was not so much one of pathology or defect but *rigidity*, the idea that people get "stuck" by failing to use a range of skills, competencies, and learnings that they have but are not applying:

> Patients have problems because their conscious programming has too severely limited their capacities. The solution is to help them break through the limitations of their conscious attitudes to free their unconscious potential for problem solving. (Erickson et al., 1976, p. 18)

Various interventions are thus designed to get people to have experiences that put them in touch with their latent or overlooked abilities—a "reassociation of experience" (Erickson & Rossi, 1979, p. 9; Erickson, 1980, vol. 4, p. 38).

Even a simple and relatively direct approach can have Ericksonian elements. Taking into consideration how little can actually be conveyed through a single case presentation (including tone, timing, and nonverbal communication), consider the following report (adapted from Hoyt, 1995a).

THE CASE OF THE BASEBALL FAN

Sam was a 67-year-old man when I met him sitting in a wheelchair next to his wife in the waiting room of the HMO psychiatry department. He had been referred by his internist: "Post-stroke. Fear of falling." When I introduced myself and shook hands I could see that he was a pleasant and engaging man. He had not shaved in a few days and was casually dressed, wearing an Oakland A's baseball cap. His wife immediately began to talk (a lot) and quickly told me that Sam could walk but was afraid. He had come into the building on his own, then gotten into the wheelchair. She was nice and trying to be helpful, but I sensed that it would be useful to have some time with the patient alone, so I asked: "Do you want to walk or ride to my office?" He replied: "I'll take a ride, at least this time."

As I pushed him around the corner and down the corridor, we talked baseball—about a recent trade and how the game had gone that day. His remarks showed a good knowledge of the game and an alert, up-to-date interest. I asked questions, and we connected as we talked. At my office door I stopped and asked him to take a few steps into my office and use a regular chair, so that I would not have to move the furniture around—an indirect approach that used his natural courtesy to bypass discussion of his need for the wheelchair.

He obliged. When we sat down I asked, "So, what's up?" I learned that he was a retired mechanic and printing pressman. He had suffered a stroke 3 years earlier, with a residual partial paralysis of one arm and leg. He had grown "too damn dependent" on his wife, he said, but could no longer drive and had considerable difficulty walking. "I sure miss Dr. Jarrett," he interjected, referring to his former internist who had himself retired a few years earlier. When he told me what Dr. Jarrett would have said to get him moving, I "borrowed" the good doctor's mantle of authority and replied: "Took the words right out of my mouth."

Sam went on to tell me that he wanted to go to an upcoming A's game his sons had invited him to, but he first had to overcome his great fear of falling: "I get so worried and down that I freeze up." He knew how to fall safely (protecting his head and softening the fall) but was fearful: "I'm not sure what would happen to me if I fell and no one was around. I might not be able to get back up."

(By coincidence, I had the night before read my then 4-year-old son a story [Peet, 1972] about a series of animals that each gets stranded, culminating with an elephant stuck on his back until an ant he befriended rescues him with the help of an ant hoard.)

Sam was a practical man with a predicament. After ascertaining that he was not worried about safety or embarrassment, I suggested: "I'll tell you what. Let's do a little experiment. I'll be you, you be the coach, and teach me how to get up." I then proceeded to sort of throw myself on the floor in front of him. He got right into it, advising me, "No, turn the other way, get up first on three points," and so forth. I said, "Let's try it with my arm not working," and held it limply against my side. For the next 8–10 minutes I repeatedly got down on the floor and Sam instructed me on how to get myself up again.

Back in my chair, I asked if he wanted to "try it" there in my office or wait until he got home—an "illusion of alternatives" (Watzlawick, 1978), with the underlying implication that he would perform the action. He chose to wait until he was home but offered to show me "some exercises I can still do." I watched and then asked him to "stand and do a little walking just so I can see how you do." I opened the office door and we proceeded into the corridor. We slowly made our way up and down the hallway, with my remarking a couple of times, "Good," and "Nice, better than I expected." As we went up and down the hallway I switched back to baseball, asking Sam about the game he was planning to attend with his sons. "Where are you going to park? Which ramp will you take?" I painted aloud a vivid picture of father and sons entering the baseball stadium as we made our way up and down the hallway a couple of times.

Back in my office Sam expressed concern about his wife. She was trying to be helpful but was wearing out both herself and Sam with her watchfulness. "Maybe you could talk to her, too," he asked. I said I would be glad to "when you begin to do more walking on your own, so that I'll really be able to convince her to back off." He understood and agreed to practice his falling and getting up, and we playfully bargained about how many times he would do it a day, settling on twice a day to start, then three times a day until I saw him in 2 weeks.

Before he left my office I added, "You know, I think it's really important that you go to that game with your sons if you can. I know you want to, but I think it will be even more important for them. Someday they will look back and remember going to the game with you, you know what I mean?" Sam did not know exactly how baseball was in my blood, my history of going to games with my father, but he knew I was saying something heartfelt and important. It spoke to him: "I'm sure going to give it my best."

Follow-Up and Comment. When next I saw Sam, he proudly walked into my office, slowly. He had been practicing and was eagerly anticipating going to the game the next week with his sons. I then brought his wife into the session, and we talked about ways she could help by both doing things and ways she could help by not doing things. Two weeks later, Sam told me about going to the game and his plans to go to another one. He also expressed the desire for more activity, and I suggested attending an older adults' therapy group, as well as some other outings with neighbors and former coworkers. He followed through on these suggestions, and I remained available if and when he might again request to meet with me.

Sam's worries about falling were taken seriously. The approach here was highly pragmatic, strategies being directed toward quickly getting the patient walking. It was helpful and felt natural to reverse roles temporarily, with Sam becoming the teacher/coach rather than the humbled stroke patient. This was morale restoring and opened possibilities for change. The hallway walk into the ballpark was hypnotic and future oriented. His desire for assistance in managing his wife was used to further promote treatment compliance. Part of effective brief therapy is deciding what paths *not* to take. Exploring Sam's concerns about failing powers and limited mortality were issues that might be worthwhile (and would be addressed in the older adults' group), but first helping Sam to regain his confidence in walking and being able to get up when he fell enhanced the quality of his life and put him in a stronger position to appraise his future options realistically. This is what Sam and his wife wanted. Being alert to and using whatever resources are available in the service of the patient's therapeutic needs—including the therapist's own personal experiences with baseball, inverted elephants, and father–son relations—is what I take Erickson and Rossi (1979) to mean when they suggest: "To initiate this type of therapy you have to be yourself as a person. You cannot imitate somebody else, but you have to do it in your own way" (p. 276).

Strategic Therapy: Jay Haley and the Mental Research Institute

Jay Haley was studying communication with Gregory Bateson's group at the VA in Menlo Park, California, in the early 1950s when he and John Weakland began to visit Erickson. (Many of their conversations are transcribed [Haley, 1985]). Inspired by Erickson and brilliant in his own right, Haley (e.g., 1969, 1977) went on to author a number of important books about the therapeutic use of strategy and power. An early member of the Mental Research Institute (MRI) in Palo Alto, California, founded by Don Jackson, who had consulted with the Bateson group and was one of the originators of family therapy, Haley coauthored the famous "double-bind" paper (Bateson, Jackson, Haley, & Weakland, 1956), in which they described the effects of giving a person two conflicting messages. Haley later moved to the Philadelphia Child Guidance Clinic, then cofounded the Family Therapy Institute of Washington, DC. He then spent the last two decades based in La Jolla, California, where he continued to teach, write, and make training videotapes until his death in 2007.

Although Haley's approach covers a wide variety of clinical situations, there are certain common features:

- An interactional view—the minimum unit of consideration is two people, with a symptom serving some function in their relationship.
- Each clinical situation is unique, and the focus is on what the client brings in.

- Therapeutic influence is seen to be inevitable, so the therapist takes responsibility for directing the action and making something useful happen.
- Language is appreciated, but the focus is on observable (concrete) behavior—on what people *do* more than what they *say*.

Haley makes clear his preference that the therapist take charge, asserting that "Therapy can be called strategic if the clinician initiates what happens during therapy and designs a particular approach for each problem" (1973, p. 1). Haley uses common sense and plain talk to make explicit the shift toward *solvable interactional problems* rather than putative intrapsychic complexes, noting:

> This is not a therapy where relationships are changed by talking about relationships but by requiring new behavior to solve a problem. . . . Giving directives, or tasks, to individuals and families has several purposes. First, the main goal of therapy is to get people to behave differently and so to have different subjective experiences. Directives are a way of making those changes happen. (1977, pp. 27, 49)

Meanwhile, intercurrent with Haley's work, at the Brief Therapy Center of the MRI, Weakland, Fisch, Watzlawick and Bodin (1974) published a paper entitled "Brief Therapy: Focused Problem Resolution." This was followed by two seminal books, *Change: Principles of Problem Formation and Problem Resolution* (Watzlawick, Weakland, & Fisch, 1974) and *The Tactics of Change: Doing Therapy Briefly* (Fisch, Weakland, & Segal, 1982). Taking a systemic perspective, they focused on what maintained the problem that brought the patient to therapy. They observed that sometimes the attempted solution actually perpetuates the problem, such as when someone with insomnia tries to force him- or herself to go to sleep, or when someone tries to bring a romantic partner closer by pointing out his or her faults. The basic action-oriented MRI question is thus: "*Who* is doing *what* that presents a problem, to *whom*, and *how* does such behavior constitute a problem?" (Fisch et al., 1982, p. 70; emphasis in original).

Their treatment approach, which is generally offered as a 10-session package (although patients can finish early and keep sessions "in the bank" for possible later use), follows from this conceptualization:

> A problem may be solved by behavioral changes—ceasing the attempted solution—or sometimes by a reevaluation of the original focus of complaint as "no problem," just one of life's daily difficulties. . . . Such interventions mainly involve suggestions for behavioral changes in the real world outside the therapy room. Usually, however, these are not direct prescriptions but depend on reframing the problem situation, avoiding argument, and utilizing the clients' own preexisting ideas about people and problems—speaking the client's "language"—so as to make different problem-handling behavior appear logical and appropriate to them. Since our aim is specific behavioral change rather than intellectual understanding (which may produce no change in actual daily behavior), we do not devote much effort to clarifying and discussing the overall interactional system to those involved. (Weakland & Fisch, 1992, p. 309)

Watzlawick et al. (1974, p. 95) explain what they call "the gentle art of reframing":

> To reframe, then, means to change the conceptual and/or emotional setting or viewpoint in relation to which a situation is experienced and to place it in another frame which fits

the "facts" of the same concrete situation equally well or even better, and thereby changes its entire meaning. . . . What turns out to be changed as a result of reframing is the meaning attributed to the situation, and therefore its consequences, but not its concrete facts.

Rohrbaugh and Shoham (2001, p. 66; emphasis in original) describe the Palo Alto model as "based on identifying and interrupting *ironic processes* that occur when repeated attempts to solve a problem keep the problem going or make it worse," and suggest this approach may be well suited for change-resistant clients. Bonchek (2009), for example, reports an interesting "prescribing the symptom" strategic approach to remedy the high noncompliance and dropout rate observed when using the standard cognitive-behavioral therapy technique of exposure and response prevention with patients with obsessive–compulsive disorder. Outlining careful guidelines, he presents several successful cases of what he calls "exposure and response repetition," instructing patients who say that they cannot resist or prevent performing their problematic behavior (e.g., compulsive handwashing or praying) to continue their behavior and actually *add* additional repetitions beyond that which they do regularly. Fraser and Solovey (2007, p. 39) also provide a sample list of strategic interventions that all are evidence-based yet seemingly counterintuitive:

- A therapist, working with a client who has panic attacks, asks her client to bring on panic during the session.
- Another therapist, working with someone who has been recurrently depressed, teaches his client to allow depressing thoughts to pass through her mind without needing to respond to those thoughts.
- Still another therapist asks a quarreling couple to pick a fight with one another when they are not mad.
- A sex therapist prohibits a couple from having intercourse despite prescribing arousing exercises.
- Another client is told that there may be good reasons not to change.
- A parent, needing to regain control of her child's behavior, is taught to take charge by not directly taking charge.
- Another therapist tells his client that he can't blame her for wanting to harm herself when she becomes emotionally frustrated. He then asks her to experience more emotional frustration while considering other ways to react to it.

Solution-Focused (and Solution-Oriented) Therapy

Solution-focused brief therapy (SFBT) was developed in the late 1970s and 1980s by Steve de Shazer (1982, 1985, 1888, 1994) and his colleagues (see Berg, 1994; Berg & Miller, 1992) at the Brief Family Therapy Center in Milwaukee, Wisconsin. de Shazer was influenced by the work of the MRI group, which in turn had been influenced by the work of Milton Erickson—especially Erickson's ideas about strategic intervention and the fuller utilization of clients' submerged competencies. However, whereas the MRI group focused on how clients create and resolve problems, including how efforts to solve a problem sometimes actually perpetuate the problem, de Shazer and his Milwaukee-based group took a somewhat different view. They focused instead on those times (which they called "exceptions") when the presenting problem was not present, as expressed in the title of their signal counterpaper, "Brief Therapy: Focused Solution Development" (de Shazer et al., 1986).

Initially, the SFBT approach emerged in an inductive manner, from study of what clients and therapists did that preceded clients declaring problems "solved" (or "resolved," "dissolved," or "simply no longer problems"). It was found that this happened when clients began to engage in new and different perceptions and behaviors vis-à-vis the presenting difficulty (Hoyt & Berg, 1998). This recognition led to de Shazer's "basic rules" of solution-focused therapy:

- If it ain't broke, don't fix it.
- Once you know what works, do more of it.
- If it doesn't work, don't do it again; do something different. (de Shazer, quoted in Hoyt, 1996a, p. 68)

The basic premise is deceptively simple: Increase what works; decrease what doesn't work. What are the "exceptions" to the problem? What is the patient doing differently at those times when he or she is not anxious, depressed, quarreling, and so on? What has worked before? What strengths can the patient apply? What would be a useful solution? How to construct it?

Behind these apparently simple questions is a profound paradigmatic shift: Competencies, not dysfunctions, are the focus; the quest is to access latent capacities, not latent conflicts. Consistent with its nonpathologizing perspective, rather than asking "How is the client stuck?" solution-focused therapists ask "What is the client doing when he or she is *not* stuck?" There is usually a "future focus," with the therapist helping the client to break out of painful, recurring traps by drawing attention toward what the clients have been doing and will be doing differently when he or she has achieved a desired outcome or solution (Gustafson, 2005). The orientation is toward the future and toward the fuller appreciation and utilization of human abilities. Questions are designed to evoke a self-fulfilling map of the future (Penn, 1985; Tomm, 1987). Indeed, the language of SFBT is sometimes hypnotic, collapsing time, conflating present with future. The language presupposes change ("After the miracle . . .") and excites positive expectations (Battino, 2006), with a focus on what *will* be different when the solution is achieved. The approach is not just technical, but when taken to heart epitomizes the belief that with skillful facilitation, people have within themselves the resources necessary to achieve their goals.

Solution-focused therapy is perhaps the best known of a variety of competency-based, collaborative, future-oriented approaches. Another well-known variant is called *solution-oriented* therapy (O'Hanlon & Wilk, 1987). All these various competency-based approaches are "in search of solutions" (O'Hanlon & Weiner-Davis, 1989). Clients are assisted to develop new awarenesses—not insights of buried pains and sorrows, but of underappreciated, overlooked, perhaps forgotten hopes, skills, and resources. The focus is on enhancing what I call "solution sight" (Hoyt, 2002). In solution-focused and solution-oriented therapy, there is no preset length of treatment. Appointments are usually made one at a time. de Shazer (1991b) reported average length of treatment at the Brief Family Therapy Center to be 4.7 sessions; in 1996, he indicated (in Hoyt, 1996b, p. 61; also see Macdonald, 2003) that the average had dropped to three. While the therapist–client relationship may fluctuate among *customer, complainant,* and *visitor* (Berg, 1989; Shoham, Rohrbaugh, & Patterson, 1995, p. 153), the concept of *resistance* is vitiated by the therapist taking responsibility for finding ways to work with the client's current motivation, experience, goals, ideas, values, and worldviews (de Shazer, 1984). The emphasis is on *solution talk*, not *problem talk*.

Therapists ask certain kinds of questions to help clients focus on and "see" solutions. Here are just a few, each of which the therapist might follow-up with additional questions to expand clients' "solution sight" (for further discussion and an extensive list of different types and numerous examples of each, see Berg & de Shazer, 1993; De Jong & Berg, 1997; Hoyt, 2002, 2009; Ziegler & Hiller, 2001):

- *The Skeleton Key Question* (to elicit information about presession change or improvement): "Between now and the next time we meet, I would like you to observe, so that you can describe to me next time what happens in your [pick one: family, life, marriage, relationship, etc.] that you want to continue to have happen." (de Shazer, 1985, p. 137)

- *The Miracle Question* (to enchant and orient the client toward the positive and to identify the goal of treatment): "Suppose that one night, while you were asleep, there was a miracle and this problem was solved. How would you know? What would be different?" (de Shazer, 1988, p. 5)

- *Exceptions Questions* (to identify times the presenting problem has not been present): "When in the past might the problem have happened but didn't (or was less intense or more manageable)?"

- *Endurance (or Coping) Questions* (to acknowledge difficulties and pains while still focusing on strengths and competencies): "Given all you've been through, how have you managed to keep going as well as you have?"

- *Agency (Efficacy) Questions* (to identify the client's abilities to make a difference in the desired direction): "How did you do that?" or "How did you get that to happen?"

- *Scaling Questions* (to "measure the client's own perception, to motivate and encourage, and to elucidate goals and anything else that is important to the individual client" [Berg & de Shazer, 1993, p. 9]): "On a scale from 1 to 10, with 1 being absolutely no [pick one: hope, motivation, progress, etc.] and 10 being complete [hope, motivation, etc.], what number would you give your current level of [hope, motivation, etc.]? What will tell you that you have gone up one level?"

The following excerpts from a couple therapy case (adapted from Hoyt, 2002) illustrate how some of these solution-focused ideas might be applied in action.

THE CASE OF PETER AND PAULA

The receptionist's intake appointment note gave the clients' names, indicated their ages (29 and 30 years, respectively) and simply read, "Four months pregnant—not getting along."

When we got into my office, I remarked: "Welcome. The purpose of our meeting is to work together to find a solution to whatever brings you here today. What's up?" They mentioned that they had known each other a couple of years, were pregnant but not married, and had gotten along pretty well until recently. They then began to bicker and argue, each accusing the other of having a "bad attitude" and not doing enough. I quickly interrupted:

THERAPIST: Wait a minute! You came here because you want things to be better, don't you? (*They both nodded affirmatively.*) That's why you're here. You used to get along, so you know *how* to—it seems you came here because you want some help figuring out how to get back to being happy together, right?

PETER AND PAULA: Well, yeah . . .

THERAPIST: Then let me ask you, each of you—and don't get into an argument over this—on a scale of 1 to 10, how would you say your relationship is now, where "1" is "Horrible—it sucks" and "10" is "Great—couldn't be better"?

PETER: A 2.

PAULA: Yeah, like that—a 2.

THERAPIST: OK. That gives us some room to work. Without getting into complaining, what would it take for you to think things have moved up to a 3, or even a 4? What will each of you, and the other person, be doing differently when things are getting better?

PETER: I don't know.

PAULA: I don't know, either.

THERAPIST: Oh. OK. Let me ask you this: Suppose tonight, while you're sleeping, a miracle happens . . . and the problems that brought you here are solved! But you're sleeping, so you don't know it . . . until you wake up. Tomorrow, when you wake up, what would be some of the things you'd notice that would tell you, "Hey, things are better"?

Paula laughed, and then Peter laughed. They then sat there looking dumbfounded, then laughed again, together. Paula spoke first:

PAULA: We'd be getting along better, not hassling.

PETER: Yeah, we'd talk, and she wouldn't get so mad at me.

Before the window of opportunity closed, I quickly asked: "You'd be getting along—what would you be saying and doing? How about you, Paula—what would you be doing if you and Peter were getting along? And you, Peter—how would you respond to Paula, and what would you be saying to build on the positive?"

I had been quite active, interrupting them in order to direct them toward the positive. Once they were going more in the direction they said they wanted to go, I became much less directive, although I still actively elicited details and specifics that "thickened" their positive story. I inquired about "exceptions," asking about times when they had achieved some of the togetherness they sought. Whenever they began to slip back toward arguing, I gently redirected them but did not presume to know what details and events would make their story positive. Drawing from their recall of happier times in the past and their imagination of a positive future, they seemed to be discovering and remembering—and began using—important relationship skills they already knew. They began to see each other more beneficently, slowly shifting figure and ground, moving from problem to solution.

At the end of the session, I offered a homework suggestion:

"You've come up with some very good ideas about how to make things better. Between now and when we meet in a couple of weeks—and even after that—please pay attention and notice whatever you do and whatever the other person does to make things better. It may not be perfect, but try to keep track of whatever positives you or your partner do or attempt to do. When we meet, I'll ask you about what you noticed."

Over the next several sessions, we focused on ways they were working better together. In one session, Peter acknowledged, "Sometimes my feelings get hurt, and then I withdraw and she gets even madder." I asked their ideas about how they could handle such tense situations better ("You know yourselves and each other better than I ever could—what do you think would work for the two of you?"). Paula and Peter both suggested alternatives, and I also proffered a few ideas. We discussed back and forth what would make sense that they would be willing to try, and they playfully rehearsed a couple of options.

Whenever they reported any success, I asked for details ("Wow! How did you do that?"). They also brought up frustrations and difficulties, of course, which we discussed. I was very careful, however, to keep the focus on their goals and resourcefulness. Borrowing some of Gottman's (1994) ideas about "Finding the Glory in Your Story" and Ziegler and Hiller's (2001) ideas about "Re-creating Partnership," several times I asked Peter and Paula questions ("What are some examples of ways you have compromised successfully?" "How did you make up?" "During difficult times, what are some of the things that have told you the relationship is worth pursuing?" "What did you do differently during those times you coped constructively with your frustration?") that would help highlight whatever they were doing in the direction they wanted to go. I also suggested they consider activities (e.g., a fun outing) that would build on the positive.

After several sessions, when Paula rated their relationship as a "9" and Peter gave it a "10," I congratulated them on their good teamwork and commented (alluding to the baby): "Since you're going to be together for at least the next couple of decades, it's nice to see that you're working on the "Peter *and* Paula Story" rather than the "Peter *or* Paula Story."

In the fifth session, our last (by their choice), we reviewed their progress and how they had achieved it. We also spent a few minutes talking about challenges that were sure to come, and how they could cope:

THERAPIST: Would it be OK if I ask you a hard question?

PETER AND PAULA: Sure—go for it.

THERAPIST: I'm glad that you're doing so well and that you're working as partners, but imagine a time in a few months after the baby's born, and you're both tired and stressed. . . . How are you going to remember then to work as a team?

PETER: I'm sure that will happen.

PAULA: Yeah.

THERAPIST: So, how are you going to deal with it? It could be easy to get back into fighting a lot.

PETER AND PAULA: We'll have to remember why we're together.

THERAPIST: How will you do that?

PETER: We know we'll have difficulties, but we also know that we can solve our problems.

PAULA: Yeah. Now when we start to have an argument, we stop and remember that we're "Peter *and* Paula," and that helps us not to get into "Me *versus* You." And sometimes we talk about what we've talked about in here—how to use what you called "solution talk," how we used to fight, and how we know how to treat each other respectfully, and how to take a time-out if we need it, and how to listen to each other, and stuff like that.

Follow-Up and Comment. "Fast-forwarding" to a solution by asking the "Miracle Question" (de Shazer, 1988) does not really create a miracle, of course. Rather, it serves to disrupt a persistent negative narrative and stimulate the imagination toward creative solutions. It shifts the discourse. Patients get enchanted by the question and, with or without prompting, draw on their own wisdom and experience to create answers that are hopeful, uniquely theirs, and thus more likely to occur. Various methods can then be used to promote continued changes. In solution-focused therapy, the therapist's "prime directive" is to recognize that the "client is the expert" and to help clients better access their own expertise to solve their problems (Hoyt & Berg, 1998). Every case is considered to be unique, a nonnormative view that emphasizes the use of language in the social construction of reality.

EVEN ONE SESSION (OR LESS) MAY BE ENOUGH (FOR NOW)

Therapy should not be "long term" or "short term." It should be sufficient, adequate, and appropriate, "measured not by its brevity or length, but whether it is efficient and effective in aiding people with their complaints or whether it wastes time" (Fisch, 1982, p. 156). Many people solve psychological problems without professional consultation. For some others, the "light touch" of a single visit may be enough, providing experience, skills, and encouragement to help them get "unstuck" and continue in their life journey. If used appropriately, such "ultrabrief" treatments can promote patients' sense of self-empowerment and autonomy (vs. dependency), conserve limited resources, and serve as an entree for those truly requiring longer treatments.

Considerable evidence indicates that single-session therapy—one visit without further contact—is de facto the modal or most common length of treatment, generally occurring 20–50% of the time. While most traditional psychotherapy training suggests that stopping after one visit is "dropping out" or "premature termination," scattered throughout the literature are many anecdotal reports by leading practitioners of varying theoretical perspectives suggesting the utility of single-session therapy (SST) with selected patients. There are also several published systematic studies on the frequency and potential effectiveness of SST:

1. Medical utilization was found to be reduced 60% over 5-year follow-up after a single session of psychotherapy in a study at the Kaiser Permanente Health Plan (the nation's largest HMO) by Follette and Cummings (1967). A second study (Cummings & Follette, 1976; also see Mumford, Schlesinger, Glass, Patrick, & Cuerdon, 1984) found the benefits of SST still in effect after 8 years and concluded that decreased medical utilization was due to a reduction in physical symptoms related to emotional stress.

2. Significant symptom improvement years later was noted by Malan, Heath, Bacal, and Balfour (1975) in 51% of "untreated" psychotherapy patients who had only an intake interview (which served to increase their insight and sense of personal responsibility) at the Tavistock Clinic in London, and half of those patients were also judged to have made important personality modifications.

3. Patients and therapists agreed that a single treatment visit had been sufficient in 58.6% (34 of 58) of sessions in another study conducted at Kaiser Permanente in Northern California by Hoyt, Rosenbaum, and Talmon (reported in Talmon, 1990). The other patients continued meeting with their therapists. On 3- to 12-month follow-ups, 88% of the SST-only patients reported either "much improvement" or "improvement" in their presenting symptoms since the session.

4. One session of motivational interviewing (Miller & Rollnick, 2002), which nonconfrontationally calls clients' attention to their choices and values, was found to reduce drug

consumption and perceptions of drug-related risk and harm among young people in a multisite randomized trial in London (McCambridge & Stang, 2004).

5. A 3-year review by Weir, Wills, Young, and Perlesz (2008) at community health counseling services in Victoria, Australia, involving more than 100,000 patients, found that 42% of those seen chose to have only a single session, even when more sessions were offered. Recognizing that this pattern is the preference of many clients, Weir et al. reported the development of a single-session implementation plan that has been widely accepted by counselors there.

6. Several investigators have reported studies favoring solution-focused, competency-based approaches with patients who benefited by being allowed simply to walk in or "drop in" without a scheduled appointment when they wanted to meet with a therapist, whether for family problems, child/adolescent problems, or general adult difficulties (e.g., Campbell, 1999; Perkins, 2006; Perkins & Scarlett, 2008; Slive & Bobele, 2010).

There is no single method or goal for attempting SST other than being with patients and using the skills that patient and therapist bring to the endeavor. Treatments may be as varied as the patients (and therapists) and what they wish to accomplish. SSTs, like all forms of psychotherapy, can occur either by default (usually when the patient stops unilaterally) or by design (when patient and therapist mutually agree that additional sessions are not then indicated). The choice of a single session (or more, or less) should, whenever possible, be left to the patient. "Let's see what we can get done today," is much more "user-friendly" and likely to succeed than the resistance-stimulating "We're only going to meet one time." Most effective SST is thus strictly *not* time-limited therapy. It is open-ended, the therapist mentions the possibility of one session perhaps being enough, and the patient elects to stop after one visit.

Although SST is obviously neither a panacea nor even appropriate for everyone, the following brief examples describe some instances in which a single visit promoted enhanced coping and growth. In each case, the patient made the choice (with the therapist's assent) to complete treatment with the one session and agreed to return for additional treatment when desired.

Case 1. A ceremony was used as part of an elaborate production to help a woman "emotionally divorce" her abusive father (see Talmon, Hoyt, & Rosenbaum, 1990, pp. 45–47, for a truncated report of the case). To help consolidate her gains and demarcate a before-and-after change of status, the patient (with her husband attending) read an extraordinary autobiographical plaint, played carefully selected music, and burned her father's photograph in my office. Hypnotherapeutic "inner child" work was also done. At the end of the session and on follow-up the patient felt considerable relief in regard to her relationship with her father, but she also continued to have other psychological problems that might have benefited from additional therapy.

Case 2. A woman with nightmares of someone chasing her sought help. I described to her a research study I had read (Kellner, Neidhardt, Krakow, & Pathak, 1992) in which 23 patients were successfully treated with one session of desensitization or rehearsal instruction. In both conditions, I explained, the patients were taught progressive relaxation. Half the patients were then instructed to practice imagining the nightmare while relaxed, and the other half were instructed to write down a recent nightmare, change it, and write down a modified, "happy ending" version, then practice rehearsing the changed version in imagery while in a relaxed state. In both conditions, patients were seen once and were to practice at home. I then asked her, "Which approach do you think would be best for you?" (Offering choice promotes self-empowerment, "buy in," and follow-through.) Like most patients in my experience, she chose the latter option of authoring a new ending. She developed a short scenario of being chased but finding a way to escape and never be bothered again. In the office, she then learned the relaxation method and rehearsed the new, favorable ending several times. When she felt she could do it comfortably, I said, "Now go home and practice this twice a day for a couple of weeks, and let me know how well it works." Two weeks later she reported that the nightmares were gone.

Case 3. A couple came in with their 19-year-old son, a college freshman, who lived at home with them. As they had been for some time, they were all arguing about curfews, discipline, "respecting the rules of the house," and the like. When they asked if I had any children, I gestured to a photograph of my son on the desk, "who's still little and dependent, since he's only 5." I went on to talk about a bird's nest we had seen on a windowsill at home and how smart Mother Nature was the way she designed things, like how it worked that a little bird would stay in its nest, but when it got big enough to make things crowded in the nest, it was big enough to fly on its own; and how its readiness to go was built in and signaled by its size, and neither the grown-up birds nor the grown-up bird needed to be told or could help it, since it was natural, and so on. I prattled on for a bit, sort of like an ornithological Lt. Columbo, then finally stopped myself. I shifted around in my chair, seemingly pulling myself together and returning to the topic at hand. "It's nice to see such a loving, close family. So who's going to finally give in?" I asked, and pursued a line of questioning that only escalated the fight and demonstrated the intractability of the conflict. A follow-up phone call 6 weeks later revealed that 1 week after the session, everyone had agreed that it would be best if the son lived elsewhere. He had moved (to a college dorm), and everyone was happy. We'll never know for sure, but the bird's nest metaphor, with its various embedded suggestions, seemed to prefigure and guide their conflict resolution in a developmentally appropriate direction. The "empty nest syndrome" was better than the "overcrowded nest syndrome" (reported in Hoyt, 1995a).

SOME STORIES ARE BETTER THAN OTHERS

All therapists, regardless of theoretical persuasion, use their power and authority to influence clients to change their "stories" in directions thought to be helpful. Indeed, this is why they are paid. Even therapists, such as the psychodynamic drive theorists, who may believe they are "unlocking the unconscious" and "revealing the underlying truth," are selling a story. (They may also be revealing "The Truth" and "unlocking the unconscious"—at least that's their story of what they're doing.) Some therapists see themselves (their story of themselves) as Experts, wielding special knowledge ("insight") and power. Others may not believe they know the one "Truth," but believe they have expert knowledge regarding what the client needs, and they use their power to direct situations that lead the client to what the therapist believes is needed (e.g., an emotional catharsis, a changed sense of self, a different family relationship pattern). Still others also see themselves as having expertise but eschew the role of Expert—instead seeing their role largely as the skillful asking of questions and the arranging of contexts to help clients recognize their own expertise.

Messer and Warren (1995) also provide an interesting discussion of what they term "the context of visions of reality." Without being able to do justice to their thoughtful discussion in this limited space, they contrast four "visions":

- The *romantic*, in which life is an adventure or quest in which the person as hero transcends the world of experience, achieves victory over it, and is liberated from it.
- The *ironic*, an attitude of detachment, challenging cherished beliefs, traditions, and (romantic) illusions; like the tragic vision, it emphasizes the inherent difficulties of life; there are multiple perspectives possible, so nothing is ever really complete.
- The *tragic*, inwardly directed, is full of struggle and distrust of happy endings, acknowledging the limitations of life; the clock cannot be turned back; in this view, quiet acceptance of a certain degree of despair produces wisdom.
- The *comic*, in which life is familiar and can be controlled; effective problem solving and outward action move things from bad to better; in this view, conflict is largely between people and their situation, not within the people, and increased capacity to perform social roles more adequately is the desired resolution.

As Messer and Warren note, psychoanalytic and psychodynamic brief treatment approaches would seem to have the most affinity with the tragic and ironic. Strategic and systemic approaches, I would add, might be situated more in the realm of the comic and perhaps the ironic. Solution-focused (and other narrative-based) approaches may be more consistent with the romantic and comic (and perhaps ironic) vision of reality. Life has its painful and tragic moments, its funniness, its adventures, and its twists. All are inevitable, but the one(s) you most prefer—the "lenses" (Hoffman, 1990) you like to wear (or at least are trained or accustomed to looking through)—may do a lot to influence your preference for certain ways of "storying" rather than others. One's story about one's role as therapist—as one who uses power and authority to "treat" and "fix" patients, as an operator who directs and stages contexts, as a facilitator who asks questions to promote clients' self-healing, and so forth—may also go a long way toward determining which approach(es) one resonates with and chooses to apply.

A LONG FUTURE FOR BRIEF THERAPY

Brief therapy has a long history, beginning with Freud, and it appears that it will have a long future as well. The convergence of market forces, the desire of most persons for rapid relief from psychological distress, and the development of new treatment technologies augur well for the further expansion of brief treatment. What is clear is that consumers, insurers, and health care professionals all increasingly recognize the importance of providing psychotherapeutic services that are as efficient as possible. Brief therapy methods are becoming increasingly attractive, both as treatments of choice and for their value in resource conservation. Although *brief therapy* (various approaches to time-effective treatment) antedates and is not the same as *managed care* (a term that refers to various forms of health care delivery administration), as noted earlier, combining increased attention to the study and practice of brief therapy with the fiscal imperatives of health care reform may help to satisfy consumers' preferences for effective and efficient treatments, and may also provide resources for patients who would otherwise go without to receive the benefits of professional mental health care. Although specific training in brief therapy still lags far behind need (Levenson

& Evans, 2000), we can hope that greater appreciation of various brief therapy approaches will lead to their more widespread application.

CODA

Brevity is the soul of wit.
—WILLIAM SHAKESPEARE,
Hamlet (Act II, Scene 2, line 90)

The goal of brief psychotherapy, regardless of the specific theoretical approach or technical method, is to help the patient to resolve a problem, to get "unstuck," and to move on. Techniques are specific, integrated, and as eclectic as needed. Treatment is focused, the therapist is appropriately active, and the patient is responsible for making changes. Each session is valuable, and therapy ends as soon as possible. Good outcome, not good process, is most valued. More is not better; *better* is better. The patient carries on and can return to treatment as needed. The simple truth is that most therapy *is* brief therapy and will be increasingly so; for the sake of our patients and our profession, we should learn to practice it well.

SUGGESTIONS FOR FURTHER STUDY

Recommended Reading: Research Reviews

Lambert, M. J. (2005). Early response in psychotherapy: Further evidence for the importance of common factors rather than "placebo effects." *Journal of Clinical Psychology, 61*(7), 855–869.—Documents that many clients respond quickly, even in therapies not specifically designed or planned to be brief; also provides evidence supporting the importance of "common factors" rather than specific techniques.

MacDonald, A. J. (2003). Research in solution-focused brief therapy. In B. O'Connell & S. Palmer (Eds.), *Handbook of solution-focused therapy* (pp. 12–24). London: Sage.—Compendium of research studies on the process and outcome of SFBT.

Messer, S. B. (2001a). What allows therapy to be brief?: Introduction to the special series. *Clinical Psychology: Science and Practice, 8*(1), 1–4.—Editor's introduction and the following six papers describe different brief therapy models (e.g., psychodynamic, cognitive-behavioral, family/couples, experiential) and review pertinent research.

DVDs: Clinical Demonstrations

Carlson, J., & Kjos, D. (Series Hosts). (2000). *Brief therapy: Inside out.* Phoenix, AZ: Zeig, Tucker & Theisen.—Excellent video series (each approximately 95 minutes) of 14 leading practitioners, each explaining their approach, then working with a client, and then answering questions.

Goulding, M. M., & Goulding, R. L. (1986). *Redecision therapy.* San Francisco: International Transactional Analysis Association (*www.itaa-net.org*).—The originators work with various clients, then discuss their methods.

Haley, J., & Richeport-Haley, M. (1993). *Milton H. Erickson, M.D.: Explorer in hypnosis and therapy.* New York: Brunner/Mazel.—Fascinating hourlong introduction with many clinical excerpts.

Messer, S. B. (2008). *Brief dynamic therapy* (Systems of Psychotherapy Video Series). Washington, DC: American Psychological Association.—Demonstrates how to find an appropriate focus for short-term psychodynamic therapy and determine appropriate candidates for such therapy.

REFERENCES

Alexander, F., & French, T. M. (1946). *Psychoanalytic therapy: Principles and applications*. New York: Ronald Press.

American Psychiatric Association. (2000). *Diagnostic and statistical manual of mental disorders* (4th ed., text rev.). Washington, DC: Author.

Andreas, S. (2006). *Six blind elephants: Understanding ourselves and each other* (Vols. 1 & 2). Moab, UT: Real People Press.

Appelbaum, S. A. (1975). Parkinson's Law in psychotherapy. *International Journal of Psychoanalytic Psychotherapy, 4*, 426–436.

Balint, M., Ornstein, P. H., & Balint, E. (1972). *Focal psychotherapy*. London: Tavistock.

Bandler, R., & Grinder, J. (1982). *Reframing: Neurolinguistic programming and the transformation of meaning*. Moab, UT: Real People Press.

Barten, H. H. (Ed.). (1971). *Brief therapies*. New York: Behavioral Publications.

Bateson, G., Jackson, D. D., Haley, J., & Weakland, J. H. (1956). Toward a theory of schizophrenia. *Behavioral Science, 1*, 251–264.

Battino, R. (2002). *Metaphoria: Metaphor and guided imagery for psychotherapy and healing*. Norwalk, CT: Crown House.

Battino, R. (2006). *Expectation: The very brief therapy book*. Norwalk, CT: Crown House.

Berg, I. K., & de Shazer, S. (1993). Making numbers talk: Language in therapy. In S. Friedman (Ed.), *The new language of change: Constructive collaboration in psychotherapy* (pp. 5–24). New York: Guilford Press.

Berg, I. K., & Miller, S. D. (1992). *Working with the problem drinker*. New York: Norton.

Berne, E. (1961). *Transactional analysis in psychotherapy*. New York: Grove Press.

Berne, E. (1964). *Games people play*. New York: Grove Press.

Berne, E. (1972). *What do you say after you say hello?* New York: Grove Press.

Bibring, E. (1954). Psychoanalysis and the dynamic psychotherapies. *Journal of the American Psychoanalytic Association, 2*, 745–770.

Binder, J. L., & Strupp, H. H. (1991). The Vanderbilt approach to time-limited dynamic psychotherapy. In P. Crits-Christoph & J. P. Barber (Eds.), *Handbook of short-term dynamic psychotherapy* (pp. 137–165). New York: Basic Books.

Bloom, B. L. (1992). *Planned short-term psychotherapy*. Boston: Allyn & Bacon.

Bloom, B. L. (2001). Focused single-session psychotherapy: A review of the clinical and research literature. *Brief Treatment and Crisis Intervention, 1*(1), 75–86.

Bonchek, A. (2009). What's broken with cognitive behavior therapy treatment of obsessive–compulsive disorder and how to fix it. *American Journal of Psychotherapy, 63*(1), 69–86.

Brehm, J. (1966). *A psychological theory of reactance*. New York: Appleton-Century-Crofts.

Breuer, J., & Freud, S. (1893–1895). Studies in hysteria. *Standard Edition, 2*, 1–319. London: Hogarth Press, 1955.

Budman, S. H., Friedman, S., & Hoyt, M. F. (1992). Last words on first sessions. In S. H. Budman, M. F. Hoyt, & S. Friedman (Eds.), *The first session in brief therapy* (pp. 345–358). New York: Guilford Press.

Budman, S. H., & Gurman, A. S. (1988). *Theory and practice of brief therapy*. New York: Guilford Press.

Budman, S. H., Hoyt, M. F., & Friedman, S. H. (Eds.). (1992). *The first session in brief therapy*. New York: Guilford Press.

Campbell, A. (1999). Single session interventions: An example of clinical research in practice. *Australian and New Zealand Journal of Family Therapy, 20*(4), 183–194.

Carlson, J., & Kjos, D. (Series Hosts). (2000). *Brief therapy inside out* [Videotapes/DVDs]. Phoenix, AZ: Zeig, Tucker & Theisen.

Carlson, J., & Sperry, L. (Eds.). (2000). *Brief therapy with individuals and couples*. Phoenix, AZ: Zeig, Tucker & Theisen.

Cummings, N. A. (2000). *The collected papers of Nicholas A. Cumming: Vol. 1. The value of psychological treatment* (J. L. Thomas & J. L. Cummings, Eds.). Phoenix, AZ: Zeig, Tucker & Theisen.

Cummings, N. A., & Follette, W. T. (1976). Brief therapy and medical utilization. In H. Dorken (Ed.), *The professional psychologist today* (pp. 176–197). San Francisco: Jossey-Bass.

Davanloo, H. (Ed.). (1978). *Basic principles and techniques in short-term dynamic psychotherapy*. New York: Spectrum.

Davanloo, H. (Ed.). (1980). *Short-term dynamic psychotherapy*. New York: Aronson.

Davanloo, H. (1991). *Unlocking the unconscious: Selected papers*. New York: Wiley.

De Jong, P., & Berg, I. K. (1997). *Interviewing for solutions*. Pacific Grove, CA: Brook/Cole.

de Shazer, S. (1982). *Patterns of brief family therapy*. New York: Guilford Press.

de Shazer, S. (1984). The death of resistance. *Family Process, 23*, 79–93.

de Shazer, S. (1985). *Keys to solution in brief therapy*. New York: Norton.

de Shazer, S. (1988). *Clues: Investigating solutions in brief therapy*. New York: Norton.

de Shazer, S. (1991a). Foreword. In Y. M. Dolan, *Resolving sexual abuse* (pp. ix–x). New York: Norton.

de Shazer, S. (1991b). *Putting difference to work*. New York: Norton.

de Shazer, S. (1994). *Words were originally magic*. New York: Norton.

de Shazer, S., Berg, I. K., Lipchik, E., Nunnally, E., Molnar, A., Gingerich, W., et al. (1986). Brief therapy: Focused solution development. *Family Process, 25*, 207–227.

Ellis, A. (1962). *Reason and emotion in psychotherapy*. New York: Stuart.

Erickson, M. H. (1980). *Collected papers* (Vols. 1–4; E. Rossi, Ed.). New York: Irvington.

Erickson, M. H., & Rossi, E. (1979). *Hypnotherapy: An exploratory casebook*. New York: Irvington.

Erickson, M. H., Rossi, E., & Rossi, S. (1976). *Hypnotic realities*. New York: Irvington.

Everstine, D. S., & Everstine, L. (1983). *People in crisis: Strategic therapeutic interventions*. New York: Brunner/Mazel.

Ferenczi, S., & Rank, O. (1925). *The development of psychoanalysis*. New York: Nervous and Mental Disease Publication Co.

Fisch, R. (1982). Erickson's impact on brief psychotherapy. In J. K. Zeig (Ed.), *Ericksonian approaches to hypnosis and psychotherapy* (pp. 155–162). New York: Brunner/Mazel.

Fisch, R. (1990). The broader implications of Milton H. Erickson's work. *Ericksonian Monographs, 7*, 1–5.

Fisch, R. (1994). Basic elements in the brief therapies. In M. F. Hoyt (Ed.), *Constructive therapies* (pp. 126–139). New York: Guilford Press.

Fisch, R., Weakland, J. H., & Segal, L. (1982). *The tactics of change: Doing therapy briefly*. San Francisco: Jossey-Bass.

Follette, W. T., & Cummings, N. A. (1967). Psychiatric services and medical utilization in a prepaid health care setting. *Medical Care, 5*, 25–35.

Frances, A., & Clarkin, J. F. (1981). No treatment as the prescription of choice. *Archives of General Psychiatry, 38*, 542–545.

Fraser, J. S., & Solovey, A. D. (2007). *Second-order change in psychotherapy: The golden thread that unifies effective treatments*. Washington, DC: American Psychological Association.

Freedheim, D. K. (Ed.). (1992). *History of psychotherapy: A century of change*. Washington, DC: American Psychological Association.

Freud, S. (1919). Lines of advance in psycho-analytic therapy. *Standard Edition, 17*, 157–168. London: Hogarth Press, 1955.

Freud, S. (1937). Analysis terminable and interminable. *Standard Edition, 23*, 209–254. London: Hogarth Press, 1953.

Furman, B., & Ahola, T. (1992). *Solution talk: Hosting therapeutic conversations*. New York: Norton.

Gill, M. M. (1954). Psychoanalysis and exploratory psychotherapy. *Journal of the American Psychoanalytic Association, 2*, 771–797.

Gilligan, S. (1997). Living in a post-Erickson world. In W. J. Matthews & J. H. Edgette (Eds.), *Current thinking and research in brief therapy: Solutions, strategies, narratives* (pp. 1–23). New York: Brunner/Mazel.

Gottman, J. M. (1994). *Why marriages succeed or fail . . . and how you can make yours last*. New York: Fireside/Simon & Schuster.

Goulding, M. M. (1990). Getting the important work done fast: Contract plus redecision. In J. K. Zeig & S. G. Gilligan (Eds.), *Brief therapy: Myths, methods, and metaphors* (pp. 303–317). New York: Brunner/Mazel.

Goulding, M. M. (1997). Childhood scenes in redecision therapy. In C. E. Lennox (Ed.), *Redecision therapy: A brief, action-oriented approach* (pp. 87–94). Northvale, NJ: Aronson.

Goulding, M. M., & Goulding, R. L. (1979). *Changing lives through redecision therapy.* New York: Grove Press.

Goulding, M. M., & Goulding, R. L. (1986). *Redecision therapy* [Videotape/DVD]. San Francisco: International Transactional Analysis Association. (*www.itaa-net.org*)

Goulding, R. L. (1983). Gestalt therapy and transactional analysis. In C. Hatcher & P. Himelstein (Eds.), *Handbook of Gestalt therapy* (pp. 615–634). New York: Aronson.

Goulding, R. L., & Goulding, M. M. (1978). *The power is in the patient.* San Francisco: TA Press.

Gurman, A. S. (2001). Brief therapy and family/couple therapy: An essential redundancy. *Clinical Psychology: Science and Practice, 8*(1), 51–65.

Gustafson, J. P. (1986). *The complex secret of brief psychotherapy.* New York: Norton.

Gustafson, J. P. (2005). *Very brief psychotherapy.* New York: Routledge.

Haley, J. (1969). *The power tactics of Jesus Christ and other essays.* New York: Avon.

Haley, J. (1973). *Uncommon therapy: The psychiatric techniques of Milton H. Erickson, M. D.* New York: Norton.

Haley, J. (1977). *Problem-solving therapy.* San Francisco: Jossey-Bass.

Haley, J. (1984). *Ordeal therapy: Unusual ways to change behavior.* San Francisco: Jossey-Bass.

Haley, J. (Ed.). (1985). *Conversations with Milton H. Erickson, M.D.* (Vols. 1–3). New York: Triangle Press.

Haley, J. (1994). *Jay Haley on Milton H. Erickson.* New York: Brunner/Mazel.

Haley, J., & Richeport-Haley, M. (1993). *Milton H. Erickson, M.D.: Explorer in hypnosis and therapy* [Videotape/DVD]. New York: Brunner/Mazel.

Hoffman, L. (1990). Constructing realities: An art of lenses. *Family Process, 29*, 1–12.

Horowitz, M. J., Marmar, C., Krupnick, J., Wilner, N., Kaltreider, N., & Wallerstein, R. (1984). *Personality styles and brief psychotherapy.* New York: Basic Books.

Hoyt, M. F. (1985). Therapist resistances to short-term dynamic psychotherapy. *Journal of the American Academy of Psychoanalysis, 13*, 93–112.

Hoyt, M. F. (1989). Psychodiagnosis of personality disorders. *Transactional Analysis Journal, 19*, 101–113.

Hoyt, M. F. (1990). On time in brief in therapy. In R. A. Wells & V. J. Giannetti (Eds.), *Handbook of the brief psychotherapies* (pp. 115–143). New York: Plenum Press.

Hoyt, M. F. (1995a). *Brief therapy and managed care: Readings for contemporary practice.* San Francisco: Jossey-Bass.

Hoyt, M. F. (1995b). Contact, contract, change, encore: A conversation with Bob Goulding. *Transactional Analysis Journal, 25*(4), 300–311.

Hoyt, M. F. (1996a). Solution building and language games: A conversation with Steve de Shazer (and some after words with Insoo Kim Berg). In M. F. Hoyt (Ed.), *Constructive therapies* (Vol. 2, pp. 60–86). New York: Guilford Press.

Hoyt, M. F. (Ed.). (1996b). *Constructive therapies* (Vol. 2). New York: Guilford Press.

Hoyt, M. F. (2000a). *Some stories are better than others: Doing what works in brief therapy and managed care.* Philadelphia: Brunner/Mazel.

Hoyt, M. F. (2000b). The last session in brief therapy: How and why to say "when." In *Some stories are better than others* (pp. 237–261). Philadelphia: Brunner/Mazel.

Hoyt, M. F. (2002). Solution-focused couple therapy. In A. S. Gurman & N. S. Jacobson (Eds.), *Clinical handbook of couple therapy* (3rd ed., pp. 335–369). New York: Guilford Press.

Hoyt, M. F. (2006). The temporal structure of therapy: Key questions often associated with different phases of sessions and treatments (plus twenty-one helpful hints). In W. O'Donohue, N. A. Cummings, & J. L. Cummings (Eds.), *Clinical strategies for becoming a master psychotherapist* (pp. 113–127). San Diego: Elsevier/Academic Press.

Hoyt, M. F. (2009). *Brief psychotherapies: Principles and practices.* Phoenix, AZ: Zeig, Tucker & Theisen.

Hoyt, M. F., & Berg, I. K. (1998). Solution-focused couple therapy: Helping clients construct self-fulfilling realities. In F. M. Dattilio (Ed.), *Case studies in couple and family therapy: Systemic and cognitive perspectives* (pp. 203–232). New York: Guilford Press.

Hoyt, M. F., & Miller, S. D. (2000). Stage-appropriate change-oriented brief therapy strategies. In J. Carlson & L. Sperry (Eds.), *Brief therapy with individuals and couples* (pp. 289–330). Phoenix, AZ: Zeig, Tucker & Theisen.

Hoyt, M. F., Rosenbaum, R. L., & Talmon, M. (1992). Planned single-session psychotherapy. In S. H. Budman, M. F. Hoyt, & S. Friedman (Eds.), *The first session in brief therapy* (pp. 59–86). New York: Guilford Press.

Hoyt, M. F., & Talmon, M. (1990). Single-session therapy in action: A case example. In M. Talmon, *Single-session therapy* (pp. 78–96). San Francisco: Jossey-Bass.

Johnson, L. D. (1995). *Psychotherapy in the age of accountability.* New York: Norton.

Kellner, R., Neidhardt, J., Krakow, B., & Pathak, D. (1992). Changes in chronic nightmares after one session of desensitization or rehearsal instruction. *American Journal of Psychiatry, 149,* 659–663.

Lambert, M. J. (2001). Early response in psychotherapy: Further evidence for the importance of common factors rather than "placebo effects." *Journal of Clinical Psychology, 61*(7), 855–869.

Lankton, S. R. (1990). Ericksonian strategic therapy. In J. K. Zeig & W. M. Munion (Eds.), *What is psychotherapy?: Contemporary perspectives* (pp. 363–371). San Francisco: Jossey-Bass.

Lankton, S. R., & Lankton, C. (1983). *The answer within: A clinical framework for Ericksonian hypnotherapy.* New York: Brunner/Mazel.

Lankton, S. R., & Lankton, C. (1986). *Enchantment and intervention in family therapy.* New York: Brunner/Mazel.

Lankton, S., & Lankton, C. (1998). Ericksonian emergent epistemologies: Embracing a new paradigm. In M. F. Hoyt (Ed.), *The handbook of constructive therapies* (pp. 116–136). San Francisco: Jossey-Bass.

Lazurus, A. A., & Fay, A. (1990). Brief psychotherapy: Tautology or oxymoron? In J. K. Zeig & S. G. Gilligan (Eds.), *Brief therapy: Myths, methods, and metaphors* (pp. 36–51). New York: Brunner/Mazel.

Leichsenring, F., Rabung, S., & Leibing, E. (2004). The efficacy of short-term psychodynamic psychotherapy in specific psychiatric disorders. *Archives of General Psychiatry, 61,* 1208–1216.

Levenson, H. (1995). *Time-limited dynamic psychotherapy: A guide to clinical practice.* New York: Basic Books.

Levenson, H., & Evans, S. A. (2000). The current state of brief therapy training in American Psychological Association-accredited graduate and internship programs. *Professional Psychology: Research and Practice, 31,* 446–452.

Luborsky, L., & Crits-Christoph, P. (1990). *Understanding transference: The CCRT method.* New York: Basic Books.

Macdonald, A. J. (2003). Research in solution-focused brief therapy. In B. O'Connell & S. Palmer (Eds.), *Handbook of solution-focused therapy* (pp. 12–24). London: Sage.

Malan, D. H. (1963). *A study of brief psychotherapy.* London: Tavistock.

Malan, D. H. (1976). *The frontier of brief psychotherapy.* New York: Plenum Press.

Malan, D. H. (1980). The most important development in psychotherapy since the discovery of the unconscious. In H. Davanloo (Ed.), *Short-term dynamic psychotherapy* (pp. 13–23). New York: Aronson.

Malan, D. H., Heath, E. S., Bacal, H. A., & Balfour, H. G. (1975). Psychodynamic changes in untreated neurotic patients: II. Apparently genuine improvements. *Archives of General Psychiatry, 32,* 110–126.

Mann, J. (1973). *Time-limited psychotherapy.* Cambridge, MA: Harvard University Press.

Mann, J., & Goldman, R. (1982). *A casebook in time-limited psychotherapy.* New York: McGraw-Hill.

McCambridge, J., & Strang, J. (2004). The efficacy of single-session motivational interviewing in reducing drug consumption and perceptions of drug-related risk and harm among young people: Results from a multi-site cluster randomized trial. *Addiction, 99,* 39–52.

McCullough, L. (2000). Short-term therapy for character change. In J. Carlson & L. Sperry (Eds.), *Brief therapy with individuals and couples* (pp. 127–160). Phoenix, AZ: Zeig, Tucker & Theisen.

McCullough-Vaillant, L. (1997). *Changing character: Short-term anxiety regulating psychotherapy for restructuring defenses, affects, and attachments.* New York: Basic Books.

McNeel, J. (1976). The Parent interview. *Transactional Analysis Journal, 6,* 61–68.

Messer, S. B. (2001a). What allows therapy to be brief?: Introduction to the special series. *Clinical Psychology: Science and Practice, 8*(1), 1–4.

Messer, S. B. (2001b). What makes brief psychodynamic therapy time efficient. *Clinical Psychology: Science and Practice, 8*(1), 5–22.

Messer, S. B., & Abbass, A. A. (2010). Evidence-based psychodynamic therapy with personality disorders. In J. Magnavita (Ed.), *Evidence-based treatment of personality dysfunction: Principles, methods and processes* (pp. 79–111). Washington, DC: American Psychological Association.

Messer, S. B., & Warren, C. S. (1995). *Models of brief psychodynamic therapy: A comparative approach.* New York: Guilford Press.

Miller, W. R., & Rollnick, S. (2000). *Motivational interviewing: Preparing people to change addictive behavior* (2nd ed.). New York: Guilford Press.

Mumford, E., Schlesinger, H., Glass, G. V., Patrick, C., & Cuerdon, B. A. (1984). A new look at evidence about reduced cost of medical utilization following mental-health treatment. *American Journal of Psychiatry, 141,* 1145–1158.

O'Hanlon, W. H., & Hexum, A. L. (1990). *An uncommon casebook: The complete clinical work of Milton H. Erickson, M. D.* New York: Norton.

O'Hanlon, W. H., & Weiner-Davis, M. (1989). *In search of solutions: A new direction in psychotherapy.* New York: Norton.

O'Hanlon, W. H., & Wilk, J. (1987). *Shifting contexts: The generation of effective psychotherapy.* New York: Guilford Press.

Peet, B. (1972). *The ant and the elephant.* Boston: Houghton Mifflin.

Penn, P. (1985). Feed-forward: Future questions, future maps. *Family Process, 24,* 289–310.

Perkins, R. (2006). The effectiveness of one session of therapy using a single-session therapy approach for children and adolescents with mental health problems. *Psychology and Psychotherapy: Theory, Research and Practice, 79,* 215–227.

Perkins, R., & Scarlett, G. (2008). The effectiveness of single session therapy in child and adolescent mental health. Part 2: An 18-month follow-up study. *Psychology and Psychotherapy: Theory, Research and Practice, 81,* 143–156.

Perls, F. S., Hefferline, R. F., & Goodman, P. (1951). *Gestalt therapy.* New York: Julian Press.

Pinsker, H., Rosenthal, R., & McCullough, L. (1991). Dynamic supportive psychotherapy. In P. Crits-Christoph & J. P. Barber (Eds.), *Handbook of short-term dynamic psychotherapy* (pp. 220–247). New York: Basic Books.

Prochaska, J. O., DiClemente, C. C., & Norcross, J. C. (1992). In search of how people change. *American Psychologist, 47,* 1102–1114.

Ritterman, M. (2005). *Using hypnosis in family therapy* (2nd ed.). Phoenix, AZ: Zeig, Tucker & Theisen.

Rohrbaugh, M. J., & Shoham, V. (2001). Brief therapy based on interrupting ironic processes: The Palo Alto model. *Clinical Psychology: Science and Practice, 8*(1), 66–81.

Rosen, S. (1982). *My voice will go with you: The teaching tales of Milton H. Erickson.* New York: Norton.

Seligman, M. E. P. (1995). The effectiveness of psychotherapy: The *Consumer Reports* study. *American Psychologist, 51,* 1072–1079.

Shoham, V., Rohrbaugh, M. J., & Patterson, J. (1995). Problem- and solution-focused couple therapies: The MRI and Milwaukee models. In N. S. Jacobson & A. S. Gurman (Eds.), *Clinical handbook of couple therapy* (2nd ed., pp. 142–163). New York: Guilford Press.

Short, D. (1997, Summer). Interview: Steve de Shazer and Insoo Kim Berg. *Milton H. Erickson Foundation Newsletter, 17*(2), 1, 18–20.

Short, D., Erickson, B. A., & Klein, R. E. (2005). *Hope and resiliency: Understanding the psychotherapeutic strategies of Milton H. Erickson, M.D.* Norwalk, CT: Crown House.

Sifneos, P. E. (1972). *Short-term psychotherapy and emotional crisis.* Cambridge, MA: Harvard University Press.

Sifneos, P. E. (1987). *Short-term dynamic psychotherapy: Evaluation and technique* (rev. ed.). New York: Plenum Press.

Sifneos, P. E. (1992) *Short-term anxiety-provoking psychotherapy: A treatment manual.* New York: Plenum Press.

Slive, A., & Bobele, M. (Eds.). (2010). *When one hour is all you have: Effective therapy for walk-in clients.* Phoenix, AZ: Zeig, Tucker & Theisen.

Strupp, H. H., & Binder, J. L. (1984). *Psychotherapy in a new key: A guide to time-limited dynamic psychotherapy.* New York: Basic Books.

Sullivan, H. S. (1954). *The psychiatric interview.* New York: Norton.

Talmon, M. (1990). *Single-session therapy.* San Francisco: Jossey-Bass.

Talmon, M. (1993). *Single session solutions.* Reading, MA: Addison-Wesley.

Talmon, M., Hoyt, M. F., & Rosenbaum, R. (1990). Effective single-session therapy: Step-by-step guidelines. In M. Talmon, *Single-session therapy* (pp. 34–56). San Francisco: Jossey-Bass.

Ticho, E. A. (1972). Termination of psychoanalysis: Treatment goals, life goals. *Psychoanalytic Quarterly, 41,* 315–333.

Tomm, K. (1987). Interventive interviewing: I. Strategizing as a fourth guideline for the therapist. *Family Process, 26,* 3–13.

Watzlawick, P. (1978). *The language of change: Elements of therapeutic communication.* New York: Norton.

Watzlawick, P., Weakland, J. H., & Fisch, R. (1974). *Change: Principles of problem formation and problem resolution.* New York: Norton.

Weakland, J. H., & Fisch, R. (1992). Brief therapy—MRI style. In S. H. Budman, M. F. Hoyt, & S. Friedman (Eds.), *The first session in brief therapy* (pp. 306–323). New York: Guilford Press.

Weakland, J. H., Fisch, R., Watzlawick, P., & Bodin, A. H. (1974). Brief therapy: Focused problem resolution. *Family Process, 13,* 141–168.

Weir, S., Wills, M., Young, J., & Perlesz, A. (2008). *The implementation of single-session work in community health.* Brunswick, Australia: Bouverie Centre, La Trobe University.

Weiss, J., Sampson, J., & the Mt. Zion Psychotherapy Research Group. (1986). *The psychoanalytic process: Theory, clinical observations, and empirical research.* New York: Guilford Press.

Westen, D. (1986). What changes in short-term psychodynamic psychotherapy? *Psychotherapy, 23,* 501–512.

Wolberg, L. R. (Ed.). (1965). *Short-term psychotherapy.* New York: Grune & Stratton.

Wolpe, J. (1958). *Psychotherapy by reciprocal inhibition.* Stanford, CA: Stanford University Press.

Wolpe, J., & Lazarus, A. A. (1966). *Behavior therapy techniques.* New York: Pergamon.

Yapko, M. D. (1990). Brief therapy tactics in longer-term psychotherapies. In J. K. Zeig & S. G. Gilligan (Eds.), *Brief therapy: Myths, methods, and metaphors* (pp. 185–195) New York: Brunner/Mazel.

Zeig, J. K. (1992). The virtues of our faults: A key concept of Ericksonian therapy. In J. K. Zeig (Ed.), *The evolution of psychotherapy: The second conference* (pp. 252–266). New York: Brunner/Mazel.

Zeig, J. K., & Gilligan, S. G. (Eds.). (1990). *Brief therapy: Myths, methods, and metaphors.* New York: Brunner/Mazel.

Ziegler, P. B., & Hiller, T. (2001). *Recreating partnership: A solution-oriented, collaborative approach to couples therapy.* New York: Norton.

CHAPTER 12

Integrative Approaches
to Psychotherapy

George Stricker
Jerry Gold

HISTORICAL BACKGROUND

The term *psychotherapy integration* encompasses a philosophical, conceptual, and clinical orientation to the study and practice of psychotherapy. This perspective is defined by openness to understanding the convergences and commonalities among the vast array of sectarian psychotherapies, and by an interest in promoting dialogue among therapists of all orientations. Psychotherapy integration is defined also by a willingness to learn from all therapies and therapists rather than to declare exclusive loyalty to one school or model of psychotherapy. Our preference is for a process of integration that guides psychotherapy rather than any single product or integrative psychotherapy that might become yet another sectarian approach, with all the limitations attendant upon that status (Stricker, 1994). It is impossible to discuss any single integrative psychotherapy as the definitive version, as these approaches are highly varied and, optimally, are in a continuous state of evolution. In this chapter we discuss those contemporary integrative approaches that generally are considered most influential, and we attempt to describe the commonalities and consistencies among these models when possible.

The first precursor to contemporary integrative approaches to psychotherapy occurred when French (1933) alerted psychoanalysts to the need for psychoanalytic theory and practice to account for the findings of Pavlov in the area of classical conditioning. This would have anticipated developments in behavior therapy and produced an early version of theoretical integration. A second seminal contribution was Rosenzweig's (1936) introduction of the hypothesis that the many varieties of psychotherapy shared a limited number of essential effective ingredients, or *common factors*. This article is the forerunner of contemporary versions of common factors integration.

During the 1940s and 1950s, several efforts at integrating then-current versions of psychoanalytic theory and learning theory were proposed. The most extensive, influential, and long-lasting contribution was made by Dollard and Miller (1950), who integrated central psychoanalytic ideas about unconscious motivation and conflict with concepts drawn from the learning theories of Hull, Spence, Tolman, and Mowrer (Klein, 2009). Although both orthodox psychoanalysts and learning theorists often were scornful and dismissive of this model, thinkers who were open to contributions from other theories and from empirical research found inspiration in Dollard and Miller's unique synthesis.

Another highly important influence on many integrative clinicians, although not specifically integrative, was *Psychoanalytic Therapy* (Alexander & French, 1946). This volume introduced the concept of the *corrective emotional experience*, referring to an event that takes place between therapist and patient. During the course of the therapeutic interaction, certain attitudes, emotions, and behaviors of the therapist were found to modify, powerfully and immediately, unconscious assumptions and perceptions derived from the patient's early development and interpersonal history. For example, the formulation of the corrective emotional experience, and its prescriptive perspective on interventions, expanded the psychoanalyst's role from the provision of insight via interpretation to the inclusion of behavioral interaction and the provision of new experience as valid therapeutic endeavors.

The seminal contribution of Frank (1961) was influenced by several disciplines, such as psychology, anthropology, and sociology. It sought commonalities in the change process initiated by a variety of interventions ranging from psychotherapy to faith healing. As such, it provided the foundation for works investigating the common factors in psychotherapy.

In the 1960s, the first explicit attempts at integrating two or more psychotherapeutic systems were published. Most of these focused on combining concepts and methods drawn from behavioral and psychoanalytic models. An early and neglected classic of this type was the marriage of Freud and Skinner proposed by Beier (1966), who described the role that reinforcement and operant conditioning processes played in the shaping, maintenance, and extinction of unconscious conflict and motivation.

In the next decade there were several efforts that crossed the boundaries of the traditional psychotherapies and created integrative, or eclectic (as they were more often known at that time), psychotherapies. Examples of these explorations were the papers published by Marmor (1971) and by Feather and Rhodes (1973), who found that unconscious issues could be treated through the use of behavioral methods such as being desensitized to one's core conflict. Lazarus's (1976) multimodal therapy laid the foundation for the technical integration approach to psychotherapy integration, which combines techniques from several different theoretical approaches without allegiance to any of them.

This trend culminated in the publication of *Psychoanalysis and Behavior Therapy: Toward an Integration* (Wachtel, 1977), which has been perhaps the single most important and influential work on the theoretical integration of various psychotherapies. This book, and the positive response it generated, opened the floodgates in the field of psychotherapy integration. During the 1980s, many prominent psychotherapy scholars and clinicians explored the technical, theoretical, and philosophical possibilities of integrating therapies in a newly invigorated and enthusiastic way (Arkowitz & Messer, 1984). The Society for the Exploration of Psychotherapy Integration (SEPI; *sepiweb.com*), founded in the early 1980s, began to publish the *Journal of Psychotherapy Integration* in 1991. Two thorough handbooks on psychotherapy integration, which included many of the most important integrative therapies then available, were published in the early 1990s (Norcross & Goldfried, 1992; Stricker & Gold, 1993). They demonstrated that integrative thinking had progressed beyond an exclusive focus on the synthesis of psychoanalytic and behavioral models. More recently, a second edition of the handbook (Norcross & Goldfried, 2005) and a detailed casebook

(Stricker & Gold, 2006a) have been published. Current integrative therapies combine cognitive, humanistic, experiential, and family systems models and techniques in ever more complex permutations.

Why is it that psychotherapy integration as a perspective, and integrative psychotherapies as therapeutic models, became so widely accepted in the last 15 to 20 years? Most students of the history of psychotherapy integration suggest (Gold & Stricker, 2006) that the failure of any traditional model of psychotherapy to "win all the prizes" and to establish itself as clearly superior to the others had much to do with this change. Another important group of factors was external to psychotherapeutic practice but affected psychotherapists most profoundly. These factors included the rise of biological models of psychopathology; the introduction of new generations of increasingly effective psychiatric drugs; and new requirements by the public, the government, and insurance companies for therapists to demonstrate the effectiveness of their methods. Suddenly, the "enemy" was no longer the psychoanalyst, the cognitive-behaviorist, or the Gestalt therapist across the road or in the next state. As people have always done when under siege, therapists put aside their differences and began to work together and to learn from each other.

Other, more positive events may be responsible for the rapid rise of interest in integrative therapies. Most of the founding schools of psychotherapy had their origins 50 to 100 years ago. The founders and founding generations are gone, and the succeeding generations may be more confident in crossing boundaries and assimilating new, "foreign," ideas than were those early therapists struggling to establish a new therapeutic position. As the world has become smaller and more integrated, dissemination of ideas and communication among contributors occurs more rapidly. The decades of the 1960s, 1970s, and 1980s saw a questioning of traditional authority in academics and in politics, integration in the social realm, as well as the cross-fertilization of many aspects of Western culture, including music, visual arts, literature, sports, and science.

A recent trend that has emerged in psychotherapy integration may in fact mark the end of psychotherapy integration as we know it. Magnavita (2008), Anchin (2008), and Wolfe (2008) proposed that the larger field of psychotherapy is undergoing a paradigmatic shift in theorizing, one that may have been brought about in large part by the movement toward integration. This shift in thinking, they argued, is characterized by an interest in the *unification* of many forms of psychotherapy rather than the integration of elements of single-school therapies. These authors, and others, have begun the task of describing and fleshing out the theoretical scaffolding and clinical methods that might be contained within a unified psychotherapy. It is too early to tell whether they are correct or whether they will be successful, but their argument may yet have merit, though it has been countered by other psychotherapy scholars (Messer, 2008).

Whatever the reasons may be for the rise in psychotherapy integration, and whatever the future of psychotherapy integration may be, it is an approach that has increased contemporary importance. For decades, the single most frequently endorsed approach to psychotherapy has been integrative–eclectic (Norcross, Karpiak, & Lister, 2005). A recent survey (Thoma & Cecero, 2009) has the integrative–eclectic approach second in frequency to cognitive-behavioral therapy (CBT). However, it also showed that many techniques were used by all practitioners, regardless of orientation. In addition, practitioners of each of the pure form techniques (CBT, psychodynamic, humanistic) used a great many techniques derived from approaches other than theirs. The former finding is consistent with common factors and the latter, with assimilative integration. Among expert practitioners of psychotherapy integration, it was not unusual for a single approach to be salient, but it was common to draw upon more than that single approach in practice (Hickman, Arnkoff, Glass, & Schottenbauer, 2009).

Currently there are four commonly accepted modes or forms of psychotherapy integration (Gold & Stricker, 2006). These modes, which define general ways in which theory and technique have been integrated, are known as *technical eclecticism*, the *common-factors approach, theoretical integration*, and *assimilative integration*. The ongoing process of psychotherapy integration relies on these modes, and each established integrative approach to psychotherapy can be considered an example of one of these modes, although the boundaries between them occasionally are fuzzy.

Models of Psychotherapy Integration

Technical Eclecticism

Technical eclecticism is the most clinical and technically oriented form of psychotherapy integration but involves the least amount of conceptual or theoretical integration. Clinical strategies and techniques from two or more therapies are applied sequentially or in combination, usually following a broad and comprehensive assessment of the patient. This assessment describes the interconnections between the problems to be addressed and the cognitive, behavioral, emotional, and interpersonal characteristics of the patient. Techniques are chosen on the basis of the best clinical match to the needs of the patient, as guided by clinical knowledge and research findings, regardless of their theoretical origin. It is important to note that this may not actually be a form of integration, as techniques often are merely combined rather than integrated, and have a synergistic rather than an integrative impact.

The most important examples of this type of integrative psychotherapy are (1) *multimodal therapy* (Lazarus, 1976, 2006), (2) *transtheoretical psychotherapy* (Prochaska & DiClemente, 2002), and (3) *prescriptive psychotherapy and systematic treatment selection* (Beutler & Hodgson 1993).

MULTIMODAL THERAPY

Multimodal therapy grew out of Lazarus's dissatisfaction with traditional behavior therapy and relies on supplementing behavioral interventions with cognitive, imagery-based, and experiential techniques. Lazarus (2006) assesses seven areas of each patient's biopsychosocial functioning (BASIC ID, which is an acronym for Behavior, Affect, Sensation, Imagery, Cognition, Interpersonal relations, and Drugs/biology), and develops a treatment plan that targets any of those areas for intervention, selecting the particular techniques on the basis of the empirical literature, clinical guidelines, and clinical experience.

TRANSTHEORETICAL PSYCHOTHERAPY

Transtheoretical psychotherapy (Prochaska & DiClemente, 2002) is a broadly studied, empirically validated, and widely applied framework for identifying the best match of the patient's characteristics and specific therapeutic models and techniques. In particular, patients are assessed for their readiness for change, and for the unique processes of change that will work best for them. These authors have identified *10 change processes* that predominate in the majority of therapies: consciousness raising, dramatic relief, self-reevaluation, environmental reevaluation, self-liberation, social liberation, counterconditioning, stimulus control, reinforcement management, and the helping relationship. They also have been able to demonstrate that every patient arrives in therapy at one of *six stages of readiness to change*, which include precontemplation, contemplation, preparation, action, maintenance, and termination. Someone who begins therapy at the stage of precontemplation is not even ready to think about change, while at the stage of contemplation he or she can imagine changing but is not yet ready to do anything to change. In the next stage (preparation) he or she is gathering energy and resources to alter his or her life, while in the action stage the patient makes overt use of therapy. The last two stages are focused on making sure that new ways of living are permanent (maintenance), and then in ending therapy (termination). This system also includes an assessment of the *levels of change* that are necessary for each patient. This idea refers to the particular domains of psychological problems from which the patient suffers. Assessment of the necessary levels of change in this model includes the *areas of symptoms and situational problems, maladaptive cognitions, current interpersonal conflicts, family and system conflicts,* and *intrapersonal conflicts.* Once the patient is assessed in these three domains—levels of change, stages of change, and processes of change—via specifically designed self-report scales, an individualized treatment plan drawn from all potential psychotherapeutic techniques can be developed (Prochaska & DiClemente, 2002).

PRESCRIPTIVE PSYCHOTHERAPY

Prescriptive psychotherapy does not limit the schools of therapy from which it draws its techniques, aiming similarly at the best match of therapist, strategies, and techniques to the patient's problems and characteristics. Variations on four dimensions of the wide range of psychotherapies are considered in relation to each patient's attributes. These therapeutic dimensions include (1) the necessary intensity of the therapy; (2) a focus in the therapy on insight or on skill and behavior change; (3) the degree to which the therapist is directive; and (4) changes in the ways in which the patient's emotions are managed within sessions. The patient is assessed on several dimensions. The patient's level of impairment determines the intensity of the therapy. His or her coping style is addressed by a relative emphasis on behavioral change or on insight. Internalizing styles are better matched with a more insight-oriented approach, while impulsive or externalizing styles have been found to respond more positively to more behavioral methods. Low levels of reactance on the patient's part encourage the use of a more directive stance by the therapist, while greater indications of reactance are matched with relatively more nondirective interactions. Finally, positive motivation for participation in therapy and for change is encouraged by the selection of techniques that modulate and maintain the patient at an optimal (moderate) level of emotional arousal and distress (Beutler, Harwood, Bertoni, & Thomann, 2006).

Common-Factors Approaches to Integration

Common-factors approaches start with the identification of effective ingredients that are practiced in common across many therapies. This way of thinking has its origins in Rosenzweig's (1936) seminal discovery that all therapies shared certain change processes, despite their idiosyncratic theories and techniques. J. Frank's (1961) observation, central to common-factors thinking, was that all systems of psychological healing share certain common, effective ingredients, such as socially sanctioned rituals, the provision of hope, and the shaping of an outlook on life that offers encouragement to the patient. Messer and

Wampold (2002), on the basis of several research studies and meta-analyses, concluded that there is a far more convincing argument for common factors as being critical to therapeutic change than for the treatment effects of any specific ingredients of individual therapies.

Integrative therapists who use a common-factors approach try to identify which of the several known common factors will be most important in the treatment of a particular individual. Once the most salient common factors are selected, the therapist reviews the array of interventions and psychotherapeutic interactions to find those that have been found to promote and contain those ingredients. The integrative therapies that result from this process are structured around the goal of maximizing the patient's exposure to the unique combination of therapeutic factors that will best ameliorate his or her problems. Garfield's (2000) common-factors integrative therapy, which relies on the combination of insight, exposure, and the provision of new experience and hope through the therapeutic relationship, is one well-known form of common-factors integration.

Theoretical Integration

Theoretical integration is the most complex, sophisticated, and difficult mode of psychotherapy integration. Psychotherapies that are theoretically integrated rely on a process of synthesizing aspects of varied personality theories, combining models of psychopathology, and integrating various mechanisms of psychological change from two or more traditional systems. These novel integrative theories may indicate the mutual influence of environmental, motivational, cognitive, and affective variables.

Theoretically integrated systems of psychotherapy use interventions from each of the component theories, as well as propose original techniques that may be added to the technical selection of the traditional therapeutic schools that are the basis of this new approach. Wachtel's (1977) cyclical psychodynamic theory and its integrative therapy was the first fully developed form of theoretical integration. He developed a psychodynamically based model of personality, psychopathology, and change that acknowledged and used reinforcement and social learning principles, along with traditional psychoanalytic exploration. The usual model of exploration leading to understanding and then change was supplemented by the idea that behavioral change, produced by behavioral interventions, might lead to increased understanding. For example, changing impulsive behavior may not require prior understanding, but understanding might follow from impulsive behavior change.

Assimilative Integration

Assimilative integration has been the focus of much recent interest (Messer, 2001b; Stricker & Gold, 1996) and can be seen as a derivative of both theoretical integration and technical eclecticism. Messer (1992) introduced this concept into the field of psychotherapy integration when he noted that all actions are defined and contained by the interpersonal, historical, and physical context in which those acts occur. As any therapeutic intervention is a highly complex interpersonal action, therapeutic interventions are defined, and perhaps even re-created, by the larger context of the therapy. Certain theoretically integrative approaches may be understood to be assimilative as they incorporate new techniques into an existing conceptual model of therapy. When techniques are applied clinically within a theoretical context that differs from the context in which they were developed, the meaning, impact, and use of those interventions may be modified in powerful ways. For example, when interventions such as the use of systematic desensitization are assimilated into client-centered therapy, their nature may be altered by this new context and by the alternative purposes of the therapist. Thus, a behavioral method such as systematic desensitization may mean something entirely different to a patient whose ongoing therapeutic experience has been defined by experientially oriented exploration than that same intervention would mean to a patient in traditional behavior therapy. The psychodynamically based integrative therapy proposed by Stricker and Gold (1996; Stricker, 2006) is an example of this form of integrative therapy. In this approach, therapy proceeds according to standard psychodynamic guidelines, but methods from other therapies, such as the two-chair technique from Gestalt or process–experiential therapy, are used when called for, and they may advance certain psychodynamic goals indirectly at the same time as being effective in treating the target problem.

Newman, Castonguay, and their colleagues (Newman, Castonguay, Borkovec, & Molnar, 2004; Newman, Castonguay, Borkovec, Fisher, & Nordberg, 2008) have described an ambitious and highly successful research program that has aimed at testing and validating an assimilative integrative treatment for generalized anxiety disorders. Their integrative model is based on CBT and integrates experiential and interpersonal concepts and methods. These authors suggested that the outcome of standard cognitive-behavioral protocols can be surpassed when the patient's emotional process is addressed directly through experiential techniques. Furthermore, they pointed out that the painful work of addressing anxiety symptoms, and the cognitive precursors of those symptoms, often will provoke ruptures and strains in the therapeutic relationship, which are most effectively addressed through interpersonal exploration. When this therapy was compared to a standard cognitive-behavioral approach, it was found to have a greater positive impact on patients' symptoms, and a longer lasting and more noticeable effect on both symptoms and interpersonal problems.

Bringing the Body into Psychotherapy Integration

Certain recent developments in psychotherapy integration do not fit neatly within the framework of the models we described earlier. These new models share a concern with and a focus on integrating various forms of psychotherapy *with interventions that have direct impact on the body*. The developers of these integrative approaches share certain assumptions about the relationship of the brain, the body, and central psychological processes such as cognition and emotion. Most importantly, all of these models are built upon the hypothesis that psychological variables can be changed, and psychological suffering can be alleviated, by directly utilizing or intervening in physiological processes. Some, but not all, of these integrationists also believe that most, if not all, forms of psychopathology have concurrent bodily manifestations, and that if these correlates are addressed directly and simultaneously, the effectiveness of psychological interventions is increased markedly.

Eye movement desensitization and reprocessing (EMDR; Shapiro, 1997) has emerged as an important and somewhat controversial method for the treatment of trauma and of posttraumatic stress disorder. Shapiro serendipitously discovered that the deliberate, simultaneous linkage of rapid eye movements with the emergence of disturbing thoughts and images led to a dramatic reduction in the emotional impact of those cognitions, as well as lessening the time during which those ideas and images remained in the patient's mind. EMDR therefore can be understood to be an integrative therapy that is based on the behavioral change principle of exposure, but that incorporates other active physical interventions and both psychodynamic and cognitive concepts and methods. Among the chief modifications that EMDR utilizes is the therapist's active elicitation of the patient's eye movements during the exposure phase of the therapy. This is accomplished by instructing the patient to follow the therapist's hand, a wand, or some other stimulus as it is moved laterally and rapidly in front of the patient's face. At the same time, the patient is instructed to recall a traumatic memory and to describe all of the associated memories, thoughts, feelings, and bodily sensations that are connected to and stimulated by the memory. After this phase is completed, the clinician attempts to link or to *install* new and positive ways of thinking about traumatic experiences. The EMDR therapist operates from the assumption that successful exposure and desensitization now allows the patient to consider and to adopt more useful and adaptive ways of thinking about past events. The installation is conducted as was the exposure: The patient is instructed to think about the traumatic event in a new way while undergoing the eye movement procedure.

EMDR has been evaluated in a very large number of studies and found to be as effective as other cognitive and behavioral therapies for the treatment of trauma (Seidler & Wagner, 2006). However, other writers (Prochaska & Norcross, 2009) have suggested that what is effective in EMDR is its imagery-based exposure component, and that there is no evidence that the eye movements add any benefit to the therapy. As EMDR has become more widely known and accepted within the general psychotherapeutic community, a trend toward assimilating its techniques into longer, more traditional therapies, including client-centered, psychodynamic, and systems approaches, has emerged (Shapiro, 2002).

Other new versions of integrative psychotherapy use *direct bodily interventions* to influence psychological states and their physical manifestations. Berg, Sandell, and Sandahl (2009) described an integrative model in which psychodynamic psychotherapy is combined with massage and physiotherapy. This approach, tested on patients with generalized anxiety disorders, has been found to be effective for that population. Similarly, Cartwright (2007) has reported on an integrative model that synthesizes a client-centered therapeutic approach with techniques and concepts drawn from meditation and from the practice of yoga. He argued that this integration allows the expansion of the usual goal of psychotherapy to include a focus on the body and on bodily processes in emotional functioning, work toward enhancement of emotional experience at the physical and psychological level, and work on the centering of self-experience in the body.

THE CONCEPT OF PERSONALITY

Personality as an explanatory or organizing construct (i.e., as an implicit or inferred set of psychological constructs and behaviors) is very much a part of certain integrative psychotherapies. Other systems of psychotherapy integration barely acknowledge the notion of personality or exclude it completely. *Attention to personality is omitted from most integrative models that are based on common-factors integration or on technical eclecticism.* The prescriptive focus of these psychotherapies, in which symptoms and targeted problems are matched with therapeutic ingredients (common factors) or with assumed effective techniques (technical eclecticism), results in the therapist using a narrower lens to understand the patient and his or her behavior and experience. An inferred conceptual system or model of personality presumably would add little to the effectiveness of the prescriptive power of these psychotherapies and might, in fact, serve as an intellectual distraction for the therapist.

Personality is a much more important concept in those integrative psychotherapies that are based on theoretical or assimilative integration. Assimilative integration has a single personality theory and theory of therapy as its organizing feature. Theoretical integration involves the synthesis of two or more independent personality theories into a novel model of personality. A critical assumption behind this theoretical amalgamation is that this new, integrative personality theory is an improvement over the component theories in its ability to inform the therapist's understanding of psychological development, psychopathology, and, most importantly, the best and most efficacious choice of interventions.

Integrative theories of personality are employed in two ways, the first of which is similar to the manner in which traditional theories of personality are used in pure forms of psychotherapy: as a guide in the identification of psychological structures (e.g., schemas and defense mechanisms) and other features (e.g., anxiety, unconscious motivation, and affect) that need to be influenced and changed by therapy. Second, and uniquely, these theories posit and explain the relationship between psychological phenomena that are ignored or considered irrelevant by traditional theories. Such explanations illustrate an extremely important and singular characteristic of integrative models of personality: *Integrative theories substitute circular conceptualizations of causation for the linear views of causation that are typical of traditional personality theories.* Circular views of causation suggest that there are no levels or areas of psychological life that are unimportant, or that should be understood merely as superficial, as may result from the more narrow views inherent in older models of personality.

Gold (1996) has pointed out that the personality theories that support contemporary integrative approaches share a number of common assumptions and emphases, regardless of deviations in the specific terminology used in each contribution. Integrative personality theories share a deep concern for the way the individual comes to understand his or her experience, and for those core meaning structures that compose the person's sense of self and representation of significant relationships.

The most comprehensive and influential integrative theory of personality is *cyclical psychodynamics* (Wachtel, 1977, 2008). Cyclical psychodynamic theory presented a model of personality that emphasized the mutually and reciprocally determining nature of behavior, interpersonal relationships, and unconscious motivation and conflict, demonstrating that a clinically viable and conceptually elegant synthesis of psychoanalytic and learning theories could be achieved. The theory assisted therapists in understanding how changes in psychodynamics could both lead to and follow from changes in behavior and in interactions with others. The latest iteration of cyclical psychodynamics has expanded the theory to include concepts drawn from family systems theory, relational psychoanalysis, experiential theories, and cognitive theory.

The procedural sequence object relations model (Ryle & McCutcheon, 2006) is another integrative approach to personality. This model informs cognitive analytic therapy (CAT) and is a synthesis of concepts drawn from cognitive psychology, cognitive therapy, and psychoanalytic object relations theory. The theory describes the complex interrelationships between the way that the individual consciously processes information about the self and others and the unconscious developmental antecedents of the person's cognitive structures, beliefs, assumptions, and role definitions. The therapist presents this understanding of functioning and motivation to the patient, and they then work together to modify it using both cognitive-behavioral and psychodynamic techniques.

A final example of this type of integrative personality theory, proposed by Greenberg, Rice, and Elliott (1993), integrates ideas from client-centered, cognitive, and experiential therapies. These authors see personality as the meaning-retention and meaning-generation structures through which persons come to understand, remember, and respond to the world. This theory serves as a foundation for therapeutic interventions drawn from the three aforementioned source therapies, all of which can address the modification of pathological meanings.

PSYCHOLOGICAL HEALTH AND PATHOLOGY

Few integrative approaches specifically offer a comprehensive psychological model of health, and the "disease orientation" is true of the majority of psychotherapies (Bohart & Tallman, 1999). Most integrative therapies contain within them the definition and conceptualization of health and pathology that derive from the specific component therapies that are amalgamated. However, many integrationists share certain critical assumptions about the nature and appearance of psychological health.

Psychological health seems to consist of freedom from psychological constraints on the perception and construction of meaning and experience (Bohart, 1992; Greenberg et al., 1993); repetitive, dysfunctional patterns of thought and of the organization of cognitive data (Guidano & Liotti, 1983); redundant and maladaptive ways of engaging and relating to others (K. Frank, 1999); and the unwitting repetition and maintenance of developmental traumas, conflict, and attachments (Gold & Stricker, 2001). Thus, integrationists seem to characterize psychological health as the ability to define one's goals; successfully jettison, modify, or retain goals depending on their (individual and social) adaptive benefit; develop plans to obtain and actively seek out these goals; learn from self-generated and other-generated feedback; and attain them without intrapersonal or interpersonal interference.

It stands to reason, then, that an integrative perspective on the development and maintenance of psychopathology would focus on those psychological and environmental factors that inhibit the individual's freedom of experience and responsiveness, and eventuate in psychological and behavioral redundancy. Most integrative theorists work from a developmental framework in that they emphasize the role of childhood and adolescent events in laying down the foundations of perception, thinking, and motivation that lead to psychopathology (Wachtel, 2008). Essentially, these theorists posit that negative, painful, anxious, and defeated familial and social interactions are internalized and become part of the patient's cognitive and emotional representational systems. This negatively toned representational system, which consciously and unconsciously leads to ongoing predictions and construal of danger (shame, guilt, humiliation, abandonment, etc.) in many, if not most, important interpersonal situations, cannot help but lead the patient into avoidant, defensive, and ultimately self-defeating and self-replicating patterns of construing reality and of social relatedness (Allen, 1993; Wachtel, 1977). These "vicious circles" (Wachtel, 2008) are central and critical variables in most integrative accounts of psychopathology.

Most integrative theories of psychopathology operate within what Messer (1992) has identified as the "ironic vision"; that is, things come out badly and redundantly despite the person's best efforts to achieve a new result or experience (Wachtel, 2008). Few persons are aware of the restricting power of their representational systems, or of the ways in which we unwittingly reproduce past hurts and disappointments in the present. We are aware, however, of the cognitive, emotional, and interpersonal sequelae of those hurts, and it is this distress that often eventuates in the decision to enter therapy.

The various models of integrative psychotherapy rely on several diagnostic systems, some of which are generic (i.e., fourth edition of *Diagnostic and Statistical Manual of Mental Dis-*

orders [DSM-IV; American Psychiatric Association, 1994]) and others of which are uniquely associated with the particular psychotherapy that is used. We have already described the diagnostic model (BASIC ID) that is at the heart of multimodal therapy (Lazarus, 2006). In transtheoretical psychotherapy (Prochaska & DiClemente, 2002) the patient is evaluated on a three-dimensional matrix. Ryle's (1997; Ryle & McCutcheon, 2006) CAT is built around a detailed and formal assessment of the patient's cognitive functioning or procedural sequences, with particular attention paid to "traps" (dysfunctional assumptions and beliefs), "dilemmas" (polarized alternative conceptualizations of experience), and "snags" (aims that are abandoned due to the anticipation of negative consequences).

THE PROCESS OF CLINICAL ASSESSMENT

Assessment in most integrative approaches is based on the methods that are typical of the component therapies that make up each integrative method. This is most often the case for those integrative therapies that are exemplars of either theoretical or assimilative integration, as these therapies tend to be more long term and more concerned with "deeper" or more complex changes (e.g., in personality structure and representational systems).Thus, an integrative therapy that leans heavily on a psychodynamic foundation, such as cyclical psychodynamics (Wachtel, 2008) or assimilative psychodynamic psychotherapy (Gold & Stricker, 2001), for example, assesses patients initially and primarily with regard to psychodynamic issues such as conflict, character, resistance, and object representations. These therapies also include ongoing, process-oriented assessments, as do traditional psychodynamic treatments: The patient is evaluated, and the therapist's understanding is revised and reformulated on an ongoing basis throughout therapy, based on the patient's responses and form of participation.

The integrative assessment is expanded to include evaluation of the person's functioning at the cognitive, experiential, and behavioral levels, and the mutual influence of those levels on each other and with psychodynamic issues and structures. Similarly, a theoretically integrated therapy that primarily is behaviorally based, such as Fensterheim's (1993) behavioral psychotherapy, would assess the usual behavioral variables in a context that includes an ongoing evaluation of the variables that are considered critical from the additional and integrated therapeutic orientation. Where integrative assessment differs from a traditional assessment is in the therapist's awareness of, and attention to, the possibility and advantage of using an intervention from another therapeutic system (e.g.,, a psychodynamic therapist may use techniques from CBT or experiential therapy, among others). The parameters of assessment are expanded to include an ongoing evaluation of the benefits and limitations of the "home" or foundation therapy, and of the patient's individualized needs, goals, strengths, and weaknesses, all of which may best be met by an integrative shift. Certain integrationists (Bohart, 2000; Duncan & Miller, 2000; Gold, 2000) advocate the ongoing assessment of the patient's conscious assessment of the therapy, and his or her ideas about which techniques and strategies would be most helpful.

Because most integrative therapies are oriented to the individual, the "unit" of assessment is the individual person, with awareness that this person cannot be understood separately from the interpersonal context in which he or she is located. There are, however, exceptions to this individual focus, as certain writers have made important contributions to the integration of individual therapy with couple, family, and group psychotherapies (Lebow, 2006). In these therapies, assessment is directed toward individual and systemic functioning, and particularly toward the interaction and mutual influence of the two levels upon each other.

The focus of integrative assessment usually is broader and deeper than assessment in any single, pure-form therapy, and includes interest in intrapsychic, cognitive, behavioral, experiential, and interpersonal variables. The emphasis on each class of variables is determined by the component therapies. Interest in assessing the individual within a contextual framework is an intrinsic part of many integrative approaches. Assessment of context includes an evaluation of past and current interpersonal relationships and the ways in which others in the patient's life become *neurotic accomplices* (Wachtel, 1977). This term refers to the way in which significant persons contribute to the maintenance and exacerbation of patients' problems by confirming their fears and their problematic representational processes. Assessment of context has been extended by some to include much broader issues as well. Wachtel (1989) has illustrated the need to account for the effect of racial discrimination, poverty, and social disenfranchisement on individual psychology and psychopathology. Gold (1992) extended Wachtel's (1989) cyclical psychodynamic thinking to include evaluation of the effects of gender discrimination and political disempowerment on psychological suffering and psychotherapy.

Most integrative therapists explicitly describe an assessment of patients' strengths as an integral part of their work. These strengths often become the basis of interventions, as patients are helped to take on challenges and areas of weakness by using and extending skills in which they are already proficient. As noted earlier, certain theorists (e.g., Bohart, 2000; Duncan & Miller, 2000) have suggested that patients often know best what they need, and may even have the skills to change but are unaware of the ways in which those skills could be best applied or in which situations these efforts would be most productive.

Certain integrative approaches that are examples of technical eclecticism or of common-factors integration are based on an immediate, comprehensive assessment of the patient that leads directly into the selection of therapeutic interventions. These therapies are almost entirely driven by this assessment. We have already discussed several examples of this type of integrative therapy: multimodal therapy (Lazarus, 2006); transtheoretical therapy (Prochaska & DiClemente, 2002); and systematic treatment selection (STS; Beutler et al., 2006). These approaches frequently use standardized psychological tests to conduct assessments. For example, Beutler and colleagues mention such specific instruments as the STS Clinician Rating Form, the Patient Compliance Scale, and the STS Therapy Process Rating Scale as essential and regular sources of data that inform the process through which prescriptive treatment plans evolve. Variables such as the stages of change and processes of change are assessed in transtheoretical therapy through the use of self-report measures (the URICA, or University of Rhode Island Change Assessment, and the POC, or Processes of Change measure; Prochaska & DiClemente, 2002). Few integrative systems based on theoretical integration include such heavy reliance on standardized tests, though individual therapists may use some at their discretion.

Few integrative therapies rely heavily on formalized psychiatric typologies such as DSM-IV. Those that do typically use psychiatric diagnosis as a starting point for a more intensive and psychologically oriented assessment. An example of this approach is cognitive-behavioral analytic system of psychotherapy (CBASP), an integrative therapy developed for the treatment of dysthymic disorder (depression) by McCullough (2001). In this model, the psychiatric diagnosis is the entry point, which indicates that this therapy is appropriate for this patient. However, the assessment that is crucial to the progress of the treatment goes beyond diagnosis and into the spheres of cognition, behavior, and interpersonal skills.

THE PRACTICE OF THERAPY

There is considerable variation in the basic structure of therapy across the many varieties of integrative psychotherapies. As has been stressed in this chapter, the characteristics of each approach are determined largely by its component therapies. Thus, as a general rule, though one with more than enough exceptions, those integrative therapies that are more heavily psychodynamic are longer term (2 or more years) and tend to meet at least on a weekly basis, with two or even three sessions per week being far from unknown. Integrative approaches that give more emphasis to cognitive-behavioral and experiential schools tend to be shorter in length and meet once a week or even less frequently. Typically sessions last from 45 minutes to 1 hour.

Several integrative therapies that have been described are specifically identified as *short term*. These include time-limited dynamic psychotherapy (Levenson, 1995), accelerated experiential–dynamic psychotherapy (Fosha, 2000), and short-term restructuring psychotherapy (Magnavita & Carlson, 2003), among others. These integrative therapies are designed to be completed in 20 to 30 weekly sessions. Most integrative therapies are individually focused; therefore, attendance in sessions is limited to patient and therapist. However, there is a great deal of flexibility in this arrangement. As mentioned earlier, certain integrative therapies merge individual and systems approaches, and hold sessions with individuals, couples, families, subsystems within families, and groups, as dictated by clinical necessity. The degree to which any session is structured or governed by a predetermined agenda is a function of the theoretical slant of the specific integrative model. Therapies that lean heavily on humanistic, experiential, or psychoanalytic foundations are less likely to be highly structured than those that are more cognitive-behavioral in orientation. For example, CBASP (McCullough, 2001) resembles standard cognitive-behavioral approaches much more than other integrative therapies in its extensive use of homework assignments and goal setting for each session, and in the therapist's active direction of the content and process of each session.

The various integrative therapies differ significantly with regard to the nature and specifics of the goals determined for each patient. Those approaches that are based on a psychoanalytic or humanistic–experiential foundation posit that most patients can benefit from certain broadly defined changes, regardless of the particular presenting problems. These universal goals include changes in underlying meaning or representational structures, character structure, getting in touch with one's feelings, feeling freer to act, and the patient's ability to be open to the symbolization and integration of new experiences. Those therapies that are more prescriptive or shorter term tend to avoid such general, shared goals and to focus more specifically on what ails this particular person at this specific time.

Most integrative models stress that goal setting is best accomplished through a process of collaboration in which the therapist may take the lead through the assessment process but is open and respectful of the patient's needs, wishes, and ideas, particularly as these may reflect the patient's efforts to revise or reject the therapist's formulation and treatment plan. Most integrative therapists emphasize overt discussion of some, if not all, therapeutic goals. This is an essential part of establishing trust, respect, and a therapeutic alliance. Goals that are more likely to be discussed are those that are connected to the patient's overt behavior, conscious thoughts and feelings, and relationships. For example, discussion of the wish to deal with uncomfortable affect or the problem caused by repetitive difficulty in relationships may provide clear goals for the patient and the therapist. Goals that may guide the therapist, but which refer to psychic processes and structures, probably are discussed less frequently with patients. It is possible to place the many integrative therapies on a continuum of goals that, at one end, would be described as therapist-driven, and at the other, patient-driven. Those therapies that are found at the patient-driven end are typically concerned with resolution of the presenting problem and give less emphasis to inferred intrapsychic issues. This patient-specific approach to goals is most evident in the model of client-directed therapy developed by Miller, Duncan, and Hubble (2002), in which patient and therapist collaborate in developing therapeutic strategies and selecting interventions based on the patient's theory of change, and his or her plan for achieving those changes.

Advocates of psychotherapy integration argue emphatically that one of the main advantages of this attitude is that *integrative models allow goals to be established at any level*, or in any realm of psychological experience: relational, behavioral, cognitive, affective, motivational, and characterological. Goals do not have to be excluded, overlooked, or characterized as "shallow" or inconsequential due to a preordained theoretical position. Of course, integrative therapies have their limits, broad as they may be. For example, Lazarus (2006) has made it clear that patients who understand their problems as reflecting unconscious psychosexual conflicts, and who wish to work on such issues, would be best referred to a therapist who could concur with those goals.

Almost any form of conventionally accepted therapeutic intervention may be used when deemed clinically appropriate. The choice of intervention may combine the theoretical perspective of the therapist and the needs of the patient (in theoretical or assimilative integration) or may reflect the therapist's clinical assessment of the patient's needs and the process of matching (as in technical eclecticism and common-factors integration). Interpretation of unconscious processes is used in those therapies that integrate psychodynamic principles, when the therapist hypothesizes that insight into unwitting motives, conflicts, resistances, and self- and object representations would be helpful to the patient.

Integrative therapists also use cognitive restructuring, skills-building interventions, and exposure techniques from cognitive-behavioral approaches; experiential techniques, such as the empty chair and two-chair dialogue methods from Gestalt therapy; and empathy, prizing, and reflection of feeling from client-centered therapy, to name just a few of the more prominent types of interventions. At one point in a session the patient may work on tolerating anxiety generated by a feared confrontation with a boss (imaginal desensitization), practice a conversation with someone he or she would like to date (assertiveness training), or work on resolving a long-standing grief reaction by conversing with a deceased parent who has been "placed" in the empty chair across the room. At other times during a session, or in later sessions, the focus might be on alleviating the patient's overly harsh self-criticism by pointing out the "shoulds" and "musts" that dominate his or her thinking, and by helping the patient to keep track of these thoughts and to substitute more soothing and realistic ideas. Had these interventions been selected in the context of a therapy defined as technically eclectic or as a common-factors approach, the selection would have been guided by the central, pressing clinical need and by identification of the technique that would best meet that need. Selection of that technique in a theoretically or assimilatively integrated theory would be based also on the effect of that technique on recognition of the meaning of the psychological experience, as well as on the problem.

Homework is a central feature of most integrative therapies, even those that have a psychodynamic foundation (Stricker, 2006). Sometimes the homework assignments, which usually are developed collaboratively, are traditional applications of cognitive, behavioral, or experiential exercises in the context of another theoretical orientation: Patients whose in-session work leads to psychodynamic insights about their avoidant behavior challenge themselves to face new social situations or to modify the thoughts that drive the anxiety. Other instances of homework are more assimilative and integrative in nature: Homework exercises are used to provoke changes in areas of psychological life other than those with which they usually are associated. For example, patients may be taught relaxation techniques not only because these methods lead to the expected reduction in anxiety but also because successfully lessening those symptoms lead to changes in their self-image and perception of the therapist as willing to be helpful (Gold & Stricker, 2001). Patients might be asked to evaluate the effects of the relaxation when entering situations in which they are ordinarily fearful (e.g., going through a tunnel in a train) and to see whether lessened anxiety might lead to increased awareness about feelings, thoughts, memories, and conflicts associated with that event.

Perhaps the most critical strategic and technical questions in any integrative psychotherapy are when to move from one technique to the next and, correspondingly, when to shift orientations and strategies from the behavioral to the experiential to the psychodynamic, and so on. The answers are easier and more straightforward in those technically eclectic and common-factors based integrative models that feature a comprehensive and specific assessment geared to prescriptive matching. In these therapies a shift in technique occurs when the clinical focus changes. For example, as the patient gains certain skills with a behavioral intervention, other issues of a cognitive or emotional nature may emerge. After patient and therapist agree on the next issue to be addressed, the process of prescriptive matching is reapplied and may occur many times until the completion of therapy.

Knowing when to make an integrative shift in a theoretically or assimilatively integrated therapy is more difficult and usually is guided by immediate process observations made by the therapist, often as a reflection of his or her subjective experience of the therapeutic relationship and alliance. K. Frank (1999), Gold and Stricker (2001), and Marcotte and Safran (2002) all have suggested some guidelines for such integrative shifts. Essentially, these writers agree that movement from one orientation and set of therapeutic techniques to another (perhaps from the psychodynamic to cognitive-behavioral) is indicated when the initial way of working has become uncongenial to the patient, overtaxes the patient's ability to cope or cooperate with therapy, requires skills that the patient has not yet developed, or unwittingly is damaging to the patient.

Gold and Stricker (2006), among others, have suggested that certain patients, especially those who are more fragile, less trusting, and less psychologically sophisticated, often make more rapid progress in therapy when the first techniques used are more concrete and pragmatic (i.e., more cognitive-behavioral). These patients seem to make better use of psychodynamic exploration when it is introduced after presenting problems have been ameliorated to some degree, and after the therapist has been established as helpful and trustworthy. A shift away from a psychodynamic to a more immediately pragmatic form of therapy often may help patients avoid or alleviate feelings of being confused, mystified, and frustrated by the more subtle goals and methods of psychodynamic therapy and can give these individuals a critically important boost in self-esteem when they have used a cognitive, behavioral, or other technique to solve a problem.

Resistance to change in integrative therapies is conceptualized as resulting from a single factor or a combination of psychological and social factors. The psychodynamic component of many models suggests that resistance occurs when the patient feels frightened of some internal state that is about to emerge into awareness, or is pained, guilty, or ashamed about some past experience, or about the prospect of leaving old ways of living and for-mer attachments behind. The cognitive and behavioral contributions to understanding resistance allow therapist and patient to look at the contribution of each member of the dyad. Has the therapist asked too much of the patient, or has he or she underestimated the impact of a suggestion or intervention? On the patient's side, resistance may arise from a lack of understanding of the tasks that are posed, an unwillingness to be open to the thera-pist's suggestions and interventions, or a lack of investment in actively changing. Resistance shows itself in myriad forms, from the subtle, characterological patterns with which psy-chodynamic therapists are familiar to the more overt types of reactance or noncompliance described by cognitive-behavioral therapists (Dowd, 1999). Examples of the former are the patient consistently missing a few minutes of the session; engaging the therapist in an over-compliant, hostile, or idealizing manner; or avoiding certain key subjects by substituting others. On the more obvious side is a failure to keep appointments, a disregard for agreed-on homework assignments, and an unwillingness to participate fully in active interventions of whatever type.

Resistance is resolved clinically by exploration of the meaning of the problem at any level that is necessary (interpersonal, psychodynamic, systemic, cognitive, affective, or behavioral), shifting an interpretation, altering the tone and stance of the therapeutic rela-tionship, or rethinking the choice and intensity of the interventions that are suggested. Integrative therapists who understand individual functioning in a contextual, interper-sonal context are acutely aware of "accomplices in neurosis," that is significant individuals who unwittingly or knowingly interfere with the patient's progress in therapy (Wachtel, 1977). Integrative therapists may work directly with these significant others on occasion, while at other times the therapeutic focus is on helping the patient to develop the necessary interpersonal skills to overcome the influence of an accomplice, or to end the relationship, if all else fails.

The most common therapist errors that are unique to integrative models are the fail-ure to make an integrative shift when it is called for and the too rapid use of an integrative shift when ongoing work within one theoretical and technical framework is a better fit. The first type of error seems to occur frequently because of the somewhat vague guidelines for timing shifts, and sometimes when the therapist is still bound up by loyalties and anxieties about his or her allegiance to one therapy school. Overly rapid shifting, or the overuse of integration, may also occur due to (countertransferential) anxiety on part of the therapist. For example, the therapist may feel too uncomfortable to continue working with a particu-lar issue and may therefore suggest a shift in strategy or technique.

Psychotropic medications are often a part of integrative therapy (Beitman & Saveanu, 2005). The therapist who is a psychiatrist or psychopharmacologist may integrate biologi-cal and psychological components of the therapy, or may refer the patient to a colleague for a medication consult. Otherwise, medication is handled much as it is in any traditional therapy.

Termination of therapy usually results from a mutual decision by patient and therapist that the treatment has reached its end. Some of the specifically short-term integrative mod-els mentioned earlier specify a number of sessions at the start. Other integrative therapies do not, particularly those that have a significant psychodynamic component. In this latter group of therapies, termination often is considered a significant event that is explored for several weeks or months, with particular concern for evoked developmental issues around separation and loss.

THE THERAPEUTIC RELATIONSHIP AND THE STANCE OF THE THERAPIST

The therapeutic relationship is one of the central common factors that produces changes in virtually all forms of psychotherapy (Rosenzweig, 1936; Weinberger, 1993). On this point, most therapists of most orientations agree. Where and how the various therapies deviate from each other is in their relative emphasis on the many effective ingredients of the therapeutic relationship that make it so potentially potent, and on how to maximize the impact of the relationship.

The therapeutic relationship is central to most integrative psychotherapies as well. The central theme of this chapter is highly applicable here: Integrative therapies aim to expand the therapeutic relationship as fully as possible to make that relationship as effective as possible. Again, the particular conceptualization of the relationship in each specific integrative therapy is guided by the way the relationship is construed and used in the major component therapies. Thus, an integrative therapy that is heavily interpersonal (Safran & Segal, 1990), psychodynamic (K. Frank, 1999; Wachtel, 1977), or client-centered (Greenberg et al., 1993) will emphasize, respectively, identifying and resolving enactments of the client's problems with the therapist; the interpretation of transference; or prizing, empathy, and warmth. These are considered the most important variables in producing change. Integrative therapies that are more cognitive-behavioral or systemic in orientation (Fensterheim, 1993; Pinsof, 1995) do not ignore the therapeutic relationship and its effectiveness but see it as one factor among several that can lead to change, and as a platform for the active learning that takes place in the more technical parts of the therapy. A major difference is that the latter approach uses the relationship as the foundation of care, whereas the former approach uses it as the vehicle of change.

Many integrative forms of therapy converge around the concept of the therapeutic alliance, as most integrative approaches are founded on the view that effective change occurs best when patient and therapist are bonded in a mutually agreed-on set of goals, within the context of a positively toned and perceived interaction. The process of integration, and the notion of the integrative shift in particular, seems to some integrative writers (Gold & Stricker, 2001; Marcotte & Safran, 2002) to be particularly effective in establishing an alliance firmly and quickly, and is a way to reestablish or repair the alliance when it has been strained or ruptured. K. Frank (1999) noted that the inclusion of cognitive and behavioral techniques in a psychoanalytic therapy constitutes not only a technical shift but also an interpersonal communication to the patient, one that in effect says, "I'm aware of your suffering with these thoughts, actions, and feelings, and I will try actively to help. I won't let you sit there alone." Along these same lines, Gold and Stricker (2001) point out that skills-building techniques, such as assertiveness training, and self-soothing cognitive techniques may enhance self-esteem and can assist the patient in overcoming negatively toned perceptions of his or her experience in therapy, thus enhancing the therapeutic alliance.

Some of the strengths of integrative therapy also carry the seeds of potential shortcomings. For example, the flexibility and creativity that can be exercised by the integrative therapist also open the door to more undisciplined approaches, particularly when there is no theoretical rationale for the intervention. Messer (2006) has also presented a significant challenge to integration. He has spelled out what he refers to as *visions of reality*, taking the terminology from literary criticism. Different visions characterize different therapeutic orientations, and sometimes different versions of the same orientation. For example, an extended psychodynamic treatment can be described as "tragic" because of its recognition of human limitations, whereas briefer psychodynamic therapy and behavioral approaches are more readily described as "comic" because of the focus on a happy ending. An integrative therapist often shifts from one approach to another, but with the shift in technique there also is a shift between what may be incompatible visions of the nature of reality.

Integrative therapists sometimes take active control of the sessions. This is the case when the therapist suggests an integrative shift, or a homework assignment. The therapist shifts from an exploratory, facilitative role when he or she introduces an active intervention into psychodynamic or experientially oriented psychotherapy. Certainly, therapists who identify themselves as multimodal or prescriptive, and those who work from a common-factors perspective, often are active and directive in sessions. However, active and directive does not mean dictatorial and authoritarian. The key phrase a few sentences ago was, "the therapist suggests." Most integrative therapists view their patient or client as a collaborator and partner. (In fact, we think all good therapists share this perspective, regardless of orientation.) Thus, the patient's sense of what will work for him or for her, the patient's own theory of change (Duncan & Miller, 2000), and the patient's right to refuse a suggestion must be respected. It is the therapist's task to provide the conditions in which change is most likely to occur. It is the therapist's responsibility to know and to offer the patient a variety of ideas, experiences, tasks, and resources that may lead to change. It is the patient's task and opportunity to attempt to make use of these conditions and experiences to see if he or she can and will change. The therapist may work with those issues (anxiety, resistance, neurotic accomplices, or lack of skill) that interfere with the patient's ability to change, but, ultimately, progress comes from the patient's efforts (Bohart, 2000).

The therapist's own history as a person and professional and his or her experience of the patient obviously enter into any therapy to some degree. As well versed as any clinician may be in theory and technique, ultimately, he or she will understand the patient and his or her situation and needs from a personal point of view. Once again, we must reiterate that how an integrative therapy makes use of issues such as therapeutic self-disclosure, counter-transference, and the "person" of the therapist varies from system to system. These issues are most evident in models that are concerned with interpersonal issues such as *enactment*: an event within the therapeutic relationship where the therapist is "hooked" into replaying with the patient the kinds of interactions that affected the patient negatively in the past, or that currently are dysfunctional (K. Frank, 1999; Safran & Segal, 1990). There is no way to know that an enactment is occurring without examining one's feelings, thoughts, and experiences, and often these must be shared with the patient before the enactment can be resolved.

As therapy progresses, and especially as termination of therapy nears, most integrative models suggest that the therapist turn responsibility for decision making about the sessions, homework, and integrative shifts over to the patient. This reinforces autonomy and a sense of self-efficacy, minimizes the patient's anxiety about life after therapy, and allows the patient to practice the "self-therapy" he or she will need in the future.

It is daunting to work as a therapist in any form of therapy. It may be more daunting and personally demanding to work as an integrative therapist. The integrationist must be able intellectually to master the concepts and methods of two or more systems. He or she also must be able to stay free of the common human desire to align with one school of thought, and to tolerate the ambiguity that lurks in all psychotherapies. The therapist must be able to straddle the roles of authority, participant, collaborator, and follower, and must neither idealize nor devalue his or her technical, interpersonal, and experiential expertise. Along this line, integrative therapists might consider following a suggestion for family therapists, originally made by Liddle (1982), that they engage in a periodic epistemological declaration by means of which they regularly review factors such as their theoretical position, therapeutic goals, and methods of treatment evaluation.

CURATIVE FACTORS OR MECHANISMS OF CHANGE

Integrative psychotherapies explicitly are designed to include as many relevant change factors as possible, and therefore to broaden the likelihood that patients are exposed to those factors that best meet their needs. Any change mechanism that has been described consistently in the psychotherapy literature may be found to play a prominent role in one version or another of integrative psychotherapy. Most integrative models stress some combination of the following: insight into, or increased awareness of, conscious and unconscious psychological processes; exposure to anxiety-generating stimuli; learning of new behavioral skills and correction of behavioral dysfunctions, cognitive restructuring, and modification of deep meaning structures (schemas, object representations, models of attachment, etc.); enhancing one's capacity to put experience into words and to experience emotion by directing the focus of inquiry in this direction; provision of an explanation for the troublesome behavior or relational pattern; and bringing about change in repetitive and destructive patterns of interpersonal relatedness. This last mechanism includes the provision of new experiences within the therapeutic relationship through the "corrective emotional experience" (Alexander & French, 1946) or through relational conditions such as prizing, warmth, and genuineness on the part of the therapist.

The particular emphasis given to each of the several mechanisms of change is determined by the specific nature of the integrative model, and by the theories and methods combined in that model. For example, as we have discussed previously, therapies based on technical eclecticism or on common-factors integration attempt to match the patient's problems with those curative factors that have been demonstrated to be most effective. Theoretical integration and assimilative integration add to this prescriptive focus a certain number of a priori assumptions about which of the many change factors are likely to be most important, stemming from the home theory.

For example, psychodynamically influenced integrative therapies proceed from the assumption that insight is an important change factor but expand the therapy to include other change factors, such as direct exposure, learning new interpersonal skills, and direct intervention in the patient's family system. Wachtel's (1977) cyclical psychodynamic therapy and Gold and Stricker's (2001) assimilative psychodynamic therapy are examples of this way of thinking. In addition, virtually all integrative therapists agree that there are "many roads to Rome": that several types of interventions can lead to the same change factor becoming operative, and that change factors can be linked. Wachtel has discussed the important observation that insight often follows behavioral change rather than always preceding it. Similarly, Safran and Segal (1990) base their cognitive-interpersonal therapy on the premise that important cognitive structures can and will change only after the ongoing interpersonal patterns that maintain them have changed. The notion of a cyclical rather than a linear direction of change is an important one.

Because change in interpersonal skills is considered crucial to change at every level of psychological life, any legitimate technique may be applied. Certain integrative approaches emphasize change within the therapeutic relationship, asserting that the most problematic interpersonal patterns and skills deficits will appear in the therapeutic interaction. Not surprisingly, these therapies tend toward the interpersonal, humanistic, and psychodynamic. Didactic instruction in interpersonal functioning tends to be more typical of models that slant toward the cognitive-behavioral, though these boundaries frequently are crossed, as is the wont in integrative therapies. It often is the case that changes will be experienced first in the therapeutic relationship but then be generalized, with the active assistance of the therapist, to relationships outside therapy.

Most integrative therapies include as significant change factors the impact of the therapist's personality and of the therapeutic relationship. The many lists of common factors that are available (Weinberger, 1993) always prominently include these variables. Integrative therapies that are based heavily on person-centered therapy (e.g., Bohart's [1992] experiential approach to integration) stress the classical Rogerian conditions of unconditional positive regard, accurate empathy, and warmth as critical change factors, though not to the exclusive degree that Rogers did. In many ways, a unifying goal of psychotherapy integration is the attempt to go beyond the therapeutic relationship and the impact of the therapist as a person by identifying and including technical interventions that have positive influence as well.

In this regard, integrative therapists have stressed client or patient factors as a central element in change more clearly and frequently than has any single school of psychotherapy. Bohart and Tallman (1999) suggested that client involvement and effort is the single most important factor in any form of psychotherapy, reporting that research indicates up to 30% of change may be accounted for by the client's active participation. Bohart (2000), Duncan and Miller (2000), and Gold (1994, 2000) have discussed this curative factor in the context of several different forms of integrative therapy, ranging from therapies based on strategic models to experientially and humanistically oriented approaches, to a model that is psychodynamically informed.

To summarize, there is little about curative factors in psychotherapy integration that is unique, almost by definition, because the integrative process draws on other approaches to treatment. Some approaches to integration, such as the common-factors approach, are composed entirely of general change factors rather than unique factors. Technical eclecticism is made up entirely of interventions drawn from different approaches. Both theoretical and assimilative integration are based on a home theory and at least one other major approach. They not only share a view of change with the home approach but also show a willingness to incorporate constructs or interventions from other approaches, indicating an expanded view of change. *The uniqueness of psychotherapy integration rests in the breadth of the process rather than in any theoretical or technical aspect of the treatment.*

TREATMENT APPLICABILITY AND ETHICAL CONSIDERATIONS

Goldfried (1999), drawing on an earlier informal communication from Stricker, illustrated both conceptually and visually the dilemma of the psychotherapy patient in a cartoon that he included with an article concerned with the advantages of psychotherapy integration. This cartoon depicts the first meeting of a therapist and a patient. While this duo is shaking hands in greeting, the thoughts of both are revealed in a bubble above the head of each person. The patient privately frets, "I wonder if he can treat what I have?" The therapist, equally troubled, ponders the question, "I hope he has what I treat!"

In large part, interest in psychotherapy integration, and in specifically integrative therapies, evolved in order to solve this problem. Integrative psychotherapies, at least in theory, seem to be uniquely suited to the needs of patients with diverse backgrounds and problems, those whose lives, personalities, and psychopathology deviate from the "ideal types" most easily treated by one of the sectarian therapies. Among the most obvious and important characteristics of successful integration are the flexibility of the therapist and of the therapeutic approach, and the overarching concern for the uniqueness of the patient. Several integrative systems, such as the transtheoretical model and STS, are geared toward developing the most efficacious patient–technique match possible. Common-factors integration, theoretical integration, and assimilative integration, although not based on explicit prescriptive matching, still guide the therapist toward interventions that are broader and more individualized than is possible in any traditional psychotherapeutic system. There is a broad spectrum of patient populations, psychological problems, and psychopathological disorders to which these methods have been successfully applied. As the basic premise of integrative psychotherapy is using the best of what works, any therapeutic approach to any problem, at least in theory, may be improved by the addition of active ingredients from other models.

Integrative approaches have been applied to panic and anxiety disorders (Wolfe, 1992) and to obsessive–compulsive disorder (McCarter, 1997). Although these contributions differ, they share a concern with the provision of behaviorally oriented exposure techniques, and psychodynamically and experientially oriented interventions. In this way, these integrative therapies go further than traditional therapies in ensuring that "all the bases are covered" with regard to the level of psychological activity implicated in this group of disorders.

Depression in its acute and chronic forms has been the focus of much effort on the part of integrationists. For example, Klerman (Klerman, Weissman, Rounsaville, & Chevron, 1984) has an integrative, interpersonal psychotherapy for depression. Arkowitz (1992) described a common factors-based integrative approach to depression. Hayes and Newman's (1993) integrative treatment for depression combined techniques from cognitive therapy, behavior therapy, interpersonal therapy, psychodynamic therapy, experiential therapy, and biological psychiatry. McCullough's (2000) integrative CBASP model is the most effective therapy for chronic depression that has been introduced to date.

More severe forms of psychopathology that often are refractory to traditional psychotherapies also have been treated with integrative therapies. Linehan's (1987) dialectical behavior therapy for borderline personality disorder is a prominent example. Gold and Stricker (1993) explored the integration of cognitive-behavioral and psychodynamic therapies for the treatment of personality disorders, an effort that strongly resembled Ryle's (1997) application of CAT to borderline and narcissistic disorders. More recently, Hilsenroth and Slavin (2008) reported on an approach to the treatment of comorbid depression and borderline personality disorder that combined psychodynamic, behavioral, and cognitive methods, and was supported by research findings as well. Cummings (1993) offered an integrative psychotherapy for substances abusers. Knack (2009) described an approach that integrated psychodynamic psychotherapy and 12-step work in the treatment of alcoholism. Tobin (1995) used an integrative therapy for bulimia, and Hellkamp (1993) and Zapparoli and Gislon (1999) explored integrative therapies for schizophrenia.

This description of wide applicability may make the integrative therapies seem to be the treatment of choice for all patients. Although integrative therapy may be more widely applicable than any other single approach, because it can go beyond that single approach, no treatment can be all things to all people. The type of integration that is practiced, and the presenting problem and goal of the patient establish the limits of the integrative therapies. For example, a patient who is interested solely in self-exploration and has no focal symptom would be best treated by a person with a psychodynamic or a humanistic orientation. On the other hand, a patient who has a focal symptom and no interest in self-exploration or change beyond the presenting problem would be best treated by a person with a behavioral or cognitive-behavioral orientation. Of course, the patient who presents with one and only one interest, be it self-exploration or symptom alleviation, is unusual. Comorbidity is more likely than unidimensional problems, and the integrative therapies, because of their breadth and flexibility, have much to recommend them.

Several integrative therapists also have developed models of therapy that account specifically for the unique goals, experiences, needs, and perspectives of particular patient populations. Integrative models have been developed for persons of color who live in the United States (Franklin, Carter, & Grace, 1993) and for patients who are members of traditional African societies. Madu (1991) and Pelzer (1991) introduced integrative models that combined traditional African modes of healing with Western psychotherapies. Other integrative approaches are aimed at patients for whom spirituality and religion are important (Sollod, 1993). Wachtel (1989), Gold (1992), and Butollo (2000) have demonstrated how an understanding of the economic, political, and ethnic situations in which patients live can be incorporated in therapies that also integrate psychodynamic, cognitive-behavioral, and systems components. Van Dyk and Nefale (2005) also have described an integrative therapy that is sensitive to, and incorporates, indigenous ideas and methods of healing into the framework of standard psychodynamic psychotherapy. Their model, based on their experiences working in rural areas of South Africa, is meant to address the needs of patients who live within the complex, multicultural environment of that nation and of much of Africa.

Integrative models have been developed for virtually all age groups and for individuals, couples, and families. Coonerty (1993) described an integrative therapy for children that synthesizes behavioral, family systems, and psychodynamic elements. Several integrative approaches focus on adolescents and their families [e.g., adolescents with anxiety disorders and depression (Fitzpatrick, 1993); high-risk adolescents (Alexander & Sexton, 2002); adolescent substance abusers (Rowe, Liddle, McClintic, & Quille, 2002)]. Papouchis and Passman (1993) described an integrative model of psychotherapy specifically designed to meet the needs of geriatric patients, involving a judicious integration of cognitive-behavioral techniques into a psychodynamically oriented psychotherapy. Additionally, Pinsof (1995) and Gerson (1996) have described their integrative work with families, and Gurman (2008) has offered an integrative model for work with couples.

RESEARCH SUPPORT

Research supporting integrative approaches to psychotherapy is reviewed in detail in an excellent recent summary by Schottenbauer, Glass, and Arnkoff (2005). Using criteria somewhat more stringent than those of a traditional evidence-based approach (Chambless & Ollendick, 2001), Schottenbauer et al. (2005) concluded that there was substantial support for the efficacy of psychotherapy integration in nine studies, some support in 13 studies, and preliminary support in seven studies.

Chambless, Goldstein, Gallagher, and Bright (1986) described an integrative approach to treating agoraphobia that combined behavioral, systemic, and psychodynamic theories and techniques, without the use of drugs. They found that their integrated model led to marked or great improvement for almost 58% of the patients. Specific treatment effects included lessened avoidance, depression, social phobia, and agoraphobic symptoms and enhanced assertiveness for their patients. This integrative therapy had a much lower drop-out rate than traditional approaches to agoraphobia, but there was no direct comparison of effectiveness with any other treatments.

Linehan (1987) developed an integrative therapy known as dialectical behavior therapy (DBT), which is aimed at alleviating the symptoms of borderline personality disorder. DBT is an amalgam of skills training, cognitive restructuring, and collaborative problem solving from CBT with relationship elements (e.g., warmth, empathy, and unconditional positive regard) from client-centered therapy, and with Buddhist meditative practices, especially mindfulness. DBT has gained wide acceptance among clinicians in recent years due in great part to the research support for its effectiveness. Patients who received DBT demonstrated better treatment retention, had fewer suicide attempts and episodes of self-injury, fewer hospitalizations, decreased anger, greater social adjustment, and more improved general adjustment compared with those who received standard therapies as practiced in the community (Linehan, 1987). A series of studies conducted since 1987 have confirmed and expanded these findings, yielding a solid foundation of empirical support for the efficacy of DBT (Schottenbauer et al., 2005) as one of several effective approaches to borderline personality disorder.

Research on Beutler's Systematic Treatment Selection (STS) (Beutler et al., 2006) demonstrated the validity of the strategy of matching patient characteristics and specific therapeutic interventions. Cognitive therapy was most effective for those patients who externalized responsibility for their depression, whereas patients with an internal locus of control showed the greatest improvement in insight-oriented focused expressive psychotherapy. Patients with higher levels of defensiveness and greater resistance to authority were helped most by a self-directed therapy—that is, one in which the patient was given a variety of cognitive-behavioral and experiential exercises from which to choose.

Transtheoretical therapy (Prochaska & DiClemente, 2002), which also focuses intensively on prescriptive matching, has repeatedly been demonstrated to be a highly effective form of therapy with a variety of populations. The use of the stage-of-change model is an important addition to a treatment program and is helpful in predicting change.

Empirical evaluations of integrative psychotherapies that combine psychodynamic components with behavioral, cognitive, or experiential interventions have yielded positive results. Klerman et al. (1984) found that an integrative, interpersonal psychotherapy for depression repeatedly outperformed medication and other psychological interventions. Shapiro and Firth-Cozens (1990) studied the impact of two sequences of combined CBT and psychodynamic therapy for depression: dynamic work followed by active intervention, or vice versa. Patients in the dynamic–behavioral sequence obtained the greatest improvement and reported the most comfortable experiences of treatment. Patients in the behavioral–dynamic sequence more frequently deteriorated in the second part of the therapy and did not maintain their gains over time as often as did patients in the other group. However, this sequencing effect may depend on the presenting problem and be different with patients who present with nonfocal problems (i.e., those who are more disturbed or personality disordered).

Similarly, Ryle (1995) found that CAT was more effective than purely psychodynamic or behaviorally oriented approaches, although random assignment was not part of the research design. Safran and his colleagues have conducted a number of studies on brief relational therapy, which is an integration of cognitive, experiential, and psychodynamic psychotherapies. In these studies (Marcotte & Safran, 2002) preliminary support was found for the effectiveness of this model with a variety of patient populations, including those with generalized anxiety disorder, borderline personality disorder, and major depression.

Another theoretically integrated approach that has been tested empirically is process–experiential therapy, an integration of principles and methods derived from client-centered, Gestalt, and cognitive therapies (Greenberg et al., 1993). This therapy has been found to be more efficacious than behavior therapy (Greenberg et al., 1993). This integrative model has been demonstrated to be more effective with individuals on a short-term basis for problems such as anxiety and depression, than client-centered therapy or CBT alone (Greenberg et al., 1993).

CBASP (McCullough, 2001) is the first psychotherapy that has been demonstrated empirically to be effective for treating dysthymic disorder. It has been found to be as effective as antidepressant medication and traditional forms of psychotherapy in alleviating the symptoms and interpersonal problems involved in chronic depression. The results from this integrative therapy are more enduring and more resistant to relapse than are other treatments.

The effectiveness of acceptance and commitment therapy (Hayes, Strosahl, & Wilson, 1999), an approach that combines cognitive, behavioral, and experiential techniques, has been demonstrated in eight controlled studies in which this model was tested with several patient populations (Schottenbauer et al., 2005), including depression, substance abuse, anxiety, and psychosis.

CASE ILLUSTRATION

In our assimilative psychodynamic model of integrative psychotherapy (Gold & Stricker, 2001; Stricker & Gold, 1996) we base our assessment and interventions on an expanded, psychoanalytically oriented framework we call the *three-tier model*. We consider detailed evaluations of behavior and social interactions (Tier 1) and of cognitive activity and emotional experience (Tier 2), and we share the traditional psychoanalytic concern with unconscious processes, mental representations, and character traits (Tier 3). We also assess interactions among issues at these three levels of experience in an attempt to understand the vicious circles (Wachtel, 1977) and relationship patterns that maintain problems at any of the tiers. This three-tier approach guides our understanding during assimilative psychodynamic psychotherapy integration. We conduct psychotherapy according to psychodynamic principles of exploration, clarification, confrontation, and interpretation, and are especially concerned with observing the interaction between patient and therapist, and identifying transference phenomena. However, we often intervene directly at the levels of Tier 1 and Tier 2, when it is clinically advantageous to do so. We use interventions from many therapies, including cognitive-behavioral, humanistic, and systems approaches, within an assimilative perspective: We include these interventions for their direct utility in changing behavior, thinking, and emotion; for their possible effects on unconscious sources of resistance, transference, conflict; and effects on unconscious representational systems. We also believe that it is critical to help the patient extricate him- or herself from those relationships and situations that exert a reinforcing influence on the patient's psychopathology.

Integrative interventions are assimilated carefully into the therapy. We always suggest an integrative shift in a tentative way, as an experiment for the patient to try out, evaluate, retain, or toss away, as he or she deems best. We also attend to cognitive, emotional, and dynamic reactions to an integrative shift, and to the success or failure of the technique after the fact. As Wachtel (1977) and other integrative therapists have noted, the impact of the technique on the therapeutic relationship and on the transference–countertransference situation must be continuously monitored.

Ms. F, a 36-year-old woman, was referred to psychotherapy by her internist because of chronic anxiety punctuated by periodic panic attacks and episodes of depression. Her DSM-IV Axis I diagnoses were generalized anxiety disorder (300.02), panic disorder without agoraphobia (300.01), and major depression (296.3). She also described ongoing discomfort in social situations and a pattern of managing that discomfort by maintaining superficial and distant relationships, especially with men, that met the criteria for an Axis II diagnosis of avoidant personality disorder (301.82).

Ms. F reported that she had experienced depression and anxiety since early childhood, and that these symptoms had worsened during the last year, with the addition of panic attacks. During this period she had changed careers and had experienced the death of her mother after a lingering illness. Ms. F worked in a professional field that had required graduate education, and she enjoyed her work, though it was demanding of her time and energy and was not well paid. She was forced to share an apartment with a roommate due to financial considerations and experienced this relationship as a constant source of irritation and tension. Ms. F had not had any previous experience in psychotherapy. Her internist had recommended that she consider making use of psychiatric medication in addition to psychotherapy, but she had not followed up on this recommendation.

Ms. F was the youngest of several children and had been academically talented. Her mother was described as passive, depressed, and demanding of much of Ms. F's time and attention. Ms. F reported that her mother seemed concerned only about Ms. F's professional successes and had little interest in her social life, hobbies, or other interests. She stated that she had been involved in her mother's care during her illness, and that she herself had not "felt much" about her mother's death at the time or during the ensuing period. Her father was described as a distant man who "never had much to say to or about his children." He had been a shadowy figure during his wife's illness and after her death, had offered little in the way of support to Ms. F, and rarely called or visited her.

In the initial assessment of this patient at Tier 1 (behavior and social interactions), the most prominent issues were her avoidant behaviors and interpersonal anxiety that led to the lack of supportive and satisfying friendships, and of the intimate heterosexual relationship that she desired. Tier 2 phenomena (cognitive and social spheres) included preoccupation and overconcern with the minutiae of her work, which provoked intrusive thoughts of being unable to cope with her responsibilities and of losing her job. This pattern of thinking evoked considerable conscious anxiety and periodic experiences of panic. At a more unconscious level (Tier 3, which includes unconscious phenomena, mental representations, and character traits), Ms. F seemed to be afflicted with an image of herself as unlovable and as unworthy of love. She had a wish to please an implacable mother and unattainable father, resulting in mental representations of others as demanding, impossible to please, and selfishly unconcerned. Deeply felt but disavowed pools of anger, resentment, loss, grief, and deprivation were evoked by these representations of self and others.

Ms. F's familial and professional relationships also were involved in the evocation and reinforcement of these problems. Her coworkers, siblings, and father relied on her "to fill in all of the gaps," which she always did, fearing a loss of their already unreliable esteem and interest were she not to do so. Her overt anxiety, rigidly avoidant interpersonal style, and disavowed anger and resentment kept other people at a distance and limited their ability to sympathize with her plight. These reactions fed into Ms. F's unconscious sense of vulnerability and her perceptions of others as unavailable, hateful, and incapable of responding to her needs. They also added to her image of herself as unloved, and to the smoldering anger and resentment that seemed to be at the foundation of her depression. These vicious circles had also kept alive her unhappy and anxiety-fraught relationships with her parents.

Ms. F's therapy began, as do most psychodynamic therapies, with an exploration of the patient's present and past life, and of the unconscious motivations, conflicts, fears, and residues of past relationships that contribute to current problems. Ms. F was encouraged to talk as freely as she could; to report dreams, fantasies, and idle thoughts; and to examine her interaction with the therapist as well. The therapist listened closely, asked Ms. F questions, and occasionally offered interpretations of the unconscious processes to which Ms. F's communications might be alluding.

These standard psychodynamic methods, however, were supplemented by integrative work at Tiers 1 and 2. The therapist targeted those behavioral, cognitive, experiential, and interpersonal variables that might benefit from integrative intervention. These integrative efforts always were considered with at least a dual purpose: to assist Ms. F to change an ineffective, problematic issue in Tiers 1 and 2, and potentially to resolve unconscious conflict and to change her ways of experiencing herself and other people at Tier 3.

Two central types of integrative work in Tiers 1 and 2 were used during Ms. F's therapy. The first was employed during the early weeks of the therapy, when it became obvious how weighed down Ms. F was by her insistence on "filling in the gaps" left by those people in her life who shirked important responsibilities, knowing that Ms. F would take over. These internal demands, which manifested themselves in the form of thoughts such as "I should be able to do more without complaining" or "If I don't take over here, they'll be angry" (Tier 2), were modified by standard cognitive techniques of recording one's thoughts, evaluating the evidence for them, and refuting or modifying that way of thinking based on this examination. Changing these thoughts was seen as advantageous and important by the therapist for several reasons. First, change in this way of thinking obviously would reduce Ms. F's experience of being overwhelmed, of always being behind in things, and would lessen her anxiety and make her less prone to panic. Second, this reduction in suffering might stabilize a rather shaky therapeutic relationship in which Ms. F had been having some difficulty letting go of her transferential reactions to the therapist, whom she experienced as a parent who expected her to meet everyone else's needs. Third, it had become clear that the pain and preoccupation caused by these deeply familiar and ingrained thoughts and behavioral patterns had become defenses against the anger, resentment, and neediness they continued to evoke. In the sessions, these issues had become resistances that precluded any exploration of such psychodynamic meanings and origins.

This integrative intervention accomplished much. Ms. F became less anxious and prone to panic as she learned to "stop filling in." At the same time, she achieved important insight into her history and its transference manifestation in the therapy. This technique helped her to experience her therapist as someone who wanted her to take on less and to get more out of life, therefore enabling Ms. F to make a crucial discrimination between her transference and her real experience of the therapist. As she saw in a deeply felt way how she had come to perceive the therapist as someone from her past, she began to explore the ways in which these transference perceptions influenced her relationships outside therapy, specifically with regard to the frequency with which she cast potential friends and lovers in the role of her hurtful siblings and parents. Finally, as her need "to fill in" became less pressing and less frequent, Ms. F was able to relax her resistance against exploring these issues. Her new understanding of her unconscious fear of being unlovable, and of the resulting self-hatred that this self-perception had generated, allowed Ms. F the chance to reevaluate those mental representations. In addition, as she more frequently took the chance of saying "no," she learned that her worst fears of abandonment sometimes were not confirmed. It is impossible to determine how much of Ms. F's transference was based solely on her expectations as a function of historical factors and how much on the experience of the active therapist in the relationship. Had the therapist been more silent, the same issue probably would have arisen but would likely have been construed in a traditional way: as reflecting a past relationship brought into the present, rather than an active and current way of experiencing long wished for and previously absent nurturance by the therapist.

These new experiences helped Ms. F free herself from many of the interpersonal vicious circles that had fueled her anger and resentment, and allowed her to find a few new friends and to begin to go out on dates. These new experiences had an impact on her at all three tiers. New and more assertive behavior was accepted and therefore tacitly reinforced by new friends. Her progress in modulating her conscious fears and concerns about "filling in" also were supported. And, at the psychodynamic level, these new relationships gradually helped Ms. F to integrate the anger, sadness, and resentment that she had disavowed through most of her life. As a result, her anxiety, panic, and depression gradually abated.

As Ms. F's therapy continued, her dreams and the contents of her conversation in sessions began to coalesce around the death of her mother and the unresolved grief connected with that loss. Psychodynamic work did not seem helpful. Ms. F noted that although she had attained a much greater intellectual appreciation of the effects of her unresolved grief, she could not feel much about this event or its aftermath. Attempts to analyze her defenses against her grief led to nothing but frustration and dejection.

This impasse indicated that an integrative shift might be helpful. The therapist suggested an experiential, Gestalt-therapy-influenced exercise in which Ms. F imagined herself in conversation with her mother as they sat together in the therapist's office. Ms. F hesitantly, and with considerable embarrassment, began but soon fell into the dialogue more naturally. After a couple of sessions she found herself experiencing and expressing the sadness, fear, anger, and guilt that she had disavowed since her mother's death.

In addition to these important changes, some other gains accrued from this integrative intervention. These changes were of immediate conscious benefit to the patient, and they also aided the psychodynamic work of the therapy. Ms. F found that her painful dialogue with her mother had led to a new sense of confidence and more acceptance of her own needs, wishes, and anger. She decided that she would give more weight to relationships with people who were open to knowing about her feelings, positive and negative, and Ms. F began to describe herself as "throwing her weight around a little" with her siblings, and with her father on his rare visits. She also reported that the therapist's active interest in helping her to grieve, and his ability to tolerate and to empathize with the feelings that she had contacted during the Gestalt exercise, had been helpful in allowing her to test, challenge, and modify the negative view of emotional intimacy that she long had held.

Ms. F's therapy lasted about 20 months and was conducted on a once-weekly basis. Approximately 65–75% of the sessions might be identified as psychodynamically oriented exploration, whereas the remaining time was spent working in the active, integrative way described previously. Ms. F decided to end therapy after this period, because she felt she had come as far as she could and needed a break to consolidate her gains and all that she had learned. She had been free from any major depressive episodes and from panic attacks for over 6 months. Her ongoing level of anxiety had improved, though she noted that it was her hope to have more anxiety-free hours and days in the future. Her relationship with her roommate had improved to the point that they had developed a casual friendship, occasionally sharing a meal or going to a movie together, and Ms. F's level of irritation and tension about sharing her home had diminished. She had made a couple of other female friends and was hopeful that her relationship with one of these women could become a closer and more enduring friendship. She continued to date and to feel guardedly optimistic about marrying, though she had not yet established the serious intimate relationship with a man that she wanted.

CURRENT AND FUTURE TRENDS

The integrative therapies constitute a heterogeneous group of approaches and, as such, future trends must be considered in a differentiated way. First, we make some general comments that pertain to all the integrative therapies, then we consider trends that are more specific to different approaches to psychotherapy integration.

There is a paucity of supportive research, a problem that certainly is not restricted to the integrative therapies. Some approaches do have research support (e.g., Linehan, 1987) and others rely on research for the specifics of intervention (e.g., Beutler, Alomohamed, Moleiro, & Romanelli, 2002). However, the majority of the integrative therapies do not have much, if any, support, and this clearly is an area for future development. There is awareness in the integrative community of both the research that has been produced and this need (Glass, Arnkoff, & Rodriguez, 1998; Schottenbauer et al., 2005), and we hope that the future will provide more documentation of effectiveness.

It is important to recognize the breadth of research efforts that are possible. Efficacy research, with its emphasis on randomized assignment of cases to the therapy of interest and to control groups, is not a promising design, because the nature of integration includes the ongoing innovation that makes the required manualization of treatment difficult to achieve. Effectiveness research, which studies therapy as it is practiced in the field, is more likely to be suitable to the integrative therapies, because they are less rigid in their approach to specific interventions and would be difficult to standardize, as is required by efficacy research. This concern probably is true of most therapies, but it is particularly problematic for the integrative therapies. There is a growing sense that research focusing on the process of psychotherapy will contribute more than research that remains concerned with outcome. In addition, when outcome research is done, the focus should be more on the client and the relationship than on the theory and the technique.

Psychotherapy integration is "a growth industry," because it captures what most therapists actually do rather than what they were trained to do. There are many indications of its growth. The SEPI's *Journal of Psychotherapy Integration* and its predecessors have now been in existence for more than two decades. Important compilations of developments in psychotherapy now routinely include chapters on psychotherapy integration. For example, a four-volume handbook of psychotherapy devoted an entire volume to integrative–eclectic approaches (Lebow, 2002).

It is likely that theory will play an increasing role in the development of the integrative therapies. For example, the well-documented observation of the critical role of common factors may lead to development of a theory of common factors (e.g., Arkowitz, 1992). Regarding technical eclecticism, those approaches with a systematic underpinning that guides the eclecticism (e.g., Beutler et al., 2002) are likely to prove more appealing than those guided according to the immediate preferences, preferably empirically based, of the psychotherapist. Both theoretical integration and assimilative integration have theory at their center, and the further developments of these approaches also rest on theoretical advances.

Some well-developed assimilative systems have been presented (e.g., Gold & Stricker, 2001; Stricker & Gold 1996), and we can anticipate that more will follow. However, the challenge for each of these systems is how not only to assimilate techniques from other systems but also to make accommodations in the theory to reflect the value of the imported techniques (Gold & Stricker, 2001; Wolfe, 2001). Despite the interest in separating the four approaches to psychotherapy integration, it also has been noted that the boundaries between the types have become blurred (Stricker & Gold, 2006b).

Finally, we would like to close by reiterating a distinction between psychotherapy integration and integrative therapies. This chapter has focused on the integrative therapies, but our preference remains the process of psychotherapy integration rather than the product per se. Safran and Messer (1997) reach a similar conclusion by endorsing pluralism, emphasizing the dialogue among proponents of the various approaches rather than an ultimate goal of achieving a single, correct system of psychotherapy. We see the future of psychotherapy integration as lying within an ongoing consideration of the challenges of psychotherapy without regard to disciplinary boundaries, whether those boundaries are established by traditional sectarian approaches or by newer integrative approaches. We applaud all the gains made by stretching these boundaries, as indicated by the innovative integrative therapies. However, we hope that these do not become frozen, but remain open to consideration by the therapist, functioning in a thoughtful and creative way, and also by the results of ongoing psychotherapy research.

SUGGESTIONS FOR STUDY

Recommended Reading

Messer, S. B. (2000). Applying the visions of reality to a case of brief therapy. *Journal of Psychotherapy Integration, 10,* 55–70.—An application of the perspectives of a number of therapeutic outlooks to a case example.

Beutler, L. E., Consoli, A. J., & Lane, G. (2005). Systematic treatment selection and prescriptive psychotherapy: An integrative eclectic approach. In J. C. Norcross & M. R. Goldfried (Eds.), *Handbook of psychotherapy integration* (2nd ed., pp. 121–143). New York: Oxford University Press.—A summary of a research based approach to technical integration.

Schottenbauer, M. A., Glass, C. R., & Arnkoff, D. B. (2005). Outcome research on psychotherapy integration. In J. C. Norcross, & M. R. Goldfried (Eds.), *Handbook of psychotherapy integration* (2nd ed., pp. 459–493). New York: Oxford University Press.—An extensive review of the empirical support for many of the approaches described in this chapter.

Wachtel, P. L. (1997). *Psychoanalysis, behavior therapy, and the representational world.* Washington, DC: American Psychological Association.—An expanded edition of a classic in psychotherapy integration that remains the most complete and influential version of theoretical integration.

DVD

Stricker, G. (2009). *Psychotherapy integration over time* (Psychotherapy in Six Sessions Video Series). Washington, DC: American Psychological Associatio.—A DVD illustrating the practice of assimilative integration.

REFERENCES

Alexander, F., & French, T. (1946). *Psychoanalytic therapy.* New York: Ronald Press.

Alexander, J. F., & Sexton, T. L. (2002). Functional family therapy: A model for treating high-risk, acting out youth. In J. Lebow (Ed.), *Comprehensive handbook of psychotherapy: Vol. 4. Integrative–eclectic* (pp. 111–132). New York: Wiley.

Allen, D. M. (1993). Unified psychotherapy. In G. Stricker & J. R. Gold (Eds.), *Comprehensive handbook of psychotherapy integration* (pp. 125–138). New York: Plenum Press.

American Psychiatric Association. (1994). *Diagnostic and statistical manual of mental disorders* (4th ed.). Washington, DC: Author.

Anchin, J. (2008). Pursuing a unifying paradigm for psychotherapy. *Journal of Psychotherapy Integration, 18,* 310–349.

Arkowitz, H. (1992). Integrative theories of therapy. In D. K. Freedheim (Ed.), *History of psychotherapy: A century of change* (pp. 261–303). Washington, DC: American Psychological Association.

Arkowitz, H., & Messer, S. (Eds.). (1984). *Psychoanalytic therapy and behavioral therapy: Is integration possible?* New York: Plenum Press.

Beier, E. G. (1966). *The silent language of psychotherapy.* Chicago: Aldine.

Beitman, B. D., & Saveanu, R. V. (2005). Integrating pharmacotherapy and psychotherapy. In J. C. Norcross & M. R. Goldfried (Eds.), *Handbook of psychotherapy integration* (2nd ed., pp. 417–436). New York: Oxford University Press.

Berg, A., Sandell, R., & Sandahl, C. (2009). Affect-focused body psychotherapy in patients with generalized anxiety disorder: Evaluation of an integrative model. *Journal of Psychotherapy Integration, 19,* 67–85.

Beutler, L. E., Alomohamed, S., Moleiro, C., & Romanelli, R. (2002). Systematic treatment selection and prescriptive therapy. In J. Lebow (Ed.), *Comprehensive handbook of psychotherapy: Vol. 4. Integrative–eclectic* (pp. 255–272). New York: Wiley.

Beutler, L. E., Harwood, T., Bertoni, M. & Thomann, J. (2006). Systematic treatment selection and prescriptive psychotherapy. In G. Stricker & J. Gold (Eds.), *A casebook of psychotherapy integration* (pp. 29–42). Washington, DC: American Psychological Association.

Beutler, L. E., & Hodgson, A. B. (1993). Prescriptive psychotherapy. In G. Stricker & J. R. Gold (Eds.), *Comprehensive handbook of psychotherapy integration* (pp. 151–163). New York: Plenum Press.

Bohart, A. C. (1992). An integrative process model of psychopathology and psychotherapy. *Revista de Psicoterapia, 9,* 49–74.

Bohart, A. C. (2000). The client is the most important common factor: Clients' self-healing capacities and psychotherapy. *Journal of Psychotherapy Integration, 10,* 127–150.

Bohart, A. C., & Tallman, K. (1999). *How clients make therapy work.* Washington, DC: American Psychological Association.

Butollo, W. (2000). Therapeutic implications of a social interaction model of trauma. *Journal of Psychotherapy Integration, 10,* 357–374.

Cartwright, B. (2007). *Integral psychotherapy.* Albany: State University of New York Press.

Chambless, D., Goldstein, A., Gallagher, R., & Bright, P. (1986). Integrating behavior therapy and psychotherapy in the treatment of agoraphobia. *Psychotherapy, 23,* 150–159.

Chambless, D. C., & Ollendick, T. H. (2001). Empirically supported psychological interventions: Controversies and evidence. *Annual Review of Psychology, 52,* 685–716.

Coonerty, S. (1993). Integrative child therapy. In G. Stricker & J. R. Gold (Eds.), *Comprehensive handbook of psychotherapy integration* (pp. 413–426). New York: Plenum Press.

Cummings, N. (1993). Psychotherapy with substance abusers. In G. Stricker & J. R. Gold (Eds.), *Comprehensive handbook of psychotherapy integration* (pp. 337–352). New York: Plenum Press.

Dollard, J., & Miller, N. E. (1950). *Personality and psychotherapy.* New York: McGraw-Hill.

Dowd, E. T. (1999). Why don't people change? What stops them from changing?: An integrative commentary on the special issue on resistance. *Journal of Psychotherapy Integration, 9,* 119–131.

Duncan, B. L., & Miller, S. D. (2000). The client's theory of change: Consulting the client in the integrative change process. *Journal of Psychotherapy Integration, 10,* 169–188.

Feather, B. W., & Rhodes, J. W. (1973). Psychodynamic behavior therapy: I. Theory and rationale. *Archives of General Psychiatry, 26,* 496–502.

Fensterheim, H. (1993). Behavioral psychotherapy. In G. Stricker & J. R. Gold (Eds.), *Comprehensive handbook of psychotherapy integration* (pp. 73–86). New York: Plenum Press.

Fitzpatrick M. (1993). Adolescents. In G. Stricker & J. R. Gold (Eds.), *Comprehensive handbook of psychotherapy integration* (pp. 427–436). New York: Plenum Press.

Fosha, D. (2000). *The transforming power of affect.* New York: Basic Books.

Frank, J. (1961). *Persuasion and healing.* Baltimore: Johns Hopkins University Press.

Frank, K. (1999). *Psychoanalytic participation.* Hillsdale, NJ: Analytic Press.

Franklin, A. J., Carter, R. T., & Grace, C. (1993). An integrative approach to psychotherapy with Black/African Americans. In G. Stricker & J. R. Gold (Eds.), *Comprehensive handbook of psychotherapy integration* (pp. 465–482). New York: Plenum Press.

French, T. M. (1933). Interrelations between psychoanalysis and the experimental work of Pavlov. *American Journal of Psychiatry, 89,* 1165–1203.

Garfield, S. (2000). Eclecticism and integration: A personal retrospective view. *Journal of Psychotherapy Integration, 10,* 341–356.

Gerson, M.-J. (1996). *The embedded self.* Hillsdale, NJ: Analytic Press.

Glass, C., Arnkoff, D., & Rodriguez, B. (1998). An overview of directions in psychotherapy integration research. *Journal of Psychotherapy Integration, 8,* 187–210.

Gold, J. (1992). An integrative–systemic approach to severe psychopathology in children and adolescents. *Journal of Integrative and Eclectic Psychotherapy, 11,* 67–78.

Gold, J. (1994). When the patient does the integrating: Lessons for theory and practice. *Journal of Psychotherapy Integration, 4,* 133–154.

Gold, J. (1996). *Key concepts in psychotherapy integration.* New York: Plenum Press.

Gold, J. (2000). The psychodynamics of the patient's activity. *Journal of Psychotherapy Integration, 10,* 207–220.

Gold, J. R., & Stricker, G. (1993). Psychotherapy integration with personality disorders. In G. Stricker & J. R. Gold (Eds.), *Comprehensive handbook of psychotherapy integration* (pp. 323–336). New York: Plenum Press.

Gold, J., & Stricker, G. (2001). Relational psychoanalysis as a foundation for assimilative integration. *Journal of Psychotherapy Integration, 11,* 47–63.

Gold, J., & Stricker, G. (2006). An overview of psychotherapy integration. In G. Stricker & J. Gold (Eds.), *A casebook of psychotherapy integration* (pp. 3–16.) Washington, DC: American Psychological Association.

Goldfried, M. (1999). A participant–observer's perspective on psychotherapy integration. *Journal of Psychotherapy Integration, 9,* 235–242.

Greenberg, L. S., Rice, L. N., & Elliott, R. (1993). *Facilitating emotional change.* New York: Guilford Press.

Guidano, V. F., & Liotti, G. (1983). *Cognitive processes and emotional disorders: A structural approach to psychotherapy.* New York: Guilford Press.

Gurman, A. S. (2008). Integrative couple therapy: A depth-behavioral approach. In A. S. Gurman (Ed.), *Clinical handbook of couple therapy* (pp. 383–423). New York: Guilford Press.

Hayes, A., & Newman, C. (1993). Depression: An integrative perspective. In G. Stricker & J. R. Gold (Eds.), *Comprehensive handbook of psychotherapy integration* (pp. 303–322). New York: Plenum Press.

Hayes, S. C., Strosahl, K. D., & Wilson, K. G. (1999). *Acceptance and commitment therapy: An experiential approach to behavior change.* New York: Guilford Press.

Hellkamp, D. (1993). Severe mental disorders. In G. Stricker & J. R. Gold (Eds.), *Comprehensive handbook of psychotherapy integration* (pp. 385–400). New York: Plenum Press.

Hickman, E. E., Arnkoff, D. B., Glass, C. R., & Schottenbauer, M. A. (2009). Psychotherapy integration as practiced by experts. *Psychotherapy: Theory, Research, Practice, and Training, 46,* 486–491.

Hilsenroth, M., & Slavin, J. (2008). Integrative dynamic therapy for comorbid depression and borderline conditions. *Journal of Psychotherapy Integration, 18,* 377–409.

Klein, S. B. (2009). *Learning: Principles and applications* (5th ed.). Thousand Oaks, CA: Sage.

Klerman, G., Weissman, M., Rounsaville, B., & Chevron, E. (1984). *Interpersonal psychotherapy of depression.* New York: Basic Books.

Knack, W. (2009). Psychotherapy and alcoholics anonymous: An integrated approach. *Journal of Psychotherapy Integration, 19,* 86–109.

Lazarus, A. A. (1976). *Multimodal behavior therapy.* New York: Springer.

Lazarus, A. A. (2006). Multimodal therapy: A seven point integration. In G. Stricker & J. Gold (Eds.), *A casebook of psychotherapy integration* (pp. 17–28). Washington, DC: American Psychological Association.

Lebow, J. (Ed.). (2002). *Comprehensive handbook of psychotherapy: Vol. 4. Integrative–eclectic.* New York: Wiley.

Lebow, J. (2006). Integrative couple therapy. In G. Stricker & J. Gold (Eds.), *A casebook of psychotherapy integration* (pp. 211–224.) Washington, DC: American Psychological Association.

Levenson, H. (1995). *Time-limited dynamic psychotherapy.* New York: Basic Books.

Liddle, H. A. (1982). On the problems of eclecticism: A call for epistemologic clarification and human-scale theories. *Family Process, 21,* 243–250.

Linehan, H. (1987). Dialectical behavior therapy for borderline personality disorder. *Bulletin of the Menninger Clinic, 51,* 261–276.

Madu, S. (1991). Problems of "Western" psychotherapy practice in Nigeria. *Journal of Integrative and Eclectic Psychotherapy, 10,* 68–75.

Magnavita, J. (2008). Toward unification of clinical science: The next wave in the evolution of psychotherapy? *Journal of Psychotherapy Integration, 18,* 264–291.

Magnavita, J., & Carlson, R. (2003). Short-term restructuring psychotherapy. *Journal of Psychotherapy Integration, 13,* 264–299.

Marcotte, D., & Safran, J. D. (2002). Cognitive-interpersonal psychotherapy. In J. Lebow (Ed.), *Comprehensive handbook of psychotherapy: Vol. 4. Integrative–eclectic* (pp. 273–294). New York: Wiley.

Marmor, J. (1971). Dynamic psychotherapy and behavior therapy: Are they reconcilable? *Archives of General Psychiatry, 24,* 22–28.

McCarter, R. (1997). Directive activity and repair of the self in the cognitive behavior treatment of obsessive compulsive disorder. *Journal of Psychotherapy Integration, 7,* 75–88.

McCullough, J. P., Jr. (2001). *Skills training manual for diagnosing and treating chronic depression: Cognitive-behavioral analysis.* New York: Guilford Press.

Messer, S. B. (1992). A critical examination of belief structures in integrative and eclectic psychotherapy. In J. C. Norcross & M. R. Goldfried (Eds.), *Handbook of psychotherapy integration* (pp. 130–168). New York: Basic Books.

Messer, S. B. (Ed.). (2001). Assimilative integration [Special issue]. *Journal of Psychotherapy Integration, 11,* 1–4.

Messer, S. B. (2006). Psychotherapy integration using contrasting visions of reality. In G. Stricker & J. Gold (Eds.), *A casebook of psychotherapy integration* (pp. 281–291). Washington, DC: American Psychological Association.

Messer, S. B. (2008). Unification in psychotherapy: A commentary. *Journal of Psychotherapy Integration, 18,* 363–366.

Messer, S. B., & Wampold, B. E. (2002). Let's face facts: Common factors are more potent than specific therapy ingredients. *Clinical Psychology: Science and Practice, 9,* 21–25.

Miller, S. D., Duncan, B. L., & Hubble, M. A. (2002). Client-directed, outcome-informed, clinical work. In J. Lebow (Ed.), *Comprehensive handbook of psychotherapy: Vol. 4. Integrative–eclectic* (pp. 185–212). New York: Wiley.

Newman, M., Castonguay, L. G., Borkovec, T., & Molnar, C. (2004). Integrative psychotherapy. In R. Heimberg, C. Turk, & D. Mennin (Eds.), *Generalized anxiety disorder* (pp. 320–350). New York: Guilford Press.

Newman, M., Castonguay, L. G., Borkovec, T., Fisher, A., & Nordberg, S. (2008). An open trial of integrative therapy for generalized anxiety disorder. *Psychotherapy: Theory, Research, Practice and Training, 45,* 135–147.

Norcross, J. C., & Goldfried, M. R. (1992). *Handbook of psychotherapy integration.* New York: Basic Books.

Norcross, J. C., & Goldfried, M. R. (2005). *Handbook of psychotherapy integration* (2nd ed.). New York: Oxford University Press.

Norcross, J. C., Karpiak, C. P., & Lister, K. M. (2005). What's an integrationist?: A study of self-identified integrative and (occasionally) eclectic psychologists. *Journal of Clinical Psychology, 61,* 1587–1594.

Papouchis, N., & Passman, V. (1993). An integrative approach to the psychotherapy of the elderly. In G. Stricker & J. R. Gold (Eds.), *Comprehensive handbook of psychotherapy integration* (pp. 437–452). New York: Plenum Press.

Pelzer, K. (1991). Cross-cultural psychotherapy in an African context. *Journal of Integrative and Eclectic Psychotherapy, 10,* 75–80.

Pinsof, W. (1995). *Integrative problem-centered therapy.* New York: Basic Books.

Prochaska, J. O., & DiClemente, C. C. (2002). Transtheoretical therapy. In J. Lebow (Ed.), *Comprehensive handbook of psychotherapy: Vol. 4. Integrative–eclectic* (pp. 165–184). New York: Wiley.

Prochaska, J. O., & Norcross, J. C. (2009). *Systems of psychotherapy: A transtheoretical analysis.* Belmont, CA: Brooks/Cole.

Rowe, C., Liddle, H., McClintic, K., & Quille, T. (2002) Integrative treatment development: Multidimensional family therapy and adolescent substance abuse. In J. Lebow (Ed.), *Comprehensive handbook of psychotherapy: Vol. 4. Integrative–eclectic* (pp. 133–164). New York: Wiley.

Rosenzweig, S. (1936). Some implicit common factors in diverse methods of psychotherapy. *American Journal of Orthopsychiatry, 6,* 412–415.

Ryle, A. (1995). *Cognitive analytic therapy: Developments in theory and practice.* Chichester, UK: Wiley.

Ryle, A. (1997). *Cognitive analytic therapy and borderline personality disorder.* New York: Wiley.

Ryle, A., & McCutcheon, L. (2006). Cognitive analytic therapy. In G. Stricker & J. Gold (Eds.), *A casebook of psychotherapy integration* (pp. 121–136). Washington, DC: American Psychological Association.

Safran, J. D., & Messer, S. B. (1997). Psychotherapy integration: A postmodern critique. *Clinical Psychology: Science and Practice, 4,* 140–152.

Safran, J. D., & Segal, Z. (1990). *Interpersonal process in cognitive therapy.* New York: Basic Books.

Schottenbauer, M. A., Glass, C. R., & Arnkoff, D. B. (2005). Outcome research on psychotherapy integration. In J. C. Norcross & M. R. Goldfried (Eds.), *Handbook of psychotherapy integration* (2nd ed., pp. 459–493). New York: Oxford University Press.

Seidler, G. H., & Wagner, F. E. (2006). Comparing the efficacy of EMDR and trauma-focused cognitive-behavioral therapy in the treatment of PTSD: A meta-analytic study. *Psychological Medicine, 36,* 1515–1522.

Shapiro, D., & Firth-Cozens, J. (1990). Two year follow-up of the Sheffield Psychotherapy Project. *British Journal of Psychotherapy, 151,* 790–799.

Shapiro, F. (1997). EMDR in the treatment of trauma. Pacific Grove, CA: EMDR Institute.

Shapiro, F. (Ed.). (2002). *EMDR as an integrative psychotherapy approach.* Washington, DC: American Psychological Association.

Sollod, R. N. (1993). Integrating spiritual healing approaches and techniques into psychotherapy. In G. Stricker & J. R. Gold (Eds.), *Comprehensive handbook of psychotherapy integration* (pp. 237–248). New York: Plenum Press.

Stricker, G. (1994). Reflections on psychotherapy integration. *Clinical Psychology: Science and Practice, 1,* 3–12.

Stricker, G. (2006). Using homework in psychodynamic psychotherapy. *Journal of Psychotherapy Integration, 16,* 219–237.

Stricker, G., & Gold, J. R. (Eds.). (1993). *Comprehensive handbook of psychotherapy integration.* New York: Plenum Press.

Stricker, G., & Gold, J. R. (1996). An assimilative model for psychodynamically oriented integrative psychotherapy. *Clinical Psychology: Science and Practice, 3,* 47–58.

Stricker, G., & Gold, J. (Eds.). (2006a). *A casebook of psychotherapy integration.* Washington, DC: American Psychological Association.

Stricker, G., & Gold, J. (2006b). Overview: An attempt at a metaintegration. In *A casebook of psychotherapy integration* (pp. 293–302). Washington, DC: American Psychological Association.

Thoma, N. C., & Cecero, J. J. (2009). Is integrative use of techniques in psychotherapy the exception or the rule?: Results of a national survey of doctoral-level practitioners. *Psychotherapy: Theory, Research, Practice and Training, 46,* 405–417.

Tobin, D. (1995). Integrative psychotherapy for bulimic patients with comorbid personality disorders. *Journal of Psychotherapy Integration, 5,* 245–264.

Van Dyk, G., & Nefale, M. (2005). The split-ego experience of Africans: *Ubuntu* therapy as healing alternative. *Journal of Psychotherapy Integration, 15,* 48–66.

Wachtel, P. L. (1977). *Psychoanalysis and behavior therapy:Toward an integration.* New York: Basic Books.

Wachtel. P. L. (1989). *The poverty of affluence.* New York: Free Press.

Wachtel. P. L. (2008). *Relational theory and the practice of psychotherapy.* New York: Guilford Press.

Weinberger, J. (1993). Common factors in psychotherapy. In G. Stricker & J. R. Gold (Eds.), *Comprehensive handbook of psychotherapy integration* (pp. 43–58). New York: Plenum Press.

Wolfe, B. (1992). Integrative therapy of the anxiety disorders. In J. C. Norcross & M. R. Goldfried (Eds.), *Handbook of psychotherapy integration* (pp. 373–401). New York: Basic Books.

Wolfe, B. E. (2001). A message to assimilative integrationists: It's time to become accommodative integrationists: A commentary. *Journal of Psychotherapy Integration, 11,* 123–131.

Wolfe, B. E. (2008). Toward a unified conceptual framework of psychotherapy. *Journal of Psychotherapy Integration, 18,* 292–300.

Zapparoli, G., & Gislon, M. (1999). Betrayal and paranoia: The psychotherapist's function as an intermediary. *Journal of Psychotherapy Integration, 9,* 185–198.

CHAPTER 13

Group Psychotherapies

Virginia Brabender

Group psychotherapy is a modality that is highly efficient and effective for the treatment of a wide range of psychological problems. To address the great array of difficulties that people present, contemporary therapy groups include a tremendous variety of formats. Yet all of them that have potential for fostering substantial positive change have critical attributes that capitalize upon the unique features of this modality. This chapter describes the rich differences among groups, as well as the underlying commonalities.

HISTORICAL BACKGROUND

In the early 1900s, both the events and intellectual currents of the times favored the emergence of group psychotherapy as a distinct modality. During the first three decades of the century, large-scale events affecting vast segments of society inspired health care professionals to recognize the potential usefulness of bringing people together for the purpose of therapy.

The Beginnings

The first documented group occurred in response to the epidemic of tuberculosis. Joseph Pratt (1905), a Boston internist, after seeing one tubercular patient after another, began to suspect that his patients might be a source of mutual comfort. He also reasoned that meeting as a group would provide his patients with a respite from the loneliness that accompanies the characteristically long periods of convalescence of the tubercular patient. To explore this possibility, Pratt convened thought-control classes, which he and "a friendly visitor" led (Pratt, 1907, p. 29). Although Pratt provided minilectures on the characteristics of the disease and techniques for coping with them, he felt that much of the benefit of attendance was a bolstering of morale and positive emotions: "One [member] confided to the friendly visitor that the meeting was her weekly picnic. Made up as our membership is of widely different races and different sects, they have a common bond in a common disease. A fine spirit of camaraderie has been developed" (p. 29). Pratt encouraged members to record information, such as time spent outdoors and weight gain.

The Concept of the Group and Its Application to Group Psychotherapy

As the century progressed, the simmering tensions in Europe, culminating in World War I, drew attention to the large-scale destruction that could be wrought by a gathering of large groups. The writings of the late 19th-century thinker Gustav LeBon (1895/1985) had resonance for many 20th-century scholars. LeBon wrote about the potential of large groups to regress to a primitive level of functioning, in which emotions and impulses gain dominance over rational thought. Within the group, the phenomenon of *contagion* can occur, wherein group individuals adopt the emotional states exhibited by others, so that feelings travel through a group with great rapidity. William McDougall (1923), who had direct experiences with aggression in World War I, having served in both the French and British armies, acknowledged the destructive capacity of groups described by LeBon (1895/1985). At the same time, he saw groups as having the capability for exceedingly constructive action. McDougall posited the controversial notion of a *group mind*, suggesting that individuals in their collectivity show distinctive patterns of behavior.

In *Group Psychology and the Analysis of the Ego* (1921/1955), Sigmund Freud catapulted the study of groups by raising the question, "What is a group?" This required grappling with the fundamental issue of how a group becomes a group. He answered it by highlighting the important role of identification as a process that distinguished a true group from a mere collection of individuals. According to Freud, members of a group identify with one another through their shared attachment to the leader. He saw members' yearning for an exclusive relationship with the leader as a process akin to falling in love, in which members substituted their own values and principles (*ego ideal*) with those of the leader. The notion of the centrality of the leader to the forging of member connections and the very existence of the group itself proved to be a key tenet of most developmental models of group life, and a resource employed by group psychotherapists in assisting members in achieving therapeutic goals.

In Triggant Burrow's (1928/1992) work, we see in a particularly clear way, the influence of a major intellectual current upon group theory—*American pragmatism*. For Burrow, the group situation is one that addresses problems in living within society. In consonance with the pragmatic supposition that the value of knowledge is in its ability to enhance adaptation, Burrow believed that groups offer an individual the ability to correct conceptualizations of self and other in a way that improves communication and ultimately, strengthens the individual's capacity to forge constructive relationships within society. Burrow emphasized the importance of attending to process, recognizing the latent content of communications, and understanding that the process phenomena exist at the level of the "group as a whole," a term Burrow coined that was destined to have great importance in group theory.

The interest in groups shifted in a very practical direction both during and following World War II. This chain of events created the necessity of treating a large number of military personnel efficiently. Group psychotherapy was a natural choice as a means to accommodate this demand. The phenomena observed in these military-based groups were seen through the lens of the sociopolitical context that created their need. Group thinkers continued to work on the problem of the characteristics of the group as a whole and what distinguished group behavior from actions of individuals operating in isolation. Wilfred Bion (1959), a military psychiatrist who both conducted psychotherapy groups and administered a group program in a London military hospital, provided an account of the regressive aspects of group life that has been enormously influential in subsequent theory construction about groups in general and psychotherapy groups specifically.

Bion (1959) differed from Freud (1921/1955) in that he believed group phenomena transcend the cumulative identification members experience in their common relation to the leader (Schermer, 2000). Bion, influenced by object relationist Melanie Klein, distinguished between the *basic assumption groups*, representing primitive modes of cognition and affect, and the *work group*, representing a more mature, adult mode of functioning.

Bion (1959) held that the anxieties stimulated by group membership invite the emergence of *basic assumption states*, in which the group is in the thrall of some fantasy that temporarily inoculates it against the anxieties stimulated by group membership. He identified three basic assumption states, each of which was associated with a belief about the group. In the *basic assumption dependent state*, the group behaves as though it believes it will be rescued by an all-capable, all-knowing leader who will eradicate members' difficulties. In the *basic assumption fight–flight state*, the group acts as if its survival is in jeopardy and it needs a leader who will either lead group members away from the danger or mobilize the group to obliterate the threat. In the *basic assumption pairing state*, the group behaves as though a messiah will be the issue of the union between two members. When a basic assumption has taken hold of the group, members exhibit minimal appreciation of reality, as most people perceive it, and behavior dominated by emotions and urges. Contrasting with the basic assumption configurations is the work group, in which members' behavior is goal-directed and reality-oriented. Bion's delineation of these different psychological states was important: It furthered the notion that group phenomena exist beyond the psychology of individual members.

During the war and postwar periods, other important theorists articulated processes whereby alterations in the group can change individuals. Kurt Lewin, whose ideas are explored in a subsequent section in the context of field theory, talked about the group and the individual moving toward a state of *mutual adaptation*—a notion that explains how the group can be used to change the individual. S. H. Foulkes (1975/1986) proposed the notion of the *group matrix*, the unique web of communications built by a group. Foulkes posited that the group process provides members with an invaluable resource to achieve communications that are more direct, and broader and richer in expression. Ezriel (1973), in highly specific terms, focused on how the dynamics of the individual interface with those of the group. He believed that it was important for the therapist to identify for each member the type of relationship for which he or she longed, the type he or she feared, and the calamity the member imagined would occur if the yearned-for relationship were achieved. All of these individuals helped therapists to understand the importance of attending to both group-level phenomena and the individual's internal and external activity within the group.

The Popularization of the Psychotherapy Group

Beginning in the 1960s, group psychotherapy transitioned from a modality used in specialty contexts to one that pervaded most segments of society. In the United States, the burgeoning of community mental health centers, due to the Community Mental Health Center Act of 1963, saw the availability of reasonably affordable group psychotherapy virtually everywhere. Some of these groups had a more structured character than had past groups, with methods of intervention tailored to help members meet highly specific goals. Once again, we see large-scale wars having an enormous influence on group psychotherapy. The Vietnam War bred mistrust of authority, the consequence for group psychotherapy being the embrace of groups without a clear authority figure (Scheidlinger, 2000). Groups came to be used for purposes of personal growth rather than the amelioration of psychological difficulties, a development anticipating the current positive psychology movement (Seligman & Csikszentmihalyi, 2000). This expansion in purpose led to an enormous increase in the number of individuals participating in group psychotherapy, either as group leaders or members. Many individuals who took on leadership roles were not adequately trained to assume this responsibility. Moreover, some individuals who were accepted into the group lacked the personality strengths to cope with the feelings and impulses stimulated by the group, a problem intensified when the leader was minimally trained. The upshot of these circumstances was that many widely publicized casualties occurred and bred skepticism in the public about group psychotherapy.

This skepticism was an impetus to conduct research on the effectiveness of group psychotherapy. Although research programs were initiated in the 1960s, it was not until the next decade that studies possessed sufficient rigor to permit the drawing of conclusions about the value of this modality (Fuhriman & Burlingame, 1994). Most studies yielded findings supportive of group psychotherapy relative to no treatment, alternate types of groups, and individual therapy. A related event during the 1970s was the publication of Yalom's (1970) seminal text *The Theory and Practice of Group Psychotherapy*. Not only did this book describe an interpersonal approach to group psychotherapy but also, building on others' efforts (especially Corsini & Rosenberg's review, 1955), it provided a rich discussion of the process factors that account for the change effected by participation in a psychotherapy group. This work was the impetus for many studies on therapeutic factors. This careful attention to process is a feature that has characterized the history of research on group psychotherapy.

Group Psychotherapy in Context

In the last several decades, group psychotherapy has been affected by a sociocultural and economic environment that has created an emphasis on efficiency and effectiveness of treatment. Group psychotherapy is inherently efficient, because it involves the treatment of multiple individuals simultaneously by one or two professionals. The efficiency of group psychotherapy was enhanced further by the development of brief and short-term frameworks for various types of settings, such as Budman and Gurman's (1988) outpatient model and Yalom's (1983) inpatient model for ongoing groups, or Brabender's (1985) model for closed-ended groups (those in which all members begin and end group participation during the same sessions). Short-term models for the treatment of homogenous populations (e.g., individuals with depression, anxiety, or eating disorders) are increasingly available (Scheidlinger, 2000). Effectiveness continues to be assessed by meta-analytic reviews that examine trends across studies and have the potential of revealing patterns that might not be evident otherwise. This meta-analytic work is considered later in the chapter.

Another trend concerns the training of group psychotherapists. A long-term problem in the delivery of effective group psychotherapy services is that therapists conducting the groups have frequently not been adequately trained. Increasingly, the group psychotherapy community recognizes that formal academic programs in colleges and universities do not emphasize training in the theories and techniques of group psychotherapy (Brabender, 2010; Brabender, Fallon, & Smolar, 2004). Consequently, professional organizations have taken on this responsibility and provided organized curricula. For example, the American Group Psychotherapy Association has developed a core curriculum that trainees can pursue using diverse resources, some of which may be accessed within their academic programs or at conferences and regional workshops. Along with this intensified interest in training is a focus on the ethical and legal issues that attend group psychotherapy (see special series on ethics; Brabender, 2006). Finally, much greater attention has been given in the last decade to the topic of diversity, that is, how the practice of group psychotherapy must take into account ethnicity, sexual preference, age, gender, and so forth.

CONCEPTIONS OF PERSONALITY, HEALTH, AND PSYCHOPATHOLOGY

L. Cody Marsh (1931), one of the first group psychotherapists, said, "By the crowd have they been broken; by the crowd shall they be healed" (p. 330). This famous quote reveals the thread that runs through theoretical perspectives on group psychotherapy and its relationship to the individual's personality. It suggests that personality is forged through interaction with others, and that personality is, in large part, defined by an individual's relational patterns. When we say a person is "outgoing," "shy," "stubborn," "rebellious," "domineering," or "passive," we are talking about attributes that are aspects of both personality and interpersonal relations. The theoretical approaches that inform the practice of group psychotherapy subscribe to the notion that personality is rooted in, and defined by, interpersonal relations.

Four theoretical strains have had a large influence on group psychotherapy practice— interpersonal theory, psychodynamic theory, systems theory, and action-oriented approaches. Three of these were identified by Robert Dies in his 1992 review of theory in group psychotherapy. However, developments since that time warrant the addition of systems theory as a major class of model. Each of these models has somewhat different views on personality, health, and psychopathology. Particular models frequently involve some combination of these four theoretical orientations.

Interpersonal Orientation

The founder of the interpersonal school, Harry Stack Sullivan (1940, 1953), held that personality has its foundation in the longing of the child to establish a secure attachment with others. The child both perceives his or her interpersonal world and acts in that world in such a way as to enable him or her to feel a strong sense of connection to and acceptance by others, especially the parents. Whatever perceptual and behavioral patterns the child establishes during his or her early years become *formative*—that is, basic features of personality.

Suppose a child, Peter, must contend with the difficulty of establishing an emotional bond with a parent whose affect toward him ranges between indifference and hostility. Peter may respond to this challenge by reinterpreting the parent's hostility as concern (a phenomenon Sullivan labeled a *parataxic distortion*) and engage in behavior to evoke concern (hostility) and avoid indifference. While Peter is a child, his reinterpretation has adaptive value in that it enables him to gratify his longings for attachment. Yet when Peter reaches adulthood, the selective perception of feelings and behaviors attached to this misperception is no longer adaptive. It might, for example, lead Peter to strive to evoke hostility in others, thereby preventing him from enjoying authentically positive emotional interactions.

The interpersonal view of personality is highly compatible with group psychotherapy, because this modality provides a venue wherein parataxic distortions can be corrected by the individual's access to the observations of group members. Members in the group have the opportunity to obtain feedback on others' perceptions of their behaviors, and the reactions members have to those behaviors. In an interpersonally oriented group, Peter would achieve greater acuity in reading others' feelings toward him, because the group culture would promote members' speaking about their feelings with greater openness than what Peter would encounter in his life outside the group. This information would allow him to disentangle anger, indifference, and affection. He would also come to identify what relational patterns elicit these different feelings in the other members and, by extension, those outside of the group. This idea that the learning a member achieves with the group is transferable outside involves another concept critical to interpersonal theory: the *group as a microcosm* (or little world). From an interpersonal perspective, individuals manifest their interpersonal style wherever they go. Particularly conducive to the manifestation of different aspects of this style is a circumstance in which the individual must interact with a great range of personalities. The psychotherapy group is just such a situation: Inevitably within the group, those behaviors that create difficulties for members in their everyday lives will appear and evoke responses characteristic of those reactions of others outside of the group.

Psychodynamic Orientation

Highly compatible with an interpersonal perspective of personality is a psychodynamic orientation. Within this orientation, many more specific theoretical approaches, such as self psychology, ego psychology, and object relations theory, have emerged. However, they all place an emphasis on the formative role of early experience in shaping personality. From a psychodynamic perspective, personality development takes place across a sequence of stages. Within each stage are conflicts and tasks, and how the child addresses them will affect the individual's adult personality. Impediments to resolving conflicts and completing tasks create a vulnerability to particular types of psychopathology.

The psychodynamic account sees personality as constituting not only those features and processes that can be consciously accessed but also those that reside outside of conscious awareness (McLeod & Kettner-Polley, 2004). A psychodynamic perspective holds that in the course of development, individuals develop mechanisms of defense to keep out of awareness psychological contents (e.g., fantasies, impulses, affects) that are felt to be intolerable to the person.

For the psychodynamic therapist, the group provides a useful medium, because, like the individual, the group proceeds through stages of development. Although the development of the group has its own unique character, it nonetheless evokes the conflicts that may have been insufficiently addressed and resolved in individual development. Group psychotherapy provides the opportunity to redress those conflicts more satisfactorily. As part of this process, some defense modification can occur: Those members who enter the group with primitive defenses that distort reality are enabled to develop more mature defenses that do not run roughshod over reality as most people know it, and that can be used flexibly in concert with other defenses.

Psychodynamic group psychotherapy is a general term covering a variety of more specific theories, such as drive theory, ego psychology, object relations theory, self psychology, relational theory, and intersubjectivist approaches. Each provides a unique view of both personality and psychopathology, and the means by which the latter should be addressed in group psychotherapy. Object relations theory serves here as an example.

Like interpersonal theory, object relations theory sees the individual as, above all, relationship seeking. As the infant and then the child interacts with others, the object relations position holds, he or she forms templates of experiences that then guide future interactions. The infant's organization of experiences is influenced by his or her developmental status. Early on in development, the infant uses splitting to organize internal representations, separating those associated with pleasure versus pain. As the infant matures, the capacity to integrate positive and negative representations increases. This integration is crucial to the individual's capacity to see the self and others realistically—as an admixture of characteristics both positive and negative. Yet to accomplish this feat and sustain it, the child must have a sense that the positive dimension of experience prevails over the negative. Without this sense, the child reverts back to a position in which splitting is used as a core defense, thereby hindering him or her from seeing others and the self in a holistic and balanced way. However, once achieved, the child can move into a position in which other types of relationship issues—for example, Oedipal conflicts—can have their shaping role upon the personality.

The object relations approach is especially helpful in understanding how group psychotherapy can address difficulties of individuals with severe psychopathology. The basic principle is that if individuals have sustained experiences with other human beings that are incongruous with their representations, eventually those representations can be modified. The psychotherapy group provides a special atmosphere in which individual members have the opportunity to have interactions that represent a substantial departure from those of the past. This circumstance provides the opportunity for revision of templates.

This special atmosphere is characterized by several features. First, predictability and accompanying safety are created by stable boundaries—constancy of time, place, and membership. Second, the therapist fosters the norm of understanding reactions rather than acting on them. Certainly, members' honoring of this injunction is itself a developmental process. However, consistently, the therapist fosters the goal of identifying impulses and feelings, and understanding rather than acting upon them. This emphasis interrupts the often downward spiral that occurs when one member responds to another's unbridled expression of negative affect (Kibel, 1981). Third, the therapist incorporates as one of his or her core leadership functions the support of members in managing their negative reactions. Many of members' most intense negative reactions during the early life of the group are directed toward the therapist, because, early in its development, the group is highly absorbed with authority issues. Members may attempt to rid themselves of angry feelings by projecting them upon the therapist. For example, suppose Alicia becomes enraged at the group psychotherapist because he will not tell her whether she should confront her stepfather about childhood sexual abuse. She alleges that the therapist's withholding of counsel is a hostile gesture due to the therapist's envy because Alicia was better able than he to help the other members. The therapist listens with sensitivity to Alicia's complaint and empathizes with the deprivation she and other members experience when they feel they are left to make such critical decisions on their own. By responding in a nonretaliatory way and by maintaining his therapeutic bearing, the therapist contains Alicia's hostility (Bion, 1959). Rather than dispute the projection concerning the hostility and envy, the therapist merely accepts it until Alicia can reown these affect states. When Alicia does reown the projected content, she also internalizes the therapist's capacity to retain control in the presence of affect, and thereby achieves greater control of affective life—a degree of control that expands her tolerance of affect.

Systems Theory

Lewin (1951) characterized the group as a force field residing within an environment or life space. As the group moves toward its goals, forces inside both the group and the life space drive the group toward its goals, and other forces restrain the group from achieving its goals. For example, in an inpatient group, constant interruptions of group sessions by a broken fire alarm would be a *restraining force*, as would the group therapist's frequent cancellation of sessions. On the other hand, the treatment team's support of members' arriving at the session in a timely way would be a *driving force*, as would group members' development of a norm to remain within the session until it is over. Whether a group achieves its goals depends upon the relative weight of driving and restraining forces. Each group member can also be understood as a force field existing within the broader life space of the group. Just like the group at large, each individual member has goals, the pursuit of which is affected by driving and restraining forces. The goals, driving forces, and restraining forces all constitute aspects of personality. Psychological health is achieved when a system can continue to grow in consonance with its values, while achieving a relationship with the environment that is mutually sustaining.

Psychopathology, within this framework, is understood in a way that is largely compatible with psychodynamic theory: It is an imbalance between driving and restraining forces in the direction of the latter. For example, a group member who was unable to fulfill the goal of separating from her parents during her early adulthood may be stymied by the restraining force of her dependency on her parents for the regulation of her self-esteem. Within the group, she may show a relatively high dependence on the approval of the therapist and, concomitantly, demonstrate a lack of interest in connecting with peers. Her goal would be to lessen the restraining forces of reliance upon caretakers, so that her drives toward development would be unleashed.

Another historical influence on systems applications of group psychotherapy was the open systems theory of von Bertalanffy (1950), which provided further illumination of the interrelationships among the group, the individual members, and the broader environment. Von Bertalanffy described a *system* as a concatenation of elements that affect and are affected by all of the other elements in a system. Any system comprises subsystems, and is itself a subsystem of a larger system in which it resides. Within this scheme, the group is a system that comprises individual members or subsystems; each member also comprises subsystems; the group is embedded in progressively broader systems, such as an inpatient unit, the hospital, and the society. Systems and their subsystems, which can be represented pictorially as a progressive series of concentric circles, share structural and functional features. Von Bertalanffy referred to these shared features as *isomorphies*.

Dynamically, the systems and subsystems within a hierarchy are related, in that the boundary between a subsystem and the broader system is porous: It allows for the constant exchange of information between the subsystem and system. Indeed, this exchange of information creates the basis for the existence of isomorphies, in that whatever elements exist within a given system tend to be exported to its subsystems and the broader system in which it is embedded. As an example, if an inpatient unit is characterized by a high level of authoritarianism on the part of the staff, that leadership stance is likely to enter the psycho-therapy group, because both members and leaders will come to see it as the customary way for patients and staff to interact.

The permeability of group boundaries provides a conceptual hook by which we can understand how, by addressing group-level phenomena, the therapist can support the advancement of individual members. For example, many writers (e.g., Bennis & Shepard, 1956) have noted that at any period in the life of a group, the group's activity is organized around one or more conflicts. The resolution of each conflict creates an environment in which a new conflict can emerge. For instance, early in the life of a particular group, members were struggling with the issue of whether to become a group or to avoid the perils of involvement by remaining a mere collection of individuals—a conflict characteristic of this developmental phase of the group. The position of members in relation to this conflict varied. Some members manifested an eagerness to connect, denying the very real dangers that attend forging connections with others. Others demonstrated a marked hesitancy about sharing information and getting to know the other members. Underlying these behaviors were exaggerated worries about the likely outcomes of group members. The therapist, viewing the system holistically, recognized that individuals were grappling with the issue of whether or not to come together as a group.

The therapist articulated this conflict and pointed out how different members expressed one side of it or another. This intervention led those members who had not yet shared their reactions to any prior topic, to declare themselves in one camp or another. Two members said they felt split between the two positions. These members indicated that, on the one hand, they recognized that some dangers existed, but on the other hand, they did not consider them sufficiently significant to warrant giving up the benefits the group could hold. One member was particularly uninvolved, and the therapist wondered whether this member was holding on to a reaction that was not yet expressed. In response, the member brought up a concern about confidentiality. The therapist reminded members of the con-fidentiality rule and the consequences for its violation. Members who had expressed fears about involvement then recounted the difficulties in earlier relationships that had made them wary. In fact, these disclosures were more significant than those of members denying any ambivalence about group involvement, and they prompted others to speak about disap-pointments in certain past relationships. At several points, the therapist noted how natural it was for members to have reluctance about immersing themselves in their relationships with one another given these difficult past experiences.

In this example, the therapist performs a function critical to the systems therapist, which is the *management of the group boundaries* (Skolnick, 1992). For the systems therapist, the group functions optimally when the boundaries between members and the group as a whole, and between the group as a whole and the broader environment, are carefully monitored and maintained at an optimal level of permeability. In attending to a silent member, the systems therapist is ensuring that each member's boundaries are permeable to the group. This intervention both fosters the member's openness to input regarding what he or she needs to change, and ensures that no member by his or her silence will provide a mechanism for suppressing some psychological content whose exploration is critical to the group's progress. The therapist also bolstered the boundary between the group and the external environment by reminding members of the confidentiality rule. Lessening the permeability of the group's boundary increases the porousness of the boundaries between members; that is, knowing that their confidentiality is protected, members can feel suffi-ciently safe to disclose personal material to one another.

The systems therapist sees the thoughts, feelings, and urges expressed by members as residing not simply within themselves but within the group. Different members give expression to different facets of their shared experience. For example, all members in a new group are likely to have some misgivings and worries about what this experience might bring; the member expressing these concerns may simply be more aware of these reactions. In making an interpretation at the level of the group-as-a-whole, the systems therapist is bringing all of the resources of the group to bear upon the psychological challenge of how to integrate different sides of the conflict between wishes to join and to remain insular. Furthermore, the therapist, by using a group as a whole formulation, is conveying the notion that these different impulses are simply the reactions that human beings have. This communication assists members in being tolerant of whatever aspects of themselves they have found objectionable. The cultivation of a tolerance for the multiple psychological facets that constitute a human being increases the permeability of the boundaries between different subsystems of the self. Rather than using personal resources to keep psychological content out of awareness, the individual can deploy them in the enterprise of making contact with others.

Action-Oriented Theory

This family of approaches rests upon the notion that to effect internal change, individuals must behave differently. A variety of group models employ components of action. For example, cognitive-behavioral group psychotherapy typically involves behavioral experiments in which members are given the assignment to test out certain beliefs they have either within the session or between sessions. Social skills training involves members' practicing the microsteps of a particular skill, such as initiating social interactions (Mueser, Bellack, Douglas, & Wade, 1991).

Although action within the psychotherapy group is a common element, no approach provides the depth of theoretical justification and technical development as *psychodrama*, a theoretical approach founded by Jacob Moreno (1969); psychodrama is truly the exemplar of an action-oriented approach. From a psychodramatic standpoint, action in therapy is vital, because when a group member merely verbalizes the way one does in the traditional group psychotherapy session, he or she leads with the adult self, a self in which many aspects of the person have been submerged in the process of becoming an adult. In contrast, bodily activity within the session provides the participant with access to more child-like parts of the person that enrich the self (Blatner, 2000). Calling these less mature elements to the fore enables the client's integration of all facets of his or her person.

The particular type of action this theoretical approach employs is the drama: the individual creates a play to dramatize his or her challenges. This medium, Moreno (1969) believed, is so powerful because, regardless of the origin of the individual's difficulties—whether in childhood or the individual's current life—it brings it into the here and now. By bringing his or her life circumstance into the immediacy of the group, the individual, using all of the resources of the group, approaches it with an inventiveness, vigor, and freshness that enables him or her to change. Drama enables the individual to experiment with new ways of being within a safe environment. Psychodrama is a holistic approach in that it restores the balance among the various systems that make a person—cognitive, affective, and motoric. It affords the opportunity not merely to resolve problems but also to bring dreams, aspirations, and fantasy into reality.

Critical to psychodramatic theory is the concept of *role*. A role is the individual's way of relating to others and to the self. Personality is the set of roles available to the person.

Psychopathology is a severe limitation in one's range of roles, or the fixity of a particular role. Psychological health is the capacity to deploy a wide range of roles, so that one can respond with spontaneity to the present situation and move toward the realization of one's dreams. The goal of psychodrama is to increase one's spontaneity and dream seeking, and, hence, one's psychological health.

Although variations exist on how psychodrama is delivered, typically, this approach entails a highly structured session involving a warm-up in which psychodramatic techniques are practiced; transition to the drama, entailing selection of the protagonist and individuals who will take key roles; the psychodrama itself; and sharing and closure involving the actors and audience. The following brief example illustrates how a psychological problem might be addressed psychodramatically and a few of the techniques involved in this process.

Eunice, a heterosexual female, struggled with social anxiety, which led her to have difficulty placing herself in situations in which she could meet men whom she might date. She felt abjectly self-conscious about her body. Although she was only slightly overweight, she described herself as "grotesquely fat." Her mother had been extremely perfectionistic in relation to her daughter's physicality and would become quite distraught when her daughter fell short of her standards of beauty. This heightened attention had bred insecurity and anxiety, especially in circumstances where Eunice saw her attractiveness as relevant to her ability to be successful. When she entered a situation with candidates for dating, she would begin a conversation with a man, become overwhelmed with anxiety, make a quick excuse, then flee the situation. She joined a psychodrama group of 15 members—larger than the traditional psychotherapy group, but not at all unusual for a psychodramatic group. The current session followed 1 month of participation, during which time Eunice played roles in other members' psychodramas.

After a warm-up in which Eunice and other members practice various exercises both to create the necessary group atmosphere and to develop the skills needed for the psychodrama, the group moves into a transitional phase. Selected to be the protagonist of the drama by the director (therapist), Eunice indicates that it would be useful to enact a drama in which she encountered a man and held a conversation. She in turn chooses her auxiliaries—the individuals who play the other roles. She picks Harold to play the role of a man who approaches her at a social event. She also chooses a *double*, a figure who dramatizes some facet of her internal world. As Pio-Abreu and Villares-Oliveira (2007) note, the double "develops activities [the protagonist] is unable to do" (p. 129). Eunice selects a member to play her mother's voice within her. Another double plays a more confident part of herself, to which Eunice has easy access whenever she is not in this critical situation.

The drama begins with Harold walking up to Eunice:

HAROLD: So, do you come here often?

EUNICE: No, this is my first time.

The director asks Eunice to deliver a soliloquy—to tell members what is in her mind during this encounter:

EUNICE: What is going to be my exit strategy? He is very good looking and I think he is beginning to notice that I am overweight. I'm a big fat pig. I'm going to tell him I'm going to the ladies' room.

The director then motions to the mother to add her commentary:

MOTHER: You never tried hard enough to lose weight. You have no control. No one will ever be interested in you if you don't lose weight.

CONFIDENT EUNICE: That is rubbish! I am extremely successful, and people constantly compliment me on my discipline. And I have many friends.

MOTHER: Then why don't you have any dates?

DIRECTOR: (*to Eunice*) See if you can answer her.

EUNICE: Because I think he's looking at me with the same intensity and criticalness that you do, and so I run. But, of course, no one could possibly do that. When I'm running from him, I'm running from you. But he's not you, so I'll stay right here.

The psychodrama continues, with Eunice carrying on a conversation with Harold. Both the Mother and Confident Eunice are active in providing opposing appraisals of the situation, but as the psychodrama progresses, Eunice is increasingly able to dispute her mother's narrative about her.

In the sharing and closure stage that follows the drama, members of the audience express anger toward Eunice's mother and also explore how their own parents' judgmental attitudes unnecessarily limit their pursuits in various areas of life. Some members wonder whether the parental criticism is really an effort to discourage separation.

Like all action-oriented approaches, psychodrama offers a rich set of techniques for effecting progress toward therapeutic goals. Many group psychotherapists who identify themselves as being affiliated primarily with an alternate theory incorporate these techniques into their approach (Kipper & Matsumoto, 2002).

Many other action-oriented approaches are available to group psychotherapists. For example, dialectical behavior therapy (DBT; Linehan, 1993) is a multicomponent therapeutic package designed to meet the treatment needs of individuals with borderline personality disorder. One component is group therapy, which entails the cultivation of four classes of skills. Group members practice skills in affect regulation, mindfulness, interpersonal effectiveness, and negative affect tolerance. A strength of this approach is that it addresses not only the member's motivation to change but also the therapist's motivation to treat a difficult patient population.

THE PROCESS OF CLINICAL ASSESSMENT

In creating a group, the therapist must determine not merely who would *not* benefit from group but also who are the best possible candidates. In recent years, tools have been developed and tested for this purpose. Two particularly promising instruments are the Group Therapy Questionnaire (GTQ; MacNair & Corrazzini, 1994) and the Group Selection Questionnaire (GSQ; Davies, Seamam, Burlingame, & Layne, 2002). Both instruments primarily identify individuals who are likely to do poorly in group psychotherapy—not those who will do relatively well. Increasingly, clinicians are being called upon to find evidence that their methods are producing favorable outcomes (Burlingame & Beecher, 2008). Accordingly, group psychotherapists need the means of assessing what their group members derive from their participation in the group. Moreover, in order for the therapist to improve the group continually, he or she needs to link progress to processes in the group. Both outcome and process measures are provided by the *Clinical Outcomes REsults Standardized Measures* (CORE) battery (Burlingame et al., 2006).

In determining whether a candidate is appropriate for a given group, the therapist should consider the composition of the group. If the potential member is to increase the heterogeneity of the group on some dimension, the therapist must consider how the group is likely to respond to that member's outlier status. For example, if the member operates at a lower level of ego functioning, such as having greater difficulty with reality testing or affective control, the therapist considers whether the model employed can accommodate that level of heterogeneity. The therapist must also consider the group's likely response to that which distinguishes the member from other members. What is the risk that that candidate's qualities would make him or her a scapegoat, that is, a figure on whom group members project unwanted impulses and affects?

A candidate's suitability for group may be affected by identity-related variables such as race, culture, socioeconomic status, sexual orientation, and age. For example, if the therapist proceeds to accept candidates who may have social concerns that hinder them from accomplishing their therapeutic goals, it is incumbent upon that therapist to address these concerns either in the preparation or early on in the course of the group. A truism worth stating is that no individual should be accepted for group psychotherapy who does not have a high likelihood of deriving benefit from it.

THE PRACTICE OF THERAPY

Basic Structure of the Therapy

In designing a psychotherapy group, the therapist must think about each structural element carefully, because every variable has an influence on the process and progress of the group. A typical group psychotherapy session lasts between 45 minutes and 2 hours, although psychodrama groups tend to be longer to accommodate all of the steps of the method. Hence, one consideration in establishing the length of the session is to determine the requirements of the model. A second factor is the level of functioning of the group members. Lower-functioning members generally use the group optimally when sessions are brief (Brabender & Fallon, 1993).

Another temporal variable is the anticipated length of member participation. Will the therapy be brief (1–11 sessions), short term (12–24 sessions), or long term (beyond 24 sessions)? The relationship between member goals and length of participation is bidirectional. When the length of group participation is prescribed by some entity external to the therapist–client relationship, the length determines the goals. For example, in an inpatient group, a member may remain for only two to three sessions not because he or she cannot benefit from further group work but because the third-party payer will not provide coverage for a longer duration of hospitalization. However, when an external factor does not create a limit, the goals and motivation of the client play a role in determining the length of group involvement. Short-term group therapy has been demonstrated to produce a reduction in symptoms over a short period of group participation. In fact, most of the outcome research on group psychotherapy—research that has been resoundingly favorable—has been carried out on short-term groups.

Nevertheless, when the individual is seeking interpersonal change that is far-reaching, a longer course of group participation is necessary. What the long-term situation affords the individual is the opportunity to proceed with the other group members through the stages of group development, each one of which offers the member an opportunity to do significant interpersonal work (Bernard et al., 2008). Stage 1 provides members the opportunity to explore basic conflicts about being involved with others. In Stage 2, members examine conflicts related to authority figures—the wish to depend on authority and the longing for self-sufficiency. This stage is likely to emerge most clearly in the relatively unstructured groups in which members' frustration with the leader becomes palpable. In action-oriented group psychotherapy, the therapist's directive stance does not create the latitude for members' feelings toward authority to emerge in as salient a way as in the other approaches. In Stage 3, members begin to explore issues related to intimacy, and in Stage 4, they approach the conflict of how to maintain one's individuality within the context of an intimate relationship. Stage 5 allows members to address issues that pertain to loss and approaching the future. Each of these stages requires time, and individual groups vary in the length of time they spend within each stage.

The size of the typical psychotherapy group ranges from seven to 10 members. The number of group members is an important factor in a group's functioning. Too few members deprive the group of the needed multiplicity of perspective and interactional styles. If the number is extremely low, members may fear the dissolution of the group (Rutan, Stone, & Shay, 2007). Having too many members hinders each member from being active in the group, and the therapist from adequately monitoring each member's progress.

Sessions vary greatly in terms of level of structure. Generally, the psychodynamic, interpersonal, and social systems models require relatively unstructured sessions in which members can interact spontaneously with one another. The action-oriented approaches, such as psychodrama and cognitive-behavioral therapy, tend to demand a much more structured session composed of different segments, with each directed by the therapist.

Combined Therapy

Group psychotherapy is frequently used in concert with other modalities. The individual may be in individual therapy, family therapy, pharmacotherapy, or an alternate intervention. In general, the incorporation of other modalities besides group psychotherapy enhances the effectiveness of treatment (Parloff & Dies, 1977). The person may be in individual therapy and group psychotherapy, either with the group therapist (an arrangement referred to as *combined therapy*) or another professional. The presence of both modalities has innumerable advantages. Raps (2009) provided a case illustration of Gary, a hospitalized Vietnam War veteran who had sexually abused his daughter. Within the individual treatment, the client approached difficult topics, such as his experiences in combat, and eventually his shame and guilt in relation to his daughter, which at that juncture he would not have considered sharing in the group. After a year, however, the client himself noted that something was missing. The therapist accepted the client into his psychotherapy group, in which his difficult self-disclosures led to acceptance. Raps writes, "Regarding guilt, the group had come to function as an external, kinder superego for Gary" (p. 81). This experience in turn led him to deepen his explorations in individual therapy. In this example, each modality intensified the other (see Special Series on Combined Psychotherapy [Billow, 2009] for further discussion).

Group psychotherapy may be used in conjunction with medication. The value of adding either treatment to the other is an area of active empirical inquiry, and preliminary findings with certain populations suggest that the combination of medication and group psychotherapy may be more beneficial than medication by itself. Hellerstein, Little, Samstag, Batchelder, Muran, et al. (2001) randomly assigned dysthymic (characterologically depressed) patients who had received 8 weeks of medication either to continued medication only or to 16-week manualized group psychotherapy with medication. They found that participants assigned to the combination therapy had an advantage in the area of interpersonal functioning at the termination of treatment.

Goal Setting

The task of the group psychotherapist during the evaluation phase is different from that of the individual therapist, in that the group design involves the establishment of certain goals. Whereas the individual therapist has great flexibility to set goals for a given client, the group psychotherapist must ascertain whether the individual's goals broadly fit into the goals that have been established for the group. However, very often, the goal that the candidate states initially may not be what is most important to him or her.

LaToya was referred by her physician to a group psychotherapist for the treatment of her depression. The group the psychotherapist had been conducting was a long-term outpatient group, geared to address members' interpersonal problems. Most members remained in the group for 2 years. When the therapist asked LaToya why she was interested in participating in group, she said that she wanted to feel less depressed. The therapist then asked why she was depressed, and she said she had no friends. She talked about having built her social life around her much more outgoing sister, who had moved to another state 2 years ago. She lacked the confidence and the skills to build her own life.

In an instance such as this one, which is by no means atypical, the formulation of the candidate's goal changes during the assessment process. However, another feature the therapist assesses is the candidate's motivation. Were the candidate to have the willingness to participate only in a short-term group experience, then the group psychotherapist must apprise the candidate of both the options within that time frame and the consequences of pursuing any given option.

In accepting a member into his or her group, the therapist is enlisting an individual with more than a diagnosis or a set of psychological problems. Each member has an identity that is informed by a host of factors, such as cultural background, gender, race, sexual preference, religious beliefs, and socioeconomic status. The therapist, by virtue of his or her own identity and range of experiences, may have a limited grasp of the worldview of an incoming member. In such instances, the therapist has a professional obligation to become educated on how these factors affect the experiences and behaviors of the group member. Furthermore, the therapist must have a grasp of how that individual's culture might influence his or her social behaviors. For example, if a female group member comes from a culture in which women are expected to be passive, she may have a longer, more challenging course of pursuing the goal of becoming more assertive than a woman from a different culture. With this knowledge, the therapist can help the member to take microsteps en route to her group goal.

In contemplating any member's goals, the therapist might usefully distinguish between the ultimate goals of treatment and intermediate goals. The therapist in the previous example who identifies microsteps is recognizing the intermediate steps between the member's psychological status upon entering the group and the desired change upon his or her departure and posttreatment. However, sometimes the intermediate steps are achieved not merely by the individual but by the group as a whole. Earlier, I described the stages of group development. Each stage requires the accomplishment of a goal, the resolution of a conflict, or the accomplishment of a task for the group to progress to the subsequent stage of development. From this perspective, the completion of each stage is an intermediate goal.

THE THERAPEUTIC RELATIONSHIP AND THE STANCE OF THE THERAPIST

In addressing the role of the therapist, this section focuses on the common qualities of effective group psychotherapists regardless of their theoretical orientation, the implications of the leadership structure, and the role of countertransference in the therapist's work.

Essential Qualities

Probably the most important research on group leadership was carried out in the 1970s, and concerned not psychotherapy groups but encounter or experiential groups. So influential was this study that it was featured in the recently promulgated practice guidelines of the American Group Psychotherapy Association (Bernard et al., 2008). This study (Lieberman, Yalom, & Miles, 1973) was extraordinary in terms of the range of groups studied, process variables tracked, and outcome variables measured. Individuals participated in one of 18 encounter groups. Many of the participants were involved in these groups as part of their matriculation in a "Race and Prejudice" course. Experienced clinicians observed the groups as they took place, and a factor analysis of the observations yielded four leadership functions: executive, caring, meaning attribution, and emotional stimulation. These functions were then linked to outcome. What is helpful about this study is that it identifies those functions that are important to consider across theoretical models.

- The *executive function* comprehends those structural activities that enable the group to run. A partial list of executive activities includes recruiting members, goal setting, directing members' actions, and enforcing rules. The investigators found that a moderate level of executive function is optimal. A group with a low level of executive function lacks clear direction. A high level can deprive members of the necessary leeway to show their typical social behaviors. Even models that require the therapist to take a highly directive role, such as cognitive-behavioral therapy and psychodrama, to be optimally effective must accord members the freedom to build in latitude for members to reveal their social selves.

- The *caring function* entails the leader's demonstration of affection toward and protection of the group member. As Lieberman et al. (1973) describe it, "Stylistically, such leaders express considerable warmth, acceptance, genuineness, and a real concern for other human beings in the group. The style is characterized by the establishment of specific, definable, personal relationships to particular group members who [*sic*] the leader works with in a caring manner" (p. 238). These investigators found that the more caring the leader, the more favorable the group outcomes.

- *Meaning attribution* is the provision of structures that enable members to make sense of their experiences. Many of the theoretical models make a contribution in offering the therapist a vocabulary and awareness of a set of relationships by which members can organize their reactions to group events. The relationship between meaning attribution and outcome is positive and direct: the more, the better. In a study by Lieberman and Golant (2002), professional leadership of support groups composed of cancer patients resulted in lower depression, fewer physical problems, more favorable well-being, and better functioning. Management–executive behaviors also contributed to positive outcomes.

- *Emotional stimulation* is an activity of the therapist that enhances members' engagement in the group and is often accompanied by emotional expression. For example, when the therapist calls attention to the group process a function of emotional stimulation is being served. The therapist's self-disclosure can be highly provocative and stimulating to the group. The relationship between emotional stimulation and outcome is curvilinear. A moderate level is optimal and far preferable to high and low levels of emotional stimulation. At low levels, group members are insufficiently activated, and at high levels, they are insufficiently secure. An example of a low level of emotional stimulation is a circumstance in which the therapist avoids calling attention to group process; such a circumstance reduces the group to little more than an indifferent conversation about issues, much like members would have in their lives outside the group. An example of a high level is the situation in which the therapist engages in risky self-disclosure—for example, talking about his or her own unresolved problems. The research is clear that disclosure revealing the therapist's active psychopathology is associated with poorer outcome and less activity on the part of the group members (Dies, 1977).

The popularity of Lieberman et al. (1993) four-dimension system exceeds its empirical support (Kivlighan, 2008). The original study was conducted with encounter groups, not psychotherapy groups. In one of the few empirical tests of this sytem, Tinsley, Roth, and Lease (1989) failed to replicate the four-dimension structure, but they identified eight dimensions that were consistent with their data. Kivlighan (2008) points out that within other domains of group study, such as organizational psychology, much more progress has been made in isolating those leadership dimensions that bear upon outcome and developing measures to render the dimensions operational. He notes that group psychotherapists might take advantage of the work in other areas of group scholarship to advance understanding of the effective leadership of psychotherapy groups.

Additionally, research is needed to determine the optimal target of the leader's interventions. Should interventions be targeted at the individual, dyadic, subgroup, or group-as-a-whole level? Investigating a youth support group, Kivlighan and Tarrant (2001) found that leader behavior influences group climate, which affects member outcome. The importance of group atmosphere was also demonstrated by Ogrodniczuk and Piper (2003), who studied two 12-week psychotherapy groups, one supportive and one interpretive, for participants with at least moderate symptoms of grief and social role dysfunction. The investigators found that the group atmosphere dimension of engagement in the group significantly affected outcome for both types of groups. Members' perception of a high level of engagement among members was associated with greater diminution of grief and other symptoms. When conflict was perceived to be higher, however, a lower level of engagement was associated with more favorable outcomes. This latter finding might suggest that members benefit from feeling that if they need to maintain some distance from the conflict in the session, they can. However, the broader finding is that group psychotherapists must concern themselves with how members experience the group's atmosphere.

The Significance of Countertransference

Countertransference has played an important role in group psychotherapy, but how it is understood has changed drastically over the years (Bernard, 2005). Freud contributed the notion of countertransference as the influence of the therapist's unresolved conflicts. Countertransference needed to be recognized, because, otherwise, it hindered the therapist from understanding the patient. The contribution of object relations theory fostered awareness that because countertransference has an interactive component, it provides a window into the dynamics of the group. By turning inward and reflecting upon his or her reactions to the group, the group psychotherapist can learn something about the group. In recent years, a postmodern perspective has allowed an understanding of the co-constructed character of both transference and countertransference. To elucidate the group psychotherapist's reactions, it is necessary to examine not only the members' reactions in relation to the therapist, but the therapist's reactions in relation to the members (Brabender & Fallon, 2009). With the therapist's acknowledgment of responsibility for the role he or she plays in the experiences both participants have, each member receives a validation that enables him or her also to take responsibility and to make him or herself vulnerable within the group.

Leadership Structure

Group psychotherapy may be conducted using a solo or a cotherapy format. Occasionally, three or more leaders are present, but this circumstance is fairly unusual and occurs in circumstances where the leadership is unstable (e.g., in a psychiatric hospital in which the group convenes on days particular staff are off duty) or the management issues are so significant as to require additional human resources. Whether solo or cotherapy is employed is an important design feature of the group. Solo therapy creates the greatest intensity of reactions toward the leader and provides a fertile medium for exploration of authority-related conflicts (Brabender, 2002). On the other hand, the partnership of cotherapy provides each therapist the opportunity to receive peer feedback on his or her behavior in the group. Cotherapy provides greater continuity for the group, because when one therapist is absent, the other can lead the group. Finally, in certain types of groups in which major management problems exist (as is sometimes true in inpatient groups), one therapist can be available to manage individual member issues (e.g., a member leaving the group in a state of distress) while the other remains with the group.

Cotherapy requires that the cotherapists attend carefully to their relationship. Dugo and Beck (1997) noted that cotherapists proceed through developmental stages just as members do. In order for the group to grow and flourish, the relationship between cotherapists must itself have progressed to a mature level. Cotherapists must have engaged in sufficient dialogue to embrace a common set of goals and processes, and have achieved a capacity to be candid with one another. Effective functioning as a cotherapy pair requires that members of the team regularly process their observations of, and reactions to, one another both before and after the group sessions.

CURATIVE FACTORS OR MECHANISMS OF CHANGE

Among the theoretical approaches to group psychotherapy, both overlap and variability exist with respect to understanding of how change proceeds and how positive outcomes are effected in the psychotherapy group. All of the approaches use the interpersonal aspect of the group, so those factors that have been identified by this model largely pertain to the others as well. Hence, in this section I first describe the mechanisms of change specified by the interpersonal model, then indicate those contributions of the other approaches. In the everyday practice of group psychotherapy, group psychotherapists, even if they have a primary theoretical allegiance, typically employ and integrate the change concepts of the other major approaches.

Interpersonal Approach

In 1955, Corsini and Rosenberg published what they considered a comprehensive list of mechanisms whose operation was believed to have a curative effect. These investigators reviewed 300 group psychotherapy articles, extracting 10 factors highlighted by different authors as being important to their group members' progress: acceptance, altruism, universalization, intellectualization, reality testing, transference, interaction, spectator therapy, ventilation, and miscellaneous. Although some of the factors Corsini and Rosenberg specified have received little attention and others have been combined, their effort was extremely important in that it catalyzed research on the factors that effect change. For example, only 8 years later, Berzon, Pious, and Farson (1963) proposed an alternative but similar system of nine factors based on their analysis of group members' responses to the question of what event in a given session was most critical or important to them.

Probably the most significant scheme to influence the work of both group psychotherapists and researchers was Yalom's work, which rested heavily on prior efforts and advanced those efforts. Yalom (1970) and collaborators conducted their own empirical research and came up with a similar list, which appeared in the seminal volume *The Theory and Practice of Group Psychotherapy*. The therapeutic factors included in Yalom's most recent text (Yalom & Leszcz, 2005) are the following: universality, altruism, instillation of hope, imparting information, corrective recapitulation of primary family experience, development of socializing techniques, imitative behavior, cohesiveness, existential factors, catharsis, interpersonal learning–input, interpersonal learning–output, and self-understanding.

Several points should be considered about the therapeutic factors. First, none of these factors is inherently therapeutic, but all are potentially so, depending upon the context. In fact, given certain conditions, any of these factors could have a detrimental effect upon members' progress. Second, not all groups access all types of factors. Part of developing a design for a group is identifying those factors that are expected to have the most significant role in affecting outcomes. Third, therapeutic factors have different types of relationships to one another and to outcome. Some factors, such as cohesion, may create the conditions for the operation of other factors that more directly mediate outcome.

The linchpin of the interpersonal model is the process of interpersonal learning. Critical to interpersonal learning is the notion that members' interpersonal behaviors are more stable than they would otherwise be, and the behaviors that members demonstrate within the group are representative of those they exhibit in their relationships outside. However, the group situation differs from their engagements outside the group, because in those situations, members rarely obtain information about how their interpersonal behaviors affect others. The group psychotherapy situation provides exactly this opportunity but requires that members be immersed in the here and now—in their immediate experience with one another—rather than in the more remote events outside the group. When members share their reactions to one another's behaviors, it almost invariably stimulates affect. For example, Harry's communication to Carlotta that her constant interrupting annoys him is likely to evoke feelings in her such as shame, anger, or indignation. If their engagement in this interaction progresses no further, little benefit is to be had for either of them. Members' achievement of understanding of their affective responses and interpersonal behaviors is crucial. For example, rather than berating herself for interrupting behavior, Carlotta could benefit from Harry's feedback by learning to recognize the features within a social context that elicit her interrupting behavior.

As a mechanism of change, then, interpersonal learning engages various systems of the group member. For example, cognition plays an important role in at least two respects. The individual gains information and, ultimately, he or she constructs a cognitive frame for the information. Affect is also critical, both in terms of the member's recognition of another's affect and the activation of his or her own. Affect arousal fosters a high level of interest in the present situation, which enables continued engagement and processing until significant learning has been achieved. The perceptual system is also involved, in that interpersonal learning leads to a change in how people see others and themselves. For example, Carlotta may interrupt Harry because she sees him as a threat, a perception that may be rooted in early experiences. Through their mutual exchanges, she may come to see him differently, which will in turn lessen her need to interrupt him. Sullivan (1940) would describe this development as involving the correction of *parataxic distortions*, perceptions that may have been accurate or useful at an earlier point in life but are no longer functional.

Psychodynamic Approaches

Within psychodynamic group psychotherapy are many specific approaches, such as object relations therapy, self psychology, intersubjectivity, and so on, and each provides its own descriptions of the mechanisms of change, which vary from one to another. Yet the authors of a leading text on psychodynamic group psychotherapy, Rutan et al. (2007), identify three processes that are germane to most forms of psychodynamic group psychotherapy: *imitation* (an emulation of another's behavior), *identification* (taking in a quality or attribution of another and making it part of the self), and *internalization*. This discussion focuses on the third process, internalization, which leads to the deepest and most far-reaching change, and has the most significant ramifications for the member's life outside of group.

Internalization entails an alteration in basic psychological structures, functions, or both. For example, the defense of *projective identification* involves a group member's projection of some unwanted internal content, perhaps a feeling or an urge, onto an external figure. A member might project his or her anger, for instance, onto the therapist. The member may even succeed in evoking anger in the therapist. However, the therapist will contain those feelings rather than be stimulated to retaliate or to manifest some extreme negative reaction toward the member. Over time, the group member's emotional connection to the therapist allows him or her to incorporate the therapist's capacity for control as part of his or her emotional functioning. This in turn makes the anger less toxic, and the group member's felt pressure to project this feeling increasingly diminishes. In the group member's life outside of group, a lessened tendency toward projection reduces the negative emotionality that imbues his or her interactions. Note that from a psychodynamic perspective, interactions in the group are critical to instigating intrapsychic change. Yet the processes that effect change are themselves intrapsychic.

Social Systems Approach

Within a social systems model, change occurs through the processes of the differentiation and integration of information. These processes can be best illustrated through a relatively recent development in systems theory applications to group psychotherapy—systems-centered psychotherapy, developed by Agazarian (1997) and colleagues. In a systems-centered approach, the members of a newly formed group tend to form subgroups according to stereotypic differences among members, such as different status levels in their lives outside the group. The therapist can interrupt stereotypic subgrouping by fostering *functional subgrouping*, a method by which members are assisted in forming subgroups according to the differences in their positions on basic psychological issues.

Imagine that early in the group, members are preoccupied by issues related to authority figures. The anxiety of being in a new group stimulates a desire to be cared for and protected by an authority figure, in this case, the therapist. Yet members have different stances in relation to authority. Some deny their dependent yearnings, whereas others acknowledge them freely, while ignoring their own longings for independence. The therapists assist group members in recognizing those with similar positions, and as they do so, they form a subgroup (e.g., those who have dependency yearnings). The safety of a subgroup—the absence of aloneness with a position—enables subgroup members to explore the differences among them. This potential for differentiation is especially likely to be realized if the therapist intervenes in a way that supports the individuating process. As members witness similar activity of the alternative subgroup (e.g., those who long for independence), they increasingly recognize that their positions are not so disparate from those of particular members of the opposing subgroup—in fact, they may be less disparate from the positions of certain members of their own subgroup. Members' growing identification with the positions of members in the alternative subgroup leads to the dissolution of the subgrouping structure: Cohesion is restored and members feel themselves to be one group. The dismantling of the subgroups is all important: Because members' boundaries are porous to the group as a whole, the integration of positions toward, in this example, dependency, is one in which all members participate. They thereby achieve a higher level of integration in themselves—that is, they can integrate that part of each member that wants to rely utterly on authority and that part that wants to be self-sufficient. A rigid, nonporous boundary between these two sectors of self becomes unnecessary.

Although the example here concerns functional subgrouping, all applications of systems approaches rely upon the maintenance of porous boundaries, the increasing exchange of information among subsystems of a system, and the eventual integration of information. In addition, applications of systems approaches rely upon group mechanisms that foster the development of the system and its increased harmony with the environment in which the system is ensconced.

Action-Oriented Approaches

The action-oriented approaches emphasize the transformative role that action can have in fostering a change in cognitive schemas and affects. We have seen how, in psychodrama, the experimentation with new roles—novel modes of responding to others—engenders an internal shift by which the person expands his or her cognitive–affective repertoire to accommodate the new role. In our example, Eunice's role play with Harold and others first invites her to act like a confident person who can sustain a conversation, but ultimately makes it possible for her to have the authentic confidence and attitudes to sustain such interactions in her life outside of therapy.

The group component of DBT (Linehan, 1993) is like many psychoeducational action-oriented approaches, in that it emphasizes the cultivation of skills, the acquisition of which enables members to negotiate more successfully difficult external and internal situations.

TREATMENT APPLICABILITY AND ETHICAL CONSIDERATIONS

Treatment Applicability

Given the variety in the availability of group formats, an appropriate group structure exists for individuals with a great range of personal characteristics and psychological problems. However, three characteristics of the potential group member would suggest that group therapy, regardless of the format, is not likely to be a useful modality and could in some cases even produce harm (Roback, 2000). The first is degree of cognitive intactness. If the individual has a severe neurological impairment, such as Alzheimer's disease, he or she will not be able to track the interactions among members sufficiently to derive benefit from group psychotherapy. The second contraindication is an extreme level of suspiciousness of others. Most group formats require that the individual develop in the early stage of group psychotherapy some identification with, and attachment to, the other members. A new member who sees the other group members as posing a great threat to his or her security will have difficulty constructively engaging with them. If the suspicion is reactive rather than long-standing, the person may be able to adjust to the group. In the former instance, an extended preparation for group psychotherapy may enhance the individual's receptivity to forging relationships with the other member. The third characteristic is an inability to control aggressive impulses. The concern here is the safety of other members. In some settings (e.g., forensic), special resources may exist to ensure the safety of members despite particular members' control difficulties.

As Roback (2000) points out, the therapist must always be alert to qualities that may lead a group member to assume deviant roles within the group. Such role assignments, particularly on a prolonged basis, lead that individual to be cast as a *scapegoat*, a process whereby members project their own negative feelings on to the person, then attack him or her for possessing these psychological contents. Especially in vulnerable populations, this process can lead to negative treatment outcomes.

Unique Ethical and Legal Issues That Characterize the Practice of Group Psychotherapy

These issues generally pertain to the fact that this modality involves the simultaneous, interactive treatment of individuals who generally are strangers to one another before entering the group.

Confidentiality, Privilege, and Privacy

Confidentiality is a condition of successful treatment. A client in any modality will not have the necessary trust to engage in treatment if he or she worries that material shared in sessions will be shared with others. What distinguishes group therapy from individual therapy is that the individual therapist can strictly control the flow of information. The individual therapist can absolutely guarantee that he or she will not share material from the sessions in any circumstances except those required by law (e.g., suicidality on the part of the patient). In the group situation, the therapist can offer no such assurance (Brabender, 2002). The group members are free agents; the therapist can influence their behavior but cannot completely control it. This problem confers special responsibilities upon the group psychotherapist. The first is that the therapist must establish confidentiality as a rule and do all that he or she can to elicit members' compliance. Among the therapist interventions that foster observance of confidentiality is to cultivate members' understanding of the rationale for this rule during the preparation phase. Group members can be helped to see that violations in confidentiality lead to other negative consequences for members, such as loss of relationships or employment. The second is to provide regular reminders of this member obligation throughout the course of the group. The third is to establish consequences for violations in confidentiality, which may include dismissal from the group, particularly if the violation is intentional.

Yet another responsibility that falls upon the therapist due to his or her inability to guarantee confidentiality is to make this fact clear in the informed consent. Members must understand that while the therapist will do everything he or she can to ensure that members do not discuss material shared by other members with individuals outside the group, the therapist cannot strictly guarantee it.

A related obligation concerns the legal concept of *privilege*, the guarantee that what is said within a session will not be used in a court of law without the expressed permission of the client (Slovenko, 1998). However, privilege has generally been interpreted by the court to mean a communication made exclusively to the therapist. In the group psychotherapy situation, a communication is made to a therapist and multiple nontherapists. This feature raises question as to whether communications in the group are privileged. Because the group therapist cannot answer this question definitively, the burden is placed on him or her to reveal the possible lack of privilege during the informed consent process. Members also may be told, however, that the therapist is willing to take steps to have privilege granted by the court to the client's communications during the session. The outcome of such steps depends upon multiple factors, such as the jurisdiction in which the material in question is being considered and the value of the information to the case.

With particular types of groups, special issues present themselves with respect to confidentiality and the individual's right to the privacy of his or her information. For example, groups for children and adolescents often take place in school settings. In attempting to recruit participants for theme-based groups (e.g., coping with parents' divorce), school counselors must recruit participants and conduct the group in such a way that group members and their families are not identified to the broader community as having a particular area of concern (Knauss, 2007).

Multiple Relationships

As noted previously, the benefits of group psychotherapy may be enhanced through the concomitant introduction of one or more other modalities. However, combining modalities requires the group psychotherapist to negotiate certain ethical challenges, one of which concerns the sharing of information the member discloses in a particular modality. If the therapist is the same for group and individual psychotherapies, the question is whether the therapist should ever disclose information obtained in individual therapy in the group. Group psychotherapists have taken different stances on this issue. Some group psychotherapists would argue that the therapist may need to disclose material from individual therapy to preclude the group member's use of the individual treatment as a resistance to his or her group work; that is, the member may share issues and concerns (either about the group or other matters) in the individual treatment and thereby experience a lessened need to explore this material in group. What is critical, whatever policy the therapist establishes, is that it be made explicit in the informed consent process (Brabender & Fallon, 2009). In this way, the client's autonomy is respected, and he or she is free to enter the group or not based on knowledge of this feature. Likewise, the client must agree to the intended plan for communication that occurs between the group psychotherapist and other professionals, an agreement that may be obtained at the beginning of group participation. When the group member is seeing another professional for medication on an occasional basis, the group psychotherapist must clearly indicate to that professional the limitations of the information he or she can garner in the group setting about ways medication may be affecting the group member.

An additional problem in the area of multiple relationships is the possibility of coercion. For example, when the individual therapist makes a recommendation for the client to join his or her psychotherapy group, the client may feel more compelled to do so than if he or she were referred to another practitioner's group. If the therapist practices in both modalities, the client may perceive him or herself as highly dependent upon the therapist, and this sense could influence the client's decision making about one of the modalities (Brabender & Fallon, 2009). For example, the client may wish to terminate group psychotherapy but fear the loss of the therapist in individual therapy. The therapist must be ever-alert to ensure that the multiple relationships do not place inappropriate limits upon the client's autonomy.

Qualifications of the Group Psychotherapist

Another ethical issue concerns the group psychotherapist's achievement of competence in the types of psychotherapy groups he or she runs. All practitioners have an ethical responsibility to acquire the knowledge bases and skills for their domain of practice. Group psychotherapy is a modality that, historically, has received relatively little attention during graduate training in the mental health professions (Brabender et al., 2004). For example, Weinstein and Rossini (1998) found that those PhD programs that offer group psychotherapy training are in the minority, and although most PsyD programs offer a group psychotherapy course, generally these offerings are elective. Moreover, based on their survey research, Marcus and King (2003) found that although group psychotherapy experiences are common during predoctoral psychology internship, they are also narrow in terms of the types of groups interns conduct, the time frame of the groups, and the theoretical orientation used.

This training deficit places greater responsibility in crafting an individual training program on the individual who wishes to become a competent group psychotherapist than on individuals pursuing other modalities (Brabender, 2010). A useful strategy for the individual who seeks to complete his or her training is to affiliate with a national organization associated with the advancement of group psychotherapy, such as the American Group Psychotherapy Association or the Association for Specialists in Group Work. These organizations offer an array of educational resources that enable the trainee to remedy gaps in his or her training.

RESEARCH SUPPORT AND EVIDENCE-BASED PRACTICE

Evidence of the efficacy of group psychotherapy with a range of populations and problems is overwhelming. Burlingame, MacKenzie, and Strauss (2004) undertook a review of 14 meta-analyses and 107 individual studies involving the use of a range of treatment models. In 50 of the studies, group psychotherapy was compared to individual therapy. They found that the effectiveness of group and individual therapy did not differ. Overall, group therapy produced a reliably favorable effect, regardless of whether it was used as a primary or adjunctive intervention.

Beyond knowing that group psychotherapy is effective, we need to know with whom it is effective. Burlingame, Fuhriman, and Mosier (2003), based on their review of 111 studies, found that the average recipient of group psychotherapy exhibits at termination a more favorable psychological profile than 72% of untreated controls. Among the dimensions accounting for variability in outcome, three have been identified: *diagnosis, group composition*, and *setting*. They found that group members with depression or eating disorders exhibited greater positive change than members with other diagnoses, such as anxiety disorders, stress reactions, and medical conditions. Members in diagnostically homogeneous groups had more favorable outcomes than members in heterogeneous groups, and inpatient group members showed more favorable changes than those in outpatient groups. However, as Kivlighan (2008) pointed out, this is merely one type of homogeneity, and others (e.g., interpersonal style) are in need of exploration. The usefulness of inpatient group psychotherapy was also demonstrated in the meta-analysis by Kosters, Burlingame, and Nichtigall (2006).

Although these findings provide a great deal of support for the usefulness of group psychotherapy, Burlingame et al. (2004) point out that prior empirical efforts suffer from many limitations, two of which are especially significant. First, researchers should be careful to assess durability of change by at least having follow-up assessments at the 6-month and 1-year points. Additionally, they should study retention of group members given that retention rates are highly variable. The generally positive empirical effects of group treatment can be lost if a group is subject to the disorganizing effect of high membership loss. Hence, identifying those factors that mediate retention rates would be essential to get a full picture of the effectiveness of group psychotherapy.

Most studies have focused on short-term groups; more information is needed on the effectiveness of long-term group psychotherapy. A study by Lorentzen (2005) suggests that long-term treatment may benefit a different population than does short-term treatment. In his study, the factors that are typically predictive of outcome, such as the presence of a personality disorder, negative expectations, and intensity of symptoms, had no predictive power on outcome following participation in a group in which members remained an average of 32.5 months. Instead, age was a predictive factor, with older members faring more poorly. Overall, 86% of members demonstrated recovery or significant improvement 1 year after treatment (Lorentzen, Bogwald, & Hoglend, 2002).

CASE ILLUSTRATION

The group featured in this vignette was a private outpatient group. In all cases, the members had been referred for group psychotherapy by their individual therapists. Each member had proceeded through a series of interviews with the group psychotherapist, first to ensure their suitability for the group, then to prepare them for group participation. At the point when members entered the group, they had clearly identified their personal goals and recognized the kinds of group processes they could use to pursue these goals.

The group was composed of eight group members. For the reader's tracking ease, only six of them are described. The group had been meeting for 9 months and had lost one member during the first few weeks of the group's life. The therapist's approach combines elements of systems, interpersonal, and psychodynamic theory.

Members

- *Marion*—A white woman in her early 60s and a successful business woman, whose children had children of their own and remained in her geographic area. She struggled with not only a sense of emptiness but also a constant worry about how much initiative she could take in integrating herself and her husband into her children's lives.

- *Alberto*—A Hispanic man in his early 50s whose parents had emigrated from Nicaragua to the United States when he was a child. He was a contractor who frequently defaulted on his work responsibilities because of symptoms associated with bipolar disorder.

- *Aurora*—A black woman in her mid-30s whose distress was connected to her failure to have forged a committed, long-term relationship. Aurora had a modeling career, which was waning. She felt self-recrimination for having valued career over relationships.

- *Russell*—A 32-year-old white man who entered the group after the dissolution of a 2-year relationship that he had initiated but later regretted.

- *Genevieve*—A 40-year-old white woman who had recently left her husband due to discovery of his 3-year affair. Feelings of inadequacy prevented her from engaging in activities to form new relationships.

- *Betty*—A 34-year-old white woman with three young children, who experienced severe depression following the delivery of her third child. In connection with this depression, she developed the conviction that she was no longer attractive to her husband. Her expressions of insecurity about his feelings toward her were causing her husband consternation.

Group Session

The session featured in this vignette is a composite of multiple sessions. This condensation allows readers to see how change occurs in a group. Typically, however, progress would be slower.

The members were all present when the therapist entered the room. Genevieve told Russell she had been thinking about him since the last session. She asked whether he had been brooding over his lost relationship this past week, and he confessed that he had been ruminating continuously. Aurora responded that, over the week, she had worried about Russell, and Betty revealed that she attempted to think what she could say to help him. Marion asked Russell if he had made any attempt to go out, and with a slight note of impatience, he stated that he had not.

She firmly stated, "Of course, you will never feel better unless you try to help yourself."

"OK, I'll do that just as soon as this session is over," he quipped. Betty laughed nervously. Alberto, ignoring the sarcasm, expressed agreement with Marion and asked Russell if he had thought about reestablishing ties with his parents. Russell answered in a more temperate tone that engaging with his parents at the present time would work to his detriment. Aurora agreed with Russell that in times of stress and loss, family members are the least helpful individuals. The therapist wondered aloud whether Russell doubted whether some other members were particularly helpful members of the group.

Russell muttered, "Well, maybe some are more helpful than others." With a note of anxiety in her voice, Genevieve noted that everyone tried to be helpful, but not everyone had the same experiences, so sometimes relating to one another was difficult. Marion remarked that she was sure the younger members saw her as being one of the unhelpful members. Alberto said he thought he was probably in her club. Genevieve said that it depended on the topic—sometimes a member could understand and make helpful comments, and other times he or she could not. The therapist noted that members were trying very hard to protect others' feelings.

Marion insisted that she did not want anyone protecting her feelings. She had been in the group 9 months, she noted, and felt that some members treated her like a piece of "Meissen china," and in other ways like someone who "just wasn't part of the team." She wondered whether she was too old to be in the group. Alberto said, "Then where do we draw the line? Am *I* too old?" Genevieve said she felt very uncomfortable with that idea—that someone should not be the right age to be in the group. The therapist wondered whether a focus on this difference might obscure other differences that might be causing tension. She noted that disharmony seemed to begin with the interaction between Marion and Russell, and suggested that their interaction, and others' reactions to it, might warrant further exploration.

Genevieve said she felt that Russell had spoken to Marion impatiently, almost rudely, and had she been Marion, she would have felt hurt. Yet she also recognized immediately that Russell would not appreciate Marion asking him if he went out. When asked why, she said, "When I'm at my lowest ebb, it doesn't help for people to tell me that I should be doing something, no matter how right they may be. In fact, it's because they're right that it's so irritating. But, Russell, I must say, you get irritated very easily."

Aurora said, "But I thought Russell wouldn't have gotten irritated so quickly had Marion just waited a little before she said what she said. In fact, I was getting ready to say something similar, but I was biding my time and choosing my words." A member asked her to elaborate and she responded, "I had just asked him how he was doing, and he hardly finished before Marion started pressuring him. It was just too early to do that."

Russell said, "I don't know—I just feel that if she had said what she did a few minutes later, I would have responded exactly the same way."

Alberto said, "Because she's a mom. She's going to make those kinds of comments and you're going to have the reaction you did."

Russell responded, "You know, now that you mention it, I think that's why I get so annoyed. [to Marion] You do remind me of my mother, because she needs to fix things. If I tell her something in my life that's bothering me, she can't just let me complain. She has to come up with something I could do to take it away, and I know why she does it—because she can't stand to see me unhappy. But I would feel better if she would just let me feel unhappy."

Marion said, "I probably do that with my kids. I can't stand it when they're miserable. I want something to take it away."

Aurora commented, "But they need you just to listen. I bet that's what they want from you. Anyway, that's what we want."

The therapist asked Marion how she felt to hear those reactions. Marion responded, "It makes things easier for me. If I could just accept the fact that everyone I care about is going to have troubles, I would feel freer, although I suspect I still might annoy Russell. Honestly, I'd like to know why I irritate him so much."

"Why do you say that you irritate him so much?" asked Genevieve.

"Well, I think I've been the way I have with other people in the group and they don't bite my head off like he does," Marion explained.

Alberto noted, "She has a point, man."

"I won't deny it, but I can't put my finger on it, either," Russell responded.

Aurora said, "Well, I can't say for sure what it is with you and Marion, but for me, Marion does seem more like a parent. When she told you that you had to do something for yourself, it just seemed like a reprimand."

Russell said, "Yes, Marion, I thought you were judging me, and I realize I don't know if you were. I react to you as a kind of parent, and I don't give you a chance."

The therapist asked, "What do you mean by not giving Marion a chance?"

Russell answered, "I assume she is evaluating me, without asking her what she meant or if she's feeling negatively toward me."

Alberto turned to Marion and asked, "Were you evaluating him?"

She responded, "Well, I don't think so—not this time. But I can't say that I never do that. I really judge everyone."

Betty said, "Including in here, including everyone?"

Marion responded, "Yes, I suppose I do."

[Long silence]

Genevieve responded, "I know what you mean—I find myself judging people, and I don't like that about myself but I do it anyway."

Russell protested, "I don't see you that way at all. I never hear a judgmental tone in your voice." Marion and Aurora agreed with him.

Alberto laughed and commented, "It's obvious....she was trying to lift Marion up. She thought Marion might get in trouble for telling us that she judges. So she said that she does, too. And because she's nice and kind, well, she knew we would be OK with Marion doing it if she does it too." Members were amused but acknowledged that this account might have some accuracy.

With an expression of bemusement, Genevieve shook her head. The therapist said, "Is that head shake a disagreement? Or something else?"

"It's disagreement *and* something else," Genevieve responded.

"Say, what?" Russell demanded.

"When Marion said she judges others, I *did* think the group was going to jump on her. But here's the thing: What I said is true. I see myself as a very judgmental person. I have high standards for others, and it's easy to get in trouble with me. Only one thing: I'm really good at covering it up [speaking softly, almost to herself]. I am so critical that I've had to hide it to survive."

"That is so hard to believe. You seem so accepting of everyone," said Aurora.

Russell said, "Yeah, if you think about it, no one could possibly be as accepting as Genevieve seems."

Betty remarked, "What you're saying is making me very shaky. It bothers me to think I know someone only to find out another side is lurking around."

Aurora reasoned, "I know that everyone has multiple sides, so I'm not surprised to find a new one. But somehow, with Genevieve, I find it really disturbing. I guess I count on her to be a safe harbor. If all the group is against me, she will be for me, kind of protect me. Now I'm worried that it's all been fake, and that makes me feel very alone and exposed."

Genevieve exclaimed, "Why would you think I am fake?"

Aurora responded, "If you've been having negative thoughts and expressing other thoughts—positive ones, then, that is pretty fake."

Russell said, "I don't think that means what Genevieve says is disingenuous."

Aurora injected, "Can you say that in English?" [Group members laugh.]

Russell answered, "OK—sorry, I don't feel that Genevieve is insincere and, obviously you can talk for yourself, Genevieve, but I think it's not that what you say is insincere but you hold back on reactions you have that are critical."

Genevieve responded, "That's exactly right. [to Aurora] It upsets me to think that you would think that of me."

Aurora said, "I don't know if I do really think that. I'm confused."

Betty added, "Me, too. When I think about it, I know that Genevieve is not a liar. And I have to acknowledge that I have had thoughts I haven't shared."

The therapist said, "Perhaps others can identify with holding back."

Russell responded, "Are you kidding? I don't know if I hold back per se, but I constantly water down my comments. For example, if I think something a member does in here is revolting, I might say that it is disturbing, annoying, irritating, or something mild like that."

Marion said, "I try to be diplomatic and try not to give advice, because my children hate it, but you see how I fail."

The therapist commented, "Different people have different ways of holding back. But then the question becomes: What are the fears that lead you to present only the positive or to keep certain reactions to yourself?

Genevieve responded, "Well, I worry always about hurting other people, so I do that in here. I worry about hurting Marion and Betty and Russell and, really, everyone. In fact, even with all of my inhibiting myself, I still leave here and feel guilt about different things I said, and better ways I might have said them."

"Have you said anything in the current session that might have caused you to worry?" the therapist asked.

"Just a few minutes ago," Genevieve responded. "I told Russell that he was acting rudely toward Marion."

"But it was true," noted Betty.

"Even so, I would have worried later, because I suspect it would bother Russell."

Russell commented, "Yes, you're right: It would have caused me some consternation, but I also felt relieved when you said it. Being called out on the carpet that way helps me to shift gears, so I can respond in a more constructive way. I'm telling you, I'm better if other people check me."

The session continued, with some members sharing their fears of what would occur if they were more candid with one another and other members identifying those fears, or as Russell did, offering their appraisal of the extent to which the fears were warranted in the context of members' relationships with one another. Typically, this process leads members to realize that while their fears are not altogether unwarranted, they are exaggerated, and their dominion hinders members from accomplishing their therapeutic goals.

Comment

In this vignette, we see a relatively mature group in operation. One manifestation of maturity is that Aurora leaves the group thinking about Russell, and Genevieve wonders how he is faring during the week. This process of members' maintaining an intrapsychic connection to one another outside of the session is a phenomenon that is characteristic of groups that have achieved at least a rudimentary sense of cohesion. In addition, the group members demonstrate awareness of how group psychotherapy works. They exhibit some appreciation of the process of feedback but do not yet show a facility in identifying how to use feedback to reduce interpersonal tensions.

The therapist performed the function of translating members' discussion of external figures into here-and-now terms, based on the awareness that the group had stepped away from the friction that developed among members early in the session. Genevieve exerted a leadership of another sort in reminding members of their good intentions toward one another. It is more than a Band-Aid: it bolsters members' efforts to be honest with one another. However, members avoid dealing with one another in their particularity by taking refuge in a resource that is always available to groups—*stereotypic subgrouping* (Agazarian, 1997), which occurs when members see one another in terms of demographic categories, and unite and divide based on demographic variables. The therapist's gentle challenge of the stereotypic subgrouping paves the way for members to see one another as individuals and to engage in observation and reflection—observation of others' behaviors and reflection on how those behaviors affects oneself. Members' effort to understand their experiences led them to foster Marion's awareness of her discomfort and difficulty in sitting with others' affective reactions. Behaviorally, Marion learned that her uneasiness with others' feelings leads her to interrupt their expression.

Yet, in this example, both Marion and Russell made a contribution to the disconnection between them. Had Marion not taken the initiative to explore further Russell's reactions to her, it would have been important for the therapist to encourage this investigation. In Russell, we see a member who is willing to take responsibility for his behavior, so all that was required of the therapist was to help him to be more explicit about his self-observations, so that they would be more useful to him. Had he been unable to take this responsibility, the therapist might have invited other members to reflect upon whether Marion had actually expressed judgment of Russell.

Marion, it can be seen as the session progresses, has an ability to be quite forthright in her appraisal of herself and others, a quality that is helpful to the progress of the group, but one that also leads her to earn the disapprobation of the other group members. In this instance, Marion is candid about the fact that she judges other members. During this period in the life of the group, members tend to deny negative affects and judgments except when some provocation overrides their efforts at control. Although Marion is functioning in a leadership role, Genevieve's modulation of negative reactions performs another. Her admission is threatening to the group: The person who functions as a protector is someone, they learn, who could also challenge rather than bolster self-esteem. Yet this shift in Genevieve provides a potent stimulus for members to begin to integrate all aspects of their perceptions of one another—positive and negative. It frees them up to share their reactions to others more openly—a step that is critical for each member to obtain the highly specific, individual feedback he or she requires to make substantive interpersonal change. Her admission is also threatening to herself, and the therapist works to help her pinpoint this threat, using her immediate group experience. All members appear to identify with Genevieve's self-exploration.

Although we cannot follow the trajectory of all members over the course of treatment, we can see the work Genevieve has cut out for her. Essentially, the therapeutic goal would be to diversify her repertoire of ways of relating to others, and to expand her range of awareness of her full psychic contents and to accept all of them. The therapist will assist Genevieve to reach this goal based upon the group's stage of development. Stage 1 will require very little intervention on the part of the therapist. Genevieve's self-esteem will be bolstered, because members will show appreciation of the aid she provides them in relating to one another. The therapist will merely support her in engaging in this activity. Stage 2 will be much more challenging. Genevieve's discomfort with negative affect will require that the therapist assist her in exploring her fears of expressing negative feelings toward the therapist. In part, this task will be made easier for her by the therapist encouraging Genevieve and others who share this reticence to form a subgroup. The safety of a subgroup will bolster her confidence in making the difficult investigation of her feelings toward authority. In Stage 3, Genevieve is likely to be a leader of the movement toward the eradication of group boundaries, and the therapist plays an important role in helping her and others to recognize the consequences of the loss of those boundaries. In Stage 4, in which the vignette takes place, the therapist supports members in giving Genevieve the crucial feedback she needs to modify her interpersonal style. For example, Genevieve learns in this session how vital it is to members that she remain within a particular role. In Stage 5, the greatest challenge for Genevieve is to acknowledge any disappointment in the group or particular members. The therapist's assistance in helping her to achieve an integrated experience of loss—one that takes into account the positive and negative aspects—will be crucial.

SUGGESTIONS FOR FURTHER STUDY

Recommended Reading

Motherwell, L., & Shay, J. J. (Eds.). (2005). *Complex dilemmas in group therapy: Pathways to resolution.* New York: Brunner-Routledge.—Section 1 (pp. 1–38), written by multiple contributors, provides a discussion of some of the everyday boundary problems inevitably encountered by the group psychotherapist.

Ogrodniczuk, J. S., & Piper, W. E. (2003). The effect of group climate on outcome in two forms of short-term group therapy. *Group Dynamics: Theory, Research, and Practice, 7*(1), 64–76.—This article is an exemplar of a research effort to identify those factors that mediate outcome and the variables that influence the mediators. Such work provides important information in order to identify effective models and leadership styles.

Yalom, I. D., & Leszcz, M. (2005). *The theory and practice of group psychotherapy.* New York: Basic Books.—Chapter 1 provides an extensive coverage of the therapeutic factors in group psychotherapy.

DVDs

Nelson, V., & Roller, B. (1997). *The promise of group therapy: A live video of a time-limited group.* Berkeley, CA: Berkely Group Therapy Education Foundation.—A strength of this approach is that it is an actual, unscripted group. It is composed, however, primarily of mental health professionals who, because they understand certain aspects of the psychotherapeutic process, cause the latter to appear in more muted form than would be typical.

Yalom, I. (1990). *Understanding group psychotherapy: Process and practice.* Pacific Grove, CA: Brooks/ Cole.—Vol. I presents segments of sessions with outpatients. Vol. 2, focusing on inpatient group psychotherapy, features an entire group session led by Yalom.

REFERENCES

Agazarian, A. (1997). *Systems-centered therapy for groups.* New York: Guilford Press.

Bennis, W. G., & Shepard, H. A. (1956). A theory of group development. *Human Relations, 9,* 415–438.

Bernard, H. S. (2005). Countertransference: The evolution of a construction. *International Journal of Group Psychotherapy, 55*(1), 151–160.

Bernard, H. S., Burlingame, G., Flores, P., Greene, L., Joyce, A., Kobos, J. C., et al. (2008). Clinical practice guidelines for group psychotherapy. *International Journal of Group Psychotherapy, 58*(4), 455–542.

Berzon, B., Pious, C., & Farson, R. (1963). The therapeutic event in group psychotherapy: A study of subjective reports of group members. *Journal of Individual Psychology, 19,* 204–212.

Billow, R. M. (2009). The radical nature of combined psychotherapy. *International Journal of Group Psychotherapy, 59*(1), 1–28.

Bion, W. (1959). *Experiences in groups.* New York: Basic Books.

Blatner, A. (2000). *Foundations of psychodrama: History, theory, and practice* (4th ed.). New York: Springer.

Brabender, V. (1985). Time-limited inpatient group therapy: A developmental model. *International Journal of Group Psychotherapy, 35,* 373–390.

Brabender, V. (2002). *Introduction to group therapy.* New York: Wiley.

Brabender, V. (2006). The ethical group psychotherapist. *International Journal of Group Psychotherapy, 56*(4), 395–414.

Brabender, V. (2010). The developmental path to expertise in group psychotherapy. *Journal of Contemporary Psychotherapy, 11,* 163–173.

Brabender, V., & Fallon, A. (1993). *Models of inpatient group psychotherapy.* Washington, DC: American Psychological Association Books.

Brabender, V., & Fallon, A. (2009). Ethical hot spots of combined individual and group therapy: Applying four ethical systems. *International Journal of Group Psychotherapy, 59*(1), 127–147.

Brabender, V., Fallon, A., & Smolar, A. (2004). *Essentials of group therapy.* New York: Wiley.

Budman, S. H., & Gurman, A. S. (1988). *Theory and practice of brief therapy.* New York: Guilford Press.

Burlingame, G. M., & Beecher, M. E. (2008). New directions and resources in group psychotherapy: Introduction to the issue. *Journal of Clinical Psychology: In Session, 64*(11), 1197–1205.

Burlingame, G. M., Fuhriman, A., & Mosier, J. (2003). The differential effectiveness of group psychotherapy. *Group Dynamics: Theory, Research, and Practice, 7,* 3–12.

Burlingame, G. M., MacKenzie, K. R., & Strauss, B. (2004). Small group treatment: Evidence for effectiveness and mechanisms of change. In M. Lambert (Ed.), *Bergin and Garfield's handbook of psychotherapy and behavior change* (5th ed., pp. 647–696). New York: Wiley.

Burlingame, G. M., Strauss, B., Joyce, A., MacNair-Semands, R., MacKenzie, K., Ogrodniczuk, J., et al. (2006). *Core Battery—Revised.* New York: American Group Psychotherapy Association.

Burrow, T. (1992). The basis of group analysis, or the analysis of the reaction of normal and neurotic individuals. *British Journal of Medical Psychology, 8,* 198–206. (Original work published 1928)

Corsini, R., & Rosenberg, B. (1955). Mechanisms of group psychotherapy: Processes and dynamics. *Journal of Abnormal and Social Psychology, 51,* 406–411.

Davies, R., Seamam, S., Burlingame, G. M. J., & Layne, C. M. (2002, February). *Selecting adolescents for group-based trauma treatment using a self report questionnaire.* Paper presented at the annual meeting of the American Group Psychotherapy Association, New Orleans, LA.

Dies, R. R. (1977). Group therapist transparency: A critique of theory and research. *International Journal of Group Psychotherapy, 27,* 177–200.

Dies, R. R. (1992). Models of group psychotherapy: Sifting through confusion. *International Journal of Group Psychotherapy, 42,* 1–17.

Dugo, J. M., & Beck, A. P. (1997). Significance and complexity at early phases in the development of the co-therapy relationship. *Group Dynamics: Theory, Research, and Practice, 4*(1), 294–305.

Ezriel, H. (1973). Psychoanalytic group therapy. In L. R. Wolberg & E. K. Schwartz (Eds.), *Group therapy: An overview* (pp. 183–210). New York: Intercontinental Medical Book Corp.

Foulkes, S. H. (1986). *Group analytic psychotherapy: Methods and principles.* London: H. Karnac. (Original work published 1975)

Freud, S. (1955). Group psychology and the analysis of the ego. In J. Strachey (Ed. & Trans.), *The standard edition of the complete psychological works of Sigmund Freud* (Vol. 14, pp. 243–258). London: Hogarth Press. (Original work published 1921)

Fuhriman, A., & Burlingame, G. M. (1994). Group psychotherapy, research, and practice. In A. Fuhriman & G. M. Burlingame (Eds.). *Handbook of group psychotherapy: An empirical and clinical synthesis* (pp. 3–41). New York: Wiley.

Hellerstein, D. J., Little, S. A., Samstag, L. W., Batchender, S., Muron, J. C., Fedak, M., et al. (2001).

Adding group psychotherapy to medication treatment in dysthymia: A randomized prospective pilot study. *Journal of Psychotherapy Practice and Research, 10,* 93–103.

Kibel, H. D. (1981). A conceptual model for short-term inpatient group psychotherapy. *American Journal of Psychiatry, 181*(1), 74–80.

Kipper, D., & Matsumoto, M. (2002). From classical to eclectic psychodrama: Conceptual similarities between psychodrama and psychodynamic and interpersonal group treatments. *International Journal of Group Psychotherapy, 52*(1), 111–120.

Kivlighan, D. M., Jr. (2008). Comments on the practice guidelines for group psychotherapy: Evidence, gaps in the literature, and resistance. *International Journal of Group Psychotherapy, 58*(4), 543–554.

Kivlighan, D. M., Jr., & Tarrant, J. M. (2001). Does group climate mediate group leadership-group member outcome relationships?: A test of Yalom's hypothesis about leadership priorities. *Group Dynamics: Theory, Research, and Practice, 5,* 220–234.

Knauss, L. (2007). Legal and ethical issues in providing group therapy to minors. In R. W. Christner, J. L. Stewart, & A. Freeman (Eds.), *Cognitive-behavioral group therapy with children and adolescents.* (pp. 65–85). New York: Routledge.

Kosters, M., Burlingame, G. M., & Nichtigall, C. S. (2006). A meta-analytic review of the effectiveness of inpatient group psychotherapy. *Group Dynamics: Theory, Research and Practice, 10*(2), 146–163.

LeBon, G. (1985). *The crowd.* New York: Viking. (Original work published 1895)

Lewin, K. (1951). *Field theory in social science.* New York: Harper & Row.

Lieberman, M. A., & Golant, M. (2002). Leader behaviors as perceived by cancer patients in professionally directed support group and outcomes. *Group Dynamics: Theory, Research, and Practice, 6*(4), 267–276.

Lieberman, M. A., Yalom, I. D., & Miles, M. B. (1973). *Groups: First facts.* New York: Basic Books.

Linehan, M. M. (1993). *Cognitive-behavioral treatment of borderline personality disorder.* New York: Guilford Press.

Lorentzen, S. (2005). Predictors of change after long-term analytic group psychotherapy. *Journal of Clinical Psychology, 61*(12), 1541–1553.

Lorentzen, S., Bogwald, K. P., & Hoglend, P. (2002). Change during and after long-term analytic group psychotherapy. *International Journal of Group Psychotherapy, 52*(3), 419–429.

MacNair, R. R., & Corazzini, J. (1994). Client factors influencing group therapy dropout. *Psychotherapy: Theory, Research, Practice and Training, 31,* 352–361.

Marcus, H. E., & King, D. A. (2003). A survey of group psychotherapy training during predoctoral psychology internship. *Professional Psychology: Research and Practice, 34*(2), 203–209.

Marsh, L. C. (1931). Group treatment of the psychoses by the psychological equivalent of the revival.. *Mental Hygiene, 15,* 328–349.

McLeod, P. L., & Kettner-Polley, R. B. (2004), Contributions of psychodynamic theories to understanding small groups. *Small Group Research, 35*(3), 333–361.

McDougall, W. (1923). *Outline of psychology.* London: Methuen.

Moreno, J. S. (1969). *Psychodrama* (Vol. 3). Beacon, NY: Beacon House

Mueser, K. T., Bellack, A. S., Douglas, M. S., & Wade, J. H. (1991). Prediction of social skill acquisition in schizophrenic and major affective disorder patients from memory and symptomatology. *Psychiatry Research, 37,* 281–296.

Ogrodniczuk, J. S., & Piper, W. E. (2003). The effect of group climate on outcome in two forms of short-term group therapy, *Group Dynamics: Theory, Research, and Practice, 7,* 64–76.

Parloff. M. B., & Dies, R. R. (1977). Group psychotherapy outcome research 1966–1975. *International Journal of Group Psychotherapy, 27,* 281–319.

Pio-Abreu, J. L., & Villares-Oliveira, C. (2007). How does psychodrama work?: How theory is embedded in the psychodramatic method. In C. Baim, J. Burmeister, & M. Maciel (Eds.), *Psychodrama: Advances in theory and practice* (pp. 127–137). London: Routledge.

Pratt, J. H. (1905). The home sanatorium treatment of consumption. *Boston Medical Survey Journal, 154,* 210–216.

Pratt, J. H. (1907). The organization of tuberculosis classes. *Medical Communications of the Massachusetts Medical Society, 20,* 475–492.

Raps, C. S. (2009). The necessity of combined therapy in the treatment of shame: A case report. *International Journal of Group Psychotherapy, 59*(1), 67–84.

Roback, H. B. (2000). Adverse outcomes in group psychotherapy: Risk factors, prevention, and research direction. *Journal of Psychotherapy Practice and Research, 9*, 113–122.

Rutan, J. S., Stone, W. N., & Shay, J. (2007). *Psychodynamic group psychotherapy* (4th ed.). New York: Guilford Press.

Scheidlinger, S. (2000). The group psychotherapy movement at the millennium: Some historical perspectives. *International Journal of Group Psychotherapy, 50*(3), 315–339.

Schermer, V. L. (2000). Contributions of object relations theory and self psychology to relational psychology and group psychotherapy. *International Journal of Group Psychotherapy, 50*(2), 199–217.

Seligman, M., & Csikszentmihalyi, M. (2000). Positive psychology: An introduction. *American Psychologist, 55*(1), 5–14.

Skolnick, M. R. (1992). The role of the therapist from a social systems perspective. In R. H. Klein, H. S. Bernard, & D. L. Singer (Eds.), *Handbook of contemporary group psychotherapy: Contributions from object relations, self psychology, and social systems theories* (pp. 321–369). Madison, CT: International Universities Press.

Slovenko, R. (1998). *Psychotherapy and confidentiality: Testimonial privilege communication, breach of confidentiality, and reporting dues.* Springfield, IL: Thomas.

Sullivan, H. S. (1940). *Concepts of modern psychiatry.* New York: Norton.

Sullivan, H. S. (1953). *The theory of psychiatry.* New York: Norton.

Tinsely, H. E., Roth, J. A., & Lease, S. H. (1989). Dimensions of leadership and leadership style among group intervention specialists. *Journal of Counseling Psychology, 36*(1), 48–53.

Von Bertalanffy, L. (1950). The theory of open systems in physics and biology. *Science, 3*, 23–29.

Weinstein, M., & Rossini, E. D. (1998). Academic training in group psychotherapy in cinical psychology doctoral programs. *Psychological Reports, 82*(3, Pt. 1), 955–959.

Yalom, I. (1970). *The theory and practice of group psychotherapy.* New York: Basic Books.

Yalom, I. (1983). *Inpatient group psychotherapy.* New York: Basic Books.

Yalom, I. D., & Leszcz, M. (2005). *The theory and practice of group psychotherapy* (5th ed). New York: Basic Books.

Author Index

Abbass, A. A., 398
Abelson, R. P., 8–9
Ablon, J. S., 21, 93
Abramowitz, J. S., 118
Abramson, L., 146
Acheson, D. T., 118
Ackerman, N., 298, 306
Ackerman, N. W., 346
Addington, D., 135
Addis, M. E., 107, 116, 121
Adler, A., 34, 145
Agazarian, A., 479, 489
Ahola, T., 394, 405
Aichhorn, A., 58
Ainsworth, M., 95
Alderfer, M. A., 305
Alexander, J. F., 83, 324, 337, 427, 444, 447
Allen, D. M., 435
Allen, L. B., 127, 136
Alloy, L., 146
Alomohamed, S., 453
Alsup, R., 263
Altman, N., 58, 59, 75, 92, 99
Amantea, M., 263
Amir, N., 127
Anchin, J., 428
Andersen, S. M., 94
Anderson, C. M., 328
Anderson, H., 331
Anderson, T., 251
Andersson, G., 14, 135
Andreas, S., 405
Angus, L., 251, 252
Antony, M. M., 92, 107, 108, 115, 117, 118, 119, 134, 160
Antshel, K. M., 123

Aponte, H., 320, 355
Appelbaum, S. A., 388
Arch, J. J., 147
Arkowitz, H., 427, 446, 453
Arnkoff, D., 453
Arnkoff, D. B., 429, 447
Aron, L., 88, 99
Astin, J., 125
Atwood, G. E., 74, 274
Auerbach, J. S., 95
Auerswald, E., 320
Austin, S. B., 253

Babcock, J. C., 348
Bacal, H. A., 415
Bach, P. A., 189
Bagnini, C., 355
Baker, T. B., 18, 21
Baldwin, C. M., 305
Baldwin, S. A., 377
Balfour, H. G., 415
Balint, E., 393
Balint, M., 73, 74, 92, 393
Ballinger, B., 263
Bandler, R., 405
Bandura, A., 109, 111, 123, 184, 233
Barber, J. P., 78, 93
Barkham, M., 252
Barlow, D. H., 18, 22, 108, 116, 119, 125, 127, 165
Barnes-Holmes, D., 190
Barnhardt, T. M., 94
Barnoski, R., 338
Barrett-Lennard, G. T., 224, 247
Barry, W. A., 353
Barten, H. H., 393
Baruch, D. E., 211

Baskin, T. W., 165
Batchender, S., 473
Bateman, A., 95
Bateson, G., 297, 315, 318, 408
Battino, R., 405, 411
Baucom, D. H., 123, 367, 369, 377
Baudry, F., 40
Baum, W. M., 186
Beach, S. R. H., 299, 303
Beard, C., 127
Beavers, W. R., 20, 302, 303, 305
Beck, A. P., 477
Beck, A. T., 115, 132, 145, 147, 149, 150, 151, 152, 153,
    160, 163, 165, 166, 167, 170, 171, 173, 176, 184
Becker, E., 263, 281
Becker, R. E., 123, 134
Bedard, D., 253
Beebe, B., 76, 78
Beecher, M. E., 471
Beels, C. C., 348, 355
Been, H., 14
Behar, E., 135
Behrends, R. S., 95
Beier, E. G., 427
Beitman, B. D., 441
Bell, J., 297, 306
Bellack, A. S., 107, 123, 469
Bender, M. B., 336
Benefield, R. G., 128
Benish, S., 21
Benjamin, J., 74, 76
Bennis, W. G., 468
Bennum, I., 320
Berchick, R., 165
Berg, A., 433
Berg, I. K., 410, 411, 412, 415
Bergin, A. E., 144
Bernard, H. S., 472, 475, 476
Berne, E., 393, 400, 401
Bernstein, D. A., 124
Bertoni, M., 430
Berzon, B., 478
Best, K. M., 228
Beutler, L. E., 16, 18, 429, 430, 437, 448, 453, 454
Bhaju, J., 5, 297
Bibring, E., 393
Billow, R. M., 473
Binder, J. L., 232, 397
Binswanger, L., 262, 283
Bion, W. R., 89, 462, 466
Birchler, G., 370
Bishop, D. S., 305
Bisson, J. I., 166
Biyanova, T., 225
Blackburn, I. M., 164
Blatner, A., 469
Blatt, S. J., 57, 59, 95
Blau, J. S., 119
Blechner, M. J., 86
Bloom, B. L., 387, 388, 396
Bobele, M., 388, 416
Bodin, A. H., 315, 359, 409
Boggs, S. R., 327
Bogwald, K. P., 484
Bohart, A. C., 5, 11, 223, 228, 236, 246, 249, 252, 265,
    283, 284, 285, 435, 436, 437, 443, 445
Boisvert, C., 241, 249

Bollas, C., 78
Bolton, D., 173
Bomyea, J., 127
Bonaparte, N., 6
Bonchek, A., 410
Bond, F. W., 189, 202
Borkovec, T. D., 124, 135, 165, 432
Bornstein, R. F., 55
Boscolo, L., 317
Boss, M., 262, 283
Boston, P., 320
Boszormenyi-Nagy, I., 297, 306, 309, 350
Boulanger, G., 78
Bourne, E. J., 160
Bowen, M., 297, 348, 350, 351, 352
Bowlby, J., 76, 94, 95, 145, 148, 348, 363
Boyd-Franklin, N., 298
Bozarth, J., 240
Bozarth, J. D., 243
Brabender, V., 460, 463, 464, 472, 477, 481, 482,
    483
Bracke, P., 281
Bradford, G. K., 265
Bradley, B., 364
Brandshaft, B., 274
Bratton, S. C., 250, 252
Brehm, J., 390
Brenner, C., 38, 39, 42, 50, 53
Brent, J., 74
Bressi, C., 320
Breuer, J., 24, 35, 44, 45, 392
Bright, P., 447
Brinkmeyer, M. Y., 324, 326
Brodley, B. T., 236
Bromberg, P., 76
Brondino, M., 336
Bronfenbrenner, U., 335
Brotman, M. A., 165
Brown, G., 115, 152, 153
Brown, G. K., 152
Brown, L., 263, 266
Brown, T. A., 165
Brown, W. A., 14
Buber, M., 265, 275
Buchanan, R. W., 173
Budman, S. H., 349, 388, 389, 390, 396, 404, 463
Bugental, E., 263
Bugental, J. F. T., 264, 265, 267, 268, 269, 270, 271,
    277, 278, 279, 280, 281, 282, 283
Bunting, K., 263, 282
Burlingame, G. M., 463, 471, 483, 484
Burlingame, G. M. J., 471
Burns, D., 160, 165
Burns, M., 127
Burrow, T., 461
Burton, N., 78
Butler, A. C., 132, 163, 164, 165
Butler, S., 15
Butollo, W., 447

Cahill, S. P., 118, 129
Callaghan, G. M., 108, 128, 146, 184, 196, 198, 200
Calton, T., 284
Campbell, A., 416
Campbell, C., 173
Campbell, T. L., 298
Cantor, D. W., 13

Cardemil, E. V., 107
Carlson, J., 396
Carlson, L., 125
Carlson, R., 438
Carter, B., 301
Carter, M. M., 131
Carter, R. T., 447
Cartwright, B., 433
Caspi, A., 227
Cassidy, J., 95, 364, 378
Castellani, A. M., 348, 377
Castonguay, L. G., 16, 18, 135, 251, 253, 432
Cecchin, G., 317
Cecero, J. J., 428
Celano, M. P., 5, 297, 298, 299, 339
Chaider, T., 253
Chambless, D., 447
Chambless, D. C., 447
Chambless, D. L., 16, 18, 124, 128, 135, 166
Chapman, J. E., 132, 163
Charcot, J. M., 35
Chevron, E., 446
Chevron, E. S., 80
Chiesa, M., 185
Christensen, A., 125, 348, 367, 371, 377
Christopher, M. S., 22
Churchill, S., 262
Clark, D., 165
Clark, D. A., 166
Clarke, J. C., 133
Clarkin, J. F., 25, 94, 95, 395
Cleary, A. A., 359
Clingempeel, W., 335
Cloitre, M., 127, 135
Clum, G. A., 128
Cohen, L. R., 127
Comas-Diaz, L., 266
Combs, G. C., 375
Connell, G. M., 312
Connell, J., 252
Connell, L. C., 312
Cook, J. M., 225
Coonerty, S., 447
Cooper, A., 93
Cooper, M., 245, 262
Corazzini, J., 471
Cordova, J. V., 125
Cormac, I., 173
Cornelison, 297
Corsini, R., 463, 478
Costello, E., 165
Cottraux, J., 164
Cottrell, D., 320
Cowan, P. A., 232
Cozolino, L., 15
Craske, M. G., 108, 119, 125, 129, 130, 147, 165
Crits-Christoph, P., 45, 50, 78, 93, 94, 397
Crocket, K., 373, 375
Csikszentmihalyi, M., 463
Cucherat, M., 164
Cuerdon, B. A., 415
Cuijpers, P., 14, 135
Cummings, N. A., 393, 415, 446
Cunningham, P., 335
Curtis, R., 76
Curtis, R. C., 34, 72, 75, 76, 84, 88, 91, 92, 94
Cushman, P., 75

Dahl, J., 191, 198
Dahlen, E., 166
Daiuto, A. D., 377
Dakof, G. A., 336
Davanloo, H., 397
Davidson, J., 156
Davies, J. M., 76, 78, 90
Davies, R., 471
Davis, S. D., 17, 298, 378
Davis, T. E., 108, 117
De Jong, P., 412
de Jonghe, F., 14
De Martino, R., 99
de Shazer, S., 331, 332, 373, 387, 394, 395, 405, 410, 411, 412, 414
Deacon, B. J., 118
Decker, L., 263
Deffenbacher, J., 166
Dekker, J., 14
den Boer, P. C. A. M., 127
Denniston, J. C., 119
DeRubeis, R., 165
Di Cesare, E. J., 355
Diamond, G., 336
Diamond, G. M., 309
Diamond, G. S., 309
Dickerson, F. B., 173
Dickerson, V. C., 373, 375
Dicks, H. V., 353
Dickstein, S., 305
DiClemente, C. C., 395, 429, 430, 436, 437, 448
Dienes, K. A., 9, 143
Dies, R. R., 464, 473, 476
Dilling, L. A., 173
Dimen, M., 76
Dimidjian, S., 121, 122, 371
Director, L., 78
Dirksen, C., 170
Dixon, L., 330
Dixon, L. B., 173
Doane, J. A., 327
Doherty, W. J., 346
Doidge, N., 58
Dollard, J., 24, 427
Dorman, D., 263
Dostoyevski, F., 9
Douglas, M. S., 469
Dowd, E. T., 441
Draguns, J. G., 20
Drescher, J., 76
du Toit, P. L., 149
Duberstein, P. R., 14
DuBois, D. L., 164
Dugo, J. M., 477
Dumas, J. E., 327
Duncan, B. L., 107, 374, 436, 437, 439, 443, 445
Dupuy, P., 284
Dweck, C. S., 229
D'Zurilla, T. J., 123

Eagle, M. N., 47, 49, 54, 58
Eells, T. D., 11
Ehlers, C. L., 122
Ehrenberg, D., 90
Ehrenreich, J. T., 127
Einstein, A., 72
Eisengart, S., 333

Elder, G. H., 227
Elkin, I., 164, 165
Elkins, D. N., 281, 283, 284
Elliott, R., 24, 223, 226, 231, 232, 234, 241, 247, 249, 251, 252, 253, 283, 284, 434
Ellis, A., 145, 146, 184, 393
Ellman, S., 42
Ellman, S. J., 62
Emery, G., 145, 184
Emmelkamp, P. M. G., 118
Epictetus, 144
Epp, L. R., 263, 268, 283
Epstein, L., 84
Epstein, M., 99
Epstein, M. B., 305
Epstein, N. B., 123, 153, 166, 324, 367
Epstein, R., 228
Epston, D., 331, 375
Erickson, M. H., 315, 332, 393, 394, 403, 404, 405, 406, 408, 410
Erikson, E. H., 37
Erwin, B. A., 124
Escudero, V., 4
Evans, S. A., 419
Everitt, B., 173
Everstine, D. S., 405
Everstine, L., 405
Eyberg, S. M., 324, 326, 327
Eysenck, H. J., 109
Ezriel, H., 462

Fairbairn, W. R. D., 34, 73, 74, 76, 94–95
Fairburn, C. G., 136
Fallon, A., 464, 472, 477, 482, 483
Falloon, I. R. H., 325
Fals-Stewart, W., 348
Fantozzi, B., 367
Farach, F., 126, 127, 130
Farber, B. A., 205
Farmer, R. F., 186
Farson, R., 478
Favrod, J., 173
Fay, A., 388
Feather, B. W., 427
Febrarro, G. A. R., 128
Federn, P., 59
Feldman, G., 125, 127
Feldman, L. B., 4
Feldman, S. L., 4
Fensterheim, H., 436, 442
Ferber, A., 348, 355
Ferenczi, S., 42, 73, 392, 393
Ferenschak, M. P., 166
Ferriter, M., 284
Field, C., 84
First, M. B., 115, 133
Firth-Cozens, J., 448
Fiscalini, J., 48, 78
Fisch, R., 315, 359, 362, 406, 409, 415
Fischer, C. T., 266, 267
Fish, J. M., 20
Fishbane, M. D., 15, 349, 378
Fisher, A., 432
Fisher, J. E., 116
Fishman, C., 355
Fishman, D. B., 24
Fleck, 297

Fleming, B., 166
Fleming, R. R., 21
Foa, E., 166
Foa, E. B., 118, 119, 120, 129, 166
Follette, V. M., 189
Follette, W. C., 108, 128, 146, 184, 187, 189, 415
Fonagy, P., 60, 61, 95
Fontes, L. A., 11
Ford, R. Q., 59
Forgatch, M. S., 324
Forman, E. M., 132, 163
Forsyth, J. P., 118
Fosha, D., 263, 270, 282, 438
Fosshage, J., 76, 84, 85
Foulkes, S. H., 462
Fournier, J. C., 14
Fraenkel, P., 19, 22, 346, 347, 371
Framo, J., 306
Framo, J. L., 347
Frances, A., 395
Frank, E., 122
Frank, J. B., 7, 427, 430
Frank, J. D., 7
Frank, K., 435, 440, 442, 443
Frank, K. A., 88, 92
Frankl, V., 280
Franklin, A. J., 447
Franklin, M. E., 120
Franks, C., 109
Fraser, J. S., 410
Frawley, M. G., 76, 78
Freedheim, D. K., 7, 392
Freedman, B., 125
Freedman, J., 375
Freeman, A., 9, 143, 145, 153, 166, 169
French, T., 427, 444
French, T. M., 83, 426
Fresco, D. M., 127, 135
Freud, A., 38, 53
Freud, S., 14, 23, 24, 33, 34, 35, 36, 37, 38, 41, 42, 43, 44, 45, 46, 47, 49, 51, 52, 54, 58, 73, 74, 76, 79, 86, 93, 95, 145, 232, 262, 390, 392, 396, 427, 461, 462, 476
Friedlander, M. L., 4
Friedman, M., 265, 269, 275, 281
Friedman, S., 389
Friere, E., 251
Fristad, M. A., 330
Fromm, E., 73, 74, 76, 86, 99
Fromm-Reichmann, F., 73, 74, 79, 83, 88
Frongia, P., 320
Fruzzetti, A. E., 367
Fuentes, M. A., 13
Fuertes, J. N., 20
Fuhriman, A., 463, 484
Furman, B., 394, 405
Furrow, J., 364
Fusé, T., 118

Galen, 18, 19
Gallagher, R., 447
Galvin, J., 268
Garcia-Preto, N., 298
Garfield, S., 431
Garfield, S. L., 144
Garmezy, N., 228
Gaudiano, B. A., 173

Gendlin, E. T., 223, 225, 226, 230, 234, 236, 237, 240, 241, 244, 248, 249, 251, 284
Gentile, K., 78
George, E. L., 330
Gerson, M.-J., 447
Gerson, R., 310
Gibbon, M., 115
Gibbons, C. J., 165
Gibbons, M. B. C., 78, 93
Gielen, U. P., 20
Giesen-Bloo, J., 170
Gifford, E., 196
Gifford, E. V., 185
Gil, E., 314
Gilbert, P., 128
Gill, M. M., 43, 46, 47, 73, 84, 91, 393
Gilligan, S., 404
Gilligan, S. G., 394
Gillihan, S. J., 166
Gingerich, W. J., 333
Giordana, F., 284
Giordano, J., 298
Giorgi, A., 262
Gislon, M., 446
Giyaur, K., 253
Gladding, S. T., 299
Glass, C., 453
Glass, C. R., 429, 447
Glass, G. V., 415
Glassman, N. S., 94
Gloaguen, V., 164, 165
Glynn, S., 324
Godfrey, E., 253
Goff, D., 173
Golant, M., 475
Gold, J., 4, 7, 426, 428, 429, 434, 435, 436, 437, 440, 442, 444, 445, 447, 449, 454
Gold, J. R., 427, 431, 432, 446, 449, 454
Goldfried, M. R., 5, 123, 145, 253, 283, 427, 445
Goldiamond, I., 129, 194
Goldman, A., 377
Goldman, R., 226, 397
Goldman, R. N., 231, 247, 252, 253, 363
Goldstein, A., 447
Goldstein, C. R., 127
Goldstein, M. J., 327
Goodheart, C. D., 22
Goodman, P., 226, 393
Gorall, D. M., 305
Gordon, L. B., 252
Gore, K. L., 131
Gorman, J. M., 16, 21, 116, 132
Gorsuch, R. L., 153
Gotlib, I. H., 303
Gottlieb, M. C., 19
Gottman, J. M., 349, 362, 365, 366, 367, 378, 414
Gottman, J. S., 362, 365
Gould, R. A., 165, 173
Goulding, M. M., 394, 400, 401, 402, 403
Goulding, R. L., 394, 400, 401, 402
Grace, C., 447
Grant, P., 170
Gratz, K. L., 127
Grawe, K., 284
Gray, P., 42, 48, 58
Grayson, J. B., 120
Green, L., 114

Green, M., 90
Greenbaum, P. E., 336
Greenberg, H., 79
Greenberg, J. R., 73, 74, 76, 85
Greenberg, L., 377
Greenberg, L. S., 149, 223, 226, 231, 232, 234, 235, 236, 241, 247, 249, 251, 252, 253, 284, 348, 362, 363, 434, 435, 442, 449
Greenberger, D., 160
Greene, B. L., 347
Greenson, R. R., 45, 46, 48, 49, 51, 65
Gregg, J. A., 196
Grencavage, L. M., 17
Grinder, J., 405
Grinfeld, L., 25
Grondin, J., 261
Grunebaum, J., 309
Guerney, B., 298
Guevremont, D. C., 120
Guidano, V. F., 166, 435
Gunderson, J. G., 127
Gunther, L. M., 119
Gurman, A. S., 3, 4, 5, 7, 13, 14, 19, 22, 249, 305, 312, 345, 346, 347, 348, 349, 350, 359, 370, 371, 377, 378, 388, 389, 390, 447, 463
Gustafson, J. P., 394, 395, 397, 411

Hadley, S. W., 243
Haley, J., 297, 315, 320, 348, 355, 356, 359, 393, 403, 404, 405, 406, 408, 409
Halpern, J. M., 166
Hampson, R. B., 302, 303, 305
Han, H., 127
Hanna, F. J., 284
Hardy, K. V., 298
Harper, R., 146
Harris, A., 76
Hart, J., 127
Hartmann, H., 38, 39
Harwood, T., 430
Hathaway, W. L., 20
Hawley, L., 119
Hayden, L. C., 305
Hayes, A., 446
Hayes, A. M., 125, 127
Hayes, J. A., 251
Hayes, L. J., 185
Hayes, S. A., 136
Hayes, S. C., 5, 11, 19, 112, 125, 126, 129, 130, 144, 147, 160, 185, 186, 189, 190, 202, 211, 249, 263, 282, 449
Haynes, S. N., 193
Hays, P., 144, 210
Hays, P. A., 131
Hazlett-Stevens, H., 124
Hearon, B., 93
Heath, E. S., 415
Heatherington, L., 4
Heavey, C. L., 377
Hedges, L. V., 211
Hedges, M., 19
Hefferline, R. F., 393
Heidegger, M., 262
Heimberg, R. G., 123, 124, 134
Heisenberg, W., 72
Hellerstein, D. J., 473
Hellkamp, D., 446
Hembree, E., 166

Henderson, C. E., 336
Hendricks, M. N., 240, 253
Henggeler, S. W., 335
Hepworth, J., 298
Herbener, E. S., 227
Herbert, J. D., 123
Herman-Dunn, R., 121
Hersen, M., 107
Hertel, R. K., 353
Hervis, O. E., 338
Hexum, A. L., 404, 406
Heyman, R. E., 299
Hickman, E. E., 429
Hill, C. E., 253
Hiller, T., 412, 414
Hilsenroth, M., 446
Hilsenroth, M. J., 253
Hinton, D. E., 131
Hirsch, I., 34, 72, 73
Hodgson, A. B., 429
Hoffman, I. Z., 75
Hoffman, L., 263, 281, 317, 318, 320, 418
Hofmann, S. G., 135
Hofstee, W. K. B., 8
Hogarty, G. E., 328
Hoglend, P., 484
Hohmann-Marriott, B. E., 299
Holdstock, T. L., 236
Hollon, S., 164, 165
Hollon, S. D., 14
Hoogduin, C. A. L., 128
Hooley, J. M., 303, 304
Hope, D. A., 166
Hopko, D. R., 121
Hopko, S. D., 121
Horney, K., 34, 73, 74, 76
Horowitz, M. J., 149, 397
Hovarth, A. O., 284
Howard, K. I., 253
Hoyt, M. F., 5, 7, 81, 374, 387, 389, 390, 392, 394, 395, 396, 400, 401, 406, 411, 412, 415, 416, 417
Huband, N., 284
Hubble, M. A., 374
Hulgus, Y. F., 305
Hunsely, J., 377
Huppert, J. D., 129
Husserl, E., 262

Imber-Black, E., 301
Imel, Z. E., 21
Ingram, R., 150
Ingram, R. E., 167
Invernizzi, G., 320
Ionesco, E., 5
Isaacs, L., 309
Iwamasa, G. Y., 131

Jackson, D., 315, 347, 393, 408
Jackson, D. D., 297, 346, 408
Jacobs, G. A., 153
Jacobson, E., 38, 42, 124
Jacobson, N. S., 121, 122, 125, 129, 185, 348, 367
Jaffe, J., 76
James, W., 262, 281
Jameson, J. S., 119
Janet, P., 35
Jarrett, R., 164

Jiménez, J. R., 16
Johnson, L. D., 393
Johnson, S. M., 241, 249, 348, 362, 363, 364, 377
Jones, C., 173
Jones, M. C., 108
Jung, C. G., 34, 262

Kabat-Zinn, J., 125, 147
Kachele, H., 42
Kaley, H., 58
Kalogerakos, F., 252
Kane, R., 132
Kanter, J. W., 186
Karoly, P., 121
Karpiak, C. P., 428
Kaslow, F. W., 299, 303
Kaslow, N. J., 5, 297, 298, 299
Katerelos, M., 119
Katzenstein, T., 21
Kazdin, A. E., 317
Keijsers, G. P. J., 128
Keim, J., 357, 370
Keith, D. V., 312, 313, 350
Keller, M. B., 165
Kellner, R., 416
Kelly, 95
Kennedy-Moore, E., 231
Kernberg, O. F., 25, 38, 41, 59, 94
Kettner-Polley, R. B., 465
Khan, A., 14
Kibel, H. D., 466
Kierkegaard, S., 261, 262, 272, 281
Kiesler, D. J., 226
Kihlstrom, J. F., 94
King, 265
King, D. A., 483
Kipper, D., 471
Kirby, J. S., 367
Kirsch, I., 14
Kishna, M. A., 336
Kitayama, S., 59
Kivlighan, D. M., Jr., 476, 484
Klein, M., 73, 74, 76, 89, 462
Klein, M. H., 253
Klein, R. E., 404
Klein, S. B., 427
Klerman, G. L., 80, 94, 446, 448
Klonsky, E. D., 21
Kloosterman, P., 115
Klosko, J. S., 146
Knaan-Kostman, L., 84
Knack, W., 446
Knauss, L., 482
Knoblauch, S., 78
Knox, S., 253
Koenen, K. C., 127
Kohlenberg, B. S., 129, 196
Kohlenberg, R. J., 128, 186
Kohut, H., 34, 38, 57, 74, 84, 90
Kolden, G. G., 253
Kool, S., 14
Korbei, L., 225
Korman, L. M., 253
Kornreich, M., 7, 10
Kosters, M., 484
Kotova, E., 94
Kovacs, M., 149, 151

Kozak, M. J., 129
Krakow, B., 416
Krasner, L., 109
Kreyenbuhl, J., 173
Kris, E., 38
Krug, O. T., 263, 266, 268, 270, 273, 274, 282, 284, 289
Krystal, J. H., 135
Kupfer, D. J., 122
Kurtz, M. M., 123

La Taillade, J. J., 367
L'Abate, L., 324
Lachmann, F., 76, 85
Lachmann, F. M., 76
Ladany, N., 251
Laing, R. D., 268
Lam, K. N., 131
Lambert, M. J., 16, 17, 18, 21, 388
Lammers, M. W., 128
Lang, P. J., 127
Langan, R., 99
Langs, R. J., 55
Lankton, C., 405, 406
Lankton, S., 406
Lankton, S. R., 404, 405
Lappin, J., 357, 370
LaRoche, M., 22
Larson, D., 225
Lasser, J., 19
Latimer, P., 119, 120
Lawrence, W. G., 86
Laws, K. R., 173
Layne, C. M., 471
Lazarus, A., 109
Lazarus, A. A., 109, 388, 393, 427, 429, 436, 437, 439
Leahy, R. L., 128, 161, 253
Leary, K., 99
Lease, S. H., 476
LeBon, G., 461
Lebow, J., 436, 453
Lebow, J. C., 17
Lebow, J. L., 298, 333, 334, 349, 370, 377, 378
Ledley, D. R., 118
Lee, A., 364
Lee, T., 335
Leeuw, I., 117
Leff, J., 377
Leggett, E. L., 229
LeGrange, D., 166
Leibing, E., 398
Leichsenring, F., 14, 61, 93, 398
Leitner, L. M., 283
Lejuez, C. W., 121
Lenzenweger, M. F., 25, 94
Lester, D., 153
Leszcz, M., 478
Levant, R. F., 249
Levenson, E. A., 74, 85, 86
Levenson, H., 15, 397, 418, 438
Levy, K. N., 25, 94
Levy, R. A., 21, 93
Lewicki, P., 230
Lewin, K., 4, 462, 467
Lewinsohn, P. M., 121
Lewis, K. L., 131
Liberman, R. P., 324

Lichtenberg, J. D., 76, 85
Liddle, H. A., 336, 337, 444, 447
Lidz, R., 297
Lidz, T., 297
Lieberman, M. A., 475, 476
Lietaer, G., 244, 249, 252
Lillis, J., 189, 202
Linden, D. E., 61
Lindsley, O. R., 109
Linehan, H., 446, 448, 453
Linehan, M., 125, 127, 249
Linehan, M. M., 25, 125, 135, 186, 471, 480
Linnerooth, P. N., 189
Lionells, M., 78
Liotti, G., 166, 435
Liss, A., 118
Lister, K. M., 428
Little, S. A., 473
Loewald, H., 42
Loewenstein, R. M., 38
Lorentzen, S., 484
Lorenz, A., 298
Lovibond, P. F., 133
Lovibond, S. H., 133
Luborsky, L., 21, 45, 49, 50, 93, 397
Lucksted, A., 330
Lukens, E., 330
Lundgren, T., 191
Luoma, J. B., 189, 202
Luquet, W., 370
Lushene, R. E., 153
Lynch, D., 173
Lyness, J. M., 14
Lyons-Ruth, K., 57, 78

Macalpine, I., 46
Macdonald, A. J., 411
MacKenzie, K. R., 483
MacNair, R. R., 471
Madanes, C., 315, 317, 355, 359
Maddux, R. L., 169
Madu, S., 447
Magee, L., 124
Magnavita, J., 428, 438
Mahler, M., 38, 42
Mahoney, M., 143, 247
Mahrer, A. R., 232, 272
Main, M., 95
Malan, D., 48
Malan, D. H., 390, 393, 396, 397, 415
Malone, T., 297
Manber, R., 14
Manenti, S., 320
Mann, C. H., 78
Mann, J., 388, 397, 400
Mannix, K., 84
Manus, G., 347
Marcotte, D., 440, 442, 449
Marcus, H. E., 483
Margolin, G., 348, 367
Marin, N. W., 131
Markowitz, J., 164
Markowitz, J. C., 14
Marks, I., 109, 119
Markus, H. R., 59
Marmor, J., 427
Marris, P., 95

Marsh, L. C., 464
Martell, C. R., 121, 131, 371
Marx, B. P., 196
Masten, A. S., 228
Masuda, A., 189, 202
Matano, R., 263
Matsumoto, M., 471
Mattick, R. P., 133
May, R., 261, 262, 263, 264, 265, 267, 268, 271, 272, 277, 280, 281, 282, 283
Mays, V., 173
Mazzuchelli, T., 132
McCabe, R. E., 117, 119
McCambridge, J., 416
McCann, L., 24
McCarter, R., 446
McClintic, K., 447
McCullough, 438, 449
McCullough, J. P., Jr., 437, 446
McCullough, L., 397, 400
McCullough-Vaillant, L., 397
McCutcheon, L., 434, 436
McDaniel, S. H., 298
McDougall, J., 78
McDougall, W., 461
McElwain, B., 283, 284
McFall, R. M., 18, 114
McFarlane, W. R., 328, 330
McGoldrick, M., 298, 301, 310
McHugh, R. K., 127
McKenna, P. J., 173
McLeod, P. L., 465
McMain, S., 177
McMinn, M. R., 20
McMullin, R. E., 176
McNeel, J., 403
Mearns, D., 245
Meehan, 95
Meek, L., 281
Meichenbaum, D., 146, 159
Melamed, B. G., 127
Melancon, S. M., 129
Melby, J., 305
Mellor-Clark, J., 252
Meltzoff, J., 7, 10
Mendelowitz, E., 281
Mennin, D. S., 126, 127, 130, 135
Merbaum, M., 145
Mercier, M., 165
Merleau-Ponty, M., 262, 270
Messer, S. B., 3, 4, 5, 7, 9, 10, 13, 14, 16, 18, 22, 24, 25, 40, 41, 43, 44, 49, 52, 93, 94, 285, 388, 389, 397, 398, 400, 418, 427, 428, 430, 431, 435, 442, 454
Metalsky, G., 146
Meuser, K. T., 377
Midelfort, C., 298
Miklowitz, D. J., 135, 327, 330
Miles, M. B., 475
Miller, I. J., 283
Miller, N. E., 24, 427
Miller, R. R., 119
Miller, S. D., 21, 107, 374, 394, 395, 410, 436, 437, 439, 443, 445
Miller, W., 305
Miller, W. R., 128, 249, 415
Millon, T., 149
Mineka, S., 129

Minuchin, S., 298, 320, 355
Mischel, W., 110
Mitchell, A. E., 348, 370, 371
Mitchell, C. C., 336
Mitchell, S., 34, 74
Mitchell, S. A., 73, 74, 75, 76, 83, 85, 94
Mittelman, B., 347, 353
Modell, A. H., 42
Moleiro, C., 453
Molière, 20
Molnar, C., 135, 432
Mondale, W., 10
Montalvo, B., 298, 320
Montuori, M., 263
Moodley, R., 20
Moos, B. S., 305
Moos, R. H., 305
Moreno, J. S., 469
Morin, C. M., 116
Morrison, K., 285
Moscovitch, D. A., 118
Mosher, L., 263, 284
Mosier, J., 484
Moss, D., 261, 281
Mowrer, O. H., 109, 427
Mueser, K. T., 123, 173, 324, 469
Muller, J. P., 74
Mumford, E., 415
Mundo E., 61
Munoz, R. F., 144
Muran, J. C., 50, 94, 99, 251, 473
Murray, H. A., 262
Murrell, A. R., 126
Myhr, G., 132

Najdowski, A. C., 120
Nathan, P. E., 16, 21, 116, 132
Naugle, A. E., 128
Nefale, M., 447
Neidhardt, J., 416
Neisser, U., 9
Nelson, M. M., 327
Nelson, R. O., 112
Nelson-Gray, R. O., 186
Nemeroff, C. J., 121
Newman, C., 446
Newman, M., 432
Newman, M. G., 135
Nezu, A. M., 123, 124
Nichols, M. P., 353, 363, 375, 378
Nichtigall, C. S., 484
Nietzsche, F., 262
Norberg, M. M., 135
Norcross, J. C., 4, 7, 16, 17, 19, 21, 94, 253, 395, 427, 428, 433
Nordberg, S., 432
Norton, P. J., 136

Oberndorf, C. P., 347
O'Brien, W. H., 193
O'Donohue, W., 109
O'Donohue, W. T., 116
O'Farrell, T. J., 348
Ogden, J., 253
Ogden, T., 75
Ogles, B. M., 16, 17, 21
Ogrodniczuk, J. S., 94, 476

O'Hanlon, W. H., 331, 404, 406, 411
O'Hara, M., 263, 281, 283
O'Hara, M. M., 229, 250
Ollendick, T. H., 18, 447
Olson, D. H., 303, 305
Orange, D. M., 74
Oremland, J., 48
Organista, K. C., 131, 144
Orlinsky, D. E., 253, 284
Ornstein, P. H., 393
Orsillo, S. M., 115, 125, 126, 130, 135
Otto, M. W., 135, 165

Padesky, C. A., 160
Paivio, S. C., 241
Palmer, S., 20
Panksepp, J., 15
Papouchis, N., 447
Papp, P., 318
Parkes, C. M., 95
Parks, B. K., 284
Parloff, M. B., 473
Pascual-Leone, J., 232
Passman, V., 447
Pathak, D., 416
Patrick, C., 415
Patterson, G. R., 324, 325
Patterson, J., 411
Paul, G., 194
Paul, N., 306
Payne, K., 132
Payne, L. L., 119
Peen, J., 14
Peet, B., 407
Pelzer, K., 447
Penn, P., 317, 411
Pergament, K. I., 20
Perkins, R., 416
Perlesz, A., 416
Perloff, J., 165
Perls, F., 226, 363
Perls, F. S., 393
Perls, L., 226
Persons, J., 154, 156, 165
Peterson, C., 189
Petrucelli, J., 78
Petry, S., 310
Phillips, A., 79
Phillips, J., 273
Piaget, J., 232
Pickrel, S., 336
Piers, C., 74
Pine, F., 34
Pinquart, M., 14
Pinsker, H., 400
Pinsof, W. M., 298, 334, 345, 371, 442, 447
Pinsoff, W., 226
Pio-Abreu, J. L., 470
Pious, C., 478
Piper, W. E., 94, 476
Plumb, J., 191
Pollack, M. H., 165
Pomini, V., 173
Popper, K., 5
Porcellana, M., 320
Portnoy, D., 270, 282
Pos, A. E., 253
Pote, H., 320

Powers, M. B., 118, 166
Prata, G., 317
Pratt, J. H., 460, 461
Pretzer, J., 166
Prigogine, I., 247
Prince, S. E., 131
Prochaska, J. O., 16, 19, 395, 429, 430, 433, 436, 437, 448
Prout, M., 119
Prouty, G. F., 237, 249
Puhakka, K., 284
Purdon, C., 118, 166
Purser, R., 263

Quille, T., 447
Quitkin, F., 165

Rabung, S., 14, 61, 93, 398
Rachman, S. J., 109, 119, 129
Radomsky, A. S., 119
Rait, D., 346, 370
Rand, K. L., 167
Rank, O., 262, 277, 392, 393
Rapee, R., 166
Raps, C. S., 473
Rasco, C., 17
Raskin, N. J., 224
Rastogi, M., 348, 378
Raue, P. J., 253
Rausch, H. L., 353
Ray, D., 250, 252
Rector, N. A., 170, 171, 172, 173
Redding, N., 14
Rees, C., 132
Reese, H. W., 185
Rehm, L., 159
Reich, W., 40
Reinecke, M. A., 9, 143, 153, 163, 164, 165
Reis, B. F., 309
Reiss, D., 299
Reiss, D. J., 328
Remer, R., 123
Rennie, D. L., 252, 284
Resick, P. A., 166
Reynoso, 95
Rhodes, J. W., 427
Rice, D., 263, 268, 283
Rice, L. N., 223, 226, 231, 232, 241, 251, 284, 434
Richard, J. A., 330
Richeport-Haley, M., 404
Ridsdale, L., 253
Riggs, D. S., 118
Rindskopf, D. M., 211
Riso, L. P., 149, 169
Ritterman, M., 405
Roback, H. B., 481
Robbins, M. S., 339
Roberto, L. G., 313, 314
Roberto-Forman, L., 350, 352
Roberts, J., 301
Robinson, E. A., 326
Roche, B., 190
Rodriguez, B., 453
Roemer, L., 92, 107, 115, 125, 126, 127, 130, 135, 160
Rogers, C. R., 209, 223, 224, 225, 226, 227, 228, 229, 230, 231, 233, 234, 235, 236, 238, 240, 242, 243, 244, 250, 251, 253, 363, 445
Rogers, N., 236

Rohrbaugh, M. J., 359, 410, 411
Rollnick, S., 249, 415
Romanelli, R., 453
Rombauts, J., 249
Roodman, A. A., 128
Rosen, H., 150
Rosen, S., 405
Rosenbaum, R., 415, 416
Rosenberg, B., 463, 478
Rosenthal, R., 400
Rosenzweig, S., 426, 430, 442
Rosman, B., 298, 320
Rossi, E., 405, 406, 408
Rossini, E. D., 483
Roth, G., 288
Roth, J. A., 476
Rothbaum, B. O., 118
Rounsaville, B. J., 80, 446
Rowa, K., 108, 117, 118
Rowan, J., 262
Rowe, C., 447
Rowe, C. L., 336
Rowe, M. K., 119
Rowland, M., 335
Rubin, J., 99
Ruckstuhl, L. E., 189
Rush, A. J., 145, 184
Rutan, J. S., 473, 479
Ryan, N. E., 164
Ryle, A., 434, 436, 446, 448
Rynn, M., 309

Safran, J., 149, 177
Safran, J. D., 50, 94, 99, 100, 149, 177, 440, 442, 443, 444, 449, 454
Safren, S. A., 131
Sager, C. J., 347, 353
Sampson, H., 48
Sampson, J., 397
Samstag, L. W., 94, 473
San Antonio, W., 305
Sandahl, C., 433
Sandell, R., 60, 93, 433
Sanderson, W. C., 7
Sandler, J., 50
Sano, N., 117
Santen, B., 250
Santorelli, N. T., 169
Saperia, 226
Sapirstein, G., 14
Sarbin, T. R., 185
Satir, V., 297, 312, 315, 346, 348, 362, 363
Sauer, A., 9, 143
Savard, J., 116
Savard, M.-H., 116
Saveanu, R. V., 441
Sawalani, G., 167
Saxena, S., 130
Sbrocco, T., 131
Scarlett, G., 416
Schaap, C. P. D. R., 128
Schachter, J., 42
Schafer, R., 49, 53
Schamburger, M., 78
Scharff, D. E., 353, 354
Scharff, J. S., 306, 309, 353, 354, 355
Scheidlinger, S., 463
Schermer, V. L., 462

Schiller, M., 305
Schindler, D., 377
Schlesinger, G., 55, 56
Schlesinger, H., 415
Schlesinger, S., 166
Schneider, K. J., 11, 24, 261, 263, 264, 265, 266, 267, 268, 271, 272, 277, 278, 279, 280, 281, 282, 283, 284, 289
Schneider, W. J., 348, 378
Schnicke, M. K., 166
Schoenwald, S., 335
Schottenbauer, M. A., 429, 447, 448, 449, 453
Schumer, F., 298
Schwartz, R., 353, 375
Schwartz, S., 338
Scott, J., 145
Scott, L. N., 94
Seamam, S., 471
Searles, H., 59, 79, 91
Seed, P., 253
Segal, L., 359, 409
Segal, Z., 149, 442, 443, 444
Segal, Z. V., 125, 126, 130, 144, 147, 177
Segraves, R. T., 370
Seiden, D. Y., 131
Seidler, G. H., 433
Seifer, R., 305
Seligman, M., 146, 463
Seligman, M. E. P., 189, 283, 388
Seltzer, M. H., 94
Selvini-Palazzoli, M., 317
Serby, M., 14
Serketich, W. J., 327
Serlin, I. A., 272
Sexton, T. L., 22, 337, 338, 377, 447
Shadish, W. R., 211, 377
Shafran, R., 119
Shafranske, E. P., 20
Shakespeare, W., 419
Shapiro, D. A., 165, 320, 448
Shapiro, F., 432, 433
Shapiro, S. L., 125
Sharf, J., 253
Shaver, P., 95, 364, 378
Shaw, B., 149
Shaw, B. F., 145, 184
Shay, J., 473
Shedler, J., 61, 93, 94
Sheidow, A. J., 335
Shepard, H. A., 468
Shlien, J. M., 249
Shoham, V., 18, 359, 360, 377, 410, 411
Short, D., 394, 404, 405
Shostrom, E. L., 238
Siegel, D., 15
Siev, J., 124
Sifneos, P. E., 393, 396, 397
Silveira de Mota Neto, J., 173
Silverstein, O., 318
Simmons, D. S., 346
Simon, G. M., 355, 358, 359
Simon, K., 153, 166
Simoneau, T., 330
Simpson, G. L., 19
Simpson, L., 320
Siqueland, L., 309
Sitarenios, G., 305
Skinner, B. F., 109, 111, 185, 186, 187, 427

Skinner, H., 305
Skolnick, M. R., 468
Skynner, A. C. R., 306, 353
Slavin, J., 446
Slive, A., 388, 416
Slovenko, R., 482
Smith, C. O., 299
Smith, D., 225
Smits, J. A. J., 135
Smolar, A., 464
Snow, K. N., 20
Snyder, D. K., 7, 348, 370, 371, 377, 378
Sobel, R., 298
Sokol, L., 165
Sollod, R. N., 447
Solomon, H. C., 109
Solovey, A. D., 410
Spandler, H., 284
Spence, D. P., 24, 427
Sperry, L., 20, 396
Spiegler, M. D., 120
Spielberger, C. D., 153
Spillman, A., 94
Spinelli, E., 262, 283
Spinhoven, P., 170
Spinks, S., 370
Spitzer, R. L., 115
Sprenkle, D. H., 17, 298, 339, 378
Springer, J. R., 136
Stanton, L. R., 253
Stanton, M. D., 299, 323, 357
Steckley, P., 252
Steel, C., 173
Steer, R., 153
Steer, R. A., 115, 152
Stein, D. J., 149
Steinhauer, P., 305
Steketee, G., 120
Sterba, R., 51
Sterling, M., 264, 265, 275, 276
Stermac, L., 252
Stern, D., 76
Stern, D. B., 75, 78
Stern, R., 119
Stevenson-Hinde, J., 95
Stewart, I., 191
Stewart, J., 165
Stewart, R. E., 16, 135
Stewart, S., 281
Stickle, T. R., 377
Stiles, T., 94
Stiles, W. B., 251, 252
Stolar, N., 170
Stoller, R., 76
Stolorow, R. D., 74, 274, 282
Stone, L., 42
Stone, W. N., 473
Strachey, J., 42
Strang, J., 416
Stratton, P., 320
Strauss, B., 483
Street, L., 119
Stricker, G., 4, 7, 426, 427, 428, 429, 431, 432, 435,
    436, 439, 440, 442, 444, 445, 446, 449, 454
Strosahl, K. D., 125, 186, 249, 449
Strümpfel, U., 226
Strupp, H. H., 232, 243, 397

Stuart, C., 78
Stuart, R. B., 348, 367
Stunkard, A. J., 286
Suddath, R. L., 330
Sue, D., 20, 163
Sue, D. W., 20, 163
Sullivan, H. S., 72, 73, 74, 75, 78, 79, 80, 82, 83, 94,
    387, 464, 479
Summerfeldt, L. J., 115
Suzuki, D. T., 99
Svartberg, M., 94
Swain, M. A., 353
Swinson, R. P., 117, 118, 134
Szapocznik, J., 317, 338, 339

Takuya, M., 165
Tallman, K., 228, 236, 252, 284, 285, 435, 445
Talmon, M., 388, 415, 416
Tanaka-Matsumi, J., 131
Tarragona, M., 5
Tarrant, J. M., 476
Tarrier, N., 173
Tataryn, D. J., 94
Tauber, E. S., 90
Taylor, E. T., 261
Taylor, S., 124
Teasdale, J., 146
Teasdale, J. D., 125, 130, 144
Terhune, W. S., 108
Thase, M., 164
Thase, M. E., 14
Thoma, N. C., 428
Thomann, J., 430
Thomas, C., 129
Thomas, V., 348, 378
Thompson, C., 73, 74, 76, 83
Thompson, M. G., 263
Ticho, E. A., 396
Tierney, S. C., 165
Tillich, P., 267, 281
Timmons-Mitchell, J., 336
Tinsely, H. E., 476
Tishby, O., 94
Titelman, P., 352
Toarmino, D., 11, 19
Tobin, D., 446
Todd, T. C., 323, 357, 370
Tolin, D. F., 135
Tolman, E., 145, 427
Tomm, K., 411
Tompkins, M., 156
Tonigan, J. S., 128
Torres-Harding, S., 9, 143
Traux, C. B., 226
Trexler, L., 153
Trieu, V. H., 173
Tropiano, H. L., 21
Tsai, M., 128, 186
Turner, C. W., 336
Turner, R. M., 119, 120

Ullmann, L. P., 109
Ulrich, D., 309
Ulrich, D. N., 350

Vagg, P. R., 153
Vallis, T., 149

van Aalst, G., 14
Van Balen, R., 249
van den Bosch, R. J., 127
van Dyck, R., 170
Van Dyk, G., 447
van Oppen, P., 14
van Straten, A., 14, 135
van Tilburg, W., 170
Vandenberghe, L., 210
VandenBos, G., 7
Veale, D., 166
Verducci, J. S., 330
Villares-Oliveira, C., 470
von Bertalanffy, L., 300, 467
von Goethe, J., 281
Vontress, C. E., 263, 268, 283
Voss Horrell, S. C., 144

Wachtel, P. L., 13, 14, 20, 24, 25, 88, 92, 427, 431, 434,
    435, 436, 437, 441, 442, 444, 447, 449, 450
Wadden, T. A., 286
Wade, J. H., 469
Wagner, F. E., 433
Wakefield, J., 49
Waldron, H. B., 336
Wallace, M. D., 120
Wallerstein, R. S., 34, 60
Walsh, F., 298, 302
Walsh, R. A., 283, 284
Walters, K. L., 330
Wamboldt, M. Z., 299
Wampold, B. E., 16, 18, 21, 22, 165, 265, 269, 283, 284,
    285, 289, 431
Wang, C., 253
Warkentin, J., 297
Warmerdam, L., 135
Warren, C. S., 43, 44, 52, 93, 389, 397, 398, 400, 418
Warren, W., 281
Wasserman, R. H., 94
Watson, J., 262
Watson, J. B., 185
Watson, J. C., 5, 11, 223, 226, 231, 232, 234, 244, 247,
    249, 252, 253, 265, 284
Watzlawick, P., 315, 359, 407, 409
Weakland, J., 297, 315
Weakland, J. H., 359, 408, 409
Weber, 95
Webster, 226
Weinberger, J., 442, 445
Weinberger, J. L., 17
Weiner, I. B., 55
Weiner-Davis, M., 331, 373, 411
Weinstein, M., 483
Weinstein, S. E., 324
Weir, S., 416
Weishaar, M. E., 146
Weiss, J., 48, 397
Weiss, R. L., 370
Weissman, A., 152
Weissman, A. N., 152
Weissman, M., 446
Weissman, M. M., 80
Weissman, S., 153
Wells, A., 166
Welwood, J., 272

Wertz, F. J., 262, 283
Westen, D., 80, 94, 285, 397–398
Wexler, D. A., 231, 241
Wheeler, J. G., 125
Whiffen, V. E., 348, 378
Whisman, M. A., 377
Whitaker, C., 297
Whitaker, C. A., 312, 313, 350
White, M., 331, 375
Whiteside, S. P., 118
Whiting, R., 301
Wiersma, D., 127
Wilk, J., 411
Williams, J. B. W., 115
Williams, J. M. G., 125, 144
Williams, K. E., 128
Williams, R. A., 317, 339
Wills, M., 416
Wills, R. M., 371
Wilson, G. T., 107, 116
Wilson, J., 166
Wilson, K. G., 125, 126, 186, 249, 449
Winnicott, D. W., 34, 54, 74, 75, 83, 90, 352
Winokur, M., 5, 7
Winston, A., 14, 94
Wiseman, H., 226
Wiser, S., 253
Witenberg, E., 88
Wolberg, L. R., 393
Wolf, A. W., 23
Wolfe, B., 263, 282, 446
Wolfe, B. E., 283, 428, 454
Wolitzky, D. L., 10, 33, 40, 41, 47, 49, 54, 55, 56, 58,
    93
Wolpe, J., 109, 393
Wolstein, B., 84, 89
Wood, J. K., 229
Woods, S. W., 20
Woolfolk, R. L., 9, 13
Wright, F., 165
Wright, J. H., 128
Wright, L. R., 127
Wykes, T., 173
Wynne, L., 297

Yager, J., 61
Yalom, I. D., 262, 264, 266, 267, 269, 272, 274, 275,
    283, 463, 475, 478
Yapko, M. D., 388
Yeomans, F. E., 94
Yoerger, K., 325
Yontef, G., 226
Young, J., 152, 416
Young, J. E., 146, 147, 149, 151
Young, M. E., 330

Zapparoli, G., 446
Zeig, J. K., 394, 406
Zeldow, P. B., 21, 23
Zetzel, E. R., 46, 49
Ziegler, P. B., 412, 414
Zimmerman, G., 173
Zinbarg, R. E., 129
Zlomke, K., 108, 117
Zung, W. W. K., 153

Subject Index

Page numbers followed by *t* indicate tables, by *f* indicate figures.

ABC model, 146, 192–193, 195
Acceptance, 125, 202*t*, 203, 243, 244
Acceptance and commitment therapy (ACT). *see also*
    Cognitive therapy; Integrative approaches to
    psychotherapy
    functional analytic psychotherapy (FAP) and,
        195–196
    functional contextual approaches and, 187–188
    intrapersonal and interpersonal functions and,
        201–202, 202*t*
    overview, 146–147
    relational frame theory (RFT) and, 191
    research support for, 212, 449
    techniques used in, 160
    treatment applicability and, 209–211
Acceptance-based strategies, 125–126, 130, 135–136,
    368. *see also* Behavior therapy (traditional
    approach)
Action-oriented theory, 469–471, 480
Actualizing tendency, 228, 280
Addiction, 249, 446
Agency, 252–253, 412
Aggression, 36–38, 76, 77–78
Agoraphobia, 124, 165–166, 168, 447–448
American relational theory, 34–35. *see also*
    Psychoanalysis
Anxiety
    anxiety threshold, 168
    behavior therapy (traditional approach) and,
        127–128, 130–131
    case illustration, 450–453
    cognitive therapy and, 153–154, 165–168, 172
    disease model and, 14
    exposure-based strategies and, 117–119
    psychoanalysis and, 38
    relational psychoanalytic therapy and, 94

relaxation-based strategies, 124
    response prevention and, 119–120
    self-system and, 75–76
Anxiety disorders, 166–168, 446
Applicability of treatment. *see* Treatment
    applicability
Applied psychoanalysis, 33–34
Assertion, 77, 199*t*
Assessment, clinical. *see* Clinical assessment
Assessment tools. *see also* Clinical assessment
    behavior therapy (traditional approach) and,
        112–113, 113–116
    cognitive therapy and, 152–153
    family therapies and, 299, 304–305, 325–326
    Functional Idiographic Assessment Template
        (FIAT), 198, 199*t*–200*t*
    group psychotherapies and, 471–472
    integrative approaches to psychotherapy and, 437
Assimilative integration. *see also* Integrative
    approaches to psychotherapy
    assessment and, 436–437
    current and future trends in, 454
    overview, 431–432
    personality and, 433–434
    treatment applicability and, 446
Attachment, 77, 94–95, 148–149, 306–307
Authenticity, 209. *see also* Genuineness
Autism, 130–131
Automatic thoughts
    anxiety and, 168
    cognitive distortions, 151–152, 159–160
    cognitive therapy and, 145, 168
    personality and, 148–149
    treatment planning and, 155
Autonomy, 228–229
Avoidance behaviors, 122, 199*t*, 200*t*

506

Beck Depression Inventory (BDI-II), 115, 152–153
Beck Hopelessness Scale (BHS), 153
Behavior rating scales, 152–153. *see also* Clinical assessment
Behavior therapy (functional–contextual approaches). *see also* Functional–contextual approaches
Behavior therapy (traditional approach). *see also* Behavioral activation
    assessment and, 112–116
    case illustration, 133–135
    cognitive and behavioral family therapies, 324–328
    curative factors and, 128–130
    current and future trends in, 135–136
    emotion regulation skills training, 126–127
    ethical considerations, 131–132
    exposure-based strategies, 117–119
    historical background of, 108–109
    mindfulness- and acceptance-based strategies, 125–126
    modeling, 123
    operant strategies, 120–121
    overview, 107–108, 367–370
    personality and, 110–111
    problem-solving training, 123–124
    psychoeducation, 116–117
    psychological health and pathology, 111–112
    relaxation-based strategies, 124
    research support for, 132
    response prevention, 119–120
    social and communication skills training, 122–123
    therapeutic relationship and, 127–128, 131–132
    therapist stance and, 127–128
    therapy practice and, 116–127
    treatment applicability and, 130–131
Behavioral activation, 121–122. *see also* Behavior therapy (traditional approach)
Behavioral approach tests (BATs), 113–114. *see also* Clinical assessment
Behavioral assessment, 112–113. *see also* Clinical assessment
Behavioral couple therapy (BCT), 367–370. *see also* Couple therapies
Behavioral diaries, 114. *see also* Clinical assessment
Behavioral exchange, 368
Behavioral experiments, 129
Behavioral flexibility, 189
Behavioral Marital Therapy (BMT), 348. *see also* Couple therapies
Behavioral techniques, 160–161
Behaviorism, 185, 262
Behaviour Research and Therapy, 109
Bidirectionality networks, 190–191, 199t
Biological factors, 110–111, 130, 170–171, 428
Biopsychosocial perspective, 298
Bipolar disorder, 135, 173–178
Bisexuality, 76–77, 99. *see also* Sexuality
Bodily interventions, 432–433
Borderline personality disorder, 249, 446
Boundaries, 300–301, 320–321, 468
Bowen Family Systems Therapy (BFST), 350–355. *see also* Couple therapies
Brief dynamic psychotherapy, 396–397. *see also* Brief psychotherapies

Brief psychotherapies
    beliefs that can promote or impede, 388–390, 389t
    case illustration, 398–400, 402–403, 406–408, 412–415, 416–417
    current and future trends in, 418–419
    duration of therapy and, 415–417
    evolution of psychotherapy and, 5
    historical background of, 392–394
    models of, 396–415
    overview, 52, 387–388, 419
    reasons clients come to therapy, 390–392
    research support for, 415–416
    short-term psychodynamic psychotherapies, 396–400
    structure of therapy, 394–396, 395f
    therapist stance and, 417–418
Brief strategic family therapy (BSFT), 338–339. *see also* Family therapies
Brief Strategic Therapy, 359–362
Brief therapy. *see* Brief psychotherapies

Case illustration
    behavior therapy (traditional approach) and, 133–135
    brief psychotherapies and, 398–400, 402–403, 406–408, 412–415, 416–417
    cognitive therapy and, 173–178
    existential–humanistic psychotherapies and, 285–289
    functional contextual approaches and, 212–218
    group psychotherapies and, 484–490
    integrative approaches to psychotherapy and, 449–453
    overview, 23–24
    person-centered and experiential therapies and, 253–256
    psychoanalysis, 62–68
    relational psychoanalytic therapy, 95–99
Change, 8–9, 394–396, 395f. *see also* Mechanisms of change
Circular epistemology, 318, 434
Classical conditioning, 108–109, 110–111, 145, 324
Client factors
    behavior therapy (traditional approach) and, 131
    brief psychotherapies and, 390–392
    cognitive therapy and, 148–149, 161–162
    functional contextual approaches and, 194
    overview, 17
    person-centered and experiential therapies and, 248–249, 252–253
    psychoanalysis and, 40, 58–60, 61–62
Clinical assessment. *see also* Assessment tools; Case illustration
    behavior therapy (traditional approach) and, 112–116
    cognitive therapy and, 152–153, 155, 168
    couple therapies and, 368
    existential–humanistic psychotherapies and, 265–267
    family therapies and, 299, 304–305, 310, 324, 326, 335, 336, 338–339
    functional analytic psychotherapy (FAP) and, 198, 199t–200t
    functional–contextual approaches and, 188, 192–195
    group psychotherapies and, 471–472, 474

Clinical assessment *(cont.)*
  integrative approaches to psychotherapy and,
    436–437
  overview, 10–11
  person-centered and experiential therapies and,
    235–236
  psychoanalysis and, 40–42
  relational psychoanalytic therapy and, 80
Clinical interviews, 11, 40–42, 115, 316. *see also*
    Clinical assessment
Clinical Outcomes REsults Standardized Measures
    (CORE) battery, 471
Clinically relevant behaviors (CRBs), 198, 200–201,
    205–206
Clinician rating scales, 152–153, 305. *see also* Clinical
    assessment
Cognitive and behavioral family therapies, 324–328.
    see also Family therapies
Cognitive distortions, 151–152, 159–160
Cognitive models, 129, 130
Cognitive specificity hypothesis, 148, 166–167
Cognitive therapy
  assessment and, 152–153
  assumptions of, 148
  behavioral techniques, 160–161
  case illustration, 173–178
  challenges and, 161–162
  cognitive and behavioral family therapies,
    324–328
  efficacy and effectiveness of, 163–166
  historical background of, 144–147
  homework and, 161
  overview, 143–144, 178
  personality and, 148–149
  psychological health and pathology, 149–152
  termination and, 162–163
  therapeutic relationship and, 163
  therapy practice and, 153–163
  treatment applicability and, 166–173
Cognitive-behavioral analytic system of
    psychotherapy (CBASP), 437, 449. *see also*
    Integrative approaches to psychotherapy
Cognitive-behavioral therapy (CBT). *see also*
    Cognitive therapy
  behavioral techniques, 160–161
  efficacy and effectiveness of, 163–166
  functional contextual approaches and, 185, 209
  integrative approaches to psychotherapy and, 439
  overview, 111, 143–144, 146–147
  psychotic disorders and, 170–173
  relaxation-based strategies and, 124
  research support for, 252
Collaboration, 163, 438–439
Combined therapy, 473–474
Commitment, 202*t*, 267–268
Common factors approach. *see also* Integrative
    approaches to psychotherapy
  current and future trends in, 453–454
  family therapies and, 339
  overview, 17–18, 426, 430–431
  treatment applicability and, 446
Communication skills training, 122–123, 128–129,
    368
Comorbidity, 130–131, 446
Conflict, 199*t*, 345
Confrontation, 48, 277, 278–279
Conjoint therapy, 346, 375. *see also* Couple therapies

Contemporary Freudian psychoanalysis. *see*
    Psychoanalysis
Contextualism, 18, 146, 185
Coping questions, 374, 412
Cotherapists, 310–311, 314, 477
Countertransference. *see also* Therapist stance
  family therapies and, 308
  functional contextual approaches and, 206
  group psychotherapies and, 476–477
  overview, 15
  person-centered and experiential therapies and,
    245–246
  relational psychoanalytic therapy and, 85, 89–90
  therapeutic relationship and, 49–51, 54–56
Couple therapies
  behavioral approaches, 367–370
  current and future trends in, 378
  experiential–humanist approaches, 362–367
  historical background of, 345–350
  integrative approaches, 370–373
  overview, 5, 346
  postmodern approaches, 373–377
  research support for, 377
  structural and strategic approaches, 355–362
  transgenerational approaches, 350–355
Cultural factors
  behavior therapy (traditional approach) and, 131
  cognitive therapy and, 161–162, 163
  functional contextual approaches and, 194–195,
    210–211
  overview, 10, 11, 18–19
  psychoanalysis and, 59
  relational psychoanalytic therapy and, 99–100
  therapy practice and, 12
Curative factors
  behavior therapy (traditional approach) and,
    128–130
  couple therapies and, 352, 355, 362, 365, 366–367,
    372, 374–375
  existential–humanistic psychotherapies and,
    281–282
  family therapies and, 308–309, 311–312, 314, 317,
    319–320, 323, 327, 330, 333
  functional contextual approaches and, 207–209
  group psychotherapies and, 477–480
  integrative approaches to psychotherapy and,
    444–445
  overview, 16–18
  person-centered and experiential therapies and,
    246–249
  psychoanalysis and, 56–58
  relational psychoanalytic therapy and, 91–92
Cybernetics, 298, 318, 323

Defenses
  defensive analysis, 48
  family therapies and, 307–308
  overview, 351
  psychoanalysis and, 37
  psychological health and pathology, 39
  relational psychoanalytic therapy and, 82, 84
Depression
  behavior therapy (traditional approach) and,
    130–131, 135
  behavioral activation (BA) therapy and, 121–122
  case illustration, 173–178, 212–218, 253–256,
    450–453

cognitive therapy and, 153–154, 164–165, 166–167, 172
disease model and, 14
integrative approaches to psychotherapy and, 437, 446
psychotic disorders and, 171
relational psychoanalytic therapy and, 94
Developmental factors, 83, 232–233, 301
Diagnosis. *see also* Clinical assessment
behavior therapy (traditional approach) and, 113
brief psychotherapies and, 391
family therapies and, 319, 322, 338–339
functional contextual approaches and, 193–194
group psychotherapies and, 474, 484
integrative approaches to psychotherapy and, 435–436, 437
overview, 10–11
person-centered and experiential therapies and, 235–236
psychoanalysis and, 41–42
relational psychoanalytic therapy and, 80
Diagnostic and Statistical Manual of Mental Disorders (DSM)
behavior therapy (traditional approach) and, 111, 113
brief psychotherapies and, 391
family systems and, 303
family therapies and, 299
functional contextual approaches and, 188–189
integrative approaches to psychotherapy and, 435–436
psychoanalysis and, 41
psychological health and pathology, 79
Dialectical behavior therapy (DBT). *see also* Behavior therapy (traditional approach)
functional contextual approaches and, 187–188
group psychotherapies and, 471, 480
overview, 127, 135–136
research support for, 448
treatment applicability and, 446
Diaries/journaling, 114, 159–160. *see also* Clinical assessment
Directives, 316, 357–358
Disclosure, 199*t*. *see also* Self-disclosure of the therapist
Disease model, 14, 435
Dissociated states, 76, 92, 94
Distorted thinking, 159–160
Distraction technique, 159, 405
Drive-defense model, 39. *see also* Defenses; Instinctual drives
Duration of therapy, 162–163, 415–417, 472. *see also* Termination
Dyadic Parent–Child Interaction Coding System (DPICS), 326
Dynsfunctional Attitudes Scale (DAS), 152

Eating disorders, 130–131, 446
Effectiveness of treatment, 19, 163–166. *see also* Treatment applicability
Ego, 36–38, 38, 53–56, 461
Emotionally Focused Couple Therapy (EFT), 348, 363–365. *see also* Couple therapies
Emotion-focused therapy, the process–experiential approach (PE-EFT), 223, 231–232, 235–236. *see also* Experiential approaches
Emotions, 231–232, 247–248, 284

Empathy
behavior therapy (traditional approach) and, 128
cognitive therapy and, 154
couple therapies and, 368–369
family therapies and, 310–311
functional contextual approaches and, 209
integrative approaches to psychotherapy and, 439, 445
operant strategies and, 121
person-centered and experiential therapies and, 240, 243, 244–245, 247
psychoanalysis and, 53
relational psychoanalytic therapy and, 82, 89, 90
Enmeshment, 321, 356
Escape, 199*t*, 200*t*. *see also* Avoidance behaviors
Ethical considerations
behavior therapy (traditional approach) and, 131–132
existential–humanistic psychotherapies and, 282–283
family therapies and, 299
functional contextual approaches and, 206, 209–211
group psychotherapies and, 481–483
integrative approaches to psychotherapy and, 445–447
overview, 18–20
person-centered and experiential therapies and, 249–251
psychoanalysis and, 59–60
relational psychoanalytic therapy and, 92–93
Evidence-based practice, 20–23, 132, 211–212, 483–484. *see also* Research support
Exception-finding question, 332, 412
Existential–humanistic psychotherapies
assessment and, 265–267
case illustration, 285–289
curative factors and, 281–282
current and future trends in, 289
ethical considerations, 282–283
historical background of, 261–263
person-centered and experiential therapies and, 263–265
psychological health and pathology, 263–265
research support for, 283–285
therapist stance and, 267–281
therapy practice and, 267–281
treatment applicability and, 282–283
Experiences in the moment, 87, 202*t*, 228. *see also* Mindfulness
Experiential approaches
assessment and, 235–236
case illustration, 253–256
curative factors and, 246–249
ethical considerations, 249–251
evolution of psychotherapy and, 5
historical background of, 223–227
integrative approaches to psychotherapy and, 439
overview, 223
personality and, 227–233
psychological health and pathology, 233–235
research support for, 251–253
symbolic–experiential family therapy, 312–315
therapeutic relationship and, 243–246
therapist stance and, 243–246
therapy practice and, 236–242
treatment applicability and, 249–251

Experiential–humanist approaches, 362–367
Exposure-based treatments. *see also* Behavior therapy
        (traditional approach)
    acceptance and, 125
    cognitive therapy and, 166, 172
    historical background of, 108–109
    integrative approaches to psychotherapy and, 439
    overview, 117–119, 127, 130
Expressed emotions, 284, 303–304
Expressive approach to psychoanalysis, 42
Extinction, 121, 129
Eyberg Child Behavior Inventory, 326
Eye movement desensitization and reprocessing
        (EMDR), 432–433

Family therapies
    assessment and, 304–305
    cognitive and behavioral family therapies, 324–328
    context of the family and, 299–304
    couple therapies and, 346
    historical background of, 297–299
    integrative models, 333–339, 447
    intergenerational–contextual family therapy,
        309–312
    overview, 305–306, 340
    postmodern family therapy, 330–333
    psychodynamically informed family therapy, 306–309
    psychoeducational family therapy, 328–330
    strategic family therapy, 315–317
    structural family therapy, 320–324
    symbolic–experiential family therapy, 312–315
    systemic family therapy, 317–320
Family-based preventive interventions, 298, 299. *see
        also* Family therapies
Family-of-origin experiences, 306, 311–312
Fear
    behavior therapy (traditional approach) and,
        108–109, 127–128
    cognitive therapy and, 166
    exposure-based strategies and, 117–119
    relaxation-based strategies, 124
    response prevention and, 119–120
Feedback, 277, 300
Feelings, 229–231, 247–248
Financial factors, 13–14, 116, 418–419
Flexibility, 189, 300–301, 442–443
Focusing-oriented psychotherapy, 223, 238–239,
        240–241. *see also* Experiential approaches;
        Person-centered psychotherapy
Free association method
    overview, 35, 43–44
    relational psychoanalytic therapy and, 82, 83–84
    resistance and, 46–47
Freedom, 263–265, 267–268
Freudian psychoanalysis, 33. *see also* Psychoanalysis
Functional analysis. *see also* Clinical assessment;
        Functional contextual approaches
    behavior therapy (traditional approach) and,
        112–113, 130–131
    behavioral activation (BA) therapy and, 122
    couple therapies and, 368
    functional contextual approaches and, 188
    overview, 192–193
Functional analytic psychotherapy (FAP)
    case illustration, 196–198, 201–202, 212–218
    curative factors and, 207–209
    mistakes, 204–205

    overview, 186
    research support for, 211–212
    therapeutic relationship and, 205–207
    therapist stance and, 205–207
    therapy practice and, 195–205, 199*t*–200*t*, 202*t*
    treatment applicability and, 209–211
Functional–contextual approaches. *see also* Behavioral
        techniques; Functional analysis; Functional–
        contextual approaches
    assessment and, 192–195
    case illustration, 196–198, 201–202, 212–218
    curative factors and, 207–209
    ethical considerations, 209–211
    historical background of, 184–186
    overview, 185–186
    personality and, 186–188
    psychological health and pathology, 188–192
    research support for, 211–212
    therapeutic relationship and, 205–207
    therapist stance and, 205–207
    therapy practice and, 195–205, 199*t*–200*t*, 202*t*
    treatment applicability and, 209–211
Functional family therapy, 337–338. *see also* Family
        therapies
Functional Idiographic Assessment Template (FIAT),
        198, 199*t*–200*t*
Functionality, 263–264
Functioning
    couple therapies and, 349–350
    existential–humanistic psychotherapies and, 264–265
    family systems and, 302–303
    family therapies and, 300
    person-centered and experiential therapies and,
        234–235

General anxiety disorder, 94
Generalized anxiety disorder, 165, 166–167, 168
Genetic factors, 110–111
Genuineness, 128, 209, 244–245, 284
Gestalt empty-chair exercise, 241
Gestalt therapy, 4–5, 223, 226–227, 400, 439
Global Assessment Scale of Relational Functioning,
        299
Goal setting. *see also* Therapy practice
    acceptance and commitment therapy (ACT) and, 203
    brief psychotherapies and, 391
    cognitive therapy and, 155, 172
    couple therapies and, 351, 354, 357, 360, 364,
        365–366, 368, 372, 374, 375–376
    family therapies and, 307, 310, 313, 315–316, 318,
        321–322, 328, 331, 337–338
    group psychotherapies and, 474
    integrative approaches to psychotherapy and,
        438–439
    overview, 12
    person-centered and experiential therapies and,
        238–239
    psychoanalysis and, 44–45
    relational psychoanalytic therapy and, 81–82
    structure of therapy, 325
Gottman Method Couple Therapy (GMCT), 365–367.
        see also Couple therapies
Group Psychology and the Analysis of the Ego (Freud,
        1921/1955), 461
Group psychotherapies
    assessment and, 471–472, 474
    case illustration, 484–490

curative factors and, 477–480
ethical considerations, 481–483
goal setting and, 474
historical background of, 460–464
overview, 460
personality and, 464–471
psychological health and pathology, 464–471
research support for, 483–484
therapeutic relationship and, 475–477
therapist stance and, 475–477
therapy practice and, 472–474
treatment applicability and, 481–483
Group Selection Questionnaire (GSQ), 471
Group Therapy Questionnaire (GTQ), 471
Growth, 228, 236–237

Hallucinations, 171
Health care systems, 13–14, 116, 418–419
Health problems, 130–131
Heterosexuality, 76–77, 99. see also Sexuality
Hierarchical organization, 320–321
Homeostasis, 300, 356
Homework, 159–160, 161, 172, 391, 439–440
Homosexuality, 76–77, 99. see also Sexuality
Humanistic family therapies, 312–315. see also Family
    therapies
Hypnosis, 35, 405

Id, 38, 53–56
Imaginal exposure, 118, 130. see also Exposure-based
    treatments
In vivo exposure, 117–118, 128–129, 130, 166, 172. see
    also Exposure-based treatments
Individual differences, 131
Insight, 207–208, 248
Insight-oriented approach to psychoanalysis, 42
Insight-Oriented Marital Therapy (IOMT), 348, 371.
    see also Couple therapies
Instinctual drives, 36–38, 39
Instructing octave, 270–271
Integrative approaches to psychotherapy
    assessment and, 436–437
    case illustration, 449–453
    couple therapies and, 370–373
    curative factors and, 444–445
    current and future trends in, 453–454
    ethical considerations, 445–447
    family therapies and, 298, 333–339
    historical background of, 426–433
    overview, 4, 24–25
    personality and, 433–435
    psychological health and pathology, 435–436
    research support for, 447–449
    therapeutic relationship and, 442–444
    therapist stance and, 442–444
    therapy practice and, 438–441
    treatment applicability and, 445–447
Integrative Behavioral Couple Therapy (IBCT), 367,
    370–371. see also Couple therapies
Integrative Couple Therapy (ICT), 371–373. see also
    Couple therapies
Integrative problem-centered therapy (IPCT), 334. see
    also Family therapies
Integrative–eclectic approach, 428–429. see also
    Integrative approaches to psychotherapy
Intensive short-term dynamic psychotherapy, 397. see
    also Brief psychotherapies

Intergenerational–contextual family therapy,
    309–312. see also Family therapies
Internal experiences, 130, 145, 229–231
Interoceptive exposure, 118, 130. see also Exposure-
    based treatments
Interpersonal functioning, 198, 199t–200t, 201–204,
    273–276
Interpersonal theory, 34–35, 73, 464–465, 478–479
Interpretation
    cognitive therapy and, 148
    couple therapies and, 357
    family therapies and, 307–308
    functional contextual approaches and, 208
    person-centered and experiential therapies and,
        239–240
    psychoanalysis and, 47–49
    relational psychoanalytic therapy and, 82, 86
Interventions
    acceptance and commitment therapy (ACT) and,
        203
    cognitive techniques, 155–161, 156–160
    couple therapies and, 357–358, 361, 364–365,
        365–366, 368–370, 372, 374, 376
    existential–humanistic psychotherapies and,
        268–280
    family therapies and, 298, 316, 316–317, 319, 322,
        332
    functional contextual approaches and, 193–194
    integrative approaches to psychotherapy and,
        431–432, 439
    person-centered and experiential therapies and,
        239–241
Intimacy, 199t, 210–211
Intrapersonal functioning, 11, 201–204

Journaling/diaries, 114, 159–160. see also Clinical
    assessment

Managed care organizations (MCOs), 13–14, 116,
    418–419
Marital therapy. see Couple therapies
Mechanisms of change
    behavior therapy (traditional approach) and,
        128–130
    couple therapies and, 352, 355, 362, 365, 366–367,
        369, 372, 374–375, 376–377
    existential–humanistic psychotherapies and,
        281–282
    functional analytic psychotherapy (FAP) and,
        204
    functional contextual approaches and, 204,
        207–209
    group psychotherapies and, 477–480
    integrative approaches to psychotherapy and,
        429–430, 444–445
    overview, 16–18
    person-centered and experiential therapies and,
        246–249, 252–253
    psychoanalysis and, 56–58
    relational psychoanalytic therapy and, 91–92
Medication. see also Pharmacotherapy
    behavior therapy (traditional approach) and,
        130–131
    cognitive therapy and, 155–156
    group psychotherapies and, 473–474
    integrative approaches to psychotherapy and, 441
    overview, 14

Menninger Foundation Psychotherapy Research
    Project (PRP), 60
Mental health. *see* Psychological health
Mental illness. *see* Pathology
Mindfulness, 146, 202*t*, 228, 448. *see also* Experiences
    in the moment
Mindfulness-based cognitive therapy (MBCT), 144,
    147. *see also* Cognitive therapy
Mindfulness-based strategies, 125–126, 130. *see also*
    Behavior therapy (traditional approach)
Miracle question, 332, 412
Modeling, 123, 206. *see also* Behavior therapy
    (traditional approach)
Monitoring forms, 114, 159–160. *see also* Clinical
    assessment
Motivation
    functional analytic psychotherapy (FAP) and, 204
    person-centered and experiential therapies and,
        248–249, 252–253
    psychoanalysis and, 36–38
    relational psychoanalytic therapy and, 77
Motivational interviewing, 249, 415–416
MRI approach, 359–362, 373. *see also* Couple
    therapies
Multidimensional family therapy (MDFT), 336–337.
    see also Family therapies
Multimodal therapy, 304–305, 429, 436, 437. *see also*
    Integrative approaches to psychotherapy
Multisystemic therapy (MST), 304–305, 335–336. *see
    also* Family therapies
Mutual enactment, 85–86, 273–276
Mutuality, 88–89

Narrative Couple Therapy (NCT), 375–377. *see also*
    Couple therapies
Neurobiological factors, 170–171
Neurotic accomplices, 437, 441
Noncompliance, 161–162. *see also* Resistance

Object relations couple therapy (ORCT), 352–355,
    355
Object relations theories. *see also* Psychoanalysis
    Bowen Family Systems Therapy (BFST) and, 351
    countertransference and, 90
    family therapies and, 306–307, 308
    integrative approaches to psychotherapy and, 434
    overview, 34–35, 353–354
Objective countertransference, 308. *see also*
    Countertransference
Observational assessment. *see also* Clinical
    assessment
    behavior therapy (traditional approach) and,
        113–114
    family therapies and, 305
    integrative approaches to psychotherapy and, 440
    overview, 11, 82
Obsessive–compulsive disorder (OCD), 117–120,
    166–168
Operant conditioning, 108–109, 145
Operant strategies, 120–121, 324. *see also* Behavior
    therapy (traditional approach)

Panic disorder, 128, 165–167, 168, 446
Paradoxical interventions, 158, 316, 357, 358
Parent training, 325–326, 327–328
Parent–child interaction therapy (PCIT), 326–328. *see
    also* Family therapies

Pathology
    behavior therapy (traditional approach) and,
        111–112, 130–131
    cognitive therapy and, 149–152, 166–173
    existential–humanistic psychotherapies and,
        263–265
    family systems and, 303–304
    functional contextual approaches and, 188–192
    group psychotherapies and, 464–471
    integrative approaches to psychotherapy and,
        435–436
    overview, 9–10
    person-centered and experiential therapies and,
        233–235
    psychoanalysis and, 39–40, 59
    relational psychoanalytic therapy and, 78–80
    sexuality and, 76–77
Patient Compliance Scale, 437
Personality
    behavior therapy (traditional approach) and,
        110–111
    cognitive therapy and, 148–149
    concept of, 8–9
    existential–humanistic psychotherapies and,
        263–265
    experiential approaches and, 227–233
    functional contextual approaches and, 186–188
    group psychotherapies and, 464–471
    integrative approaches to psychotherapy and,
        433–435
    person-centered and experiential therapies and,
        227–233, 249
    psychoanalysis and, 36–38
    relational psychoanalytic therapy and, 74–78
Personality disorders, 130–131, 169–170, 446
Person-centered experiential psychotherapies
    (PCEP). *see also* Person-centered psychotherapy
    assessment and, 235–236
    overview, 223
    personality and, 229
    psychological health and pathology, 233–235
    therapist stance and, 246
    therapy practice and, 236–242
Person-centered psychotherapy
    assessment and, 235–236
    case illustration, 253–256
    curative factors and, 246–249
    ethical considerations, 249–251
    evolution of psychotherapy and, 5
    functional contextual approaches and, 209
    historical background of, 223–227
    integrative approaches to psychotherapy and, 445
    overview, 223
    personality and, 227–233
    psychological health and pathology, 233–235
    research support for, 251–253
    techniques used in, 239–241
    therapeutic relationship and, 243–246
    therapist stance and, 243–246
    therapy practice and, 236–242
    treatment applicability and, 249–251
Pharmacotherapy, 155–156. *see also* Medication
Phobias, 93, 108–109, 124, 166–167
Planned brief therapy. *see* Brief psychotherapies
Positive psychology, 188–189
Positive regard, 128, 209, 284, 445
Postmodern approaches, 5, 330–333, 373–377

Posttraumatic stress disorder (PTSD), 166, 432–433
Power, 302, 321
Practice of therapy
  behavior therapy (traditional approach) and,
    116–127
  cognitive therapy and, 153–163
  couple therapies and, 350–377, 357–359, 360–362,
    364–367, 368–370, 371–373, 374–377
  existential–humanistic psychotherapies and,
    267–281
  functional contextual approaches and, 195–205,
    199t–200t, 202t
  group psychotherapies and, 472–474
  integrative approaches to psychotherapy and,
    438–441
  overview, 12–15, 42–52
  person-centered and experiential therapies and,
    236–242
  relational psychoanalytic therapy and, 80–88
Prescriptive psychotherapy, 430. see also Integrative
    approaches to psychotherapy
Presence, 266–267, 268–276, 281–282
Present in the moment. see Experiences in the
    moment; Mindfulness
Problem-solving training, 123–124, 368. see also
    Behavior therapy (traditional approach)
Process aspects of therapy. see also Therapy practice
  couple therapies and, 351–352, 354–355, 357–358,
    361, 364–365, 365–366, 368–370, 372, 374, 376
  family therapies and, 307–308, 310, 313–314,
    316–317, 318–319, 322, 328–329, 331–332
  integrative approaches to psychotherapy and, 440
  overview, 12–13
  person-centered and experiential therapies and,
    242, 252–253
  psychoanalysis and, 45–52, 61–62
  relational psychoanalytic therapy and, 82–88
  structure of therapy, 325–326
Process–experiential psychotherapy, 238–239, 449.
    see also Experiential approaches; Integrative
    approaches to psychotherapy; Person-centered
    psychotherapy
Process–experiential/emotion-focused psychotherapy
    (PE-EFT), 241, 249–253. see also Experiential
    approaches; Person-centered psychotherapy
Projective identification, 89–90, 308
Psychoanalysis
  assessment and, 40–42
  case illustration, 62–68
  curative factors and, 56–58
  ethical considerations, 59–60
  existential–humanistic psychotherapies and, 262
  goal setting and, 44–45
  historical background of, 33–36
  overview, 33
  personality and, 36–38
  process aspects of therapy and, 45–52
  psychological health and pathology, 39–40
  research support for, 60–62
  sessions in, 43–44, 49–52
  therapeutic relationship and, 53–56
  therapist stance and, 53–56
  therapy practice and, 42–52
  treatment applicability and, 58–59
  working alliance and, 49–51
Psychodynamic group psychotherapy, 466. see also
    Group psychotherapies

Psychodynamic orientation, 465–467, 479
Psychodynamically informed family therapy. see also
    Family therapies
  curative factors and, 308–309
  goal setting and, 307
  overview, 306–307
  process aspects of therapy and, 307–308
  research support for, 309
  structure of therapy, 307
  therapist stance and, 308
  treatment applicability and, 309
Psychoeducation, 116–117, 172, 328–330. see also
    Behavior therapy (traditional approach)
Psychoeducational family therapy. see also Family
    therapies
  curative factors and, 330
  goal setting and, 328
  overview, 328
  process aspects of therapy and, 328–329
  research support for, 330
  structure of therapy, 328
  therapist stance and, 329
  treatment applicability and, 330
Psychological health
  behavior therapy (traditional approach) and,
    111–112
  cognitive therapy and, 149–152, 166–173
  existential–humanistic psychotherapies and,
    263–265
  functional contextual approaches and, 188–192
  group psychotherapies and, 464–471
  integrative approaches to psychotherapy and,
    435–436
  overview, 9–10
  person-centered and experiential therapies and,
    233–235
  psychoanalysis and, 39–40
  relational psychoanalytic therapy and, 78–80
Psychopathology. see Pathology

Questioning, 172, 374, 391–392, 412

Rapport, 154, 391
Reflection, 239–240, 331, 439
Reframing, 316, 409–410
Regression, 37, 46, 92. see also Transference
Reinforcement
  functional analysis and, 192–193
  functional analytic psychotherapy (FAP) and,
    200–201, 204
  functional contextual approaches and, 194
  operant strategies and, 120–121
Relational psychoanalytic psychotherapy
  assessment and, 80
  case illustration, 95–99
  curative factors and, 91–92
  current and future trends in, 99–100
  ethical considerations, 92–93
  goal setting and, 81–82
  historical background of, 72–74
  personality and, 74–78
  process aspects of therapy and, 82–88
  psychological health and pathology, 78–80
  research support for, 93–95
  self-disclosure and, 90–91
  termination and, 88
  therapeutic relationship and, 88–91

Relational psychoanalytic psychotherapy *(cont.)*
    therapist stance and, 88–91
    therapy practice and, 80–88
    treatment applicability and, 92–93
Relational theories, 34–35, 94. *see also* Psychoanalysis
Relationships, 349–350. *see also* Family therapies
Research support. *see also* Evidence-based practice
    behavior therapy (traditional approach) and,
        132
    cognitive therapy and, 163–166
    couple therapies and, 377
    existential–humanistic psychotherapies and,
        283–285
    family therapies and, 309, 312, 315, 317, 320,
        323–324, 327–328, 330, 333
    functional contextual approaches and, 211–212
    group psychotherapies and, 483–484
    integrative approaches to psychotherapy and,
        447–449
    overview, 20–23
    person-centered and experiential therapies and,
        251–253
    psychoanalysis and, 60–62
    relational psychoanalytic therapy and, 93–95
Resilience, 228, 252–253, 302
Resistance
    cognitive therapy and, 161–162
    existential–humanistic psychotherapies and,
        276–279
    family therapies and, 307–308, 311
    functional contextual approaches and, 193
    integrative approaches to psychotherapy and,
        440–441
    overview, 12–13
    person-centered and experiential therapies and,
        242
    psychoanalysis and, 46–47, 51–52
    relational psychoanalytic therapy and, 84
Response prevention, 119–120. *see also* Behavior
    therapy (traditional approach)
Rituals, 119–120, 301, 319. *see also* Behavior therapy
    (traditional approach)
Role of the therapist. *see* Therapist stance
Roles, 301, 469–471
Routines, 301
Rules, 301, 318

Satir model, 362–363
Scaling technique, 158, 332, 374, 412
Schema construct, 8–9, 145, 150–151, 234
Schema-based therapy, 147, 151. *see also* Cognitive
    therapy
Schizophrenia
    behavior therapy (traditional approach) and, 135
    cognitive therapy and, 170–173
    existential–humanistic psychotherapies and, 284
    family therapies and, 297–298, 328–330
    relational psychoanalytic therapy and, 79
Self psychology, 34, 57, 90. *see also* Psychoanalysis
Self-actualization, 82, 228–229, 280
Self-disclosure of the therapist. *see also* Therapist
    stance
    countertransference and, 55
    couple therapies and, 368–369
    functional contextual approaches and, 205–206
    group psychotherapies and, 476
    overview, 15

    person-centered and experiential therapies and,
        240, 244
    relational psychoanalytic therapy and, 90–91
Self-instructional training, 146, 159
Self-monitoring, 127, 130
Self-report questionnaires. *see also* Clinical
    assessment
    behavior therapy (traditional approach) and, 115
    cognitive therapy and, 152–153
    family therapies and, 304–305
    integrative approaches to psychotherapy and, 437
    overview, 11, 154
Separation–individuation, 38, 395
Sessions, 43–44, 49–52. *see also* Process aspects of
    therapy
Sexuality, 36–38, 76–77, 99
Short-term anxiety-provoking psychotherapy, 396. *see
    also* Brief psychotherapies
Short-term psychodynamic psychotherapies, 396–
    400, 484. *see also* Brief psychotherapies
Single-session therapy (SST), 415–417, 416–417. *see
    also* Brief psychotherapies
Skeleton key question, 412
Skills training, 250, 348, 439
Social and communication skills training, 122–123.
    see also Behavior therapy (traditional approach)
Social anxiety disorder, 117–119, 124, 133–135,
    166–167
Social skills training, 122–123, 128–129
Socratic questioning, 172, 280
Solution-focused brief therapy (SFBT), 332, 410–415,
    412–415. *see also* Brief psychotherapies
Solution-focused couple therapy (SFCT), 373–375. *see
    also* Couple therapies
Solution-oriented therapy, 410–415. *see also* Brief
    psychotherapies
Spirituality, 20, 281
Stance of the therapist. *see* Therapist stance
State–Trait Anxiety Inventory (STAI), 153
Stimulus–organism–response–consequence model
    (S-O-R-C), 145
Stimulus–response model (S-R), 145, 185
Stimulus–response–consequence model (S-R-C),
    145
Strategic family therapy, 315–317. *see also* Family
    therapies
Strategic therapy, 17, 408–410. *see also* Brief
    psychotherapies
Strengths, 194, 437
Stress, 148, 302, 345
Stress response therapy and microanalysis, 397. *see
    also* Brief psychotherapies
Structural approaches, 320–324, 355–362. *see also*
    Family therapies
Structural–Strategic Couple Therapy (SSCT),
    355–359. *see also* Couple therapies
Structure of therapy. *see also* Process aspects of
    therapy; Therapy practice
    brief psychotherapies and, 394–396, 395*f*
    couple therapies and, 351, 360, 364, 365, 368, 372,
        374, 375
    family therapies and, 307, 310, 313, 315, 318, 321,
        328, 331
    group psychotherapies and, 472–473
    overview, 12
    person-centered and experiential therapies and,
        237–238

relational psychoanalytic therapy and, 81
structure of therapy, 325
Structured Clinical Interview for DSM-IV (SCID-IV),
115
Structured interview guides, 11. *see also* Clinical
assessment
STS Clinician Rating Form, 437
STS Therapy Process Rating Scale, 437
Subjective units of discomfort scale (SUDS), 113–114.
see also Clinical assessment
Substance abuse, 92–93, 130–131, 249, 446
Superego, 38, 53–56
Symbolic–experiential family therapy, 312–315. *see
also* Family therapies
Symptoms, 39, 52, 92–95, 170–172, 322
Systematic desensitization, 431–432
Systematic treatment selection (STS), 437, 446, 448
Systemic family therapy, 317–320. *see also* Family
therapies
Systems theory, 299–304, 340, 467–469

Technical eclecticism, 429–430, 437, 453–454. *see also*
Integrative approaches to psychotherapy
Termination
brief psychotherapies and, 395
cognitive therapy and, 162–163
curative factors and, 17
family therapies and, 308, 316–317, 319, 334
functional analytic psychotherapy (FAP) and,
205
functional contextual approaches and, 205
integrative approaches to psychotherapy and, 441,
443
psychoanalysis and, 52
relational psychoanalytic therapy and, 88
Theoretical integration. *see also* Integrative
approaches to psychotherapy
assessment and, 436–437
current and future trends in, 454
overview, 431
personality and, 433–434
treatment applicability and, 446
Therapeutic collaboration, 154
Therapeutic relationship. *see also* Working alliance
behavior therapy (traditional approach) and,
127–128, 131–132
brief psychotherapies and, 391, 395
challenges and, 161–162
cognitive therapy and, 154, 163, 169–170, 172
existential–humanistic psychotherapies and,
267–281, 284
family therapies and, 307, 339
functional contextual approaches and, 205–207
group psychotherapies and, 475–477
integrative approaches to psychotherapy and,
438–439, 442–444, 444–445
overview, 15–16
person-centered and experiential therapies and,
243–246, 252–253
psychoanalysis and, 48–49, 49–51, 53–56
relational psychoanalytic therapy and, 88–91
Therapist errors, 162
Therapist qualities. *see also* Therapist stance
behavior therapy (traditional approach) and, 128
brief psychotherapies and, 389*t*, 417–418
countertransference and, 54–56
family therapies and, 313–314

functional analytic psychotherapy (FAP) and, 204
group psychotherapies and, 475–476, 483
integrative approaches to psychotherapy and, 445
overview, 17, 206–207
person-centered and experiential therapies and,
243, 248
psychoanalysis and, 40–41
Therapist stance. *see also* Therapist qualities
behavior therapy (traditional approach) and,
127–128
brief psychotherapies and, 389*t*, 417–418
cognitive therapy and, 163
couple therapies and, 352, 355, 359, 362, 365,
366–367, 369, 372, 374–375, 376–377
existential–humanistic psychotherapies and,
267–281
family therapies and, 308, 311, 314, 317, 319, 323,
327, 329, 332
functional contextual approaches and, 205–207
group psychotherapies and, 475–477
integrative approaches to psychotherapy and,
442–444
overview, 15–16
person-centered and experiential therapies and,
243–246
psychoanalysis and, 44, 53–56
relational psychoanalytic therapy and, 88–91
Therapy practice. *see* Practice of therapy
Three-tier model, 449, 450–453. *see also* Integrative
approaches to psychotherapy
Time-limited therapy. *see* Brief psychotherapies
Traditional Behavioral Couple Therapy, 367. *see also*
Couple therapies
Transactional analysis, 4–5, 400–403. *see also* Brief
psychotherapies
Transference
cognitive therapy and, 169–170
family systems and, 302
family therapies and, 307–308, 312
interpretation and, 47–49
overview, 45–46
person-centered and experiential therapies and,
245–246
relational psychoanalytic therapy and, 82, 84–85,
94
therapeutic relationship and, 49–51, 53–54
Transference reactions, 46
Transformation, 191, 331
Transgenerational approaches, 350–355
Transtheoretical psychotherapy, 429–430, 437,
446, 448. *see also* Integrative approaches to
psychotherapy
Trauma, 76, 79, 166, 432–433
Treatment alliance, 15–16. *see also* Therapeutic
relationship
Treatment applicability. *see also* Case illustration
behavior therapy (traditional approach) and,
130–131
cognitive therapy and, 166–173
couple therapies and, 352, 355, 359, 362, 365, 367,
369, 372–373, 375, 377
existential–humanistic psychotherapies and,
282–283
family therapies and, 309, 312, 315, 317, 320, 323,
327, 330, 333
functional contextual approaches and, 209–211
group psychotherapies and, 481–483

Treatment applicability *(cont.)*
  integrative approaches to psychotherapy and,
     445–447
  overview, 18–20
  person-centered and experiential therapies and,
     249–251
  psychoanalysis and, 58–60
  relational psychoanalytic therapy and, 92–93
Treatment efficacy, 19, 163–166. *see also* Treatment
     applicability
Treatment goals. *see* Goal setting
Treatment planning, 10, 155
Trust, 273, 309, 438–439

Unconditional regard, 209, 243
Utilization technique, 405, 406

Values, 202*t*, 203
Vivification of resistance, 277–278, 279
Vulnerability factors, 153, 269–270

Warmth, 128, 243, 244–245, 445
Working alliance, 48, 49–51, 395. *see also* Therapeutic
     relationship
Working through, 51–52, 310, 395

Young Schema Questionnaire (YSQ), 152